ORTHO.

# Instructional Course Lectures

Volume XXXVI 1987

American Academy
of Orthopaedic Surgeons

# Instructional Course Lectures

Volume XXXVI 1987

Edited by
Paul P. Griffin, MD
Chief of Staff
Shriners Hospitals for Crippled Children
Chicago Unit
Chicago, Illinois

With 699 illustrations

American Academy
of Orthopaedic Surgeons

American Academy of Orthopaedic Surgeons

Instructional Course Lectures
Volume XXXVI

Senior Editor: Marilyn L. Fox, PhD
Director of Communications and Publications: Mark W. Wieting
Editor: Wendy O. Schmidt
Editorial Assistant: Alice A. Michaels

Design: James Buddenbaum Design, Wilmette, Illinois
Layout: Boldt Production, Evanston, Illinois
Typesetting: Black Dot Graphics, Chicago, Illinois
Printing: Mack Printing Company, Easton, Pennsylvania

The material presented in this volume has been made available by the American Academy of Orthopaedic Surgeons for educational purposes only. This material is not intended to represent the only, or necessarily best, methods or procedures for the medical situations discussed, but rather is intended to present an approach, view, statement, or opinion of the author(s) or producer(s), which may be helpful to others who face similar situations.

# Contributors

**George J. Alker, MD**, Professor and Chairman, Department of Radiology, State University of New York at Buffalo, Buffalo, New York

**Steven Blazar, MD**, Chief Resident in Orthopaedic Surgery, University of Massachusetts Medical School, Worcester, Massachusetts

**Carl T. Brighton, MD, PhD**, Professor and Chairman, Department of Orthopaedic Surgery, University of Pennsylvania School of Medicine, Philadelphia, Pennsylvania

**Joseph A. Buckwalter, MD**, Professor of Orthopaedic Surgery, University of Iowa Hospitals, Iowa City, Iowa

**David L. Butler, PhD**, Associate Professor, Department of Aerospace Engineering and Engineering Mechanics, University of Cincinnati, Cincinnati, Ohio

**Norris C. Carroll, MD**, Head, Division of Orthopedics, Martha Washington Professor of Orthopedic Surgery, The Children's Memorial Hospital, Chicago, Illinois

**Joseph R. Cass, MD**, Orthopaedic Surgery, Midwest Orthopaedic Center, PA, Sioux Falls, South Dakota

**John F. Connolly, MD**, Professor and Chairman, Creighton-Nebraska Universities Health Foundation, Orthopaedic Surgery Residency Training Program, Omaha, Nebraska

**William P. Cooney III, MD**, Associate Professor of Orthopaedic Surgery, Mayo Clinic and Mayo Foundation, Rochester, Minnesota

**Reginald R. Cooper, MD**, Professor and Head, Department of Orthopaedic Surgery, University of Iowa Hospitals, Iowa City, Iowa

**Charles N. Cornell, MD**, Assistant Professor of Orthopaedic Surgery, Cornell University Medical College, Attending, Metabolic Bone Disease, The Hospital for Special Surgery, Assistant Chief, Fracture Service, New York Hospital, New York, New York

**Michael J. Coughlin, MD**, Chief, Department of Orthopaedic Surgery, St. Alphonsus Regional Medical Center, Boise, Idaho

**Kenneth E. DeHaven, MD**, Professor of Orthopaedics, Head, Section of Athletic Medicine, University of Rochester School of Medicine, Rochester, New York

**William R. Dobozi, MD**, Associate Professor of Orthopaedic Surgery, Loyola University, Maywood, Illinois

**Edward J. Dunn, MD**, Chief of Orthopaedic Surgery, Worcester Memorial Hospital, Professor of Orthopaedic Surgery, University of Massachusetts Medical School, Worcester, Massachusetts

**J. William Fielding, MD**, Clinical Professor of Orthopaedic Surgery, College of Physicians and Surgeons, Columbia University, Director, Department of Orthopaedic Surgery, St. Luke's-Roosevelt Hospital Center, New York, New York

**Melvin J. Glimcher, MD**, Harriet M. Peabody Professor of Orthopaedic Surgery, Harvard Medical School, Director, Laboratory for the Study of Skeletal Disorders and Rehabilitation, The Children's Hospital, Boston, Massachusetts

**J. Leonard Goldner, MD**, James B. Duke Professor, Chief Emeritus, Division of Orthopaedic Surgery, Duke Medical Center, Durham, North Carolina

**Neil E. Green, MD**, Professor of Orthopaedic Surgery, Head, Pediatric Orthopaedics, Vanderbilt University Medical Center, Nashville, Tennessee

**Adam Greenspan, MD**, Associate Professor of Radiology, New York University School of Medicine, Associate Director, Department of Radiology, Hospital for Joint Diseases Orthopaedic Institute, New York, New York

**Edward S. Grood, PhD**, Professor of Engineering Mechanics, Noyes-Giannestras Biomechanics Laboratory, University of Cincinnati, Cincinnati, Ohio

**Ramon B. Gustilo, MD**, Chairman, Department of Orthopaedics, Hennepin County Medical Center, Professor of Orthopaedic Surgery, University of Minnesota, Minneapolis, Minnesota

**Robert F. Hall, Jr., MD**, Chairman, Division of Orthopaedic Surgery, Cook County Hospital, Assistant Professor of Orthopaedic Surgery, University of Illinois, Chicago, Illinois

**John H. Healey, MD**, Associate Professor of Orthopaedic Surgery, Cornell University Medical College, Co-Chief, Metabolic Bone Disease, The Hospital for Special Surgery, Assistant Attending, Division of Orthopaedic Surgery, Memorial Sloan-Kettering Cancer Center, New York, New York

**Kenneth D. Johnson, MD**, Associate Professor of Orthopedic Surgery, The University of Texas Health Science Center at Dallas, Dallas, Texas

**Joseph M. Lane, MD**, Professor of Orthopaedic Surgery, Cornell University Medical College, Chief, Metabolic Bone Disease, The Hospital for Special Surgery, Chief, Division of Orthopaedic Surgery, Memorial Sloan-Kettering Cancer Center, New York, New York

**Loren L. Latta, PE, PhD**, Director of Research and Associate Professor, Department of Orthopaedics and Rehabilitation, University of Miami School of Medicine, Miami, Florida

**Michael M. Lewis, MD**, Robert K. Lippmann Professor of Orthopaedics, Mt. Sinai School of Medicine, Chairman, Department of Orthopaedics, Mt. Sinai Medical Center, New York, New York

**John E. Lonstein, MD**, Clinical Associate Professor of Orthopaedic Surgery, University of Minnesota, Minneapolis, Minnesota

**Roger A. Mann, MD**, Associate Clinical Professor of Orthopaedic Surgery, University of California, San Francisco, California

**Newton C. McCollough III, MD**, Director of Medical Affairs, Shriners Hospitals for Crippled Children, Professor of Orthopaedic Surgery, University of South Florida, Tampa, Florida

**Vert Mooney, MD**, Professor and Chairman, Division of Orthopedic Surgery, University of Texas Health Science Center at Dallas, Dallas, Texas

**Alex Norman, MD**, Professor of Radiology, New York University Medical School, Chairman, Department of Radiology, Hospital for Joint Diseases Orthopaedic Institute, New York, New York

**Frank R. Noyes, MD**, Clinical Professor of Orthopaedic Surgery, University of Cincinnati, The Center for Sportsmedicine and Cardiovascular Fitness, The Deaconess Hospital, Cincinnati, Ohio

**Manohar M. Panjabi, PhD, D Tech**, Professor and Director of Biomechanical Research, Department of Orthopaedics and Rehabilitation, Yale University School of Medicine, New Haven, Connecticut

**Arsen M. Pankovich, MD**, Department of Orthopaedic Surgery, Booth Memorial Medical Center, Hospital for Joint Diseases, Long Island College Hospital, New York, New York

**Michael J. Patzakis, MD**, Associate Professor of Orthopaedic Surgery, University of Southern California, Los Angeles, California

**Donald S. Pierce, MD**, Clinical Assistant Professor of Orthopaedic Surgery, Harvard Medical School, Boston, Massachusetts

**Thomas S. Renshaw, MD**, Director, Department of Orthopaedic Surgery, Newington Children's Hospital, Associate Professor of Orthopaedic Surgery, University of Connecticut Health Center, Farmington, Connecticut

**Leon Root, MD**, Attending Surgeon, Hospital for Special Surgery and New York Hospital, Chief, Pediatric Orthopaedic Surgery, Hospital for Special Surgery, Professor of Clinical Surgery (Orthopaedics), Cornell University Medical Center, New York, New York

**Augusto Sarmiento, MD**, Professor and Chairman, Department of Orthopaedics, University of Southern California, Los Angeles, California

**David Segal, MD**, Chairman, Department of Orthopaedics, Hadassah Hospital, Jerusalem, Israel

**Hubert A. Sissons, MD**, Chairman, Department of Laboratories, Hospital for Joint Diseases Orthopaedic Institute, Professor of Pathology, New York University School of Medicine, New York, New York

**Douglas K. Smith, MD**, Resident, Department of Orthopaedic Surgery, Mayo Clinic and Mayo Foundation, Rochester, Minnesota

**Elizabeth A. Szalay, MD**, Assistant Professor, Department of Orthopaedics and Rehabilitation, Vanderbilt University School of Medicine, Nashville, Tennessee

**Augustus A. White III, MD**, Chief, Orthopaedic Surgery, Beth Israel Hospital and Harvard Medical School, Boston, Massachusetts

**Joseph B. Zagorski, MD**, Clinical Associate Professor, Department of Orthopaedics and Rehabilitation, University of Miami School of Medicine, Miami, Florida

**Robert E. Zickel, MD**, Clinical Professor of Orthopaedic Surgery, Columbia University, Attending Orthopaedic Surgeon, St. Luke's-Roosevelt Hospital Center, New York, New York

**Gregory A. Zych, DO**, Assistant Professor and Chief, Orthopaedic Trauma Service, Department of Orthopaedics and Rehabilitation, University of Miami School of Medicine, Miami, Florida

# Preface

Volume 36 of the American Academy of Orthopaedic Surgeons *Instructional Course Lectures* follows in a long and distinguished tradition. Like its predecessors, this volume contains selected topics from Instructional Course Lectures. The chapters in Volume 36 are based on material presented at the Annual Meeting of the American Academy of Orthopaedic Surgeons in New Orleans, Louisiana, in February of 1986.

Volume 36 also represents a significant departure from tradition, in that it is the first *Instructional Course Lectures* volume to be published by the American Academy of Orthopaedic Surgeons. Over the years, several publishers have produced these volumes, the most recent being The C. V. Mosby Company. In 1985, however, the Board of Directors of the Academy made the decision to assume the publishing responsibilities for these volumes. We on the Instructional Course Committee hope that Volume 36 will serve as a worthy beginning of a new tradition, as well as maintain the high standards of publishing excellence represented by past volumes.

Volume 36 covers a variety of topics, with the largest section devoted to the diagnosis and management of extremity fractures. The chapters in this section reflect a broad range of orthopaedic knowledge and offer various approaches to the management of fractures, from more traditional methods and outlooks to recently developed techniques. All of the sections, however, represent timely and important subjects in the field of orthopaedics. We think each chapter will be informative and will provide an important contribution to the orthopaedic literature.

I would like to thank all of the authors for their efforts in producing the material for this volume. I would especially like to thank the members of the Committee on Instructional Courses who worked so diligently and so long in the service of the Instructional Course Lectures presented at the 1986 American Academy of Orthopaedic Surgeons Annual Meeting.

Additional thanks are due a number of Academy staff members who assisted in the production of this volume: Marilyn L. Fox, PhD; Wendy O. Schmidt; Alice A. Michaels; Geraldine Dubberke; Mark W. Wieting; and Thomas C. Nelson.

Paul P. Griffin, MD
Chicago, Illinois
1986 Chairman
Committee on Instructional Courses

Lewis D. Anderson, MD
Mobile, Alabama

Joseph S. Barr, Jr., MD
Boston, Massachusetts

Frank H. Bassett III, MD
Durham, North Carolina

E. Shannon Stauffer, MD
Springfield, Illinois

# Contents

# Physiology of Bone

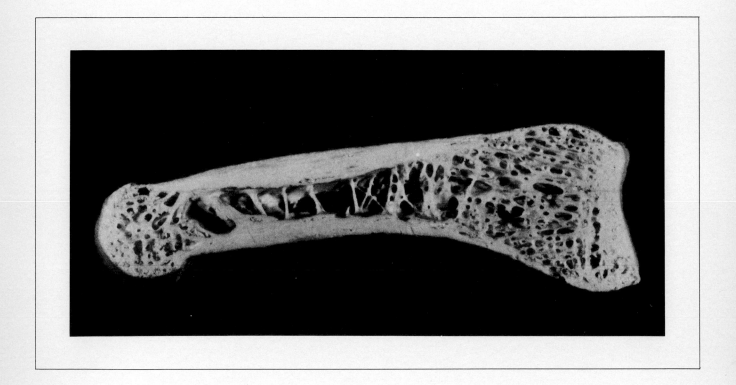

# Longitudinal Bone Growth: The Growth Plate and Its Dysfunctions

Carl T. Brighton, MD, PhD

## Introduction

Longitudinal growth of a typical long bone is confined predominantly to the growth plates located at each end of the bone. Hales[1] was the first to recognize that long bones increase in length by adding new bone at the ends, termed appositional growth, rather than by expanding from within, termed interstitial growth. He found that two drill holes placed in a chicken leg bone did not move farther apart as the bone increased in length. Later Belchier,[2] Duhamel,[3-5] and Hunter[6] conducted experiments with madder dye, which colored newly forming bone red. They concluded that bone increased both in length and width by the progressive laying down of new bone on the outer surfaces. After the advent of roentgenography, metallic markers were used to demonstrate that longitudinal growth occurred primarily at the epiphyseal growth plate, more properly called the growth plate.[7] The intent of this discussion is to explain the structure and function of the growth plate and to point out examples of its dysfunction. Only those clinical entities in which the physiologic abnormality has been fairly well documented are presented.

## Development of the Growth Plate

Early in the sixth week of human embryonic life, condensations occur in the mesenchyme that are the forerunners of the limb bones.[8] By the end of the sixth embryonic week, these mesenchymal condensations closely resemble the future long bones, and they begin to transform into cartilage. By the beginning of the seventh embryonic week, the future long bone is represented by a cartilage model, which in outline is a miniature replica of the bone-to-be. In the center of the cartilaginous anlage, the chondrocytes enlarge and become vacuolated, and the matrix between the cells begins to calcify. Near the end of the seventh week, cells in the inner layer of the perichondrium encircling the middle of the cartilaginous anlage increase in number and begin laying down a perichondrial, or, more properly, a periosteal collar of bone. The bone made by the periosteum is formed directly by osteoblasts derived from the periosteum without an intervening cartilaginous stage. This process of bone forming without a cartilage anlage is termed membranous or intramembranous ossifica-

tion. By the end of the embryonic period, or at the end of the eighth week, the periosteal bony collar is well formed.

The beginning of the fetal period in most human long bones begins with vascularization of the calcified midshaft of the cartilaginous anlage. This vascular invasion is marked by penetration of the bony collar by periosteal vascular buds.[9] These primitive buds contain mesenchymal cells that invade the calcified cartilage, differentiate into chondroclasts and osteoblasts, remove much of the matrix, and lay down bone on the remaining calcified cartilage remnants. This process of bone forming within or on cartilage is termed endochondral ossification, and it begins in the center of the cartilaginous anlage as the primary center of ossification. Once started, the primary center of ossification enlarges rapidly, and within a short time it occupies the middle two fourths of the cartilage model. By this time, endochondral ossification is confined to two structures called the growth plates at the proximal and distal ends of the primary center (Fig. 1–1). Endochondral ossification occurs in the growth plates in the same manner as it occurred originally when the primary center was formed; that is, chondrocytes enlarge and become vacuolated, the matrix is calcified, and invading cells from the metaphysis penetrate the cartilaginous base of the plate and lay down bone on calcified cartilage bars. Longitudinal growth occurs by the continued addition of cartilage at the top of the plate and the continued replacement of calcified cartilage by bone at the bottom of the plate.

As growth continues, the growth plates move progressively away from each other. At a rather definite time in each end of each long bone, in each species of animal, a secondary center of ossification appears. The secondary center of ossification, termed the epiphysis, similarly grows and expands centrifugally in all directions, although at a much slower rate than that which occurred in the primary center. As the distance between the growth plate and epiphysis gradually decreases, the portion of the epiphysis that faces the growth plate closes and becomes sealed with condensed bone, termed the terminal bone plate or simply the bone plate.[10] Thereafter, the epiphysis assumes a somewhat flattened, hemispheric appearance and slowly fills out the remaining end of the long bone. The fully developed growth plate may be divided anatomically into three different components

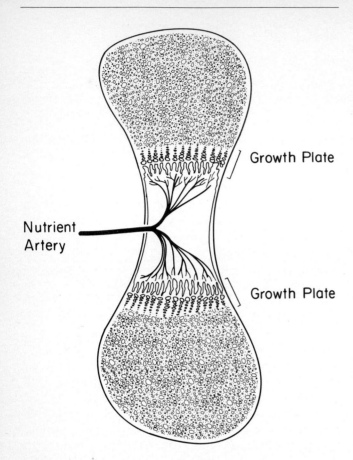

Growth Plate

Nutrient Artery

Growth Plate

**Fig. 1–1** The two growth plates of a typical long bone. Each growth plate is a peripheral extension of the original primary center of ossification that arose in the mid-portion of the cartilaginous anlage of the future bone-to-be early in the fetal period. (Reproduced with permission from Brighton CT: The growth plate. *Orthop Clin North Am* 1984;15:571.)

according to the three different tissues just cited: a cartilaginous component, itself divided into various histologic zones; a bony component or metaphysis; and a fibrous component surrounding the periphery of the plate, consisting of the groove of Ranvier and the perichondrial ring of LaCroix (Fig. 1–2). How the growth plate synchronizes chondrogenesis with osteogenesis, or interstitial cartilage growth with appositional bone growth, while it is growing in width, bearing loads, and responding to local and systemic forces and factors is a fascinating phenomenon the key features of which are only beginning to be understood.

### Vascular Supply of the Growth Plate

Each of the three components of the growth plate has its own distinct blood supply (Fig. 1–3).[11–13] The epiphyseal artery supplies the epiphysis, or the secondary center of ossification, which is not itself part of the growth plate. Small arterial branches arise at right angles to the main epiphyseal artery in the secondary

center of ossification and pass through small cartilage canals in the reserve zone to terminate at the top of the cell columns in the proliferative zone.[13] Each small arterial branch from the epiphyseal artery branches in rake-like fashion to supply the top portion of four to ten cell columns. The proliferative zone, therefore, is well supplied with blood. None of the arterial branches from the epiphyseal artery penetrates the cartilage portion of the growth plate beyond the uppermost part of the proliferative zone; that is, no vessels pass through the proliferative zone to supply the hypertrophic zone.

The metaphysis is richly supplied with blood from both the terminal branches of the nutrient artery and the metaphyseal arteries arising from the ascending cervical arteries. The nutrient artery supplies the central region of the metaphysis, supplying perhaps as much as four fifths of the metaphysis, whereas the metaphyseal vessels supply only the peripheral regions of the metaphysis. Terminal branches from the nutrient and metaphyseal arteries pass vertically toward the bone-cartilage junction of the growth plate and end in vascular loops or capillary tufts just below the last intact transverse septum at the base of the cartilage portion of the plate. The vessels turn back at this level, and venous branches descend to drain into several veins that eventually terminate in the large central vein of the diaphysis.[14,15] All[11] or most[16] of the vascular loops are closed, and microhemorrhages from the vascular loops probably do not occur. No vessels penetrate the bone-cartilage junction beyond the last intact transverse septum; that is, no vessels pass from the metaphysis into the hypertrophic zone in the fully developed growth plate.

The fibrous peripheral structures of the growth plate, the groove of Ranvier and the perichondrial ring of LaCroix, are richly supplied with blood from several perichondrial arteries.

Thus, the three components of the growth plate have their own distinct vascular supply. While the metaphysis and fibrous peripheral components have an abundant blood supply, only the proliferative zone of the cartilage portion of the growth plate is adequately supplied with blood. There are no vessels in the hypertrophic zone in the fully developed growth plate; that zone is entirely avascular. This avascularity of the hypertrophic zone has important implications concerning chondrocyte metabolism and matrix calcification.

Chung[17] studied the blood supply of the human femoral capital growth plate and found it, in general, similar to that of a typical growth plate. Epiphyseal arteries arising from the ascending cervical branches of the medial and lateral femoral circumflex arteries supplied the epiphysis in all the femoral heads studied by Chung. In 28% of the femoral heads, the epiphysis was also supplied by one or two branches of

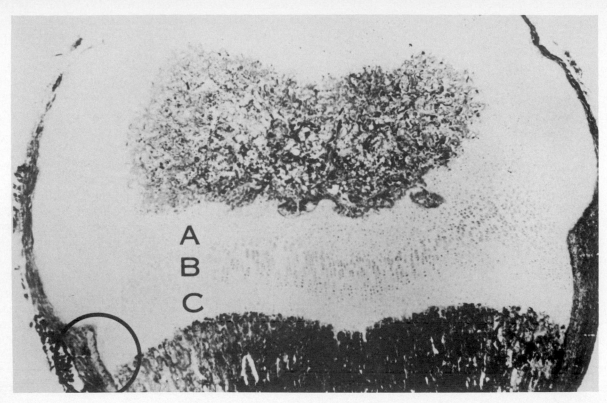

**Fig. 1–2** Photomicrograph of the distal femur of a 14-day-old rat showing the growth plate and the secondary bony epiphysis (A = reserve zone; B = proliferative zone; C = hypertrophic zone; the black ring encircles the ossification groove and the perichondrial ring) (hematoxylin-eosin, × 500). (Reproduced with permission from Brighton CT: Clinical problems in epiphyseal plate growth and development. American Academy of Orthopaedic Surgeons *Instructional Course Lectures, XXIII.* St Louis, CV Mosby, 1974, pp 105–122.)

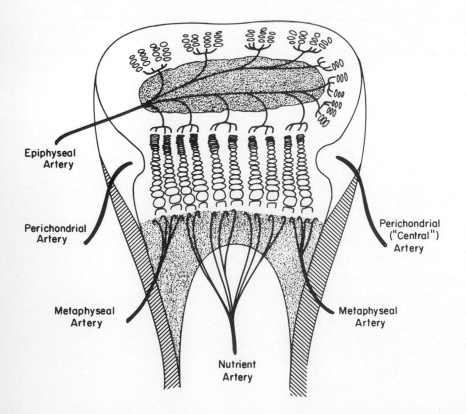

**Fig. 1–3** The blood supply of a typical fully developed growth plate. (Reproduced with permission from Brighton CT: Structure and function of the growth plate. *Clin Orthop* 1978;136:24.)

the artery of the ligamentum teres (Fig. 1–4). The metaphysis is supplied with blood from terminal branches of the nutrient artery as well as metaphyseal arteries arising from the ascending cervical arteries. The fibrocartilaginous peripheral structure of the femoral capital growth plate is richly supplied with blood from several perichondrial arteries arising from the ascending cervical arteries.

## Cartilaginous Components of the Growth Plate

The cartilaginous portion of the growth plate has been divided into various zones according to morphology or function (Fig. 1–5). It begins at the top of the reserve zone and ends with the last intact transverse septum at the bottom of each cell column in the hypertrophic zone. The reserve zone begins just beneath the secondary bony epiphysis and is followed by the proliferative zone and the hypertrophic zone. The hypertrophic zone is sometimes further subdivided into the zone of maturation, the zone of degeneration, and the zone of provisional calcification.

### Reserve Zone

The reserve zone lies immediately adjacent to the secondary bony epiphysis. Several different names have been applied to this zone, including resting zone, zone of small-sized cartilage cells, and germinal zone. However, as will be noted later, these cells are not resting, are not small in comparison with the cells in the proliferative zone, and are not germinal cells. They appear to be storing lipid and other materials and perhaps are being held in reserve for later nutritional requirements. If so, the term "reserve zone" might not be inappropriate. In any event, the cells in the zone are spherical, exist singly or in pairs, are relatively few in number compared with the number of cells in other zones, and are separated from each other by more extracellular matrix than are cells in any other zone. As stated earlier, the cells in the reserve zone are approximately the same size as the cells in the proliferative zone.[18] The cytoplasm exhibits a positive staining reaction for glycogen. Electron microscopy reveals these cells to contain abundant endoplasmic reticulum, a clear indication that they are actively synthesizing protein. They contain more lipid bodies and vacuoles than do cells in other zones[18] (Fig. 1–6) but contain less glucose-6-phosphate dehydrogenase, lactic dehydrogenase, malic dehydrogenase, and phosphoglucoisomerase.[19] The zone also contains the lowest amount of alkaline and acid phosphatase,[20] total and inorganic phosphate, calcium, chloride, potassium, and magnesium.[21]

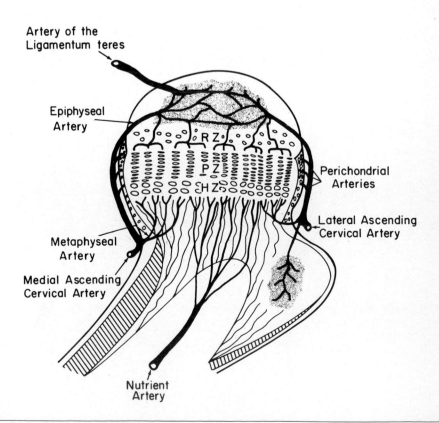

**Fig. 1–4** The blood supply of the capital femoral growth plate.

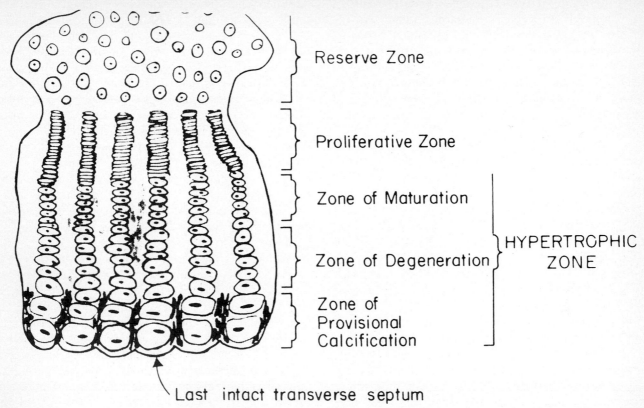

**Fig. 1–5**   The various zones of the cartilaginous portion of the growth plate. (Reproduced with permission from Brighton CT: Structure and function of the growth plate. *Clin Orthop* 1978;136:24.)

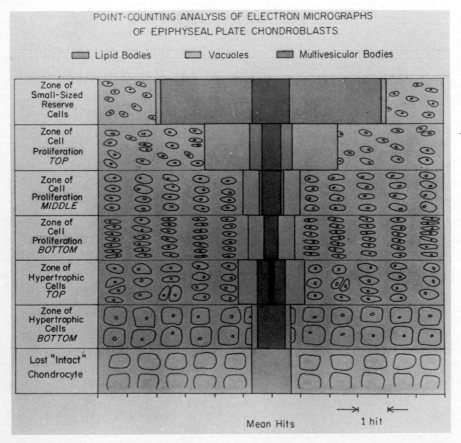

**Fig. 1–6** Content of cytoplasmic components of the various zones of the growth plate. (Redrawn with permission from Brighton CT, Sugioka Y, Hunt R: Cytoplasmic structures of epiphyseal-plate chondrocytes: Quantitative evaluation using electron micrographs of rat costochondral junctions with special reference to the fate of hypertrophic cells. *J Bone Joint Surg* 1973;55A:771–784.)

The matrix in the reserve zone contains less lipid,[22] glycosaminoglycan, protein polysaccharide, moisture, and ash[23] than the matrix in any other zone. It exhibits less incorporation of [35]S than any other zone and also shows less lysozyme activity than the other zones.[24] It contains the highest content of hydroxyproline of any zone in the plate.[22] Collagen fibrils in the matrix exhibit random distribution and orientation. Matrix vesicles are also seen, but they are fewer in number here than in other zones. The matrix shows a positive histochemical reaction for the presence of a neutral polysaccharide or an aggregate proteoglycan.

Oxygen tension measurements of the extracellular space in the different zones of the growth plate reveal that $Po_2$ is low (20.5 ± 2.1 mm Hg [2.73 ± 0.28 kPa]) in the reserve zone.[25] The blood vessels that pass through this zone in cartilage canals to arborize at the top of the proliferative zone do not actually supply the reserve zone itself.

The chondrocytes in the reserve zone either do not proliferate or do so only sporadically.[26,27] Therefore, the zone is not a germinal layer containing the so-called mother cartilage cells. As a matter of fact, the function of the zone is not clear. The high lipid, bony, and vacuole content may mean materials are being stored for later nutritional requirements, and, in this sense, the function of the zone is storage.

No known example exists in which the primary dysfunction in the growth plate is localized to the reserve zone. However, the reserve zone is affected by those abnormalities that afflict all zones of the cartilaginous portion of the growth plate, such as diastrophic dwarfism (defect in type II collagen synthesis[28]), pseudoachondroplastic dwarfism (abnormal accumulation of alternatively electron-dense and electron-lucent layers in the rough-surfaced endoplasmic reticulum in all chondrocytes of the growth plate[29] resulting from a defect in processing and transport of proteoglycans[28]), Kniest syndrome (defective processing of proteoglycans[28]), Hurler's syndrome (inborn error of metabolism in which the mucopolysaccharides chondroitin sulfate B and heparitin sulfate accumulate in chondrocytes of the growth plate[30]), Morquio's syndrome (inborn error of metabolism in which the mucopolysaccharide keratosulfate accumulates in swollen chondrocytes termed "foam cells"[31]), and cretinism (thyroid deficiency leading to abnormal mucopolysaccharide metabolism in which chondroitin sulfate polymers are thought not to be graded but instead accumulate in the chondrocytes and impair their synthetic activity[32]).

## Proliferative Zone

The spherical, single or paired chondrocytes in the reserve zone give way in the proliferative zone to flattened chondrocytes aligned in longitudinal columns, with the long axis of the cells being perpendicular to the long axis of the bone. The cytoplasm stains positively for glycogen. Electron microscopy shows the chondrocytes to be packed with endoplasmic reticulum.[18,33] Point-counting analysis shows that the percentage of the cytoplasmic area occupied by endoplasmic reticulum increases from 14.9% at the top of the zone to 40.1% at the bottom of the zone.[18] Biochemical analysis demonstrates that the zone of proliferation contains the largest amounts of hexosamine,[22,34] inorganic pyrophosphate,[20] sodium chloride, and potassium.[21] The proliferative zone shows the highest incorporation of [35]S of any zone in the growth plate, and it also has the highest level of lysozyme activity.[24]

Tritiated thymidine autoradiographic studies have indicated that the chondrocytes in the proliferative zone are, with few exceptions, the only cells in the cartilaginous portion of the growth plate that divide.[26,35] The top cell of each column is the true "mother" cartilage cell for each column, and it is the beginning or the top of the proliferative zone that is the true germinal layer of the growth plate. Longitudinal growth in the growth plate is equal to the rate of production of new chondrocytes at the top of the proliferative zone multiplied by the maximum size of the chondrocytes at the bottom of the hypertrophic zone.[26] Kember[26] showed that the average number of new chondrocytes produced daily in each column in the growth plate of the proximal tibia in the rat was five. Since the average diameter of the chondrocyte at the bottom of the hypertrophic zone is about 30 $\mu$m, the rate of growth from that particular growth plate is about 150 $\mu$m/day. Kember[36] further calculated that each division of a top cell in a cell column contributes 29 cells. This means each division of a top cell eventually contributes 0.9 mm of longitudinal growth to the rat tibia (29 $\mu$m × 30 $\mu$m = 870 $\mu$m). Forty to 50 top cell divisions would be required for the complete growth of the rat tibia. These principles (but not the absolute numbers) presumably hold true for all mammalian growth plates.

The matrix of the proliferating zone contains collagen fibrils, distributed at random, and matrix vesicles, confined mostly to the longitudinal septa. The matrix shows a positive histochemical reaction for a neutral mucopolysaccharide or an aggregated proteoglycan.

Oxygen tension is higher in the proliferative zone (57.0 ± 5.8 mm Hg [7.6 ± 0.77 kPa]) than in any of the other zones of the growth plate.[25] This is the result of the rich vascular supply present at the top of the zone. The relatively high oxygen tension in the proliferative zone, coupled with the presence of glycogen in the chondrocytes makes it apparent that aerobic metabolism with glycogen storage is occurring.

The function, then, of the proliferative zone is twofold: (1) matrix production and (2) cellular proliferation. The combination of these two functions equals linear or longitudinal growth. Paradoxically, although this chondrogenesis or cartilage growth is solely responsible for the increase in linear growth of any given long bone, the cartilaginous portion of the plate does not itself increase in length because of the vascular invasion that occurs from the metaphysis with the resultant removal of chondrocytes at the bottom of the hypertrophic zone. These events, in the normal growth plate, exquisitely balance the rate of cartilage production.

Abnormalities in the proliferative zone may affect chondrocyte proliferation or matrix production. Achondroplasia is a germ plasma defect in which endochondral bone formation is severely inhibited but membranous bone formation is normal. The basic defect may be an inability to carry on oxidative phosphorylation at normal rates.[37] The primary defect in the growth plate is in the proliferative zone where chondrocyte proliferation is decreased, cells are scanty, and column formation is poor or does not occur at all. The subsequent zones are also abnormal. The zone of hypertrophic cells is narrow and not well columnated. The metaphysis shows few calcified cores of cartilage, and trabecular new bone formation is scanty. At the bone-cartilage junction, a cellular, fibrous strip of tissue frequently appears between the cartilaginous portion of the plate and the metaphysis.[30] This so-called periosteal strip of fibrous tissue is thought to arise from the perichondrium, and at times it may effectively seal the plate. The lack of chondrocyte proliferation and the subsequent scanty matrix production result in decreased linear growth or shortening. Subperiosteal membranous bone formation is normal, however, so that the width of the shaft is normal. The metaphysis is flared as a result of the continued normal latitudinal growth from the ossification groove in the presence of decreased longitudinal growth from the zone of cell columns. The resultant clinical picture is that of an individual with severe extremity shortening (micromelia) but a trunk that is affected only slightly.

Malnutrition and protracted illness decrease chondrocyte proliferation in the proliferative zone. If severe enough or prolonged, stunting will result.[38] Chondrogenesis slows down, but bone formation in the metaphysis continues until a metaphyseal seal forms. When normal growth resumes, a dense line in the metaphysis remains as a permanent marker known as a Harris line or a growth arrest line.[39]

Irradiation of the growth plate affects the proliferative zone primarily and chondroblastic proliferation is greatly decreased. Latitudinal bone growth is not affected, and the resultant severely shortened bone of normal width resembles that seen in achondroplasia.[40] Similarly, papain depresses chondroblastic proliferation in the proliferative zone without affecting membranous bone formation. Here too, cylindrical bones are severely shortened but are of normal width.[41] Papain also releases chondroitin sulfate from the cartilage matrix by degrading the proteins to which the chondroitin sulfate is linked.

Estrogen excess and glucocorticoid excess lead to a depression of chondroblastic proliferation in the proliferative zone, whereas testosterone excess leads to an increase in chondroblastic proliferation.[42] The effect on growth is unpredictable, however, for there is a complex interrelationship among the steroid, growth, adrenal, and thyroid hormones that is not completely understood at this time. Hypergonadism, for example, may produce a temporary increase in linear growth, but early plate closure may result in a decreased total length. Hypogonadism may have the opposite effect; that is, linear growth proceeds at a slower rate, but plate closure is delayed. The net result may be an increase in total length.

An excess of growth hormone in a growing child leads to an increase in proliferation of chondroblasts in the proliferative zone. True gigantism results. A deficiency in growth hormone leads to a decrease in chondroblastic proliferation. The entire cartilaginous portion of the plate becomes thinner, and a bony metaphyseal seal appears.[39] Although there is a premature arrest in growth, the growth plates remain open for a prolonged period. Since both endochondral and membranous bone formation are depressed, the pituitary dwarf, unlike the achondroplastic dwarf, exhibits normal bodily proportions between the trunk and the extremities. Also, the cylindrical bones are not flared at the metaphyses in the pituitary dwarf, and the midshaft is not disproportionately wide when compared to total bone length as in achondroplasia.

It is obvious that any severe abnormality in chondrocyte proliferation in the proliferative zone may affect matrix production in that same zone. For the most part, these changes are quantitative rather than qualitative, at least as far as is known. Thus, in malnutrition and severe or chronic illness chondroblastic proliferation slows down, but so too does matrix production.[43] In estrogen excess and in glucocorticoid excess, both cellular proliferation and micropolysaccharide production in the proliferative zone are depressed.[42] The decrease in matrix production is secondary to the decrease in chondroblastic proliferation; that is, fewer cells produce less matrix. There are diseases, however, in which the primary abnormality is in the failure of the chondroblasts to produce a qualitatively normal matrix, such as those abnormalities affecting all zones of the growth plate (i.e., diastrophic dwarfism, pseudoachondroplastic dwarfism, Kniest syndrome, Hurler's syndrome, Marquio's syndrome, and cretinism).

### Hypertrophic Zone

The flattened chondrocytes in the proliferative zone become spherical and greatly enlarged in the hypertrophic zone. These morphologic changes are quite abrupt, and the end of the proliferative zone and the beginning of the hypertrophic zone can usually be distinguished with an accuracy of one or two cells. By the time the average chondrocyte reaches the bottom of the hypertrophic zone, it has enlarged to five times its size in the proliferative zone.[18] The cytoplasm of the chondrocytes in the top half of the hypertrophic zone stains positively for glycogen (PAS reaction coupled with diastase digestion), but near the middle of the zone the cytoplasm abruptly loses all glycogen stainability.[44,45] On light microscopy, the chondrocytes in the hypertrophic zone appear vacuolated. Toward the bottom of the zone, such vacuolation becomes extensive, nuclear fragmentation occurs, and the cells appear to be nonviable. At the very bottom of each cell column in the hypertrophic zone, the lacunae appear to be empty and are devoid of any cellular content.

On electron microscopy, the chondrocytes in the top half of the hypertrophic zone appear to be normal and contain the full complement of cytoplasmic components (Fig. 1–7).[18,46] However, in the bottom half of the zone, the cytoplasm contains holes that occupy more than 85% of the total cytoplasmic column.[18] Obviously, holes and not vacuoles account for the "vacuolation" seen on light microscopy. Electron microscopy also shows that glycogen is abundant in the chondrocytes in the top half of the zone, diminishes rapidly in the middle of the zone, and disappears completely from the cells in the bottom portion of the zone. The last cell at the base of each cell column is clearly nonviable and shows extensive fragmentation of the cell membrane and the nuclear envelope, with loss of all cytoplasmic components except a few mitochondria and scattered remnants of endoplasmic reticulum. Clearly, the ultimate fate of the hypertrophic chondrocyte is death.

Electron-dense granules appear in mitochondria on electron micrographs of growth plate chondrocytes.[47,48] These granules are not removed by microincineration[48] and, hence, are mineral. They have been shown by direct analysis to have the characteristic radiographic spectra of calcium and phosphorus[49]; they have their highest concentration in chondrocytes in the hypertrophic zone in the normal growth plate and are absent or greatly diminished in number in

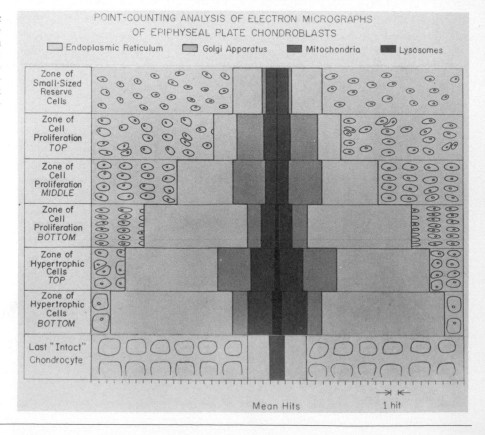

**Fig. 1–7** Content of cytoplasmic components of the various zones of the growth plate. (Redrawn with permission from Brighton CT, Sugioka Y, Hunt R: Cytoplasmic structures of epiphyseal-plate chondrocytes: Quantitative evaluation using electron micrographs of rat costochondral junctions with special reference to the fate of hypertrophic cells. *J Bone Joint Surg* 1973;55A:771–784.)

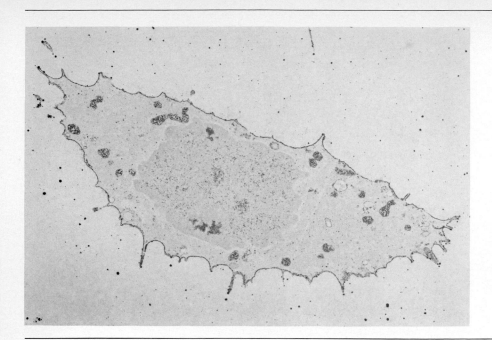

**Fig. 1–8** Electron micrograph of a cell from the top portion of the hypertrophic zone of a costochondral junction in a 21-day-old rat (potassium pyroantimonate, × 800). Note that the black antimony-calcium complex is located primarily in mitochondria and the cell membrane. (Reproduced with permission from Brighton CT: The growth plate. *Orthop Clin North Am* 1984;15: 571.)

the rachitic growth plate.[48] Histochemical localization of calcium at the ultrastructural level in the growth plate shows the mitochondria and cell membranes of chondrocytes in the top half of the hypertrophic zone to be loaded with calcium (Fig. 1–8).[50,51] Toward the middle of the zone, mitochondria rapidly lose calcium, and at the bottom of the zone, both mitochondria and cell membranes are totally devoid of calcium. All the studies cited provided circumstantial evidence that mitochondrial calcium may be involved in cartilage calcification.

Biochemical analyses of the hypertrophic zone indicate that this region, or at least the upper three fourths of it, is active metabolically. Of all the zones, it has the highest content of alkaline phosphatase, acid phosphatase, glucose-6-dehydrogenase, lactic dehydrogenase, malic dehydrogenase, phosphoglucoisomerase,[19,20] total and inorganic phosphate, calcium, magnesium,[21] moisture and ash,[23] and lipid.[22] It contains the least amount of hydroxyproline[22] and hexosamine.[34]

Oxygen tension in the hypertrophic zone is quite low (24.3 ± 2.4 mm Hg [3.2 ± 0.3 kPa]),[25] no doubt because of the avascularity of the zone.

To summarize (Fig. 1–9), in the proliferative zone, oxygen tension is high, aerobic metabolism occurs, glycogen is stored, and mitochondria form adenosine triphosphate (ATP). Mitochondria can form ATP or store calcium, but both processes cannot occur at the same place in the mitochondria at the same time[52]; that is, ATP formation and calcium accumulation are alternative processes and do not occur simultaneously. In the proliferative zone, the energy requirement for matrix production and cellular proliferation is

high, and mitochondria form ATP. In the hypertrophic zone, oxygen tension is low, anaerobic metabolism occurs, and glycogen is consumed until near the middle of the zone, where mitochondria switch from forming ATP to accumulating calcium.[50] Why this switch occurs at this level in the growth plate is not entirely clear. However, both the formation of ATP and calcium accumulation are active processes requiring energy.[53] Such energy comes from the respiratory chain in the mitochondria. In addition, ATP formation requires the presence of adenosine diphosphate (ADP), whereas calcium accumulation does not. It may well be that in the hypertrophic zone there simply is not enough ADP to allow significant ATP formation. In any event, mitochondria in the top half of the hypertrophic zone accumulate calcium and do not form ATP.

In the bottom half of the hypertrophic zone, as stated previously, glycogen is completely depleted. In this area of low oxygen tension, there is no other source of nutrition to serve as an energy source for the mitochondria. Since retention of calcium by mitochondria, as well as uptake of calcium, is an active process requiring energy,[53] as soon as the chondrocytes' glycogen supplies are exhausted, mitochondria release calcium. This released calcium may play a role in matrix calcification.

Growth plate chondrocyte mitochondria may be peculiarly adapted to accumulating and releasing calcium, especially if these processes do play a role in matrix calcification. Growth plate chondrocytes contain significantly less total mitochondrial protein per total cell protein and significantly less total mitochondrial volume per total cell volume than do liver cells,

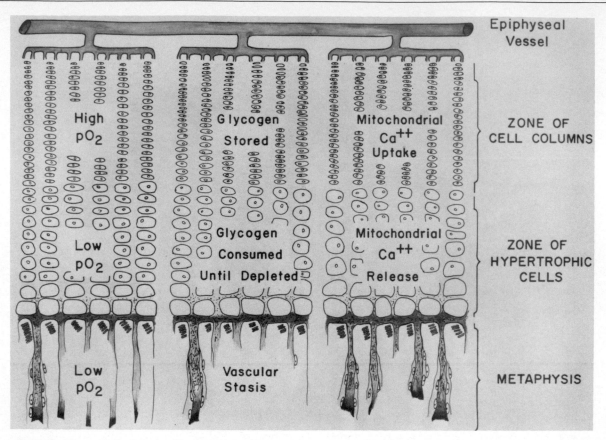

**Fig. 1–9** The growth plate showing the relative oxygen tensions in the various zones in the left-hand column, the change in glycogen storage and utilization in the center column, and the role of mitochondria in the right-hand column. (Reproduced with permission from Brighton CT, Hunt RM: The role of mitochondria in growth plate calcification as demonstrated in a rachitic model. *J Bone Joint Surg* 1978;60A:630–639.)

yet the endogenous calcium in freshly isolated chondrocyte mitochondria is significantly greater than that of liver cell mitochondria (Fig. 1–10).[54,55] Growth plate chondrocyte mitochondria also take up and release significantly more calcium than do liver mitochondria (Fig. 1–11).[55] These results suggest that the growth plate chondrocyte mitochondria are, indeed, specialized for calcium transport and provide further evidence that they may play an important role in calcification of the cartilage matrix.

Another interesting feature of growth plate metabolism is the fact that the glycerol phosphate shuttle is absent throughout all the zones of the cartilaginous portion of the plate.[56] In most normal cells, the conversion of glucose to pyruvate via the glycolytic cycle causes the constant oxidation of cytoplasmic NADH (the reduced form of nicotinamide adenine dinucleotide [NAD]) through the action of the cytoplasmic enzyme glycerol phosphate dehydrogenase. The glycerol phosphate so formed readily penetrates mitochondrial membranes resulting in a shuttle (the glycerol phosphate shuttle) that reduces equivalents from cytoplasmic NADH to the intramitochondrial

respiratory chain (Fig. 1–12). In the growth plate chondrocytes, as demonstrated in this study, there is a lack of cytoplasmic glycerol phosphate dehydrogenase (Fig. 1–13). Dihydroxyacetone phosphate cannot form glycerol phosphate but instead, reenters the glycolytic cycle eventually to form pyruvate. Cytoplasmic NADH, instead of being oxidized by dihydroxyacetone phosphate via glycerol phosphate dehydrogenase, is oxidized by pyruvate via lactate dehydrogenase to form lactate. Thus, lactate accumulates in the presence of ample oxygen concentration (aerobic accumulation) even though the Krebs cycle (tricarboxylic acid cycle) and electron transport are proceeding at normal rates.

The matrix of the hypertrophic zone, unlike that of the other zones, shows a positive histochemical reaction for an acid mucopolysaccharide or a disaggregated proteoglycan. Electron microscopy reveals that the length of proteoglycan aggregates and the number of subunits of the aggregate in the matrix progressively decrease from the reserve zone through the hypertrophic zone.[57] The distance between the subunits increases at the same time (Fig. 1–14).

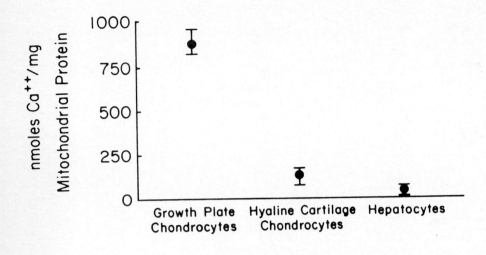

### Mitochondrial Calcium Content (Endogenous Calcium) Freshly Isolated Cells

**Fig. 1–10**  The amount of endogenous calcium in freshly isolated growth plate chondrocyte mitochondria is significantly greater than in hyaline cartilage chondrocytes or in hepatocytes.

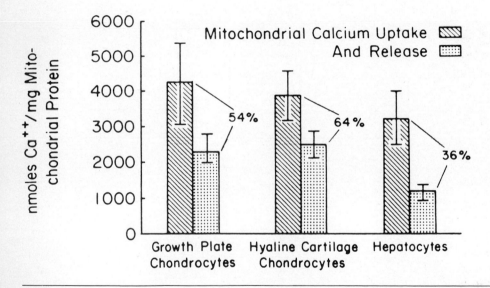

**Fig. 1–11**  The uptake and release of growth plate chondrocyte mitochondria are increased compared to those of hyaline cartilage mitochondria and liver mitochondria.

Some have speculated that the large proteoglycan aggregates with tightly packed subunits may inhibit mineralization or the spread of mineralization, whereas smaller aggregates with widely spaced subunits at the bottom of the hypertrophic zone may be less effective in preventing mineral growth.[57] Lysozyme may be involved in the disaggregation of large proteoglycan aggregates,[24,58,59] or lysosomal enzymes such as neutral proteases may degrade the proteoglycan.[60] In any event, it seems apparent that proteoglycan disaggregation or degradation must take place before significant mineralization occurs.[61,62]

The initial calcification (termed "seeding" or "nucleation") that occurs in the growth plate in the bottom of the hypertrophic zone (zone of provisional calcification) does so within or on matrix vesicles in the longitudinal septa of the matrix (Figs. 1–15 and 1–16).[63–66] Matrix vesicles are very small structures, measuring 100 to 150 nm in diameter, enclosed in a trilamellar membrane and, therefore, produced by the chondrocyte. They occur in greatest concentration in the hypertrophic zone.[65] Matrix vesicles are rich in alkaline phosphatase,[67] and this enzyme may act as a pyrophosphatase to destroy pyrophosphate, another inhibitor of calcium phosphate precipitation.[68] Matrix vesicles begin to accumulate calcium at the same level in the middle of the hypertrophic zone at which mitochondria begin to lose calcium (Figs.

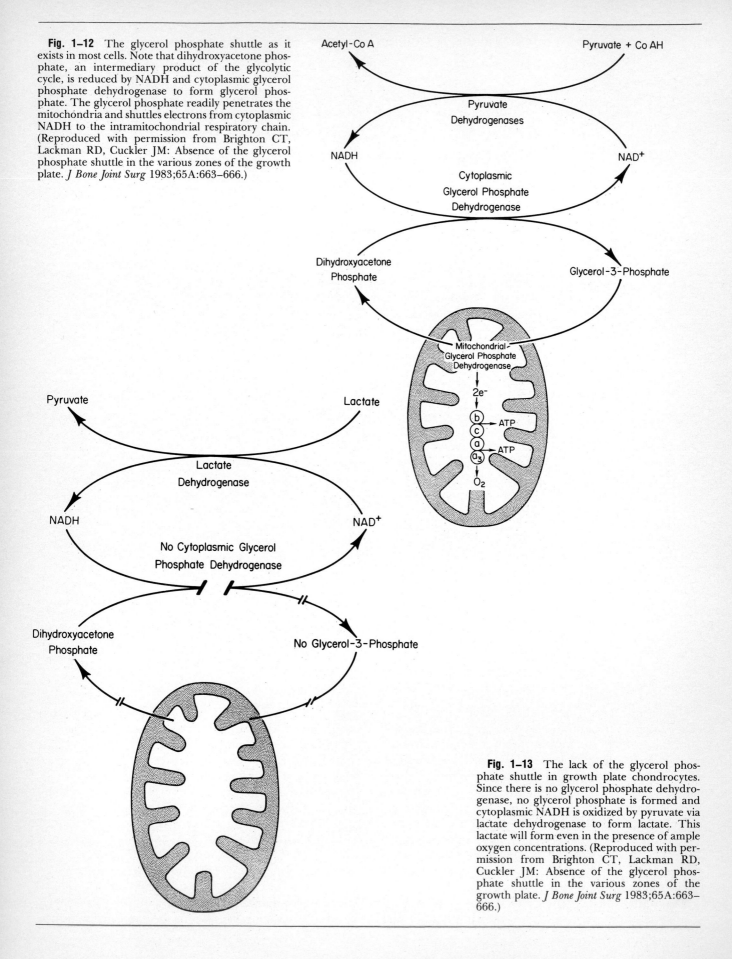

**Fig. 1–12** The glycerol phosphate shuttle as it exists in most cells. Note that dihydroxyacetone phosphate, an intermediary product of the glycolytic cycle, is reduced by NADH and cytoplasmic glycerol phosphate dehydrogenase to form glycerol phosphate. The glycerol phosphate readily penetrates the mitochondria and shuttles electrons from cytoplasmic NADH to the intramitochondrial respiratory chain. (Reproduced with permission from Brighton CT, Lackman RD, Cuckler JM: Absence of the glycerol phosphate shuttle in the various zones of the growth plate. *J Bone Joint Surg* 1983;65A:663–666.)

**Fig. 1–13** The lack of the glycerol phosphate shuttle in growth plate chondrocytes. Since there is no glycerol phosphate dehydrogenase, no glycerol phosphate is formed and cytoplasmic NADH is oxidized by pyruvate via lactate dehydrogenase to form lactate. This lactate will form even in the presence of ample oxygen concentrations. (Reproduced with permission from Brighton CT, Lackman RD, Cuckler JM: Absence of the glycerol phosphate shuttle in the various zones of the growth plate. *J Bone Joint Surg* 1983;65A:663–666.)

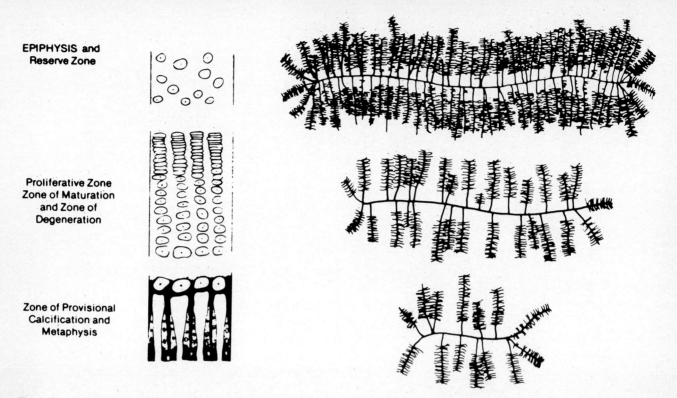

**EPIPHYSIS and Reserve Zone**

**Proliferative Zone Zone of Maturation and Zone of Degeneration**

**Zone of Provisional Calcification and Metaphysis**

**Fig. 1–14** Scaled diagram showing the average relative size and form of aggregates from the three different regions of the growth plate. Aggregates from the epiphysis and reserve zone are not only larger, but also they have much closer spacing between subunits. (Reproduced with permission from Buckwalter JA: Proteoglycan structure in calcifying cartilage. *Clin Orthop* 1983;172:207–232.)

1–17 and 1–18).[50,51] This is circumstantial evidence indicating that mitochondrial calcium is involved in the initial calcification that occurs in the growth plate.

Landis and associates[69,70] criticized the matrix-vesicle nucleation theory because of potential artifacts arising from the use of aqueous solutions in the preparation of mineralizing tissue for electron microscopy. They were unable to demonstrate any association between matrix vesicles and mineralization in the growth plate. However, Morris and associates,[71] using three different anhydrous preparatory techniques, including the methods employed by Landis and Glimcher,[69] observed the initial mineral deposition in the growth plate to be associated with matrix vesicles in all three methods of fixation. They found no evidence of mineral deposition in any other site preceding matrix-vesicle mineralization. Again, this study supported the theory that the matrix vesicle is the initial nucleating site in the cartilaginous fracture callus.

The initial calcification that occurs in the growth plate has also been described in structures other than matrix vesicles. Other possible sites of nucleation include collagen and proteoglycans. Glimcher and Krane[72] demonstrated a close relationship between collagen structure and apatite deposition. However,

Bernard and Pease[73] showed that the earliest nucleation sites have no obvious association with collagen fibrils, and certainly several other studies have supported this view.[50,51,63–66]

Shepard and Mitchell[74] demonstrated rosette-like proteoglycan structures in the growth plate when it was treated with acridine orange to stabilize proteoglycans. These rosette-like structures were quite large (as much as 1 $\mu$m in diameter) and were in the longitudinal septa of the lower portion of the hypertrophic zone after demineralization. Their location was identical to that of dense, spherical mineral clusters in undemineralized sections. The role that these proteoglycan structures play in mineralization is not yet clear. Finally, Poole and associates[75] described a calcium-binding protein, termed chondrocalcin, in the extracellular matrix of longitudinal septa that occupied the precise location at which amorphous mineral was deposited (demonstrated on electron microscopy). Since chondrocalcin has a strong affinity for hydroxyapatite, these observations suggest that chondrocalcin may represent yet another nucleating site.

The initial calcification in the matrix, regardless of the nucleating site, may be in the form of amorphous calcium phosphate[76] or, in fact, the precise nature of

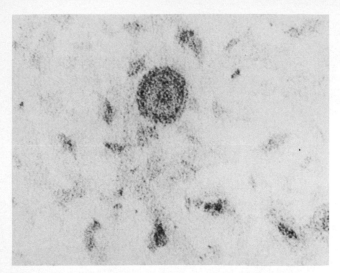

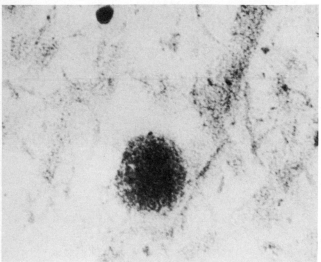

**Fig. 1–15**    Electron micrographs of matrix vesicles from the top portion of the hypertrophic zone. The matrix vesicle in the top picture was stained conventionally, and the matrix vesicle in the bottom picture was stained for calcium with potassium pyroantimonate (no calcium-stain complex is shown here) (× 240,000). (Reproduced with permission from Brighton CT: The growth plate. *Orthop Clin North Am* 1984;15:571.)

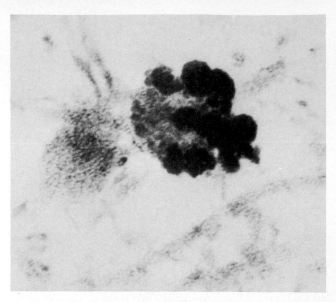

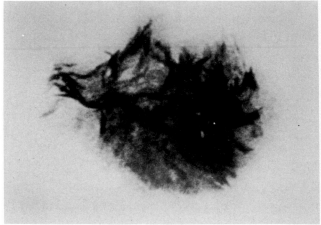

**Fig. 1–16**    Electron micrographs of matrix vesicles from the middle and the bottom of the hypertrophic zone. The matrix vesicle in the top picture is from the middle of the hypertrophic zone and exhibits large clump-like calcium-stain complex either on or within the vesicle. The matrix vesicle in the bottom picture is from the bottom of the hypertrophic zone. Note that the typical crystal formation of hydroxyapatite is present within or upon the matrix vesicle (× 240,000).

the first mineral deposited in the cartilage matrix may be unknown.[77] Regardless of the exact form of the initial calcification, it rapidly gives way to hydroxyapatite crystal formation. With crystal growth and confluence, the longitudinal septa become calcified in the bottom portion of the hypertrophic zone, a region frequently called the zone of provisional calcification.

Calcification of the matrix in the bottom of the hypertrophic zone makes the intercellular matrix relatively impermeable to metabolites. Diffusion coefficients of the various zones of the growth plate have been measured, and the hypertrophic zone has the lowest diffusion coefficient in the entire growth

plate[78] because of the high mineral content of that zone. This fact suggests that as calcification occurs, diffusion of nutrients and oxygen to the hypertrophic chondrocyte is decreased, anaerobic glycolysis with glycogen consumption occurs until all the glycogen is depleted, mitochondria release calcium, nucleation occurs in the matrix vesicles, and calcification of the matrix occurs. Thus, a cycle is established that ultimately results in the death of the hypertrophic chondrocyte (Fig. 1–19).

The functions of the hypertrophic zone seem clear; they are (1) to prepare the matrix for calcification and (2) to calcify the matrix. Although these processes are complex biophysical phenomena, it is evident from

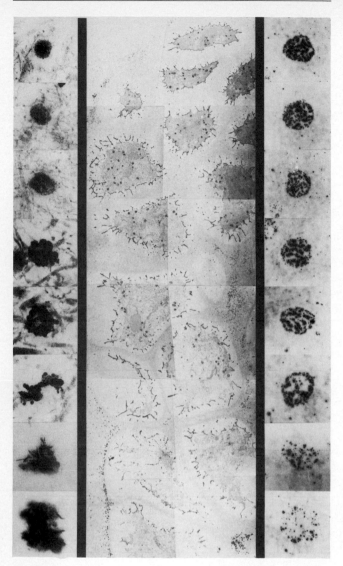

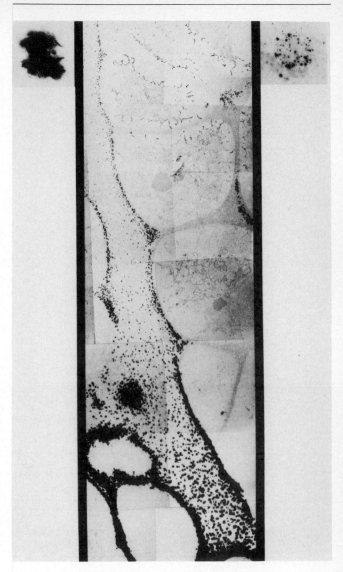

**Fig. 1–17**  Montage of electron micrographs of the upper half of the hypertrophic zone. The antimony-calcium complex is predominantly intracellular at the top of the zone but becomes progressively more extracellular farther down the zone. The inserts on the right are of mitochondria in chondrocytes at corresponding levels in the zone; note the gradual loss of antimony-calcium complex the farther down the mitochondrion is located. The inserts on the left are of matrix vesicles at corresponding levels in the zone; note the gradual accumulation of the antimony-calcium complex the farther down the zone the vesicle is located. (Reproduced with permission from Brighton CT, Hunt RM: Mitochondrial calcium and its role in calcification. *Clin Orthop* 1974;100:406–416.)

**Fig. 1–18**  Montage of electron micrograph of the lower half of the hypertrophic zone shown in Fig. 1–14. (Reproduced with permission from Brighton CT, Hunt RM: Mitochondrial calcium and its role in calcification. *Clin Orthop* 1974;100:406–416.)

the studies cited that the mechanisms and factors controlling matrix calcification are being discovered.

Abnormalities in the hypertrophic zone may be discussed in terms of the functions of that zone. Abnormalities in preparation of a calcifiable matrix include Jansen's disease, Ollier's disease, and hypophosphatasia. Jansen's disease, or metaphyseal dysostosis congenita, is a rare disease of skeletal development in which hypertrophic cartilage cells persist

down into the metaphysis. The basic defect in the disease may be the failure of hypertrophic cells to mature and degenerate, caused by a block in or deficiency of enzymes of the glycolytic cycle.[79] In some areas, the growth plate may be replaced by large accumulations of hypertrophic cartilage cells. Calcification does occur, but it is irregular, is streaky in appearance, and is not sufficient in quantity to support normal endochondral bone growth. The masses of cartilage in the metaphysis, the failure of the hypertrophic cells to degenerate, and the irregularity of calcification of the cartilage matrix all disrupt the normal sequences of endochondral bone formation, resulting in stunting.[79] The lower extremities are affected much more severely than the upper extremi-

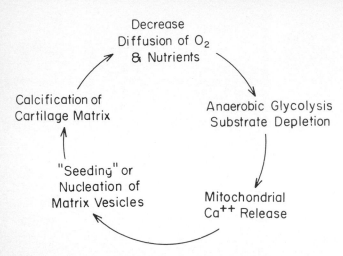

**Fig. 1–19** Events in the hypertrophic zone relating matrix calcification to decreased PO$_2$, glycogen metabolism, and mitochondrial calcium release. (Reproduced with permission from Brighton CT, Hunt RM: The role of mitochondria in growth plate calcification as demonstrated in a rachitic model. *J Bone Joint Surg* 1978;60A:630–639.)

ties. The hands of an affected patient in the standing position may almost reach the ground. Radiographic examination of the long bones show normal-appearing epiphyses, with flaring, cup-shaped metaphyses of marked irregularity containing cystic dilatations. Radiolucent areas in the metaphysis often contain punctate radiopacities, representing calcification within the cartilage clumps.

Ollier's disease (dyschondroplasia or multiple enchondromatosis) also exhibits masses of cartilage in the metaphysis and on this basis has been included as a disease of the growth plate. There is doubt as to the origin of the cartilage accumulations, however. The cartilage in the metaphysis may be immature hypertrophic cells left behind by the advancing growth plate,[80] or the cartilage cells may be derived from the cambium layer of the periosteum.[30] This last view may explain cartilage clumps in the midshaft of a long bone. In any event, if the cartilage accumulation is near the bone-cartilage junction of the growth plate, endochondral bone formation may be disrupted. Radiographic examination shows a radiolucent defect in the metaphysis of an involved bone. Frequently, the defect appears as a large cystic area that is trabeculated and irregularly calcified. Depending on the size and location of the cartilage accumulations, plate growth may be disrupted, and shortening or angulation or both may result. Usually the lesions are unilateral, and the lower extremities are affected more often than the upper extremities.

Hypophosphatasia is an inborn error in alkaline phosphatase metabolism in which either the synthesis of that enzyme is decreased or its destruction is increased. The net effect is that alkaline phosphatase concentrations in the serum, bone, growth plates, liver, kidneys, and other tissues are greatly reduced. Serum calcium levels are normal or increased. Phosphoethanolamine is present in the urine. In the normal growth plate, the highest concentrations of alkaline phosphatase are found in the zone of hypertrophic cells and in the metaphysis.[20] Alkaline phosphatase is one of a group of pyrophosphatases that degrade pyrophosphate. Pyrophosphate stabilizes bone, inhibiting either bone formation or bone resorption. When pyrophosphate is removed by alkaline phosphatase, bone formation (or bone resorption) may occur.[81] Presumably this holds true for cartilage also. If pyrophosphate is not removed, as in hypophosphatasia, the cartilage matrix fails to calcify. The zone of hypertrophic cells becomes greatly widened. Since the cartilage matrix does not calcify, a zone of provisional calcification does not form. In the metaphysis, osteoid is laid down but it is not mineralized.[82] Since serum calcium levels are normal or even increased, it seems that a calcifiable matrix has not been formed; that is, a primary spongiosa has not formed. Microscopically, the disease is similar to rickets in that the reserve zone and proliferative zone are normal, but the zone of hypertrophic cells is greatly widened and extends into the metaphysis. Calcified cartilage bars do not form, and in the metaphysis many large osteoid seams surround thin bony trabeculae. Radiographic examination demonstrates findings similar to those in rickets. There is no zone of provisional calcification, the distance between the epiphysis and the diaphysis is increased, there is mild flaring of the metaphysis, and the metaphysis may appear to be frayed. Longitudinal bone growth is usually decreased as a result of accumulations of hypertrophic cells at the bone-cartilage junction.

The primary example of an abnormality of the growth plate in which the cartilage matrix does not calcify is rickets. In hypophosphatasia a calcifiable matrix is not formed. In rickets, a calcifiable matrix is formed but the matrix does not calcify because of lack of adequate available mineral. The net effect in both diseases is the same: the primary spongiosa is not formed, and the osteoid laid down in the metaphysis is not mineralized. Microscopically these two diseases are similar if not indistinguishable. The reserve zone and proliferative zones are normal, the zone of hypertrophic cells is greatly widened, and tongues of hypertrophic cells extend down into the metaphysis. The cartilage matrix does not calcify, and wide osteoid seams are present in the metaphysis. The bone that does form is thin and sparse. Electron microscopic histochemical studies reveal that mitochondria in the bottom portion of the hypertrophic zone in phosphate-deprived rachitic rats do not release calcium,[83] the matrix does not calcify, and the normally low diffusion of the matrix in that region rises to high levels.[78] Diffusion of nutrients to the hypertrophic chondrocyte is also presumably increased. Thus, the hypertrophic cell remains alive, is not removed, and, hence, accounts for the typical increase in length of that zone seen in rickets. The radiographic view of a typical long bone in rickets is similar to that in hypophosphatasia. Laboratory findings in the two diseases are different, of course, because in rickets the serum alkaline phosphatase values are almost always increased and serum calcium values tend to be low-normal or low.

## Metaphysis

The metaphysis begins just distal to the last intact transverse septum at the base of each cell column of the cartilage portion of the growth plate (Fig. 1–20). The metaphysis ends in the region where narrowing or funnelization of the bone ceases, that is, where the wider metaphysis meets the narrower diaphysis.[80] In the first part of the metaphysis just distal to the cartilaginous portion of the plate, the oxygen tension is low ($19.8 \pm 3.2$ mm Hg [$2.6 \pm 0.4$ kPa]).[25] The low oxygen tension, as well as the rouleaux formation of the red cells frequently seen just distal to the last intact transverse septum,[84] indicates that this region is one of vascular stasis. A flocculent, electron-dense material within the lumina of vascular sprouts invading the transverse septa may similarly indicate the presence of circulatory stasis within these vessels.[85] In addition, high levels of phosphoglucoisomerase, an enzyme active in anaerobic metabolism, are found in this region and are compatible with vascular stasis.[19]

On light microscopy, in the first part of the metaphysis, the first lacuna distal to the last intact transverse septum at the base of each column of the cells is either empty or contains one or more red cells. On electron microscopy, capillary sprouts or loops lined with a layer of endothelial and perivascular cells invade the base of the cartilaginous portion of the plate.[85] Cytoplasmic processes from these cells push into the transverse septa and, presumably through lysosomal enzyme activity, degrade and remove the nonmineralized transverse septa. At this same level in the metaphysis, the longitudinal septa are partially or completely calcified. Osteoblasts, plump, oval cells with eccentric nuclei, line up along the calcified bars. Between the osteoblasts lining the calcified bars and the capillary sprouts are osteoprogenitor cells, cells with little cytoplasm but with prominent ovoid to spindle-shaped nuclei.[86] This region of vascularized calcified cartilage with little or no bone formation occurring on the calcified bars is termed the primary spongiosa.[87]

A short distance (within one or two cells) farther down the calcified longitudinal septa, the osteoblasts

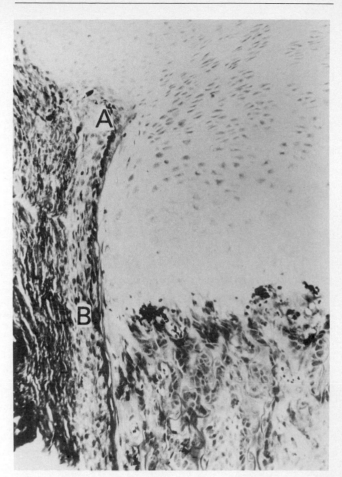

**Fig. 1–20** Photomicrograph of the periphery of the distal femoral growth plate of a 14-day-old rat showing (A) the ossification groove of Ranvier and (B) the perichondrial ring of LaCroix (hematoxylin-eosin, $\times$ 100). (Reproduced with permission from Brighton CT: Clinical problems in epiphyseal plate growth and development. American Academy of Orthopaedic Surgeons *Instructional Course Lectures, XXIII*. St Louis, CV Mosby, 1974, pp 105–122.

begin laying down bone (termed endochondral ossification, that is, bone formation within or on cartilage). The farther into the metaphysis one progresses, the more bone is formed on the calcified cartilage bars. At the same time, the calcified cartilage bars gradually diminish in thickness until they disappear altogether. This region in the metaphysis where bone is laid down on calcified cartilage bars is termed the secondary spongiosa.[87] Still further down in the metaphysis, the original fiber bone is replaced with lamellar bone. This gradual replacement of the calcified longitudinal septa by newly formed fiber bone, as well as the gradual replacement of fiber bone by lamellar bone, is termed internal or histologic remodeling.[88] Large, irregularly shaped cells with foamy, eosinophilic cytoplasm and one or more nuclei containing several nucleoli are evenly distributed throughout the entire metaphysis, except in the primary spongiosa.

These osteoclasts are also seen subperiosteally around the outside of the metaphysis at the point where it diminishes in diameter to meet the diaphysis. This narrowing or funnelization of the metaphysis is termed external or anatomic remodeling.[88]

The functions of the metaphysis are (1) vascular invasion of the transverse septa at the bottom of the cartilaginous portion of the growth plate, (2) bone formation, and (3) remodeling, both internal and histologic (removal of calcified cartilage bars; replacement of fiber bone with lamellar bone) and external or anatomic (funnelization of the metaphysis).

Abnormalities in the metaphysis, arranged according to the functions of that region, involve vascularity and vascular invasion, bone formation, and bone remodeling. In acute hematogenous osteomyelitis in the child, the infection usually starts in the metaphysis of the involved long bone. Bacteria lodge in the vascular sinusoids or loops on the metaphyseal side of the bone-cartilage junction. Why bacteria flourish in this location is not known, but possible explanations include sluggish circulation,[85] low oxygen tension,[25] and a deficiency of the reticuloendothelial system known to exist there.[89] The bacteria soon produce one or more small abscesses in the metaphysis. If untreated, the inflammatory process extends to the adjacent cortex and by means of haversian canals extends to the outer surface of the cortex where it appears as a subperiosteal abscess. In most long bones this subperiosteal abscess localizes outside the capsule of the neighboring joint. In the proximal femur, the capsule of the joint is attached to the femur near the base of the neck distal to the bone-cartilage junction. A subperiosteal abscess in this location is intracapsular, and pyarthrosis ensues. In all long bones the growth plate itself acts as a barrier to the spread of the infection. If the infection is severe enough, however, partial or total destruction of the growth plate occurs. Retardation or cessation of linear growth results, or if only one part of the growth plate is damaged, angular deformity may occur. If the osteomyelitis is not severe, actual stimulation of the growth plate may occur, leading to increased linear growth. Why growth stimulation occurs in this circumstance is not known, although traditionally it has been explained on the basis of hyperemia. Schneider[90] found that although repeated large doses of papain destroy the growth plate in experimental animals, repeated small doses stimulate it. Papain is a proteolytic enzyme, as are the enzymes released by pyogenic organisms. Perhaps mild destruction of the cartilage matrix stimulates chondroblasts to increase cellular proliferation and matrix production. Radiographic findings early in the course of acute hematogenous osteomyelitis are normal. If untreated, small areas of radiolucency appear in the metaphysis. Subperiosteal new bone may form where the periosteum has been

disturbed by an abscess. Varying degrees of osteoporosis and osteosclerosis will occur, depending on the severity of the disease, the amount of dead bone present, and the amount of new bone laid down as healing and repair occur.

Injury to the growth plate has been extensively reviewed by Salter and Harris,[91] among others, and their classification will be used in this discussion. In type I injury to the growth plate, there is a fracture or cleavage through the plate without any bone fracture. The line of cleavage may be through the zone of hypertrophic cells at the beginning of the zone of provisional calcification[91] or it may occur in a zigzag or weaving pattern through various portions of the hypertrophic zone as well as the metaphysis.[92,93] In type II injury, the most common type of growth plate injury, the fracture extends through the plate at the same level as in type I injury for a variable distance, and then extends out through a portion of the metaphysis. The triangular metaphyseal fragment is referred to as Thurston Holland's sign. In type III injuries, the fracture line extends from the articular surface of the bone longitudinally across the secondary bony epiphysis to the growth plate. The fracture then extends along the growth plate to the periphery either in the zone of hypertrophic cells or in a weaving pattern through various zones. Type IV injury is a longitudinal fracture through the distal end of the bone, extending from the articular surface through the epiphysis, across the growth plate, and down the metaphysis to the cortex near the junction of the metaphysis and diaphysis. Type V injury is a crush injury to the growth plate. In the first three types of injury to the growth plate, the metaphyseal blood supply to all or part of the cartilaginous portion of the plate is temporarily disrupted. In the first few days after injury, there is an increase in width in the zone of cell columns and especially in the zone of hypertrophic cells. This increase occurs because the normal vascular invasion of the cartilage columns temporarily cannot occur. As healing occurs and the vascular supply to the growth plate is reestablished, endochondral bone formation catches up with chondrogenesis, and the cartilaginous zones resume their normal width. The overall effect on linear growth is negligible. In types III and IV injuries, an accurate reduction of the fracture is a necessity, or bony healing of the epiphysis to the metaphysis will occur, and a mechanical block to plate growth will result. Type V injury crushes the growth plate and may irreparably damage the proliferating cells in the zone of cell columns. Complete cessation of linear growth in all or part of the plate may occur.

In rickets, vascular invasion of the cartilage columns also does not occur. Normally, matrix calcification at the bottom of the hypertrophic zone provides tunnels for the ingrowth of vascular buds that destroy the distal transverse septa and the degenerated hypertrophic cells. It has been postulated that in rickets the mineral-deficient matrix does not provide tunnels, and the invading vascular buds are turned aside.[94]

Bone formation is deficient in scurvy and in osteogenesis imperfecta. In scurvy there are at least two metabolic defects produced by vitamin C deficiency: (1) a defect in chondroitin sulfate production in the proliferative zone resulting from an enzymatic impairment of the conversion of glucose to galactosamine[6] and (2) a deficiency in collagen formation resulting from failure in the hydroxylation of proline to hydroxyproline.[95] The second defect is present in all regions of the growth plate, but it is most noticeable in the metaphysis where collagen synthesis is higher than elsewhere in the plate. On microscopic examination,[96] the cartilage portion of the plate is relatively normal, including matrix calcification at the bottom of the zone of hypertrophic cells. The metaphysis is in complete disarray, however. Calcified cartilage accumulates at the bone-cartilage junction and extends farther down into the metaphysis than it does normally. This produces the white line of Fraenkel seen on radiograph. Little osteoid is present on the calcified cartilage bars. Bony trabeculae are sparse and thin. A generalized osteoporosis exists throughout the skeletal system. The metaphyseal region is mechanically weakened, and the microfractures, hemorrhage debris accumulation, and fibrous scarring occurring in this region have led to its being called the zone of detritus or Trummerfeldzone. Collapse of the metaphysis along with continued latitudinal growth result in the formation of Pelkin's lateral spurs at the bone-cartilage junction. Growth plate dislocation may occur.

Osteogenesis imperfecta, or brittle bones, is a connective tissue disorder in which collagen throughout the body does not mature beyond the reticulin fiber stage.[97] In the growth plate apparatus, it is a disease of the osteoblasts and thus affects primarily the metaphyseal portion of the plate. The osteoblasts are not deficient in number,[98] as was formerly believed, but they elaborate an immature collagen that fails to mature. Microscopic findings are normal in the cartilaginous portion of the growth plate. In the metaphysis, however, only a small amount of bone is laid down on the calcified cartilage bars. In other words, formation of the secondary spongiosa is deficient. The bony trabeculae that do form are thin and few in number. Radiographic examination of the long bones reveals a generalized osteoporosis, thin cortices, and poor trabeculation in the metaphysis. Superimposed on these findings may be evidence of fractures in various stages of healing.

Internal or histologic remodeling is abnormal in osteopetrosis. Also termed marble bone disease or Albers-Schönberg disease, osteopetrosis is a failure of internal remodeling in that the calcified cartilage bars of the primary spongiosa are not absorbed or removed. Microscopically the growth plate shows normal zones down to the provisional zone of calcification at the bottom of the zone of hypertrophic cells. The calcified bars that begin in this region extend far down into the metaphysis and the diaphysis. Calcified bar remnants, in fact, are found throughout the entire length of the bone, including the midshaft. Primitive osseous tissue is laid down on the cartilage remnants, but, even in the midshaft of the bone, this primitive fiber bone is not converted to mature lamellar bone. Also, a true medullary cavity or canal does not form. Instead the entire interior of the bone is filled with chondro-osseous material.[99] Radiographic examination characteristically shows uniform opacity of the severely involved bones, with no discernible internal architecture. In less severely affected patients, there may be alternating darker and lighter transverse bands in the metaphysis. Occasionally a bone-within-a-bone is seen in the vertebrae or the small bones of the hands and feet. Apparently these peculiar radiographic findings represent attempts to return to normal endochondral bone formation. Also, external modeling may be affected in that normal funnelization is delayed, and metaphyseal splaying results.

External or anatomic remodeling is abnormal in Pyle's disease or familial metaphyseal dysplasia. Pyle's disease is a failure of external remodeling in the distal end of the metaphysis. The normal funnelization that occurs as the metaphysis narrows to meet the diaphysis is delayed. This failure in funnelization or constriction produces a splayed or Erlenmeyer-flask deformity of the metaphysis in affected bones. It is tempting to conclude that the failure in funnelization is caused by a deficiency in the osteoclastic resorption of bone that normally occurs subperiosteally in the metaphysis. This has not been verified histologically as yet because of the scarcity of material available for histologic study. It has been shown, however, that the fiber bone in the metaphysis persists down into what normally would be the first portion of the diaphysis,[43] that is, the secondary spongiosa is not resorbed and replaced with lamellar bone until far down in the diaphysis. Radiographic examination of an affected long bone shows metaphyseal splaying, with thinning of the cortex in that region. The metaphysis is osteoporotic. The midshaft region is normal, as are the epiphyseal regions.

## Fibrous Peripheral Structure

Encircling the typical long bone growth plate at its periphery are a wedge-shaped groove of cells, termed the ossification groove, and a ring or band of fibrous tissue and bone, termed the perichondrial ring (Fig. 1–20). Ranvier,[100] the first to describe these structures, concentrated on the cells in the groove, and the groove is now named for him. LaCroix[101] studied the perichondrial ring in detail, and this structure is frequently called after him. Although it is true that the ossification groove and the perichondrial ring are simply different parts of the same structure, they do have different functions and, for that reason alone, it is advantageous to consider them distinct entities.

The ossification groove contains round to oval cells that on light microscopy seem to flow from the groove into the cartilage at the level of the beginning of the reserve zone. For that reason and since these cells incorporate tritiated thymidine avidly, it seems that the function of the groove of Ranvier is to contribute chondrocytes to the growth plate for the growth in diameter, or latitudinal growth, of the plate.[102] In a definitive study using electron microscopy and autoradiography, three different groups of cells were identified in the ossification groove: (1) a group of densely placed cells that seemed to be progenitor cells for osteoblasts that form the bony band in the perichondrial ring; (2) a group of undifferentiated cells and fibroblasts that contribute to appositional chondrogenesis and, hence, growth in width of the growth plate; and (3) fibroblasts amid sheets of collagen that cover the groove and firmly anchor it to the perichondrium of the hyaline cartilage above the growth plate.[103]

The perichondrial ring is a dense fibrous band encircling the growth plate at the bone-cartilage junction in which collagen fibers run vertically, obliquely, and circumferentially.[89] It is continuous at one end with the group of fibroblasts and collagen fibers in the ossification groove and at the other end with the periosteum and subperiosteal bone of the metaphysis. In rodents, rabbits, and dogs, the innermost layer of the perichondrial ring consists of bone that may or may not be attached to the subperiosteal bone of the metaphysis. This cylindric sheath of bone may not be present in all species at all ages in all growth plates. For instance, it is not present in the proximal femur in humans at any age.[93] Whether or not bone is present in the perichondrial ring, there is no doubt that the perichondrial ring provides mechanical support for the otherwise weak bone-cartilage junction of the growth plate.[27,93,101,103]

Thus, the function of the ossification groove is to provide chondrocytes for the growth in width of the growth plate, and the function of the perichondrial ring is to act as a limiting membrane that provides mechanical support for the growth plate.

In the femoral capital growth plate, the functions of the ossification groove and the perichondrial ring are the same as those in any typical long bone growth plate, but the structures of these peripheral tissues are quite different. Instead of a rather distinct ossification groove and perichondrial ring, these two structures are replaced by a fibrocartilaginous structure that consists of fibrocartilage in the area occupied by both the groove of Ranvier and the perichondrial ring in other growth plates. This fibrocartilaginous structure apparently has the same functions as the groove of Ranvier and the perichondrial ring, that is, to provide for latitudinal growth of the growth plate (the top portion of the fibrocartilaginous structure) and to provide mechanical support for the growth plate (remainder of the fibrocartilaginous structure).[93]

Abnormalities of the peripheral structures include defects in both latitudinal growth and mechanical support. Multiple exostoses, or diaphyseal aclasia, is a heritable disease in which bony protuberances arise from the periphery of the metaphysis. Microscopically each exostosis is a miniature growth plate with all the zones represented. As the exostoses mature, their growth plates thin, and they close a short time after the adjacent growth plate proper closes. Several theories have been advanced as to the origin of the exostoses. Recent experiments by Rigal[104] leave little doubt but that a tear in the perichondrial ring, along with its distal displacement toward the metaphysis, is capable of producing exostoses identical to those seen clinically. In multiple exostoses, perhaps cells in the ossification groove escape laterally through holes in the perichondrial ring and form secondary growth plates, which give rise to the exostoses. Radiographic examination of an affected extremity typically shows a variable number of bony projections in the metaphysis, pointing away from the neighboring growth plate proper. The exostoses gradually become incorporated into the diaphysis as they move farther from the growth plate. Deformity, including shortening and angulation, commonly occurs in severely involved bones. Such deformity may result from dissipation of the longitudinal growth force of the neighboring growth plate in a lateral direction in the metaphysis.[105]

Germane to the discussion of the origin of exostosis in humans are the experimental findings in lathyrism. Apparently resulting from a defect in ground substance produced by the ingestion of aminonitriles, tears appear in the margins of the growth plates and give rise to exostotic protuberances.

The cause of slipped capital femoral epiphysis is unknown. The slip apparently occurs in the growth plate through the zone of hypertrophic cells as it does in any traumatic epiphyseal separation. Ponseti and McClintock[106] pointed out the similarity between epiphyseal slip in the lathyritic animal and that of slipped capital femoral epiphysis in the human. A defect in the ground substance is thought to exist in lathyrism.

Perhaps a similar defect exists in slipped femoral epiphysis in humans. If so, any mechanical support provided by the perichondrial ring at the bone-cartilage junction would be weakened, and epiphyseal slip would ensue.

The Marfan syndrome presents a body disproportion the opposite of achondroplasia; that is, the extremities are long and thin (dolichostenomelia), although the trunk is of normal length or even slightly shortened. Microscopic studies of the growth plate in this disease are lacking, but it has been suggested that the increase in bone length is caused by a lack in the binding force in the periosteum or the perichondrial ring that normally limits longitudinal growth.[97]

## References

1. Hales S: *Statistical Essays*. London, Innys, 1727, p 339.
2. Belchier JB: The bones of animals changed to a red colour by aliment only. *Phil Trans R Soc* 1736;39:287.
3. Duhamel HL: Sur une racine qui a la faculté de teindre en rouge les os de animaux vivants. *Mem Acad R Sci* 1739;52:1–13.
4. Duhamel HL: Sur le développement et la crue des os des animaux. *Mem Acad R Sci* 1742;55:354–370.
5. Duhamel HL: Cinquiéme mémoire sur ces os, dans lequel on se propose d'éclaircir par de nouvelles experiences comment se fait la crue des os suivant leur longeur, et de prouver que cet accroissement s'opère par un mécanisme tres-approchant de celui. *Mem Acad R Sci* 1743;56:87,111–146.
6. Hunter J: Experiments and observations on the growth of bones (from the papers of the late Mr. Hunter), in Palmer JR (ed): *The Transactions of a Society for the Improvement of Medical & Chirurgical Knowledge*. London, Longman, Rees, Orme, Brown, Green & Longman, 1837, vol 2, pp 315–318.
7. Dubreuil G: *C R Soc Biol* 1913;74:756, 888, 935.
8. Streeter GL: Developmental horizons in human embryos: A review of the histogenesis of cartilage and bone. *Contrib Embryol* 1949;33:149.
9. Gardner E: Osteogenesis in the human embryo and fetus, in Bourne GH (ed): *The Biochemistry and Physiology of Bone*, ed 2. New York, Academic Press Inc, 1971, vol 3, pp 77–118.
10. Siffert RS: Anatomy and physiology of the growth plate, in Rang M (ed): *The Growth Plate and Its Disorders*. Baltimore, Williams & Wilkins Co, 1969, pp 1–12.
11. Brookes M, Landon DN: The juxta-epiphyseal vessels in the long bones of foetal rats. *J Bone Joint Surg* 1963;46B:336–345.
12. Brookes M: *The Blood Supply of Bone*. New York, Appleton-Century-Crofts, 1971, pp 14–22.
13. Trueta J, Morgan JD: The vascular contribution to osteogenesis: I. Studies by the injection method. *J Bone Joint Surg* 1960;42B:98–109.
14. DeMarneffe R: Recherches morphologiques et experimentales sur la vascularisation osseuse. *Acta Chir Belg* 1951;50:681.
15. Morgan JD: Blood supply of the growing rabbit's tibia. *J Bone Joint Surg* 1959;41B:185–203.
16. Anderson CE, Parker J: Invasion and resorption in endochondral ossification: An electron microscopic study. *J Bone Joint Surg* 1966;48A:899–914.
17. Chung SMK: The arterial supply of the developing proximal end of the human femur. *J Bone Joint Surg* 1976;58A:961–970.
18. Brighton CT, Sugioka Y, Hunt R: Cytoplasmic structures of epiphyseal-plate chondrocytes: Quantitative evaluation using electron micrographs of rat costochondral junctions with special reference to the fate of hypertrophic cells. *J Bone Joint Surg* 1973;55A:771–784.
19. Kuhlman RE: A microchemical study of the developing epiphyseal plate. *J Bone Joint Surg* 1960;42A:457–466.
20. Kuhlman RE: Phosphatases in epiphyseal cartilage: Their possible role in tissue synthesis. *J Bone Joint Surg* 1965;47A:545–550.
21. Wuthier RE: A zonal analysis of inorganic and organic constituents of the epiphysis during endochondral calcification. *Calcif Tissue Res* 1969;4:20–38.
22. Irving JR, Wuthier RE: Histochemistry and biochemistry of calcification with special reference to the role of lipids. *Clin Orthop* 1968;56:237–260.
23. Lindenbaum A, Kuettner KE: Mucopolysaccharides and mucoproteins of calf scapula. *Calcif Tissue Res* 1967;1:153–165.
24. Schmidt A, Rodergerdts U, Buddecke E: Correlation of lysozyme activity with proteoglycan biosynthesis in epiphyseal cartilage. *Calcif Tissue Res* 1978;26:163–172.
25. Brighton CT, Heppenstall RB: Oxygen tension in zones of the epiphyseal plate, the metaphysis and diaphysis: An in vitro and in vivo study in rats and rabbits. *J Bone Joint Surg* 1971;53A:719–728.
26. Kember NF: Cell division in endochondral ossification: A study of cell proliferation in rat bones by the method of tritiated thymidine autoradiography. *J Bone Joint Surg* 1960;42B:824–839.
27. Rigal WM: The use of tritiated thymidine in studies of chondrogenesis, in LaCroix P, Budy AM (eds): *Radioisotopes and Bone*. Oxford, Blackwell Scientific Publications, 1962, p 197.
28. Stanescu V, Stanescu R, Maroteaux P: Pathogenic mechanisms in osteochondrodysplasias. *J Bone Joint Surg* 1984;66A:817–836.
29. Cooper RR, Ponseti IV: Pseudoachondroplastic dwarfism: A rough-surfaced endoplastic reticulum storage disorder. *J Bone Joint Surg* 1973;55A:475–484.
30. Jaffe HL: *Metabolic, Degenerative and Inflammatory Diseases of Bones and Joints*. Philadelphia, Lea & Febiger, 1972, pp 20, 200, 224, 542.
31. Ponseti IV: Morquio's syndrome, in Rang M (ed): *The Growth Plate and Its Disorders*. Baltimore, Williams & Wilkins Co, 1969, p 50.
32. Dziewiatkowski DD: Synthesis of sulfomucopolysaccharides in thyroidectomized rats. *J Exp Med* 1957;105:69–74.
33. Holtrop ME: The ultrastructure of the epiphyseal plate: I. The flattened chondrocyte. *Calcif Tissue Res* 1972;9:131–139.
34. Greer RB, Janicke GH, Mankin HJ: Protein-polysaccharide synthesis at three levels of the normal growth plate. *Calcif Tissue Res* 1968;2:157–164.
35. Sissons HA: The growth of bone, in Bourne GH (ed): *The Biochemistry and Physiology of Bone*. New York, Academic Press Inc, 1971, p 155.
36. Kember NF: Cell population kinetics of bone growth: The first ten years of autoradiographic studies with tritiated thymidine. *Clin Orthop* 1971;76:213–230.
37. Bargman GJ, Mackler B, Shepard TH: Studies of oxidative energy deficiency: I. Achondroplasia in the rabbit. *Arch Biochem Biophys* 1972;150:137–146.
38. Schneider M, Adar U: Effect of inanition of rabbit growth cartilage plates. *Arch Pathol* 1964;78:149–156.
39. Harris HA: *Bone Growth in Health and Disease*. London, Oxford University Press, 1933.
40. Rubin P, Andrews JR, Swarm R, et al: Radiation-induced dysplasias of bone. *Am J Roentgenol Radium Ther Nucl Med* 1959;82:206–216.

41. Hulth A, Westerborn O: The effect of crude papain on the epiphyseal cartilage in laboratory animals. *J Bone Joint Surg* 1959;41B:836–847.

42. Silberberg M, Silberberg R: Steroid hormones and bone, in Bourne GH (ed): *The Biochemistry and Physiology of Bone*. New York, Academic Press Inc, 1971, pp 401–484.

43. Ingalls NW: Bone growth and pathology as seen in the femur (and tibia). *Arch Surg* 1933;26:787–795.

44. Brighton CT, Ray RD, Soble LW, et al: In vitro epiphyseal plate growth in various oxygen tensions. *J Bone Joint Surg* 1969;51A:1383–1396.

45. Pritchard JJ: A cytological and histochemical study of bone and cartilage formation in the rat. *J Anat* 1952;86:259–277.

46. Holtrop ME: The ultrastructure of the epiphyseal plate: II. The hypertrophic chondrocyte. *Calcif Tissue Res* 1972;9:140–151.

47. Martin JH, Matthews JL: Mitochondrial granules in chondrocytes, osteoblasts and osteocytes. *Clin Orthop* 170;68:273–278.

48. Matthews JL, Martin JH, Sampson HW, et al: Mitochondrial granules in the normal and rachitic rat epiphysis. *Calcif Tissue Res* 170;5:91–99.

49. Suffin KV, Holtrop ME, Ogilvie RE: Microanalysis of individual mitochondrial granules with diameters less than 1000 angstroms. *Science* 1971;174:947–949.

50. Brighton CT, Hunt RM: Mitochondrial calcium and its role in calcification. *Clin Orthop* 1974;100:406–416.

51. Brighton CT, Hunt RM: Histochemical localization of calcium in growth plate mitochondria and matrix vesicles. *Fed Proc* 1976;35:143–147.

52. Lehninger AL: Mitochondria and calcium ion transport. *Biochem J* 1970;119:129–138.

53. Lehninger AL, Carafoli E, Rossi CS: Energy-linked ion movements in mitochondrial systems. *Adv Enzymol* 1967;29:259–320.

54. Stambaugh JL, Brighton CT, Iannotti JP, et al: Characterization of growth plate mitochondria. *J Orthop Res* 1984;2:235–246.

55. Iannotti JP, Brighton CT, Stambaugh JL, et al: Calcium flux and endogenous calcium content in isolated mammalian growth-plate chondrocytes, hyaline-cartilage chondrocytes, and hepatocytes. *J Bone Joint Surg* 1985;67A:113–120.

56. Brighton CT, Lackman RD, Cuckler JM: Absence of the glycerol phosphate shuttle in the various zones of the growth plate. *J Bone Joint Surg* 1983;65A:663–666.

57. Buckwalter JA: Proteoglycan structure in calcifying cartilage. *Clin Orthop* 1983;172:207–232.

58. Kuettner KE, Guenther HL, Ray RD: Lysozyme in preosseous cartilage. *Calcif Tissue Res* 1968;1:298–305.

59. Pita JC, Howell DS, Kuettner K: Evidence for a role of lysozyme in endochondral calcification during healing in rickets, in Slavkin HC, Greulich RC (eds): *Extracellular Matrix Influences on Gene Expression*. New York, Academic Press Inc, 1975, pp 721–726.

60. Sapolsky AI, Howell DS, Woessner JF Jr: Neutral proteases and cathepsin D in human articular cartilage. *J Clin Invest* 1974;53:1044–1053.

61. Howell DS: Current concepts of calcification. *J Bone Joint Surg* 1971;53A:250–258.

62. Howell DS, Pita JC, Marquez JF, et al: Demonstration of macromolecular inhibitor(s) of calcification and nucleation factor(s) in fluid from calcifying sites in cartilage. *J Clin Invest* 1969;48:630–641.

63. Ali SY: Analysis of matrix vesicles and their role in calcification of epiphyseal cartilage. *Fed Proc* 1976;35:135–142.

64. Felix R, Felisch H: Role of matrix vesicles of calcification. *Fed Proc* 1976;35:169–171.

65. Anderson HC: Vesicles associated with calcification in the matrix of epiphyseal cartilage. *J Cell Biol* 1969;41:59–72.

66. Bonucci E: Fine structure and histochemistry of calcifying globules in epiphyseal cartilage. *Z Zellforsch Mikrosk Anat* 1970;103:192–217.

67. Ali SY, Sajdera SW, Anderson HC: Isolation and characterization of calcifying matrix vesicles from epiphyseal cartilage. *Proc Natl Acad Sci* 1970;67:1513–1520.

68. Fleisch H, Neuman WF: Mechanism of calcification: Role of collagen, polyphosphates, and phosphatase. *Am J Physiol* 1962;20:671–675.

69. Landis WJ, Glimcher MJ: Electron optical and analytical observations of rat growth plate cartilage prepared by ultra-cryomicrotomy: The failure to detect a mineral phase in matrix vesicles and the identification of heterodispersed particles as the initial solid phase of calcium phosphate deposited in the extracellular matrix. *J Ultrastruct Res* 1982;78:227–268.

70. Landis WJ, Paine MC, Glimcher MJ: Electron microscopic observations of bone tissue prepared anhydrously in organic solvents. *J Ultrastruct Res* 1977;59:1–30.

71. Morris DC, Vaananen HK, Anderson HC: Matrix vesicle calcification in rat epiphyseal growth plate cartilage prepared anhydrously for electron microscopy. *Metabol Bone Dis* 1983;5:131–137.

72. Glimcher MJ, Krane SM: The organization and structure of bone and the mechanism of calcification, in Gould BS, Ramachandran GN (eds): *Treatise on Collagen: Vol 2. Biology of Collagen Part B*. New York, Academic Press Inc, 1968, pp 68–251.

73. Bernard GW, Pease DC: An electron microscope study of initial intramembranous ossification. *Am J Anat* 1969;125:271–290.

74. Shepard N, Mitchell N: Ultrastructural modifications of proteoglycans coincident with mineralization in local regions of rat growth plate. *J Bone Joint Surg* 1985;67A:455–464.

75. Poole AR, Pidoux I, Reiner A, et al: Association of an extracellular protein (chondrocalcin) with the calcification of cartilage in endochondral bone formation. *J Cell Biol* 1984;98:54–65.

76. Posner AS: Crystal chemistry of bone mineral. *Physiol Rev* 1969;49:760–792.

77. Boskey AL: Current concepts of the physiology and biochemistry of calcification. *Clin Orthop* 1981;157:225–257.

78. Stambaugh JE, Brighton CT: Diffusion in the various zones of the normal and the rachitic growth plates. *J Bone Joint Surg* 1980;62A:740–749.

79. Gram PB, Fleming JL, Frame B, et al: Metaphyseal chondrodysplasia of Jansen. *J Bone Joint Surg* 1959;41A:951–959.

80. Rubin P: *Dynamic Classification of Bone Dysplasias*. Chicago, Year Book Medical Publishers, 1964.

81. Fleisch H, Felix R, Hansen T, et al: Role of the organic matrix in calcification, in Slavkin HC, Greulich RE (eds): *Extracellular Matrix Influences on Gene Expression*. New York, Academic Press Inc, 1975, p 707.

82. Fraser D: Hypophosphatasia. *Am J Med* 1947;22:730–746.

83. Brighton CT, Hunt RM: The role of mitochondria in growth plate calcification as demonstrated in a rachitic model. *J Bone Joint Surg* 1978;60A:630–639.

84. Brighton CT: Clinical problems in epiphyseal plate growth and development. American Academy of Orthopaedic Surgeons *Instructional Course Lectures, XXIII*. St Louis, CV Mosby, 1974, pp 105–122.

85. Schenk RK, Wiener J, Spiro D: Fine structural aspects of vascular invasion of the tibial epiphyseal plate of growing rats. *Acta Anat* 1968;69:1–17.

86. Kimmel DB, Webster SS: A quantitative histological analysis of the growing long bone metaphysis. *Calcif Tissue Int* 1980;32:113–122.

87. McLean FC, Urist MR: *Bone: An Introduction to the Physiology of*

*Skeletal Tissue*, ed 2. Chicago, University of Chicago Press, 1961, p 24.

88. LaCroix P: The internal remodeling of bones, in Bourne GH (ed): *The Biochemistry and Physiology of Bone*, ed 2. New York, Academic Press Inc, 1971, vol 3, p 120.

89. Rang M (ed): *The Growth Plate and Its Disorders*. Baltimore, Williams & Wilkins Co, 1969, pp 5, 32, 78, 94.

90. Schneider M: Acceleration of longitudinal bone growth by intraosseous injection of papain protease. *Proc Soc Exp Biol Med* 1963;113:383–387.

91. Salter RB, Harris WR: Injuries involving the epiphyseal plate. *J Bone Joint Surg* 1963;45A:587–622.

92. Bright RW, Burnstein AH, Elmore SM: Epiphyseal plate cartilage: A biomechanical and histological analysis of failure modes. *J Bone Joint Surg* 1974;56A:688–703.

93. Chung SMK, Batterman SC, Brighton CT: Shear strength of the human femoral capital epiphyseal plate. *J Bone Joint Surg* 1975;58A:94–103.

94. Mankin HJ: Rickets, osteomalacia and renal osteodystrophy. Part I. *J Bone Joint Surg* 1974;56A:101–128.

95. Gould BS: Ascorbic acid-independent and ascorbic acid-dependent collagen-forming mechanisms. *Ann NY Acad Sci* 1961;92:168–174.

96. Follis RH: *The Pathology of Nutritional Disease*. Oxford, Blackwell Scientific Publications, 1948.

97. McKusick V: *Heritable Disorders of Connective Tissue*, ed 3. St Louis, CV Mosby, 1972.

98. Ramser JR, Frost HM: The study of a rib biopsy from a patient with osteogenesis imperfecta: A method using in vivo tetracycline labelling. *Acta Orthop Scand* 1966;37:229–240.

99. Cohen J: Osteopetrosis: Case report, autopsy findings, and pathological interpretation: Failure of treatment with vitamin A. *J Bone Joint Surg* 1951;33A:923–938.

100. Ranvier L: Quelques faits relatifs au développement du tissu osseux. *C R Acad Sci* 1873;77:1105.

101. LaCroix P: *The Organization of Bone*. New York, McGraw-Hill Book Co., 1951.

102. Tonna EA: The cellular complement of the skeletal system studied autoradiographically with tritiated thymidine ($H^3TDR$) during growth and aging. *J Biophys Biomed Cytol* 1961;9:813–824.

103. Shapiro F, Holtrop ME, Glimcher MJ: Organization and cellular biology of the perichondrial ossification groove of Ranvier. *J Bone Joint Surg* 1977;59A:703–723.

104. Rigal WM: Diaphyseal aclasis, in Rang M (ed): *The Growth Plate and Its Disorders*. Baltimore, Williams & Wilkins Co, 1969, p 91.

105. Jaffe HL: *Tumors and Tumorous Conditions of the Bones and Joints*. Philadelphia, Lea & Febiger, 1958, p 152.

106. Ponseti IV, McClintock R: The pathology of slipping of the upper femoral epiphysis. *J Bone Joint Surg* 1956;38A:71–83.

## Acknowledgment

This work was supported in part by Grant AM-13812 of the National Institutes of Health, United States Public Health Service

# Bone Structure and Function

Joseph A. Buckwalter, MD

Reginald R. Cooper, MD

## Introduction

The great strength and light weight of bone give vertebrates their mobility, dexterity and strength. The special material properties of bone are readily apparent. A one cubic inch block of bone can support a load of two tons. The tensile strength of bone nearly equals that of cast iron, yet it is three times lighter and ten times more flexible.

Knowledgeable treatment of patients with injuries, diseases and congenital abnormalities of the skeleton requires an understanding of bone. The mechanical function of bone clearly depends on its matrix structure while the composition of bone matrix and the activities of bone cells determine the biological behavior of bone. Failure to consider both the biological and mechanical properties of bone will compromise the most technically expert orthopaedic treatment, whereas understanding these properties will help solve the most complicated clinical problems.

Orthopaedists have learned that many injuries, deformities and diseases of bone can be treated surgically. We cut and shape it, fix one piece to another with screws, wires or plates and, unite bone with metal or plastic. In performing these procedures, we treat bone like a homogeneous inert material, similar to metal or plastic, yet it is not homogeneous and inert. In fact, bone is a dynamic living heterogeneous tissue that performs as an essential structural material and responds well to our surgical interventions because of its unique matrix and its population of specialized cells. Like most other tissues, bone is supplied by blood vessels, lymphatics and nerves, and consists of cells and an extracellular matrix. Compared with parenchymal tissues, bone has a relatively small cell population and a large matrix volume. The bone cells assume specialized forms that carry out the essential functions of bone formation, bone remodeling, mineral homeostasis and bone repair. Like tendon, ligament and fibrocartilage, bone has a large extracellular organic matrix formed primarily by collagen. Unlike these other connective tissues, the organic matrix of bone mineralizes to produce the unique integration of inorganic and organic matrix components that gives bone its great strength. The matrix of bone is so durable that it can remain unchanged for centuries after death and retain most of its strength. Yet, during life, the bone cells continually alter the matrix, and if traumatic injuries damage the elaborate structure of the matrix, the cells can restore its original form and strength without scar formation.

This discussion will review the structure and function of bone to illustrate how understanding of bone forms the basis for treating patients with skeletal disorders.

## Bone Formation

Two common mechanisms of bone formation can be identified based on the tissue in which the bone forms: enchondral ossification and intramembranous ossification. The bones of the vertebral column, the base of the skull, and the appendicular skeleton, other than the clavicle, form through enchondral ossification while most of the bones of the face, vault of the skull and most of the clavicle form by intramembranous ossification. Bones may form by both mechanisms. For example, the clavicle forms primarily by intramembranous ossification, but it also has a secondary center of ossification and a growth plate that form bone through enchondral ossification. Although the two mechanisms of bone formation differ, the ultimate structure of mature bone formed by either mechanism is the same.

### Enchondral Ossification

Formation of bones by enchondral ossification begins with the aggregation of undifferentiated mesenchymal cells to form a mesenchymal model of the bone. The aggregated mesenchymal cells then differentiate into chondrocytes, which form a hyaline cartilage model of bone. The chondrocytes hypertrophy, vascular buds invade the cartilage, and the matrix mineralizes. Osteoprogenitor cells accompanying the vascular buds differentiate into osteoblasts, which form a bone matrix on the mineralized cartilage. Osteoclasts then resorb these trabeculae of calcified cartilage and bone, and osteoblasts replace the mixed calcified cartilage and immature bone with mature lamellar bone. After forming the long bones, other than the clavicle, the short bones and the epiphyseal centers of ossification, enchondral ossification continues in the growth plates until skeletal maturity and participates in the healing of some fractures throughout life.

### Intramembranous Ossification

Aggregation of mesenchymal cells into condensed layers or membranes initiates intramembranous bone formation. The cells synthesize a loose collagenous matrix containing vessels, fibroblasts, mesenchymal cells and osteoprogenitor cells. The osteoprogenitor cells differentiate into osteoblasts, deposit a bone matrix and become osteocytes. In contrast to enchondral ossification, no cartilaginous model of the bone forms, and most of the bones formed by intramembranous ossification are flat bones. Intramembranous ossification occurs during embryonic development. Thereafter most bones formed by intramembranous ossification grow by periosteal new bone formation, which also increases the diameter of bones originally formed by enchondral ossification. Since periosteum forms successive lamellae of new bone without a preceding cartilaginous model, periosteal bone formation is often considered a form of intramembranous ossification.

### The Structure of Bone

### Size and Form

To perform their mechanical functions, bones assume a remarkable assortment of sizes and shapes. Although environmental factors exert some influence, the genome determines the ultimate size and form of any given bone. How this is accomplished remains unclear, although it is critically important for understanding congenital and developmental abnormalities of the skeleton.

Bones vary in size from the ear ossicles to the long bones of the limbs. Their wide variety of shapes can be classified into one of three groups: long bones, short bones or flat bones. Long bones, like the femur, tibia or humerus, have an expanded metaphysis and an epiphysis at either end of a thick-walled tubular diaphysis. The thick cortical walls of the diaphysis become thinner and increase in diameter as they form the metaphysis. Articular cartilage covers epiphyses where they form synovial joints. Like the larger limb bones, metacarpals, metatarsals and phalanges have the form of long bones (Fig. 2–1). Short bones are approximately the same length in all directions and have trapezoidal, cuboidal, cuneiform or irregular shapes. Examples include the tarsals, carpals and centra of the vertebrae. They have relatively thin cortices that form their external surfaces. Flat or tabular bones have one dimension that is much shorter than the other two. The larger flat bones form the cranial vault, the scapula and the wing of the ilium. The lamina of a vertebra provides an example of a smaller flat bone.

### Cortical and Cancellous Bone

Gross inspection shows that bone tissue exists in two forms: cortical or compact bone and cancellous or trabecular bone (Fig. 2–1). Cortical bone forms about 80% of the skeleton and surrounds the thin plates or bars of cancellous bone with thick lamellae. In long bones dense cortical bone forms the diaphysis, and there is little or no trabecular bone. In the metaphysis the cortical bone thins and trabecular bone occupies the medullary cavity (Fig. 2–1). Short bones and flat bones usually have thinner cortices than the diaphyses of long bones and contain more cancellous bone. Thus, the vertebral bodies, pelvic bones and metaphyses of long bones contain most of the cancellous bone surrounded by a relatively thin layer of cortical bone, and the diaphyses of long bones contain most of the dense cortical bone.

Both cancellous and cortical bone modify their structure in response to applied loads, immobilization, hormonal influences and other factors; however, they differ in their rate and manner of response. Cancellous or trabecular bone has a large surface area per unit volume, and its cell population lies primarily between lamellae and on the surface of the trabeculae. In contrast, cortical bone has approximately one-twentieth the surface area per unit volume and most of the bone cell population lies between lamellae, completely surrounded by bone matrix. Since blood vessels rarely penetrate cancellous bone, the cells receive their nourishment by diffusion from marrow vessels. On the other hand, diaphyseal cortical bone cells rely on a complex intraosseous circulatory system. Cells lying on the trabecular surfaces remodel cancellous bone while osteoclasts must resorb tunnels through cortical bone to allow remodeling. Because of this organization, that is, the large cell-covered surface area, cancellous bone usually has a higher rate of metabolic activity and remodeling and responds more rapidly to changes in mechanical loads or metabolic disease. This differential response rate can be observed in radiographs of the long bones of an immobilized limb; inspection of the images usually shows that a decrease in the density of cancellous bone, caused by resorption of trabeculae, precedes an increase in the porosity of the cortical bone, caused by formation of resorption cavities.

The material properties of cancellous bone closely resemble those of cortical bone if the differences in density and orientation are compensated for during testing. However, the compressive strength of bone is proportional to the square of its density and since cortical bone has much greater density, its modulus of elasticity and ultimate compressive strength may both be an order of magnitude greater than cancellous bone. Differences in the arrangement and amount of cortical and cancellous bone make large differences in the mechanical behavior of specific bones and parts of bones. In long bones the thicker, stiffer, tubular cortical bone of the diaphysis (Fig. 2–1) provides maximum resistance to torsion and bending. The high proportion of more flexible trabecular bone in the metaphyses (Fig. 2–1) may help distribute suddenly applied loads. The low modulus of elasticity of the trabecular bone would allow greater deformation and therefore less abrupt transmission of loads from the articular cartilage to the stiffer cortical bone of the diaphysis.

### Mineralized and Unmineralized Matrix

Light microscopic examination of bone shows both mineralized and unmineralized matrix. Initially, osteoblasts form the unmineralized organic matrix referred to as pre-bone or osteoid. In sections stained with hematoxylin and eosin, light microscopy shows osteoid as homogeneous eosinophilic seams applied to mineralized matrix on one side and covered with osteoblasts on the other. Normally osteoid mineralizes soon after it is formed, but, mineralization may be impaired in conditions such as rickets or osteomalacia while synthesis of the organic matrix continues. The increase in osteoid may be demonstrated by bone biopsy to establish the diagnosis. Since bone stiffness and strength increase with increasing mineral content, patients with decreased mineralized matrix and increased volumes of unmineralized matrix may suffer pathologic fractures or progressive bony deformity. For example, children with untreated rickets may develop a characteristic genu varum deformity while adults with moderate to severe osteomalacia may suffer pathologic fractures.

### Woven and Lamellar Bone

Microscopic examination also shows that mineralized bone exists in two forms: woven (immature, fiber, primary) bone and lamellar (mature, secondary) bone. Woven bone forms the embryonic skeleton. Normally, it is replaced by mature bone as the skeleton develops. During enchondral ossification woven bone forms on calcified cartilage. Osteoclasts and chondroclasts then resorb the woven bone and calcified cartilage. Mature lamellar bone replaces these. Small amounts of woven bone may form part of tendon and ligament attachments, the suture margins of the cranial bones, and ear ossicles. With these exceptions woven bone rarely occurs in the normal human skeleton after 4 or 5 years of age. However, it may appear at any age in healing fractures, in metabolic and neoplastic diseases or in response to inflammatory processes.

The mechanical and biological differences between the two forms of bone result from the manner in which the osteoblasts form the matrix. Woven bone has a rapid rate of deposition and turnover whereas lamellar bone is usually much less active. Compared to lamellar bone, woven bone has an irregular almost random pattern of collagen fibrils consistent with its name, and it contains approximately four times as many osteocytes per unit volume as lamellar bone.

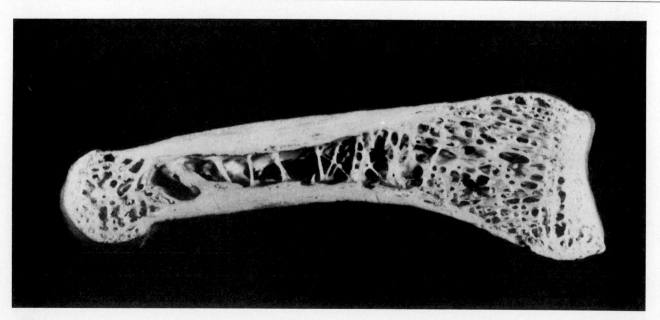

**Fig. 2–1** Longitudinal section of a human phalanx. The outer lamellae of cortical bone surround the inner cancellous bone. The metaphyses contain much more cancellous bone than the diaphysis and the thick cortical bone of the diaphysis becomes much thinner in the metaphysis. The metaphyseal trabeculae orient themselves to support the articular surface. The layer of bone under the articular surface is often referred to as the subchondral plate. Larger long bones, like the tibia, femur and humerus follow the same structural pattern.

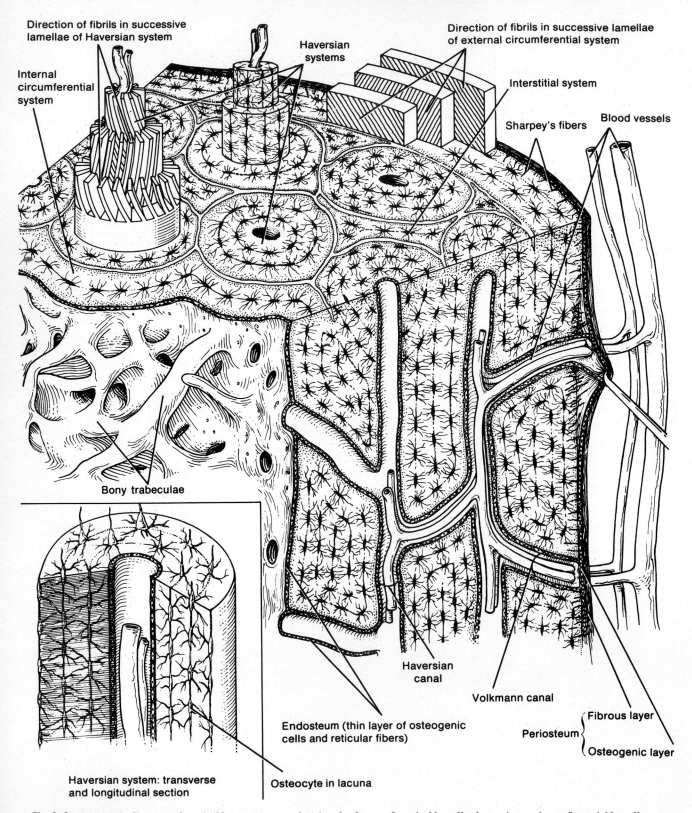

Direction of fibrils in successive lamellae of Haversian system

Haversian systems

Direction of fibrils in successive lamellae of external circumferential system

Internal circumferential system

Interstitial system

Sharpey's fibers

Blood vessels

Bony trabeculae

Haversian canal

Volkmann canal

Endosteum (thin layer of osteogenic cells and reticular fibers)

Fibrous layer

Periosteum

Osteogenic layer

Haversian system: transverse and longitudinal section

Osteocyte in lacuna

**Fig. 2–2**  Schematic diagram of cortical bone structure showing the forms of cortical lamellar bone: inner circumferential lamellae, outer circumferential lamellae, interstitial or intermediate lamellae and osteonal lamellae. The diagram also shows the intraosseous vascular system that serves the osteocytes and connects the periosteal and medullary vessels. The haversian canals spiral longitudinally through the cortex while Volkmann's canals create oblique connections between haversian canals. The periosteum covers the external surface of the bone and consists of two layers: an inner cellular layer and an outer fibrous layer. (Reproduced with permission from Kessel RG, Kardon RH: *Tissues and Organs: A Text-Atlas of Scanning Microscopy.* New York, WH Freeman and Co, 1979.)

The osteocytes of woven bone vary in size, orientation and distribution while the osteocytes of lamellar bone are relatively uniform in size and orient their principal axis parallel to other cells and to the collagen fibrils of the matrix. The mineralization of woven bone follows an irregular pattern, with mineral deposits varying in size and in their relationship to collagen fibrils. This pattern of mineralization combined with the frequent patchwork formation of woven bone creates an irregular radiographic appearance that distinguishes woven bone from lamellar bone. In contrast, the collagen fibrils of lamellar bone vary less in diameter and lie in tightly organized parallel sheets forming distinct lamellae 4 to 12 $\mu$m thick with almost uniform distribution of mineral within the matrix. This organization gives cortical lamellar bone a homogeneous radiographic appearance.

Because of its lack of collagen fibril orientation, relatively high cell and water content, and irregular mineralization the material properties of woven bone differ from those of lamellar bone. Woven bone is more flexible, more easily deformed and weaker than mature bone. For this reason restoration of normal strength in a healing fracture requires replacement of woven bone by mature lamellar bone. The importance of the differences between woven bone and lamellar bone is illustrated by the occasional deformation of fractures after they appeared to have healed radiographically. In these cases the deformation probably occurs through woven bone that has not yet been replaced by mature bone.

### Forms of Lamellar Bone

Lamellar bone appears in four general forms: the trabecular lamellae of cancellous bone, the inner and outer circumferential lamellae of cortical bone, the interstitial lamellae of cortical bone and the lamellae of osteons (Fig. 2–2). Each lamella consists of densely packed collagen fibrils. The fibrils in adjacent lamellae run in different directions similar to the alternating directions of the wood grain in plywood. The collagen fibrils frequently interconnect not only within a lamella but between lamellae. These interconnec-

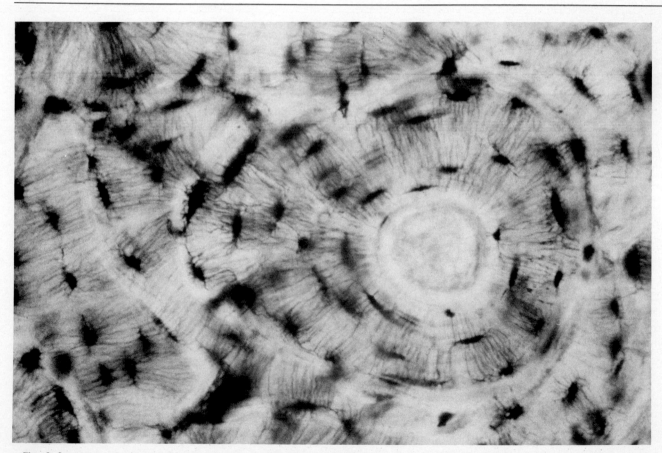

**Fig. 2–3** Light micrograph of a transverse section of cortical bone. An osteon cut transversely occupies the center of the photograph. Notice the central canal of the osteon and the dark elliptical or lens-shaped cell bodies of the osteocytes surrounded by lighter staining bone matrix. Each osteocyte sends fine, thread-like, cell processes through the matrix to contact other cell processes. The osteon remains almost a self-contained unit, since few, if any, cell process penetrate the cement line that forms the border of the osteon.

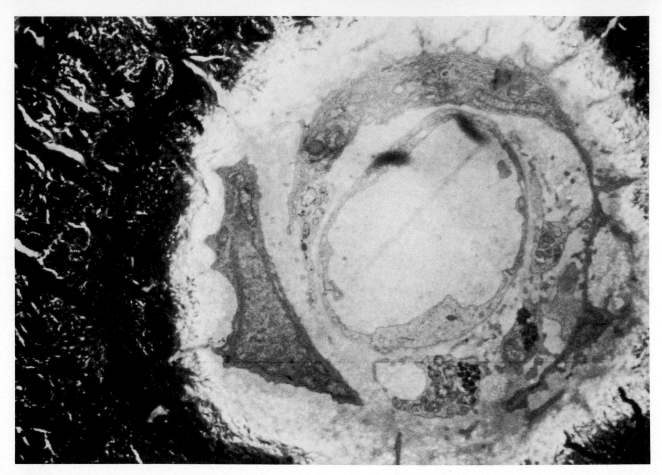

**Fig. 2–4** Electron micrograph showing the central canal of an osteon. The peripheral darkly stained regions consist of mineralized bone matrix. The central lighter staining region is the central canal containing undifferentiated cells and a central vessel. The undifferentiated cell has very little cytoplasm.

tions increase the strength of bone. Cement lines, or reversal lines, mark sites where bone resorption stopped and new bone formation began. They can be seen clearly surrounding osteons, and they contain little if any collagen. Furthermore, the lamellar collagen fibrils do not cross cement lines. This may explain why fractures tend to follow the cement lines rather than crossing osteons.

Osteons form the bulk of the diaphyseal cortical bone of the mature skeleton (Fig. 2–2). These structures consist of irregular branching and anastomosing cylinders with a centrally placed neurovascular canal surrounded by concentric lamellae (Figs. 2–3 to 2–6). A cement line defines the outer boundary of an osteon. Osteons spiral around the diaphysis running longitudinally. The central canals of osteons, frequently referred to as haversian canals, contain blood vessels, lymphatics, and occasional nerves (Figs. 2–4 to 2–6). Canaliculi containing the cell processes of osteocytes extend in a radial pattern from the central canal like spokes of a wheel (Fig. 2–3). These canaliculi connect the central canal to the osteocytes and

pass from osteocyte to osteocyte. Since diffusion of nutrients through mineralized bone matrix is limited, if it occurs at all, the cells depend primarily on the canaliculi for their metabolic needs. Like the collagen fibrils, the canaliculi rarely if ever cross cement lines; thus the cement lines separate the cells of an osteon from those just outside it. Osteons branch and anastomose and join obliquely oriented vascular canals that are sometimes referred to as Volkmann's canals (Fig. 2–2). This elaborate system of intraosseous vascular canals not only runs through the length of the bone but connects the periosteal surface with the endosteal surface. The longitudinal orientation of the osteons may explain why diaphyseal cortical bone is stronger in both tension and compression when it is loaded parallel to its long axis rather than perpendicular to its long axis.

### Periosteum

A tough connective tissue membrane, the periosteum, covers the external surface of bone (Fig. 2–2). In

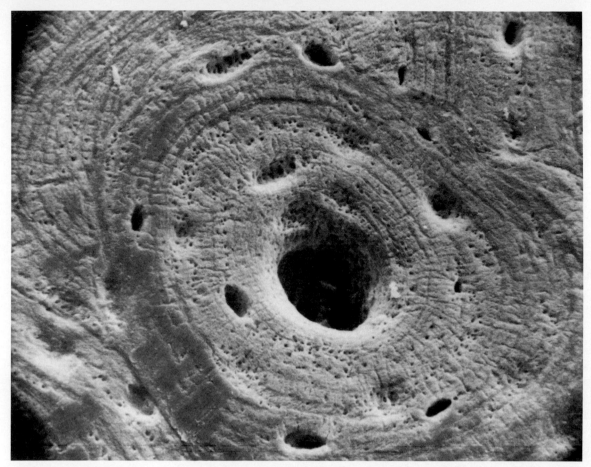

**Fig. 2–5**  Scanning electron micrograph of an osteonal system. Grooves in the bone matrix form concentric circles around the central canal and separate adjacent lamellae. Lacunae, the spaces occupied by osteocytes in living bone, appear as oval depressions. The canaliculi, which contain osteocyte processes during life, appear as small holes in the bone matrix or as grooves radiating out from the central canal like the spokes of a wheel. (Reproduced with permission from Kessel RG, Kardon RH: *Tissues and Organs: A Text-Atlas of Scanning Microscopy.* New York, WH Freeman and Co, 1979.)

most regions, the periosteum strips easily from the bone, but near the articular surfaces and at the sites of muscle, tendon, ligament and interosseous membrane insertions it attaches to bone so firmly that separating it frequently requires sharp dissection. Periosteum consists of two layers: an outer dense fibrous layer and an inner looser more vascular layer. This inner layer contains cells capable of becoming osteoblasts and thus is referred to as the cambium or osteogenic layer. The cells of this layer also form hyaline cartilage under appropriate circumstances and help form the extraosseous callus in fracture healing. During bone growth they secrete the organic matrix that enlarges the diameter of the bone. The outer fibrous layer has fewer cells and more collagen. Near joints it continues into the joint capsule and in this way connects one bone to the next. In addition some tendons and ligaments insert primarily into this fibrous layer of the periosteum.

Periosteum changes with age. The thick cellular osteogenic layer of a child's periosteum readily forms new bone. It demonstrates this capacity when osteomyelitis or severe trauma destroys the diaphysis of a child's bone and the periosteum forms an entire new shell of bone. With age the periosteum becomes thinner and its osteogenic capacity appears to decrease. At skeletal maturity the osteogenic or cambium layer has almost completely disappeared and the more superficial fibrous layer becomes thin and only sparsely cellular. Despite these changes the periosteal cells continue to form bone throughout life as demonstrated by the increasing diameter of long bone diaphyses with increasing age.

## Tendon and Ligament Insertions

Normal function of the skeletal system requires that dense fibrous tissues such as tendon, ligament and joint capsule firmly attach themselves to bone. These structures stabilize synovial joints and transmit

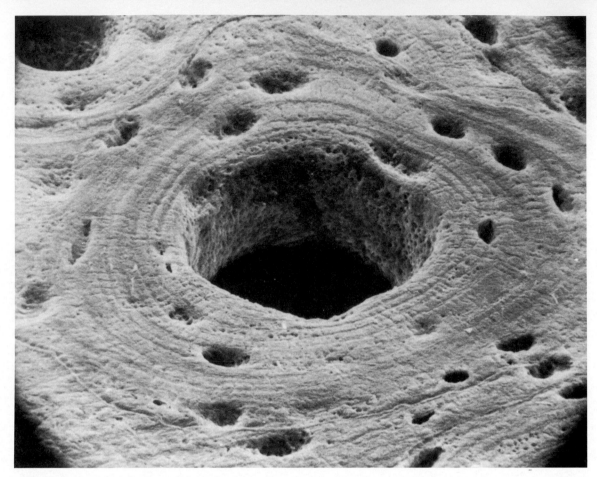

**Fig. 2–6** Scanning electron micrograph of an osteonal system showing the internal surface of the central haversian canal. Notice the multiple canaliculi that perforate the wall of the canal. These canaliculi allow osteocyte cell processes to extend from the cells to the central canal of the osteonal system and provide pathways for metabolites and gases deep within the bone matrix. (Reproduced with permission from Kessel RG, Kardon RH: *Tissues and Organs: A Text-Atlas of Scanning Microscopy.* New York, WH Freeman and Co, 1979.)

the force of muscle contraction to the skeleton. Insertions unite tissues with different material properties; that is, they must allow the transition from flexible, pliable fibrous tissue to rigid bone. They accomplish this transition by four zones of increasing stiffness: the substance of the tendon, ligament or capsule; fibrocartilage; mineralized fibrocartilage; and bone (Fig. 2–7).

As described by Havers in 1691, insertions vary in the obliquity of the angle between the collagen fibrils of the tendon, ligament or capsule and the bone as well as in the proportion of their collagen fibrils that enter the bone (Fig. 2–7). Some of the dense fibrous structures insert primarily into the fibrous layer of the periosteum (Fig. 2–7B) while others insert almost perpendicularly into the bone matrix (Fig. 2–7A). The fibers of the tendon, ligament or capsule that insert directly into bone are sometimes referred to as Sharpey's fibers. In 1856, he described such fibers as being like nails driven perpendicularly into the bone lamellae, thereby bolting adjacent lamellae together.

The medial collateral ligament of the knee illustrates the different types of insertion. The collagen fibrils of the proximal insertion penetrate the bone at an angle that lies almost perpendicular to the bone surface, while at the tibial insertion the ligament fibrils pass primarily into the fibrous layer of the periosteum. These differences may affect the mechanical behavior and biological responsiveness of the insertion. For example, Laros and associates[1] found that immobilization of the knee joint stimulated osteoclastic resorption of the tibial insertion of the medial collateral ligament and thereby decreased its strength. During the same period of immobilization, the femoral insertion remained relatively unchanged.

## Blood Supply

The elaborate organization of bone and its vascular canals insures that, even in dense cortical bone, no cell lies more than 300 $\mu$m from a blood vessel. Long bone diaphyses and metaphyses have three sources of

**A**    **B**

Ligament

Fibrocartilage

Mineralized
Fibrocartilage

Bone

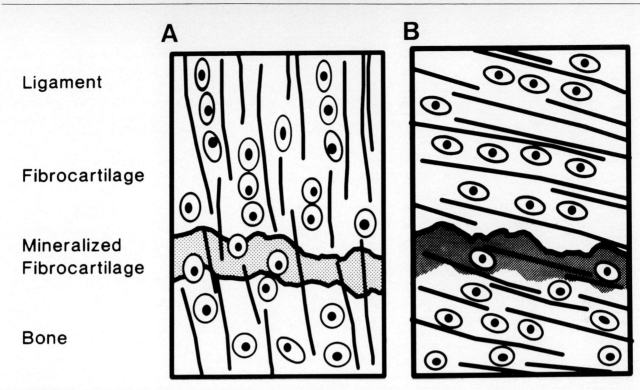

**Fig. 2–7**   Schematic illustrations of tendon or ligament insertion into bone. In the first type of insertion, the majority of the tendon or ligament collagen fibrils pass directly into bone. In the second type of insertion, many of the tendon or ligament collagen fibrils pass into the periosteum. **A:** The ligament collagen fibers pass through zones of fibrocartilage and mineralized fibrocartilage as they enter the bone. Most of the ligament collagen fibrils pass directly into the bone and lie almost perpendicular to the bone surface. **B:** The ligament collagen fibrils pass obliquely along the bone and many become part of the periosteum. In insertions of this type, the fibrocartilage and mineralized fibrocartilage zones may be poorly developed or absent.

blood supply: nutrient arteries, epiphyseal and metaphyseal penetrating arteries, and periosteal arteries (Fig. 2–8). The nutrient arteries enter the diaphysis and branch proximally and distally. These medullary arteries provide most of the blood supply to the diaphysis. The proximal and distal branches of the nutrient arteries join multiple fine branches from the periosteal and metaphyseal arteries to form the medullary arterial system. Under normal circumstances this medullary vascular system supplies most of periosteum-covered cortical bone, and therefore the primary direction of blood flow through the cortex is centrifugal. This pattern changes where dense fascial structures such as muscle or interosseous membranes insert into bone. In these areas periosteal vessels usually supply the outer third of the cortex. Prior to closure of the growth plate, medullary vessels rarely cross the physis, and the epiphyses depend on penetrating epiphyseal vessels for their blood supply. With closure of the physis intraosseous anastomoses develop between the penetrating epiphyseal arteries and the medullary arteries. However, these anastomoses may not provide sufficient blood flow to support the epiphysis without the contribution of the epiphyseal vessels.

Periosteum also has an elaborate vascular system. A vascular plexus lies over the surface of the fibrous layer and anastomoses with vessels in skeletal muscle and with the network of vessels in the osteogenic or cambium layer. The vessels of the cambium layer penetrate bone and join with the intraosseous vessels. With increasing age the periosteal vessels diminish and the contribution of the penetrating periosteal vessels to bone blood supply may decrease. Nonetheless, the periosteal vascular network remains an important part of bone circulation throughout life.

Under certain circumstances the periosteal vessels may also be an important source of blood supply for skeletal muscle. Whitesides[2] demonstrated that separating a muscle from underlying periosteum increased the probability of muscle necrosis after sectioning of the muscle's nutrient artery or crush injury to the muscle. Severing the muscle's nutrient artery with the muscle-periosteal vascular connections left intact did not significantly decrease muscle blood flow. For this reason crush injuries to muscle are less likely to cause ischemic muscle damage if the muscle-periosteal vascular connections are intact. Whitesides' work also indicates that the blood supply of the superficial and osteogenic layers of the periosteum

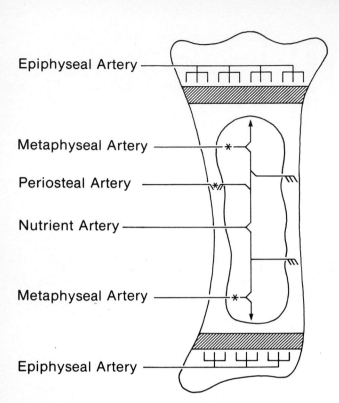

Epiphyseal Artery

Metaphyseal Artery

Periosteal Artery

Nutrient Artery

Metaphyseal Artery

Epiphyseal Artery

**Fig. 2–8** Schematic diagram showing the blood supply to a long bone. The nutrient artery enters the medullary canal and branches proximally and distally. Multiple metaphyseal arteries penetrate the cortex and anastomose with the medullary vascular system. Periosteal vessels also join with the medullary system giving diaphyseal and metaphyseal cortical bone a dual blood supply. The epiphyses receive their blood supply from vessels that enter the epiphyses directly. Vessels do not usually cross the open physis, but with physeal closure anastomoses form between the medullary vascular system and the epiphyseal system.

depends on the vascular connections with skeletal muscle. The clinical demonstration that periosteum survives and forms bone after being stripped subperiosteally, as long as the vascular connections between muscle and periosteum are not disrupted, supports these observations. Thus, disrupting the vascular connections between periosteum and muscle may adversely influence the collateral blood supply to muscle and the ability of periosteum to form new bone. On the other hand, stripping periosteum from bone deprives bone of its usual route of venous drainage and its collateral arterial supply.

The anastomoses between the medullary vascular system and the periosteal system, including the metaphyseal penetrating arteries, give the diaphysis a dual blood supply. This may be important following injuries to bone or soft tissue or in planning surgical procedures. Limited circumferential stripping of the periosteum does not decrease blood flow in the middle layers of diaphyseal cortical bone. Likewise, reaming the medullary canal, destroying the medul-

lary vascular system, does not significantly decrease blood flow in the middle layers of diaphyseal cortical bone. These observations as well as the complex anatomy of the cortical bone vascular supply, suggest that the diaphysis can receive a major portion of its blood supply from either the periosteal or the medullary systems, and that either the medullary system or the periosteal system can provide venous drainage. This dual circulatory system explains why bone remains viable and fractures heal after either medullary reaming or periosteal stripping. It also explains, in part, why segmental fractures that disrupt the medullary vascular system and have extensive soft-tissue injury or periosteal stripping may result in delayed or nonunions, and why it is best to avoid surgery that might compromise both the medullary and the periosteal blood supply.

As discussed earlier, most epiphyses have a more precarious blood supply than the diaphyses and metaphyses. Prior to closure of the growth plate the blood supply of the epiphysis depends entirely on penetrating vessels. Following fusion of the epiphysis and metaphysis, vascular channels cross the physeal scar, but their functional significance is unclear. Several experiments suggest that these anastomoses are not sufficient to supply the epiphysis following interruption of the epiphyseal arteries. Thus, while the diaphysis and metaphysis have a dual circulatory system that can only be significantly disrupted by loss of both the medullary and the periosteal system, some epiphyses depend primarily on the penetrating epiphyseal vessels. This arrangement may be partially responsible for the frequency of idiopathic necrosis in the femoral epiphysis, the epiphysis of the head of the second metatarsal and the epiphysis of the humeral capitellum. The femoral epiphysis is particularly vulnerable to loss of its blood supply since its vessels must pass along the femoral neck where they can easily be injured by dislocation of the hip, fracture of the femoral neck or surgery.

### The Composition of Bone Matrix

The remarkable mechanical properties of bone depend on the extracellular matrix. It is a composite material consisting of an organic component and an inorganic component. The inorganic component contributes approximately 70% of bone wet weight, although it may form up to 80% (Fig. 2–9). The organic component usually contributes about 22% of the weight and water contributes only 8% or 9%. The organic component, primarily collagen, gives bone its form and contributes to its ability to resist tension while the mineral component primarily resists compression. Bones that have either been demineralized or have had their organic matrix removed readily demonstrate the differences between the two matrix

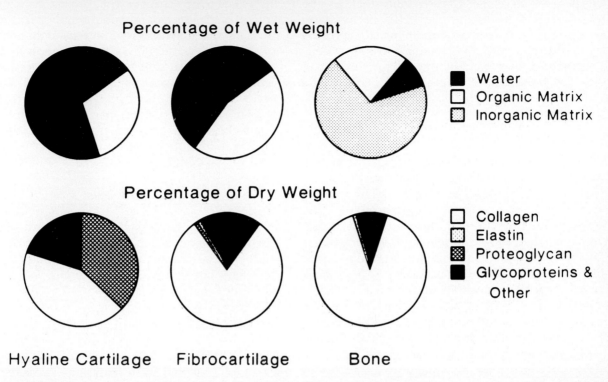

**Fig. 2–9**  Representation of the approximate compositions of bone, cartilage, and fibrous tissue. The top row of graphs illustrates the wet weight composition of these tissues. Notice that mature bone contains relatively little water and a great deal of inorganic matrix. The bottom row of graphs illustrates the relative compositions of the organic matrices and shows that the organic matrices of dense fibrous tissues and bone consist primarily of collagen. (Adapted with permission from Buckwalter JA: Cells and matrices of skeletal connective tissues, in Albright JA, Brand RA (eds): *The Scientific Basis of Orthopaedics*. Norwalk, CT, Appleton-Century-Crofts, to be published.)

components. Either of these procedures leaves the bone with its original form and size but significantly alters its mechanical properties. Demineralized bone, like a tendon or ligament, is very flexible, pliable and resistant to fracture. A demineralized long bone, such as the fibula, can be bent or even tied in a knot without fracture. In contrast, removal of the organic matrix makes bone rigid, hard and brittle; only slight deformation will fracture it, and a sharp blow will shatter it.

This composite composition of bone matrix distinguishes it from other connective tissue matrices that lack the inorganic component (Fig. 2–9). In addition, the low water content of bone differs from that of other skeletal tissues such as cartilage in which water provides 60% to 80% of the wet weight or dense fibrous tissue such as tendon, ligament and joint capsule in which water usually makes up over 50% of the wet weight (Fig. 2–9).

### The Organic Matrix

The organic matrix of bone resembles the matrix of dense fibrous tissues like tendon, ligament and joint capsule. Type I collagen makes up over 90% of the organic matrix with the other 10% consisting of noncollagenous proteins, glycoproteins and bone-specific proteoglycans (Fig. 2–9). Type I collagen is distinguished from other collagen types by its unique amino acid content, its relatively large diameter fibrils and its presence in tissues subjected to large tensile loads. Like bone, the dense fibrous tissues contain primarily type I collagen while hyaline cartilage contains primarily type II collagen.

The organic matrix of bone first appears as osteoid, but as mineralization converts osteoid into bone, the composition of the organic matrix changes. Compared to bone, organic matrix, osteoid, or pre-bone contains proportionately more noncollagenous matrix macromolecules and water. Although the matrix changes that occur during mineralization are not well understood, it is clear that as relatively insoluble mineral deposits appear, water and noncollagenous matrix molecules are lost. The absolute amount of collagen apparently remains constant. Once mineralization has occurred the organic matrix remains relatively unchanged until it is resorbed.

As previously noted, abnormalities or insufficiencies of the inorganic matrix component, like osteomalacia and rickets, can alter the material properties of bone. Abnormalities of the organic component may also cause problems. Patients with osteogenesis imperfecta have increased bone fragility that may be due to defects in the organic matrix. In this heterogeneous group of hereditary conditions, the primary bone defect frequently appears to involve the synthesis, secretion or assembly of the collagen matrix of bone. The bone lacks strength either because of a decreased amount of collagen or an abnormal collagen structure.

### The Inorganic Matrix

Deposition of mineral radically changes the material properties of the matrix. Despite extensive research, the mechanisms that initiate and control matrix mineralization remain controversial. The following sequence is perhaps the most widely accepted explanation of the events leading to matrix mineralization. Osteoblasts synthesize and secrete a unique bone matrix osteoid that can calcify. This matrix includes molecules that bind mineral and collagen, and the bone collagen has sites that can catalyze mineral nucleation and maturation of mineral crystals. To exert local control over the mineralization process, osteoblasts produce inhibitors that slow the transition of calcium and phosphate from soluble ions to relatively insoluble crystals, and the cells may concentrate calcium intracellularly and release it at the appropriate time to stimulate or facilitate mineralization. Newly mineralized bone contains a variety of calcium phosphate species that range from relatively soluble complexes to crystalline hydroxyapatite. More mature bone contains primarily hydroxyapatite although sodium, magnesium, citrate and fluoride may also be present. Investigators dispute the site of initial mineral formation, but they generally agree that in mature lamellar bone, collagen fibrils contain most of the hydroxyapatite within the structure of the fibrils. Once mineralization begins it proceeds rapidly: 60% or more of the ultimate mineral forms within hours. Following this initial phase, mineral continues to accumulate over a prolonged time, gradually increasing bone density.

Since the degree of mineralization increases with maturation the material properties of bone change as well. With increasing mineralization, bone stiffness increases, and its resistance to impact decreases. This helps explain why children's and adults' bones may differ in their patterns of fracture. When subjected to excessive load, normal adult bone usually breaks rather than deforming permanently. In contrast, children's bones may bow or buckle rather than break. Bowing of a bone is most commonly seen when an injury deforms the ulna or the fibula beyond its ability to resume its original shape. The bowing of these bones may impede reduction of associated radial or tibial fractures. In torus fractures, a compression load buckles the child's bone, usually in the metaphysis, rather than breaking it. Children may also sustain "greenstick" fractures; a bending force fractures the cortex and ruptures the periosteum on the side of the bone loaded in tension but leaves the cortex and periosteum intact on the opposite side. All three of these patterns of children's skeletal injuries, bowing, torus fractures and greenstick fractures, occur because their bones can be deformed plastically. This occurs, at least partially, because of the relatively low degree of mineralization. As the degree of mineralization increases these fracture patterns become less common.

## Bone Cells

Metabolic and neoplastic diseases of bone, the response of bone to injury, or the results of medical and surgical treatment depend on bone cells. Bone cells have been classified by their morphology, function and characteristic location into four groups: undifferentiated or osteoprogenitor cells, osteoblasts, osteocytes and osteoclasts.

### Undifferentiated Cells

Undifferentiated or osteoprogenitor cells usually reside in the bone canals (Fig. 2–4), the endosteum, or the periosteum. These small cells have an irregular form with a single nucleus and few organelles. They remain in their undifferentiated state until stimulated to proliferate and differentiate into osteoblasts. For example, in fracture healing the injury stimulates osteoprogenitor cells to proliferate rapidly and differentiate into osteoblasts.

### Osteoblasts

Osteoblasts line bone surfaces. When they are active they have a round to oval or polyhedral form, and an osteoid seam separates them from mineralized matrix. Osteoblasts synthesizing new matrix contain abundant endoplasmic reticulum, Golgi membranes and mitochondria. The surface of the cell applied to the newly formed organic matrix contains primarily endoplasmic reticulum while the nucleus is usually located in the pole of the cell opposite the endoplasmic reticulum. The cytoplasmic processes of osteoblasts extend through the osteoid matrix they have synthesized to contact osteocytes deep within the mineralized matrix (Fig. 2–10). These specialized cell contacts may help coordinate cell activities.

Active osteoblasts may follow one of two courses. They may remain on the bone surface, decrease their synthetic activity and assume a flatter form or they may surround themselves with matrix and become osteocytes (Fig. 2–10). The flattened surface osteoblasts are sometimes referred to as surface osteocytes. Both the flattened surface osteoblasts and osteocytes have less cytoplasm and fewer organelles than active

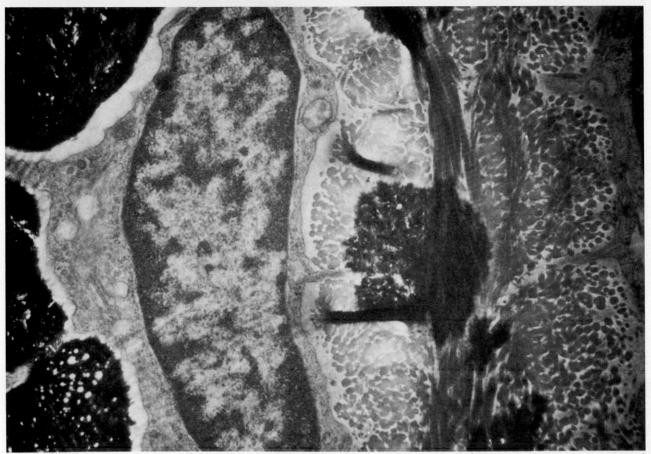

**Fig. 2–10** Electron micrograph of an osteocyte forming from an osteoblast. The cell has surrounded itself with mineralized matrix on one side and partially mineralized matrix on the other. Cell processes pass into the mineralized matrix and make contact with other cells.

osteoblasts. The principal and most obvious function of osteoblasts is the synthesis and secretion of the organic matrix of bone. They also may have a role in controlling electrolyte fluxes between the extracellular fluid and the bone fluid, and they may directly regulate the mineralization of bone matrix. Osteoblasts rarely if ever divide.

### Osteocytes

Osteocytes form more than 90% of the cells in the mature skeleton. They surround themselves with mineralized bone matrix (Fig. 2–10), and combined with the periosteal and endosteal cells, they appear to cover the bone matrix (Fig. 2–2). Osteocytes have a single nucleus and their cytoplasm varies in organelle content and volume with their activity. Long cytoplasmic processes extend from their oval or lens-shaped bodies to contact other cells within the bone matrix (Figs. 2–11 and 2–12). The surface area of these cells and their cell processes makes up more than 90% of the total surface area of mature bone matrix (Fig. 2–13). This structural arrangement gives osteocytes access to almost all of the mineralized bone matrix

surface area and may be critical in allowing cell-mediated exchange of mineral to take place between the bone fluid and the blood.

A number of experiments suggest that osteocytes are capable of resorbing and possibly forming bone. This ability to resorb and form bone of the lacunar matrix appears to help maintain serum calcium homeostasis. For example, osteocytes appear to participate in the hypercalcemic response to parathyroid hormone by removing mineral from the bone matrix that surrounds them. Although any one cell releases only a small amount of calcium from the matrix, the large number of cells and the large surface area covered by each cell magnifies the effect.

### Osteoclasts

Osteoclasts are among the largest and most unusual cells in the body. They have multiple nuclei and a large irregular form (Fig. 2–14). Mitochondria fill much of their cytoplasm to supply the great amount of energy required to resorb bone (Fig. 2–14). One of the most distinctive features of these cells is the complex folding of their cytoplasmic membrane

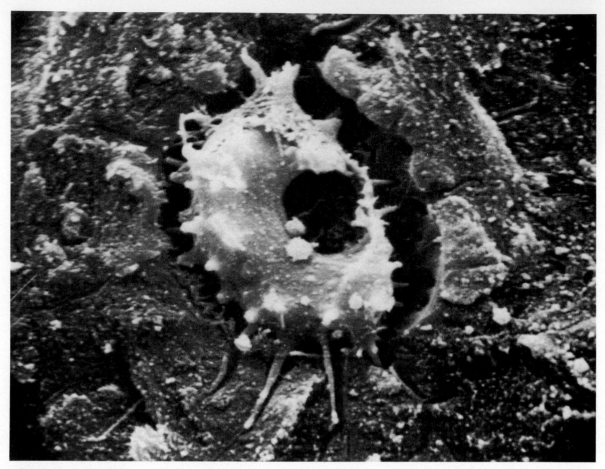

**Fig. 2–11** Scanning electron micrograph of the fractured surface of cortical bone. An osteocyte lies within its lacuna, where the cell membrane has separated from the bone matrix. Osteocyte processes extend from the cell into canaliculi, which penetrate the bone matrix. Some of the osteocyte processes ruptured when the bone was fractured. (Reproduced with permission from Kessel RG, Kardon RH: *Tissues and Organs: A Text-Atlas of Scanning Microscopy.* New York, WH Freeman and Co, 1979.)

where it is applied to the site of bone matrix resorption (Figs. 2–15 and 2–16). This ruffled or brush border appears to play a critical role in bone resorption, perhaps by increasing the surface area of the cell relative to the bone. A region of cytoplasm, almost free of organelles, referred to as the clear zone, surrounds the brush border. The clear zone may allow the brush border to move along the bone matrix surface, or it may seal off the region of bone resorption. Within the cell, deep to the ruffled border, lies a region containing membrane-bound vesicles and vacuoles (Fig. 2–15). These structures may be invaginations or infoldings of the brush border and may contain collagen and mineral. In cancellous bone, osteoclasts create a characteristic depression of the bone surface referred to as Howship's lacunae (Fig. 2–17). In dense cortical bone they lead the osteonal cutting cones that remodel the bone. Osteoclasts may move from one site of bone resorption to another, and they can gain or lose nuclei and cytoplasm.

## The Origin of Bone Cells

In the mature skeleton, osteoprogenitor cells or undifferentiated cells have the capacity to differentiate into osteoblasts after appropriate stimulation. When the osteoblast surrounds itself with bone matrix and loses much of its cytoplasm it becomes an osteocyte. The sequence is well established. However, the source of osteoclasts has been less certain. Some investigators[3] have suggested that the different bone cell types represent progressive differentiation of a single cell line. That is, primitive mesenchymal cells sequentially became preosteoclasts, osteoclasts, preosteoblasts, osteoblasts and then osteocytes and that this sequence of events forms a repeating cycle. Most bone biologists now agree that separate stem cells exist for the osteoblast and osteoclast cell lines. Several experiments have shown that blood borne monocytes can form osteoclasts and that the differentiation of osteoclasts seems to be initiated by contact between monocyte precursor cells and mineralized bone matrix.[4] These observations suggest that the special monocyte must be attracted to the bone matrix and the expression of the osteoclast phenotype depends upon proteins or glycoproteins closely associated with the bone matrix. The life span and ultimate fate of the osteoclast remains unknown.

Osteopetrosis demonstrates the adverse effects of inadequate or ineffective osteoclast function.[5] In this disorder the bone is extremely dense, hard and white. A mixture of calcified cartilage, bone and fibrous tissue replaces most of the marrow, leaving little normal marrow space. Loss of normal marrow elements may lead to severe anemia, overwhelming infection and death. Microscopic examination of the bone shows calcified cartilage cores surrounded by bone, and frequently there is no identifiable margin between cortical and cancellous bone. Although a number of abnormalities of bone cells and matrix may exist in this condition, the principal defect seems to be that the osteoclasts fail to resorb bone and calcified cartilage. This observation and those con-

cerning the origin of osteoclasts have been combined to develop a treatment for this disease. In both human and animal forms of osteopetrosis, infusion of normal donor spleen or marrow cells corrects the disorder. The infused monocytes differentiate into bone resorbing cells and remove the excessive bone and calcified cartilage and allow proliferation of the normal marrow elements and physiologic or adaptive bone remodeling.

## Bone Modeling and Remodeling

The genotype, that is the hereditary constitution of the individual, establishes the basic shape and size of each bone. Once the embryonic model of a bone forms, its ultimate shape and size have been determined; even cartilage models of bones grown in tissue culture develop their normal shapes. However, osteoclasts and osteoblasts can add and remove bone matrix, thereby changing the bone mass and aligning the matrix in accord with functional demands so that,

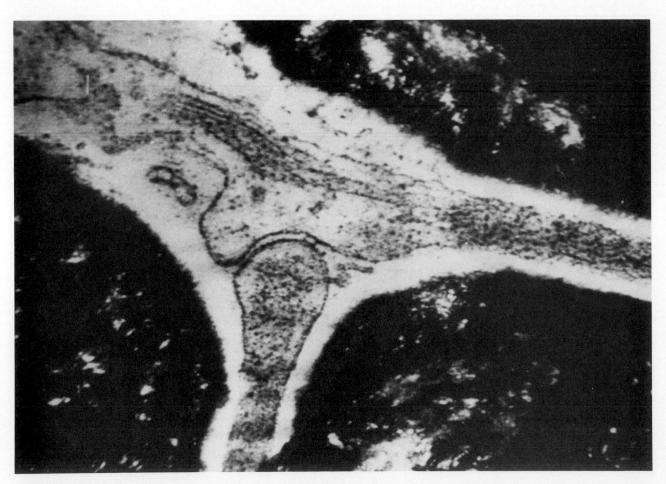

**Fig. 2–12**  Electron micrograph showing osteocyte cell processes in their canaliculi. In this micrograph two cell processes contact each other far from the cell body. Through the contact of their cell processes, osteocytes create a network of interconnecting cells. The dark material is mineralized bone matrix.

# BONE SURFACE AREA IN ADULT MAN

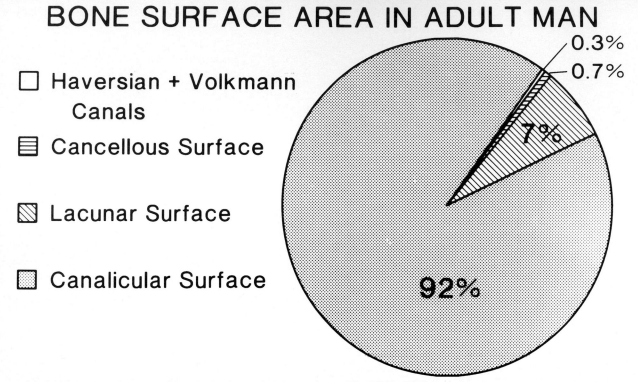

☐ Haversian + Volkmann
  Canals

▤ Cancellous Surface

▧ Lacunar Surface

▦ Canalicular Surface

0.3%
0.7%
7%
92%

**Fig. 2–13**   The distribution of bone surface area. The cell processes of osteocytes cover more than 90% of the bone matrix surface area. The cancellous surface forms less than 1% of the total bone surface area, and the periosteal surface is only a small fraction of this cancellous surface.

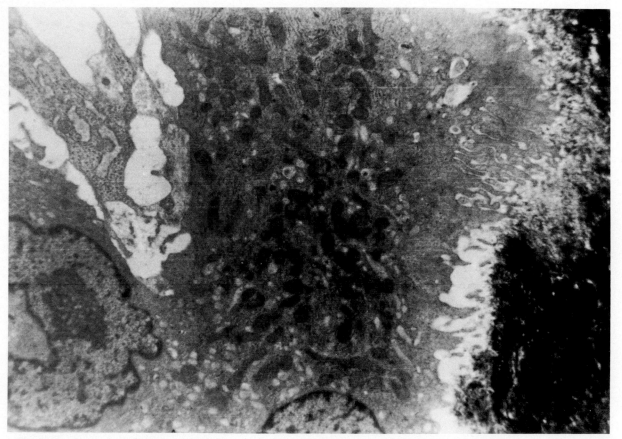

**Fig. 2–14**   Electron micrograph of an osteoclast. Notice the large number of mitochondria and the complex folding of the cell membrane at the site of bone matrix resorption.

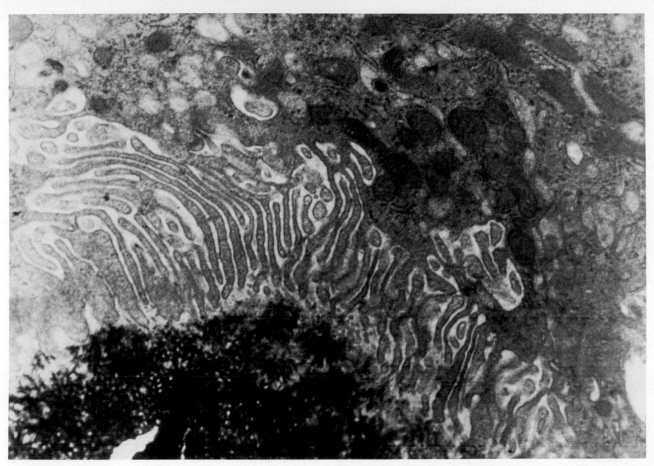

**Fig. 2–15**  Electron micrograph of an osteoclast brush border applied to mineralized bone matrix. Notice application of the folded cell membrane to the bone matrix and the large number of mitochondria.

within genetically determined limits, vertebrates can change the strength and mass as well as the form of their skeletons.

Because of their differences in structure, cortical bone and cancellous bone differ slightly in their mechanism of remodeling. Osteonal remodeling (Fig. 2–18) occurs in cortical bone. In this process osteoclasts excavate a tunnel 2 to 10 nm in length, advancing longitudinally following the long axis of the bone. This cutting cone can create large resorption cavities as successive groups of osteoclasts cut a tunnel directly through cortical bone often passing through old osteonal systems. A cement line marks the site where resorption by this cutting cone stops and new bone formation begins. Within the cutting cone, groups of spindle cells and several vessels follow the advancing group of osteoclasts. The amount of bone resorbed by one osteoclast in one day requires about 50 osteoblasts to replace it; so behind the osteoclasts, layers of osteoblasts arrange themselves along the surface of the resorption cavity and deposit successive lamellae of new bone matrix (Fig. 2–18). Subsequently the bone matrix mineralizes, successive lamellae are

added, and the tunnel size narrows to the diameter of an osteonal central canal. Physiologic osteonal remodeling continues throughout life so that cortical bone eventually consists almost entirely of osteons and the remnants of osteons that have been partially resorbed and replaced (Fig. 2–2).

Remodeling of trabecular bone resembles that of cortical bone except that the osteoclasts lie on the surface of the trabeculae (Figs. 2–17 and 2–18) and excavate a cavity or Howship's lacuna. When osteoclasts have completed their resorptive activity they move away from the site of resorption. Soon afterwards active osteoblasts begin covering the resorbed surface with osteoid seams. Approximately ten days later, mineralization of the osteoid completes the remodeling process.

Most authors distinguish bone remodeling from bone modeling. Bone modeling usually refers to the bone resorption and formation that modifies the bone during growth to create its final shape. This activity continually reshapes each bone as it grows and terminates at skeletal maturity. However, since age-related addition of periosteal new bone and re-

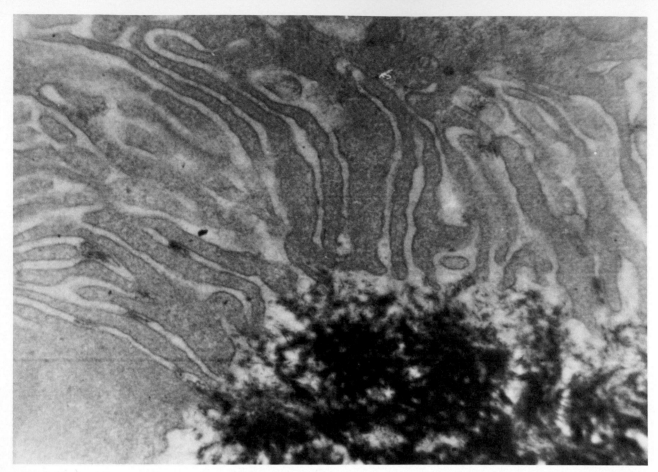

**Fig. 2–16**   A higher magnification electron micrograph showing the brush border of an osteoclast applied to mineralized bone matrix.

sorption of endosteal bone changes the shape of the diaphysis, it might be considered a form of bone modeling as well.

Removal and placement of bone at roughly the same location is referred to as physiologic remodeling. Physiologic remodeling does not affect the shape of the bone. It continues throughout life, and over a period of years can completely replace the skeleton. The purpose and control mechanism of this continual remodeling remain uncertain. It does not occur to the same extent in all animals nor is the anatomic location of physiologic remodeling necessarily related to the loading of the skeleton, so it does not seem to be activated by mechanical forces.

Remodeling may also be an adaptive response of bone to a change in loading. In 1892, Julius Wolff described how bone responded to changes in loads. He suggested that living bone adapts to alterations in mechanical loads by changing its structure in accordance with mathematical laws. Thus, the response of bone to changes in loads frequently is referred to as Wolff's law. In a simple illustration of this phenom-

enon, an eccentrically loaded long bone bends; in response cells deposit new bone on the concave or compression side and resorb bone on the convex or tension side. We frequently take advantage of this type of remodeling when we treat children's fractures. A fracture that heals with angulation may completely remodel, restoring the original alignment of the bone depending on the age of the patient, the location of the fracture, and the degree of angulation. In general the younger the patient, the closer the fracture is to a joint and the less the angulation, the more likely it is that the fracture will remodel completely. Application of a rigid metal plate to a diaphyseal fracture provides another example of adaptive remodeling. Since the plate unloads the bone, to some extent, the bone mass decreases, the cortex thins and the bone weakens. Repeated loading, as in vigorous athletic activities, produces the opposite effect: the bone mass increases and the cortex thickens.

Imbalances in remodeling can adversely affect bone strength and mass. A frequent simple example

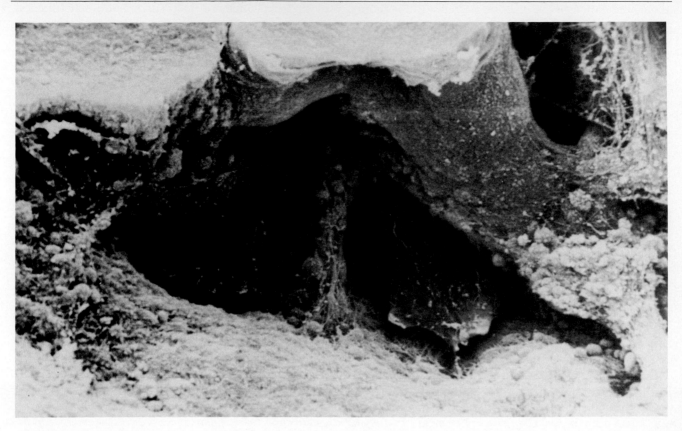

**Fig. 2–17**  Scanning electron micrographs of two osteoclasts.  They have resorbed some of the bone surface, creating resorption cavities referred to as Howship's lacunae. Notice the irregular shape of the cells and that the cavities on the bone surface have essentially the same shape as the cells. Removal of the bone mineral by the osteoclasts reveals the matrix collagen fibrils. Mineral crystals undergoing dissolution may take the form of small spheres. (Reproduced with permission from Kessel RG, Kardon RH: *Tissues and Organs: A Text-Atlas of Scanning Microscopy*. New York, WH Freeman and Co, 1979.)

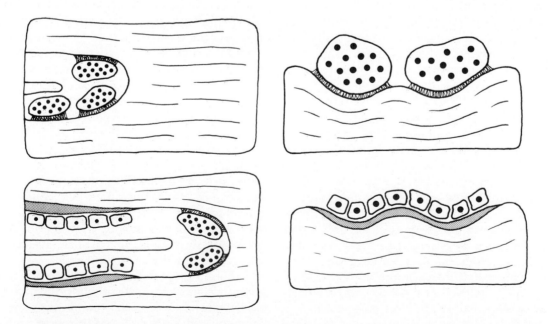

**Fig.  2–18**  Schematic diagrams of bone remodeling.  The left side of the figure shows osteonal remodeling. Osteoclasts form a cutting cone resorbing a tunnel through cortical bone. A vascular loop and loose fibrous tissue follow the osteoclasts. Osteoblasts then form new bone matrix in the resorption cavity. The right side of the figure shows trabecular remodeling. Osteoclasts remove bone from the trabecular surface producing a cavity referred to as a Howship's lacuna. The osteoclasts then leave the resorption cavity and osteoblasts form a new bone matrix.

of an imbalance between bone formation and bone resorption occurs during prolonged immobilization. When a limb is immobilized bone resorption exceeds bone formation and radiographs show increased cortical porosity, loss of trabeculae and decreased density of cancellous bone. Most metabolic diseases of bone result from disturbance of bone remodeling. In hyperparathyroidism, excessive parathyroid hormone stimulates bone resorption so that it exceeds bone formation. Occasionally this may produce large cavities within the bone filled with osteoclasts, fibrous tissue and small vessels.

With aging, bone mass steadily declines and the form of the bone changes. The degree of age-related loss of bone mass varies with sex and race. White women have much greater loss than white men or black men and women. Usually trabecular bone loss exceeds cortical loss probably because of the greater remodeling activity on the surface of trabecular bone. Commonly trabeculae decrease in number rather than thickness, and the marrow becomes less cellular and filled with fat. Radiographs show these changes as a loss of trabeculae and decreased cancellous bone density. Cortical bone is also lost with advancing age. In this process the cortex thins and expands as bone is lost from the endosteal surface while the periosteum forms new bone. However, periosteal new bone formation does not adequately compensate for endosteal bone loss. The mechanisms of these age-related changes in bone shape and mass remain unknown.

Age-related decreased bone density leads to increasing bone fragility, producing the clinical disorder of osteoporosis.[6] Currently most treatments of osteoporosis are directed toward restoring the balance between bone formation and bone resorption. For example, mechanical loading of the skeleton may help delay or halt age-related bone loss. In young individuals, bone mass increases in response to increased loads. This increase in bone mass, frequently seen in athletes and laborers, may significantly increase bone strength. However, it is not certain whether exercise can increase bone mass in older individuals including people who have osteoporosis. In particular there is some question as to whether aging produces irreversible changes in the ability of the cells to produce new bone matrix. Thus, weight-bearing activity in older persons with osteoporosis may slow the age-related loss of bone mass or even stabilize bone mass, but it has not been shown that physical activity alone can restore lost bone mass.

## Regulation of Bone Cell Function

One of the most exciting developments in bone biology has been the rapid increase in understanding of the mechanisms that control bone cell function. The ability to induce bone formation or resorption as needed would significantly improve the treatment of age-related losses of bone mass, bone diseases and skeletal injuries. In osteoporosis stimulation of bone formation or inhibition of bone resorption would help prevent the frequent and disabling fractures. The ability to initiate bone formation in specific locations would allow treatment of delayed unions and nonunions.

Control of cell function may be considered in two general categories, intracellular control and extracellular control. The genes direct cell function and it is through the repression or activation of specific genes that cells change their activities. Selective alteration of genetic material might eventually provide a method of treating inherited defects in bone cell function such as osteogenesis imperfecta and osteopetrosis.

Extracellular control of cell function may be systemic or local. Systemic factors include nutrition and the influence of hormones including parathyroid hormone, vitamin D and its metabolites, thyroid hormone, growth hormone, insulin, estrogens, testosterone, and calcitonin. Malnutrition leads to significant disturbances of bone growth and remodeling. Abnormalities of Vitamin D metabolism produce rickets and osteomalacia. Exogenous steroids can decrease the synthetic activity of osteoblasts and may interfere with the ability of osteoprogenitor cells to differentiate into osteoblasts and adversely affect calcium absorption. As a result, patients receiving corticosteroids for prolonged periods may develop severe osteopenia and multiple pathologic fractures. In postmenopausal women, use of estrogens may slow or stabilize the age-related loss of bone mass and thereby decrease the probability of fracture. Increased understanding of systemic control of bone cell function may provide other methods of preventing fractures in patients at risk for developing osteoporosis.

Local factors that influence bone cell function include oxygen tension, pH, local ion concentrations, interactions between cells, local concentrations of nutrients and metabolites, mechanical and electrical signals and interactions between cells and matrix macromolecules. The ability to exert local control over bone cell function by application of electrical fields or use of bone matrix has already begun to change the practice of orthopaedics.

Although the exact relationship between electrical potentials and bone cell function has not been fully explained, it is clear that changes in electrical environment can alter cell proliferation and synthetic activity.[7] Since bone transduces mechanical energy into electrical potentials and the electrical potentials are proportional to the strain, the responses of bone cells to changes in skeletal loading, that is, adaptive remodeling, may be mediated by changes in the electrical environment. When a bone is eccentrically loaded, creating bending forces, the concave side, which is being compressed, develops a negative electrical potential, while the convex side being subjected to tension develops a positive electrical potential. Furthermore, passing an electrical current through bone can cause bone formation around the negative electrode. This may explain why certain types of stress or loading diminish bone resorption relative to bone formation while immobilization produces the opposite effect. Remodeling of angulated fractures may occur because the electrical potentials on the concave side stimulate bone formation, while those on the convex side stimulate resorption. Correction of the angulation returns the electrical potentials to normal and restores the balance between bone formation and bone resorption. In recent years knowledge of the electrical effects on bone has been applied to the treatment of nonunions and delayed unions. Although the explanation of how electrical fields influence bone cell function remains uncertain, several trials suggest that electrical stimulation, applied either through external coils or through direct insertion of electrodes, stimulates healing.

The ability of matrix macromolecules to influence cell function also has great potential future application. Bone organic matrix contains information that can direct cell function. As mentioned earlier, bone matrix molecules apparently stimulate the transformation of monocytes into osteoclasts suggesting that the cells have specific membrane receptors that recognize the bone matrix molecules. Observations by Urist,[8] Reddi,[9] and Reddi and Anderson[10] have shown that implanted demineralized bone matrix stimulates the migration of undifferentiated cells to the region of the implanted matrix and the differentiation of these cells into chondrocytes, which synthesize cartilage. The cartilage matrix calcifies, it is invaded by vessels, and then resorbed as the cells differentiate into osteoblasts and form a bone matrix that mineralizes and subsequently remodels. Fracture healing may depend upon this sequence of events. Fractures expose the bone organic matrix like the experimental implantation of demineralized matrix. Following the fracture, mesenchymal cells migrate and proliferate, differentiate into chondrocytes and form the cartilage of fracture callus, which then mineralizes, is resorbed and is finally replaced by bone.

## Summary

Bone is a complex, living, constantly changing tissue. The architecture and composition of cancellous and cortical bone allow the skeleton to perform its essential mechanical functions. The stiffer cortical bone responds more slowly to changes in loads while cancellous bone has a much larger surface area per unit volume and a greater rate of metabolic activity. Periosteum covers the external surface of bone and consists of two layers: an outer fibrous layer and an inner more cellular and vascular layer. The inner osteogenic layer or cambium layer can form new bone while the outer layer forms part of the insertions of tendons, ligaments and muscles. The cortical bone of diaphyses and metaphyses has a dual blood supply that allows loss of one source of circulation without adversely affecting the viability of the tissue. Many epiphyses, even in adults, depend only on a single source of blood supply, the penetrating epiphyseal vessels. For this reason epiphyseal bone may infarct more easily than metaphyseal or diaphyseal bone. The bone matrix has an organic component, primarily type I collagen, which gives it tensile strength and an inorganic component, primarily hydroxyapatite, which gives it stiffness to compression. Specialized populations of bone cells form, maintain and remodel this matrix. We recognize four types of bone cells based on their locations, morphology and functions: osteoprogenitor cells, osteoblasts, osteocytes and osteoclasts. Osteoblasts develop from undifferentiated cells while osteocytes form from osteoblasts. Osteoclasts have a separate stem cell line, blood-borne monocytes. Bone matrix apparently attracts these monocytes and stimulates their differentiation into osteoclasts. The processes of bone modeling and remodeling require osteoclastic resorption of bone matrix and deposition of a new matrix by osteoblasts. Modeling shapes and reshapes bones during growth and stops at skeletal maturity. Physiologic remodeling does not change bone shape and consists of bone resorption followed by bone deposition in approximately the same location. Since it continues throughout life it appears to be important for maintenance of the skeleton, but its exact function remains obscure. Adaptive remodeling is the response of the bone to altered loads and may alter the strength, density and shape of bone. In recent years understanding of the control of bone cell function has increased significantly. The study of electrical effects on bone formation has lead to new treatments of nonunions and delayed unions. Physicians have applied understanding of matrix-induced bone formation to reconstruction of skeletal defects. Knowledge of bone cell functions and bone cell origins has led to a treatment of osteopetrosis. These examples illustrate how knowledge of bone biology contributes to the treatment of orthopaedic problems and how advances in understanding of bone structure and function will continue to improve the treatment of orthopaedic problems.

## References

1. Laros GS, Tipton CM, Cooper RR: Influence of physical activity on ligament insertions in the knees of dogs. *J Bone Joint Surg* 1971;53A:275–286.
2. Whitesides L: Circulation in bone, in Evarts CM (ed): *Surgery of the Musculoskeletal System.* New York, Churchill Livingstone Inc, 1983, vol 1, pp 51–63.
3. Rassmussen J, Bordier P: *The Physiological and Cellular Basis of Metabolic Bone Disease.* Baltimore, Williams and Wilkins Co, 1974.
4. Kahn AJ, Teitelbaum SL, Malone JD, et al: The relationship of monocytic cells to the differentiation and resorption of bone, in Kelly RO, Goetinck PF, MacCabe JA (eds): *Limb Development and Regeneration,* part B. New York, AR Liss Inc, 1983, pp 237–248.
5. Marks SC, Walker DG: Mammalian osteopetrosis, in Bourne GH (ed): *The Biochemistry and Physiology of Bone.* New York, Academic Press Inc, 1976, vol 4, pp 227–301.
6. *Osteoporosis: National Institutes of Health Consensus Development Conference Statement,* United States Department of Health and Human Services, 1984, vol 5, no 3.
7. Eriksson C: Electrical properties of bone, in Bourne GH (ed): *The Biochemistry and Physiology of Bone.* New York, Academic Press Inc, 1976, vol 6, pp 329–384.
8. Urist MR: Bone formation by auto induction. *Science* 1965;150:893–899.
9. Reddi AH: Cell biology and biochemistry of endochondral bone development. *Coll Res* 1981;1:209–226.
10. Reddi AH, Anderson WA: Collagenous bone matrix-induced endochondral ossification and hemopoiesis. *J Cell Biol* 1976;69:557–572.

# The Nature of the Mineral Component of Bone and the Mechanism of Calcification

Melvin J. Glimcher, MD

## Introduction

This discussion will be concerned principally with (1) the chemical composition and crystal structure of the solid calcium-phosphorus (Ca-P) mineral phase in bone, and the changes that occur in the mineral phase with time and maturation; (2) the ultrastructural location of the mineral phase; (3) the structural and chemical relationships between the Ca-P mineral phase and the individual components of the matrix; and (4) the mechanism and regulation of calcification.

## Biologic Functions of the Mineral Phase

The Ca-P mineral phase in bone performs two major functions, both of which depend on the size, shape, chemical composition, and crystal structure of the mineral crystallites; it acts as an ion reservoir and as an excellently designed structural material that determines in large part the mechanical properties of bone as a tissue and as an organ. The role of bone mineral as an ion reservoir can be appreciated from the fact that approximately 99% of the body calcium, 85% of the body phosphorus, and from 40% to 60% of the total body sodium and magnesium are associated with the bone crystals, which consequently serve as the major source for the transport of these ions to and from the extracellular fluids. As a result, bone crystals play a critical role in maintaining the extracellular fluid concentrations of these ions, which are critical for a variety of physiologic functions, such as nerve conduction and muscle contraction, and a number of important biochemical reactions. In addition, bone crystals maintain the serum concentrations of some ions such as calcium within a physiologically necessary narrow range.

From a structural standpoint, the impregnation of the soft, pliable organic matrix of bone tissues by the rock-like Ca-P crystals of apatite converts the soft organic matrix to a relatively hard, rigid material that now possesses the necessary mechanical properties to permit it to withstand the stresses and strains imposed on it by gait, prehension, and respiration. Moreover, this relatively inflexible and rigid material is able to preserve the shape of the organism as a whole and to protect vital organs such as the brain, spinal cord, lungs, and heart. The mechanical properties of bone depend on both the physical and chemical properties of the mineral phase, on its three-dimensional disposition within the bone, and on its ultrastructural and molecular relationships to specific components of the organic matrix.

Although not a direct function of bone mineral or of bone tissue, bone provides for another important general physiologic function: it acts as host and provides space for the precursors of the blood cells (marrow).

It is precisely because the two major biological functions of the bone mineral ultimately depend on the precise chemical composition, physical chemical properties, and crystal structure of the mineral phase that so much attention has been directed at elucidating these characteristics. It is important to keep in mind that after its initial deposition in the tissue, significant changes in both chemical composition and structure occur in the mineral phase with time. Not only must this fact be kept in mind when attempting to understand the changes in mineral metabolism as a function of organism age, but it must be taken into account when trying to explain the serum and other changes observed in healthy individuals as well as in those with metabolic bone diseases ($Ca^{47}$ uptake and disappearance). This is especially true in instances in which the rates of bone formation and resorption have been significantly altered and consequently the amount and proportion of new bone and old bone, including therefore young and old bone crystals, have also markedly changed. This alteration in turn significantly changes the population distribution of bone mineral as a function of bone mineral age and not animal age. Unfortunately, such considerations are rarely taken into account in clinical studies and may in part account for some of the discrepancies noted in metabolic studies between the predicted serum values and bone turnover rates and those actually observed.

## The Nature of the Mineral Phase in Bone and the Changes That Occur With Time

For over 150 years, bone mineral has been known by chemical analyses to contain calcium and phosphorus as its principal constituents; since 1894 it has been known to be a calcium-phosphate-carbonate.[1] The first reports of its crystal structure were published by DeJong[2] and by Roseberry and associates.[3] Both groups of investigators identified the bone mineral as a hydroxyapatite (HA) based on the reflections generated by X-ray diffraction. Unfortunately, the exact chemical composition and specific spatial arrangement of its constituents, from its initial deposition to the final mature mineral, are still not known in detail 60 years after the bone mineral was first identified as HA by DeJong.[2] The obstacles to gaining this knowledge are many—biologic, crystallographic, and technical.[4-11] In the first place, the apatite phase in bone is very poorly crystalline, generating only a few broad peaks that by themselves do not permit the assignment of a unique crystal structure or composition; i.e., X-ray diffraction and chemical composition studies cannot differentiate among a number of similar apatitic or apatite-like structures. Indeed, a number of what appear to be closely related but distinct chemical and structural Ca-P compounds give the same apatitic X-ray diffraction pattern. The poor X-ray diffraction pattern generated by the bone mineral has also precluded the detection of small amounts of Ca-P compounds other than HA that might be present in addition to HA. Bone mineral is also known by chemical and physical analyses to contain small but significant amounts of extraneous ions such as $HPO_4^{2-}$, Na, Mg, citrate, carbonate, and K; their positions and configurations are not completely known. The ideal stoichiometry (Ca/P molar ratio of 1.67) is also rarely found in bone, especially in young bone mineral, which usually has a Ca/P ratio of less than 1.67. The bone mineral has also been shown to contain strongly bound or possibly even crystalline water. The $H_2O$ cannot be a true constituent of HA since HA has the structural formula, $[Ca_{10}(PO_4)_6(OH)_2]$. Both the composition of bone mineral and its X-ray diffraction characteristics change with maturation: the mineral phase becomes more crystalline with age and maturation[12] but never approaches the highly crystalline state of naturally occurring, geologic HA, synthetic HA made by precipitation and refluxing of Ca-P in vitro, or even the HA crystals in dental enamel.

Electron micrographs of bone, which have revealed the very small size of the bone crystals [(1.5 to 3.5 nm) × (5 to 10 nm) × (40 to 50 nm)] [13,14] help to explain the poor X-ray diffraction pattern generated by the bone mineral. However, other characteristics of bone mineral such as crystal strain, vacancies, additions to (e.g., carbonate) and adsorption into the lattices of other ions (Na, Mg) also represent significant differences between bone mineral and crystalline HA and may also contribute to its specific X-ray diffraction characteristics. Most importantly, progressive changes occur in the X-ray diffraction patterns of bone mineral as a function of the age of the tissue, of the animal, and principally of the mineral itself. These X-ray diffraction changes are also accompanied by significant changes in the chemical composition of the mineral phase, namely, an increase in the Ca/P ratio, an increase in the content of carbonate, and a decrease in the concentration of $HPO_4^{2-}$ and $H_2O$.[15,16] Recognition that the mineral phase undergoes extensive structural and chemical changes after its initial formation has led investigators to explore the nature of the first solid phase of Ca-P deposited, the detailed changes that it undergoes during aging and maturation, and to search for the reasons these X-ray and compositional changes occur. There is no general agreement about the exact structure and location of all of the carbonate ions even in synthetically prepared carbonato-apatites, an indication of the technical and conceptual difficulties of determining the exact crystal structure of this class of Ca-P compounds.

Biologically, one of the major difficulties that has to be overcome in obtaining bone samples for structural and compositional studies, especially in studying the initial Ca-P solid phase deposited and the changes that occur in the mineral with time, is in the preparation of macroscopic samples homogeneous with respect to the age of the bone mineral. At any age, bone formation and resorption are continuous. Depending on both the absolute and relative rates of these two processes, a sample of bone will contain bone mineral of different ages. Since the chemistry and structure of the bone mineral change with age, sampling techniques must account for this fact if the nature of the initial mineral phase formed as well as the changes that occur in the mineral with time and maturation are to be studied. The failure of sampling techniques and the use of whole bone samples in general produce data reflecting only the average properties of a heterogeneous sample of bone mineral ranging in age from the youngest to the very oldest crystals.

## Recent Theories of the Nature of the Bone Mineral

### Amorphous Calcium Phosphate (ACP) Theory

The first recent, major new theory concerning the nature of the mineral phase in bone was provided in 1966 and in subsequent years by Aaron Posner and a group of scientists at Cornell Medical School.[17-20] In essence, they reasoned that it should be possible to determine both the chemical composition and the X-ray diffraction characteristics of synthetic Ca-P solid phases as a function of time after their precipitation in vitro. They found that the initial solid phase of Ca-P formed after in vitro precipitation of Ca and P at alkaline pH was not crystalline but rather an amorphous calcium-phosphate (ACP); the solid phase of Ca-P did not generate a coherent X-ray diffraction pattern, indicating that there was no long-range order of the Ca-P and other ions in the Ca-P solid phase.

To explore the possibility that the same sort of kinetic processes and phase changes were occurring in the bone mineral, calculations were carried out comparing the predicted X-ray diffraction intensities of bone mineral based on the Ca-P contents of the bone specimen used for X-ray diffraction, and the intensities of the X-ray diffraction reflections found experimentally. According to these calculations, it was found that a very significant amount of the Ca-P solid phase of bone was not contributing to the X-ray diffraction reflections. This observation was consistent with the conclusion that a significant fraction of the Ca-P solid phase in bone was in a noncrystalline, nondiffracting, amorphous state (amorphous calcium phosphate, ACP). Further work using bone of various ages and using other techniques such as infrared spectroscopy (later found to be of doubtful or no value) supported their hypothesis that, like the precipitation of Ca-P in vitro, the initial Ca-P solid phase deposited in bone is an ACP that gradually transforms with time to poorly crystalline hydroxyapatite (PCHA). Thus, they concluded that the initial Ca-P mineral phase in young, developing bone was ACP, and that with age the amount of ACP decreased and the amount of PCHA increased. The rate of ACP formation was postulated to be greater than the rate at which ACP was converted to PCHA so that, in young bone containing a large proportion of newly formed bone and therefore of newly deposited bone mineral, the major Ca-P solid phase was ACP. The ACP theory was a very attractive hypothesis: it accounted for the progressive change in chemical composition with age and maturation as the proportions of ACP and PCHA changed. It explained the increasing intensity of the X-ray diffraction intensities with time as more and more of the ACP, which does not generate or constitute to the intensities of the X-ray diffraction reflections at all, was converted to PCHA. The ACP formed in vitro also had a low Ca/P ratio, contained tightly bound or crystalline $H_2O$ and had other characteristics of newly deposited bone mineral. It is not surprising therefore that the ACP theory of the nature of the initial deposits of Ca-P in bone and the changes that occur in the mineral during maturation received very wide international acceptance for almost 20 years. However, as more and more experimental data were compiled, and other structural and compositional factors were taken into account and were found experimentally to reduce the X-ray diffraction intensity of a poorly crystalline substance like bone mineral, the calculated proportion of ACP decreased. Indeed, the ACP content of some samples of very young bone previously calculated to contain 60% to 70% of ACP were now recalculated to contain one half or less of this percentage. Similarly, the ACP of adult mature bone, earlier calculated to account for at least 35% of the bone mineral, was no longer even detectable within the limits of the methods used.

The critical point of the ACP theory is that the initial solid phase of Ca-P formed in bone is ACP. Consequently, it would be expected and it was experimentally found that the major Ca-P solid phase in young bone was ACP; indeed, in the very earliest bone mineral deposited in very rapidly turning over young bone, the bone mineral would be predicted to consist almost entirely of ACP. Thus, the finding that no ACP was detected in mature bone is not as significant as it might seem since it is consistent with the ACP theory: by the time this stage of maturity of the bone mineral is reached, the ACP theory would predict that all of the ACP could have been converted to PCHA.

## Problems With the ACP Theory—Alternate Theories

The increasing reservations about the ACP theory expressed by a number of research workers prompted a complete conceptual and experimental re-evaluation. Since the critical point in the ACP theory is the prediction that ACP is by far the major and in the beginning the only Ca-P solid phase in very young bone mineral, it was necessary to prepare homogeneous bone samples containing only the youngest and most homogeneous bone crystals, as well as a series of bone samples of increasing age and maturation but with each sample homogeneous as to age of the mineral phase.

The age of the mineral and the age of the animal are not synonymous, since in bone of any age both new bone formation and bone resorption are occurring simultaneously. Whole bone samples will therefore contain bone mineral of very widely different age, and data from such samples will represent values based on the average age of the bone mineral in the particular samples. In many instances, bone from animals of widely different ages will contain widely varying proportions of the youngest and oldest bone crystals, in which case the average age of the mineral phase varies considerably. Data from such animals gathered before and after long-bone growth has ceased and bone turnover has decreased will reflect qualitative differences in the age of the bone mineral per se. However, except for samples from the youngest embryonic bone, whole-bone samples cannot provide bone mineral that is relatively homogeneous with respect to age and clearly cannot provide homogeneous samples of the youngest Ca-P solid phase deposited.

Relatively homogeneous samples of young bone mineral were obtained (1) by using embryonic chick bone that was turning over so rapidly that the age of the bone mineral spanned at most 48 hours and (2) by fractionating bone powder from these embryonic bones by density centrifugation. Density centrifuga-

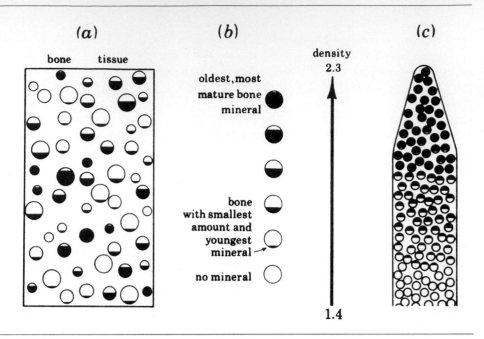

**Fig. 3–1** Schema for separating bone powder on the basis of mineral content. The younger mineral phase is in the low-density particles and the oldest mineral phase is in the highest density particles. **A:** Bone tissue is never homogeneous with respect to the age of its mineral particles. **B:** Bone tissue; the amount of bone mineral increases with increasing age and maturation. **C:** To obtain specimens of bone containing mineral particles of different ages, bone is first ground to fine powder and then separated according to its density by centrifugation. (Reproduced with permission from Glimcher MJ: Recent studies of the mineral phase in bone and its possible linkage to the organic matrix by protein-bound phosphate bonds. *Philos Trans R Soc Lond [Biol Sci]* 1984;304: 479–508.)

tion produced bone samples of different densities, different mineral content, and consequently of different bone mineral age[21] (Fig. 3–1). Not only were the ages of the bone mineral produced by this sampling technique even more homogeneous than whole bone samples, but the low-density samples from such preparations represent the youngest macroscopic samples ever obtained and studied by gross physical chemical means. This is because the samples were derived from young chick embryos of 16 to 17 days' gestation and more recently 11-day-old embryonic chicks. The young age resulted in rapid bone turnover of the whole bone mineral.

As stated earlier, the amounts of ACP in various in vitro Ca-P preparations and in bone mineral were originally determined by the Cornell group using an indirect method.[17-20] The exact amount and proportion of ACP was later found to depend on how precisely values were assigned to various chemical and structural functions. To avoid this potential pitfall, in the more recent work on embryonic chick bone, the samples were analyzed for the presence of ACP by a direct method using a procedure referred to as X-ray radial distribution function analysis (RDF).[22,23] No ACP was found in even the youngest bone mineral, at an age at which the previous studies of ACP calculated by the indirect method would predict that essentially all the solid Ca-P mineral phase should be in the form of ACP. Since no ACP was found in bone mineral of any age, the two major postulates of the ACP theory could not be substantiated experimentally: (1) that the initial Ca-P solid phase deposited and remaining in bone as the major, solid

Ca-P mineral phase was an ACP; and (2) that this ACP phase gradually transformed to PCHA.

Although failure to detect ACP in the youngest bone mineral effectively rules out the premises of the original ACP theory, ACP could occur as one of the initial solid Ca-P phases formed. The rate of ACP transformation to PCHA may be so rapid that very little or no ACP ever appears in the tissue. Under these circumstances, ACP would not be a detectable solid-phase constituent of the Ca-P mineral phase of bone. Such a concept, however, is completely different from the original ACP theory and from the calculations made from the experimental findings using this concept, namely that ACP is the major solid-phase constituent of the bone mineral in young developing bone. Indeed, if the ACP theory is applied to the bone mineral in very young chick embryos, it predicts that ACP constitutes approximately 100% of the bone mineral, when indeed none can be demonstrated.

Recent studies using $^{31}$P nuclear magnetic resonance imaging (NMR) have also failed to detect the presence of ACP.[24,25] In addition, the $^{31}$P NMR studies of both synthetic Ca-P solid phases and of bone mineral have revealed the presence of noncrystalline $HPO_4^{2-}$ groups in a brushite-$[CaHPO_4(2H_2O)]$-like configuration in addition to apatite. The amount of noncrystalline brushite decreases with the age of bone mineral. The $^{31}$P NMR spectrum of bone could be almost completely duplicated by computer modification of synthetic samples of apatite containing approximately 5% $CO_3^-$ and 5% to 10% of noncrystalline $HPO_4^{2-}$ in a brushite-like configuration.

Complementary findings were obtained from several other studies. In one comparison study, the crystallinity or crystal index of the bone mineral was studied as a function of age and maturation.[12] These data showed that from the beginning the Ca-P solid phase is a PCHA; crystallinity increases with time. However, even in the oldest bone samples studied, the PCHA remains poorly crystalline.

Hydroxyl groups have not been detected in the bone mineral of very young to very old animals by [1]H NMR and Fourier transform-infrared spectroscopy studies. What substitutes for the hydroxyl groups in these vacancies has not been determined.[26]

In summary, bone mineral can be briefly described as follows: It appears to be deposited from the beginning as a poorly crystalline type B carbonato-apatite, not a hydroxyapatite, containing approximately 5% $CO_3^-$ and 5% to 10% $HPO_4^{2-}$, the latter in a noncrystalline brushite configuration. With time, the Ca/P increases to values approximating pure apatite (Ca/P = 1.67), the content of $CO_3^-$ increases while that of $HPO_4^{2-}$ decreases slightly. The crystallinity of the apatite crystals increases but remains poor.

## Location of the Mineral Phase in Bone

The ultrastructural location of the mineral phase is important in determining its biologic functions: how it functions as an ion reservoir, its effectiveness in changing the mechanical properties of the tissue, and how and why the Ca-P crystals form at all.

Electron micrographs of osteoid and of calcified bone tissue that has been decalcified show that the space between collagen fibrils accounts for 10% to 15% of the extracellular space in most bone, up to 15% to 20% in certain bone, the remaining extracellular space being occupied by the collagen fibrils. The vast majority of the bone mineral must reside within the collagen fibrils, as there is nowhere near enough room to house the amount of bone mineral present in the tissue except within these fibrils. This has been confirmed by electron microscopy of undecalcified tissue sections, which on cross section show collagen fibrils impregnated with the mineral crystallites (Figs. 3–2 to 3–5). These electron micrographs are of the early and late stages of mineralization of fish bone. In this tissue the collagen fibrils are widely separated, thus permitting clear observation of the collagen fibrils and the extracellular space between them. The mineral phase is observed to be located almost entirely within the collagen fibrils, with the extracellular spaces between the collagen fibrils free of the mineral crystals. In some instances, in the very last stages of calcification, some mineral may be observed outside the collagen fibrils. A similar situation exists in chick bone and other species.

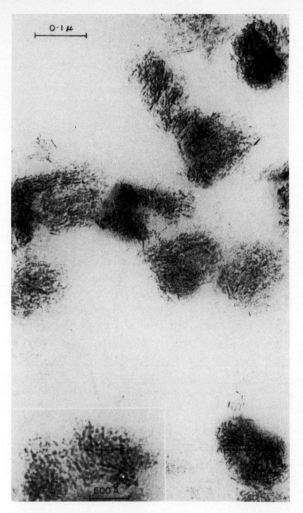

**Fig. 3–2** Unstained fish bone, which was not decalcified. The dense particles, identified by electron diffraction as Ca-P apatite crystals, are located within the collagen fibrils, which are seen primarily in cross-sectional profile. Insert shows two adjacent collagen fibrils at higher magnification. Mineral particles are located within the collagen fibrils. (Reproduced with permission from Glimcher MJ: Molecular biology of mineralized tissues with particular reference to bone. *Rev Mod Physics* 1959;31:359–393.)

The Ca-P crystals are not randomly distributed within the collagen fibrils. Electron micrographs of the early stages of mineralization have shown that the Ca-P crystals are first deposited within the hole zone region of the fibrils, essentially "staining" the fibrils to impart a 70-nm axial period to the fibrils (Figs. 3–6 and 3–7). Later, as more and more mineral is deposited within the collagen fibril, the 70-nm axial periodicity of the mineral phase is gradually lost, presumably because with increasing calcification, the crystals are also being deposited in the pores of the fibril.

Electron microscopy and electron diffraction of the mineral phase from the beginning of collagen calcification show that the long axis (crystalline c-axis) of

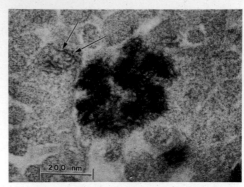

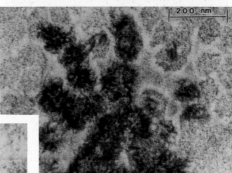

**Fig. 3–3** Successive stages of mineral deposition in herring bone tissue. Thick (1 μm) cross sections of collagen fibrils were prepared using anhydrous technique of speciman preparation. **A:** The first electron-dense deposits (arrows) occur within the boundary of the collagen fibril. **B and C:** As mineralization progresses further, no mineral particles have been deposited in the extrafibrillar spaces between the fibrils. The deposition of mineral particles in the adjacent collagen fibrils demonstrates that the nucleation of Ca-P crystals in each of the fibrils is an independent physical chemical event. (Reproduced with permission from DD Lee, unpublished).

each crystal within a single fibril is relatively parallel to the long axes of the other crystals and to the long axis of the fibril in which it is located. The localization of the earliest deposited crystals to the hole zone regions of the collagen fibrils by electron microscopy (Figs. 3–6 and 3–7)[27,28] has been confirmed by the elegant low-angle neutron and X-ray diffraction study of intact calcified turkey tendon tissue[29,30] and by reconstruction of the location of the mineral phase in collagen fibrils by optical transformation of low-angle X-ray diffraction data.[31]

Another electron microscopic observation of the early stages of calcification important in eventually formulating a hypothesis of the mechanism of calcification is that the Ca-P crystals are initiated at sites distinct from one another with unmineralized regions separating the mineralization sites, not only in adjacent fibrils but even within a single collagen fibril. The eventual deposition of the crystals within the whole length of a single collagen fibril or of groups of fibrils does not occur by propagation from one site, but rather from independent nucleation sites in the hole zone regions of the fibrils. Secondary crystal formation does occur locally and extend locally into the hole spaces and into the pores from the initial sites of Ca-P crystallization; each of the spaces corresponding to the hole zone regions is a potential independent site of heterogeneous nucleation.

## The Mechanism of Calcification

Regardless of the tissue involved (bone, dentin, enamel, cartilage), the organism involved, and the nature of the mineral phase (Ca-P, $CaCO_3$, $SrSO_4$), the formation of a solid phase from a solution phase is a phase transformation and is not a chemical reaction. Biologic mineralization, the formation of an inorganic solid phase in biologic tissues regardless of the nature of the mineral phase, can therefore be explained by the laws of thermodynamics governing the stability of phases, and with the kinetics of such phase changes. The simplest example illustrating what a phase change is and how it is distinguished

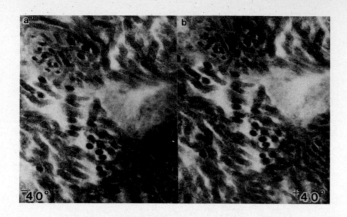

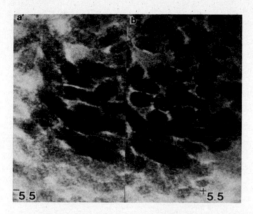

**Fig. 3–4** A pickerel fish bone prepared anhydrously seen in cross-sectional profile (top). A higher magnification of the same region (bottom) illustrating the electron-dense Ca-P particles located within collagen fibrils. Three-dimensional localization of these mineral crystallites can be fully appreciated by stereoscopic examination, eliminating the possibility that these minerals are located on the surface of the section. (Reproduced with permission from DD Lee, unpublished).

from a chemical reaction is freezing of $H_2O$: $H_2O_{(liq)} \rightarrow H_2O_{(solid)}$.[5,10,13]

No chemical reaction is occurring; there are no chemical reaction products. The $H_2O$ molecules simply change their state of aggregation from water [$H_2O_{(liq)}$] to ice [$H_2O_{(solid)}$]. To accomplish this phase transformation, the water molecules must interact to form aggregates until they reach a critical size, after which an increase in size is accompanied by a decrease in free energy and continued growth of the aggregates until a solid state is reached.[13,32] If this transformation is accomplished by gradually lowering the temperature in the absence of any external particles, a sufficient number of critically sized aggregates of $H_2O$ liquid molecules form. These "embryos" grow by the addition of more $H_2O$ liquid molecules to form critically sized embryos called "nuclei," which then grow with a decrease in free energy to form the first

particles of the new phase, ice. This process is called homogeneous nucleation. If AgI or CuI is added to the water before cooling, the process differs in several important respects from homogeneous nucleation. In the first place the extent to which the temperature must be lowered before the crystals are formed is substantially less than when AgI or CuI is present: to approximately −39 C without AgI and to only −4 to −5 C with AgI or CuI present from the start. Secondly, without AgI the ice crystals form in one mass throughout the whole vessel. With AgI present, the ice crystals begin to form on the surface of the AgI or CuI crystals. The lattice dimensions, especially of the basal planes of AgI and CuI, closely match those of ice. This complementarity of crystal lattice structure between ice and AgI allows the AgI to initiate the phase change from water to ice at a higher temperature than occurs in the absence of any particles. This process of initiating a phase change by and on an outside agent or substance is called heterogeneous nucleation and the substance that initiates the heterogeneous nucleation is termed a nucleator, nucleation agent, or nucleation substrate. For example, in order for a nucleator to initiate heterogeneous nucleation of a solid phase from a solution phase, the solution phase must be in metastable equilibrium with respect to the components in solution that will ultimately make up the solid phase. In thermodynamic terms, a fluid or any other phase may be stable with regard to adjacent states that differ infinitesimally in their intensive properties from the given state but unstable in regard to states that differ finitesimally in their intensive properties from the given state. Such a fluid remains stable with continuous changes in state but unstable with discontinuous changes in state. The fluid is in metastable equilibrium, as opposed to being in a stable or an unstable state. In metastable equilibrium, the solution phase is stable indefinitely but still has the potential to form a solid phase by the intervention of a nucleation agent. In vitro nucleation experiments with a variety of solid salts and inorganic crystals have demonstrated that even under the most careful conditions and despite every effort to remove all solid particles that might act as heterogeneous nucleators, it is virtually impossible to obtain true homogeneous nucleation. That is, even under the most stringent conditions, nucleation of the solid phase almost always takes place by the heterogeneous route. The nucleation agents such as dust and other particles, and surface defects in the vessels need not be highly specific or effective catalysts; nevertheless they are sufficiently effective to induce heterogeneous nucleation before homogeneous nucleation occurs. This fact is important in formulating any mechanism for the calcification of bone or any of the other biologically mineralized tissues. Thus, considering the complexity of any biologic tissue, which contains a

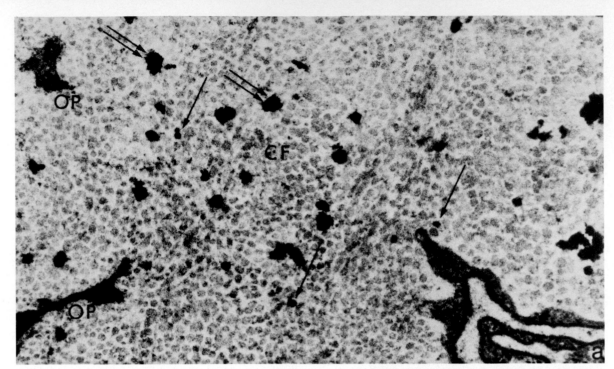

**Fig. 3–5** Early stages of calcification of embryonic chick bone. Collagen fibrils are seen in cross section. Note mineral-free collagen fibrils (c.f.) and fibrils in varying stages of mineralization impregnated with a solid phase of calcium phosphate. The spaces between the fibrils are free of mineral particles. The calcification of each of the fibrils and of the separate sites along the axial length of a single fibril is a physical chemical independent event. Two osteoblast processes (o.p.) are indicated. (Reproduced with permission from Landis WJ, Paine MC, Glimcher MJ: Electron microscopic observations of bone tissue prepared anhydrously in organic solvents. *J Ultrastruct Res* 1977;59:1–30.)

**Fig. 3–6** Electron micrograph of an unstained, longitudinal section of undecalcified embryonic chick bone. The dense mineral phase appears to "stain" the collagen fibril at regular intervals along its axial length. In some areas, the inorganic crystals can be seen on edge as dark lines. Most of the mineral phase is not resolvable into individual crystals.

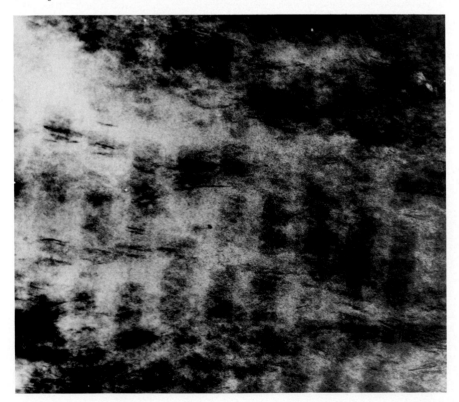

multitude of highly ordered intracellular and extracellular structures and components any or all of which can act as heterogeneous nucleators, it would hardly be possible for homogeneous nucleation of a mineral phase to occur in a biologic tissue. Instead, any one or a combination of structures or macromolecular components could and would undoubtedly serve as heterogeneous nucleators long before homogeneous nucleation could occur. Indeed, if calcification occurs according to the laws governing all other important biologic processes, the heterogeneous nucleation agent or substrate would be quite specific chemically, structurally, and spatially.

A general hypothesis of biologic mineralization has recently been proposed based on the observations that in some tissues the inorganic crystals appear to be randomly dispersed, and in some instances the crystal size and habit are similar to those observed in in vitro precipitation.[33] According to this hypothesis, biologic mineralization is divided into two general categories: (1) matrix-mediated mineralization by which certain organic matrix components (principally extracellular) induce and control the deposition of the mineral crystals, their orientation and organization, and their growth and habit; and (2) biologically induced mineralization in which the intracellular or extracellular organic (matrix) constituents do not play this role. At first glance, this subdivision has certain attractive features. However, on close inspection, both the terminology and more importantly the biologic and physical chemical concepts underlying the hypothesis can be seriously questioned. With regard to semantics, the separation of the two putative classes of biologic mineralization into matrix-mediated and biologically induced on the basis of crystal orientation and the shape and size of the crystals is misleading. Clearly, the crystals of different mineralized biologic tissues display widely varying organizational patterns: highly organized tissue in which the crystals are almost completely parallel with one another in an almost perfect two-dimensional array as opposed to crystals that appear to be essentially randomly oriented over macroscopic areas. Even so, all biologic mineralization is biologically induced, i.e., crystal nucleation by organic constituents in the tissue. Only the organic constituents that act as mediators or heterogeneous nucleators vary from tissue to tissue both intracellularly and extracellularly. Since it would hardly be possible for homogeneous nucleation of a mineral phase to occur in a biologic tissue, the critical physical chemical mechanism of mineralization in both the classes (biologically induced and matrix-mediated) is the same. No physical chemical basis exists for separating the mineralized tissues on the basis of whether the crystals are

oriented or not, which implies that orientation reflects some underlying difference in how and why the crystals are nucleated. The same is true for the size and shape (habit) of the crystals. Separation of the biologically mineralized tissues and the cellular and extracellular components of these tissues into two broad classes based on the organization, orientation, and habit of the crystals is potentially an important one, however, and investigations into the underlying bases for such phenomena are likely to shed light on the mechanism of crystal deposition and its growth and development. However, the author does not believe that there is any physical chemical, biologic, or biochemical principle according to which these morphologic differences can be used to explain the initiation of mineralization. Indeed, the failure to distinguish between crystal growth and crystal habit and to distinguish both from crystal nucleation may confuse a number of issues related to the initial mechanism of crystallization. In both cases, biologically induced and matrix-mediated calcification, the underlying mechanism of crystallization is the same: heterogeneous nucleation by a biologic substrate or nucleator. To label one group biologically induced and the other matrix-mediated based on crystal orientation or habit is to obscure this most important point and to confuse the subsequent growth and orientation of the crystals with why the crystals are formed at all.

While the crystals of many mineralized tissues are not oriented parallel to one another over any significant distance, this lack of crystal alignment does not preclude their having been initiated by the heterogeneous nucleation of an extracellular or intracellular organic matrix component or components. In general, formation of crystals by a nucleation agent or substrate in no way implies that the crystals are aligned with each other or with the nucleation substrate. While nucleation and oriented overgrowth or epitaxy overlap in some instances, they are independent processes and heterogeneous nucleation can occur with or without epitaxy of the crystals. Indeed in some cases, relatively poor nucleation substrates readily produce epitaxial growth of the nucleated crystals, i.e., the nucleated crystals grow in perfect alignment along selected planes of the heterogeneous substrate with perfect co-orientation of certain planes of the forming crystals and the nucleation substrate. Moreover, in these tissues, since the exact three-dimensional architecture of the intracellular or extracellular matrix and each of its components is not known, the nucleation sites may themselves be relatively randomly organized with respect to the three-dimensional morphology of the tissue or tissue component. In such cases, even if epitaxy did occur after heterogeneous nucleation, the inorganic crystals are still randomly organized.

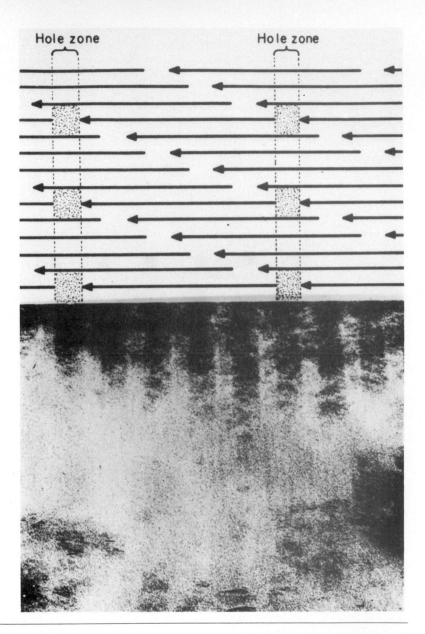

**Fig. 3–7**  The identification of the location of the mineral phase in bone collagen between the $a^3$ and $c^3$ bands places the crystals in the hole zone. (Reproduced with permission from Glimcher MJ, Krane SM: The organization and structure of bone, and the mechanism of calcification, in Ramachandran GN, Gould BS (eds): *Treatise on Collagen*. New York, Academic Press, Inc, 1968, vol 7B, pp 68–251.)

Knowledge of the orientation of the molecular or macromolecular component of the organic matrix involved and of the presumptive nucleation sites is critical in assessing the role of organic matrices on the basis of crystal disposition and orientation. For example, the collagen fibrils of newly deposited, young bone in embryonic animals that is being rapidly deposited and resorbed are almost randomly oriented, the extent depending in part on the age and rate of bone synthesis. X-ray diffraction and large-field electron diffraction studies show no preferred orientation of the crystals and routine electron microscopy likewise reveals no distinctive ordering of the crystals over long distances in relatively large regions of the tissue. However, careful high-resolution electron microscopy reveals that in local regions where only a few collagen fibrils in good longitudinal profile can be visualized, the crystals are indeed aligned with their long axes (c-axis) roughly parallel to the individual fibrils within which they are located.[13] In summary, orientation of the inorganic crystals appears to be more a matter of the state of aggregation and the orientation and organization of the organic matrix constituents, than a reflection of a basic difference in the mechanism by which the crystals are initially formed. Similarly, differences in the size and shape of the inorganic crystals in the various tissues compared with those observed in synthetic crystals made in vitro (which vary tremendously depending on the external conditions under which they are prepared) also appear to be independent of the underlying mechanism that initiates the formation of the inorganic crystals.

Another of the many possible explanations of the lack of long-range order of the crystals is that only a few nucleation sites may exist within the matrix or intracellular component where crystal formation is initiated by heterogeneous nucleation, the rest of the crystals being formed by secondary nucleation from the initial inorganic crystals formed by heterogeneous nucleation. Unless there were physical constraints within the organic matrix or its components that tended to orient crystal growth in a specific direction, the majority of the crystals formed by secondary nucleation would be randomly oriented.

Although many factors undoubtedly control crystal orientation in tissues, one of the most important appears to be the organization of the organic substrate in which the crystals are nucleated and grow. In the case of collagen or the enamel matrix and in certain invertebrate shells, the structural organic matrix molecules are themselves assembled into highly ordered macromolecular aggregates (fibrils, enamel tubules, compartments) that structurally and possibly stereochemically direct the alignment and orientation of the crystals during their growth.[27,34] If such tertiary or quaternary structure is absent, then it is probable that the crystals would be randomly oriented. Thus, the orientation of the crystals in a tissue appears to depend more on the secondary, tertiary, and possibly quaternary structure of the organic molecules composing the nucleation substrate and its state of order or disorder at the ultrastructural level, than on any basic difference in the underlying physical chemistry or biology of the basic mineralization process.

The hypothesis also suggests that the size and shape of the crystals indicate whether mineralization is biologically induced or matrix-induced. For example, in biologically induced calcification, the size and shape of the crystals closely resemble the size and shape of crystals prepared in vitro, while in matrix-mediated calcification, crystal size and shape are quite different from the size and shape of crystals prepared in vitro. While this may be true in some instances, it does not hold true of the major vertebrate calcified tissues. For example, the apatite crystals in bone, dentin, and cementum that are considered to be matrix-mediated are for the most part indistinguishable from those precipitated in the test tube, while those in enamel, which also falls into the category of matrix-mediated mineralization, contains highly oriented crystals several orders of magnitude greater than those precipitated at 37 C in vitro. In short, there is no general rule that the habit of inorganic crystals formed by heterogeneous nucleation via an organic matrix in vivo must differ from the habit of crystals formed by homogeneous nucleation in vitro or in vivo. Moreover, even in vitro, minor changes in

the solution phase can markedly alter the habit of crystals formed by either homogeneous or heterogeneous nucleation.

## Postulated Role of Collagen in Bone Calcification

Calcification of bone is a phase transformation, with calcium, carbonate, inorganic phosphate, and other ions in solution in the extracellular fluid aggregate forming a solid mineral phase of these ions; it is almost certainly initiated by heterogeneous nucleation, and data have revealed a most striking and intimate relationship between the mineral crystals and the highly ordered essentially two-dimensional liquid crystals of collagen fibrils. Based on this information, it can be hypothesized that the heterogeneous nucleation sites have a unique location in the collagen fibril, having specific physical, chemical, electrical, steric, and spatial properties.[13,28]

Experiments to test this hypothesis have been done in vitro and in vivo. In vitro, solutions of Ca-P were experimentally demonstrated to be in metastable equilibrium; for at least one month no crystals formed spontaneously. They were exposed to purified reconstituted soft-tissue collagens and to decalcified bone collagen. Both preparations nucleated apatite crystals within 24 to 48 hours.[13,32,34] A variety of other proteins failed to nucleate Ca-P crystals from identical solutions. Electron microscopy showed that the initial crystals were formed within the collagen fibrils in a very orderly pattern with an axial period of approximately 70 nm, i.e., once per collagen period. Later analyses revealed that this location within the collagen fibrils corresponded with the hole zone region similar to that found in native bone calcified in vivo.[27,28] When the collagen molecules were polymerized into fibrils in which the molecules were aggregated differently from their aggregation in the native fibrils of bone, skin, tendon, and other tissues, these fibrils were not capable of nucleating Ca-P crystals from the metastable solutions of Ca-P in vitro. This demonstrated that the ability of collagen fibrils to nucleate Ca-P crystals in vitro depended on the tertiary structure of collagen; there was something about the specific three-dimensional packing of the collagen molecules in native type fibrils (approximately 70-nm axial period) that resulted in the formation of highly specific chemical, steric, electrochemical, and spatial properties within a particular portion of the fibril (the hole zone region), which together constituted a heterogeneous nucleation site for apatite crystals. Further experimental evidence that particular regions within the collagen fibrils act as specific heterogeneous nucleation sites for apatite crystals comes from in vivo experiments in which reconstituted soft-tissue collagen fibrils prepared from the skin of animals, placed back in the peritoneal cavity and subcutaneous regions of the same animals or littermates, were found to calcify in vivo and in the same manner as they do in vitro and in native bone: the crystals are first deposited within the hole zone regions of the collagen fibrils.[35,36]

The initiation of calcification of reconstituted soft-tissue collagens both in vitro and especially in vivo is much slower than the recalcification of decalcified bone collagen fibrils in vitro. But even in vitro, the length of time between the exposure of decalcified bone collagens fibrils to a metastable solution of Ca-P and the nucleation of a Ca-P solid phase of apatite is longer than expected for a very potent nucleation substrate. This raises the possibility that while the collagen fibrils of bone and other mineralized tissues are heterogeneous nucleation substrates and are necessary for the initiation of apatite formation they may not be biologically sufficient.[10]

It is useful at this point to distinguish the chemical, structural, electrochemical, and steric factors that define a nucleation site from those ancillary factors that can control or regulate the nucleation process. The former, taken together, form the basic mechanism of calcification and the underlying basis for the initiation of calcification. The latter include factors that might facilitate or inhibit nucleation but are not part of the structural nucleation site (decreasing or increasing the lag time, for example). These factors work either directly by affecting the nucleation site or indirectly by altering the metastability of the extracellular fluids in the immediate vicinity of the nucleation substrate. Failure to make the distinction between components that are part of the nucleation site and directly related to the mechanism of nucleation, and components that regulate and control the rate of nucleation has caused a certain amount of confusion. This confusion has been especially apparent in defining the possible roles of certain tissue components in the nucleation of apatite crystals in selected tissue compartments and in the tissue as a whole, as opposed to their potential function as regulators.

In discussing some of the factors that may influence the local nucleation of apatite crystals within selected areas of the collagen fibrils, calcification of the tissue as a whole must be distinguished from calcification of specific intracellular or extracellular compartments and components within the tissue. Tissue calcification includes all the compartments and components calcified (Fig. 3–8). In addition to collagen fibrils, in which the vast majority of the bone crystals are located, Ca-P particles have been observed intracellularly in the mitochondria of osteoblasts, the chondroblasts of cartilage, and extracellularly in so-called matrix vesicles, compartments formed by the budding off of portions of the plasma membrane of osteoblasts and chondroblasts.

Lehninger,[37] Shapiro and associates,[38–41] and

**Fig. 3–8** Diagrammatic representation of bone tissue calcification and of the putative calcification of several of its intra and extracellular compartments and components. The exact and specific physical chemical roles of mitochondria and matrix vesicles in bone tissue calcification have not yet been defined. (Reproduced with permission from Glimcher MJ: Recent studies of the mineral phase in bone and its possible linkage to the organic matrix by protein-bound phosphate bonds. *Philos Trans R Soc Lond [Biol Sci]* 1984;304:479–508.)

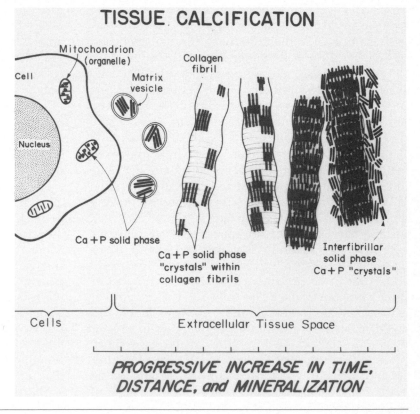

Brighton and Hunt[42] have demonstrated that the mitochondria of differentiating cartilage cells in the epiphyseal plate (chondroblasts) as well as the osteoblasts of developing bone[14] contain a significant number of dense granules composed principally of Ca and $P_i$. Using specific staining for calcium in the mitochondrial granules of epiphyseal cartilage cells, it was shown that the number of such granules decreased with increasing maturation of the cartilage cells and with the onset and progression of extracellular calcification. Because the decreasing concentration and eventual disappearance of these Ca-P granules in the mitochondria coincide with the appearance and progressive increase of extracellular calcification in the tissue, investigators[37,42] have suggested that the mitochondrial granules in some way help to initiate calcification of the extracellular matrix. For example, Lehninger[37] has suggested that the solid phase particles of Ca-P in mitochondria of bone and cartilage cells are extruded into and traverse the extracellular space, eventually becoming lodged in the hole zone regions of the collagen fibrils.[37]

Similarly, Anderson,[43,44] Morris and associates,[45] and Bonucci[46] have described plasma membrane-derived vesicles in the extracellular matrices of both bone and cartilage, many of which appear to contain crystals of HA when observed electromicroscopically.

Because calcification of these vesicles appears to occur prior to the calcification of the collagen fibrils, several hypotheses have been presented postulating that the solid-phase particles or crystals of Ca-P themselves, which are deposited in the matrix vesicles, directly cause the mineralization of the collagen fibrils.[43–49] Several different theories have been advanced as to how crystals in the matrix vesicles can induce nucleation of de novo crystals in the collagen fibrils. One proposal[44,49,50] suggests that Ca-P particles in the matrix vesicles pierce the membrane of the matrix vesicles and are extruded into the extracellular space. The extruded crystals then act as nucleation catalysts for the formation of additional crystals of Ca-P by secondary nucleation and multiplication. The continuous formation of new crystals progressively fills the extracellular tissue spaces between the collagen fibrils with inorganic crystals. When the newly forming crystals reach the collagen fibrils, the crystals enter or form only within the hole zone regions of the collagen fibrils. Later, continued secondary nucleation and multiplication within the collagen fibrils produce additional crystals within the pore spaces of the collagen. In this schema, collagen fibrils are simply a passive repository for the deposition of Ca-P crystals and subsequent secondary multiplication of Ca-P crystals, which eventually result in the almost complete impregnation of the fibrils with a solid mineral phase of Ca-P. Neither the collagen fibrils nor any of the noncollagenous macromolecules associated with them play any role in the formation of the crystals of Ca-P within the fibrils. This explanation seems completely improbable from the standpoints of both physical chemistry and electron microscopic observations.

As pointed out, calcification of the collagen fibrils consists of a large number of independent nucleation events at nucleation sites independent from each other even within the same fibril, and which therefore must clearly be completely independent of the direct influence of crystals deposited in compartments spatially separated from the collagen nucleation sites such as matrix vesicles[51] or mitochondria.[39–42]

In the matrix vesicle theory, masses of crystals would be expected to occupy the space in the extracellular fluid between the fibrils before calcification of the collagen fibrils started. However, the suggested sequence of events does not correspond to events actually observed during the calcification of bone, dentin, or cementum by electron microscopy. In extensive studies by the author and others of embryonic chick bone using nonaqueous as well as aqueous techniques for the preparation of the tissue samples[14,27,52,53] and in other published and unpublished electron micrographs, as well as in recent studies of fish bone by high-voltage stereoscopic electron microscopy, a stage of calcification in which the extracellular spaces were filled with bone mineral at a time when the collagen fibrils were unmineralized has not been observed. Indeed, even in the earliest stages of embryonic bone or dentin calcification, at a time when the collagen fibrils are just beginning to mineralize, the most common observation is of partially and completely mineralized collagen fibrils separated from one another by unmineralized space (see Figs. 3–2 to 3–5). At the stage when there are numerous well-mineralized collagen fibrils, little or no mineral phase is present between the fibrils.

Moreover, the proposal that crystals of Ca-P, formed randomly by secondary nucleation and multiplication in the extracellular spaces, are somehow able to find their way in the extracellular spaces selectively to only the hole zone regions of the collagen fibrils is improbable from both the physiochemical and biologic standpoints. Instead, if the sequence of events did occur as envisioned by the matrix vesicle theory, it would follow that during the early stages the collagen fibrils would become encrusted in random fashion by the self-propagating and multiplying mineral phase particles, which would fill the extracellular tissue spaces. Collagen fibril calcification would then proceed without the localization of the crystals to the hole zone regions of the fibrils. This does not correspond to observations by electron microscopy[27,54] and X-ray and neutron diffraction.[29–31]

Electron microscopic studies have shown that matrix vesicles are observed in only the earliest stages of embryonic chick bone development. The data from these studies are consistent with the author's own observations. Thus, the collagen fibrils of all the new bone laid down after this early embryonic bone has been resorbed[51] are calcified in the absence of matrix vesicles.[50,55] Matrix vesicles are therefore not obligatory for the calcification of bone tissue. Indeed, if they do play any role, their action must be limited to a brief period during the early stages of embryonic development, since bone synthesized afterwards calcifies in the absence of matrix vesicles.

Calcification in one compartment such as the mitochondrion or the matrix vesicle can indirectly influence the formation of solid phase mineral particles in another spatially distinct compartment. One way is dissolution of the crystals in one compartment such as the matrix vesicles or mitochondria and the pumping out and specifically directed transport of the Ca and $P_i$ ions to and within the second compartment. If sufficient amounts of Ca and $P_i$ are transported, the metastability of the fluid within the second compartment may be increased to the point that a nucleation substrate within the second compartment is capable of initiating the formation of apatite crystals by heterogeneous nucleation more easily. While this scenario is possible, it may not be likely, since the amount of mineral in either the mitochondria or matrix vesicles when dissolved is not sufficient to raise the tissue extracellular fluid concentration of Ca and $P_i$. Further work must be done. Thyberg and Friberg[56] have suggested that the matrix vesicles may function by releasing enzymes that degrade the proteoglycans surrounding the collagen fibrils. The degradation and removal of the proteoglycans, thought by many to be inhibitors of calcification, would then permit the collagen fibrils to initiate calcification.[57]

The normal calcification of turkey tendon provides further confirmation that calcification of collagen fibrils does not "spread like a wave" throughout a single fibril from a single nucleation site, but rather by nucleation of crystals at multiple, independent sites, the hole zone region within a single fibril,[58] and then by secondary nucleation within the pores.

In bone and in tendon the initial deposition of the crystals within the holes of the collagen leads to an axial periodicity of the crystals along the long axes of the fibrils identical to that of the collagen itself.[13,59] With time and with increasing mineralization, more and more crystals are deposited within the pore space eventually obliterating the initial axial periodicity of the mineral phase.

The calcifying tendon system also provides additional information. Matrix-bound mineral, presumably in vesicles can be clearly observed.[57] The mineral phase is spatially separated from the sites in the collagen where mineralization is initiated. In this tissue, the mineral crystals in the putative matrix vesicles do not play any direct role in the initiation of calcification of the collagen fibrils, the crystals in the collagen being formed at a distance from the crystals in the matrix vesicles as events totally independent of the presence of matrix vesicle crystals.

Indeed, there is no evidence of even an indirect effect of the mineral crystals of the matrix vesicles on collagen calcification; i.e., there is no evidence of a dissolution of the matrix vesicle crystals with $Ca^{2+}$ and $P_i$ ions pumped out to increase the metastability of the extracellular fluid in the close vicinity of the collagen fibrils. The crystals in the putative vesicles remain in the vesicles during the initiation of collagen calcification. Like the observations of bone, the calcification of the collagen fibrils in loci separated from one another implies that the initiation of calcification in each of the hole zone regions represents an independent event.

The fact that there is neither a physical chemical basis nor experimental evidence by electron microscopy or other techniques that solid phase particles of Ca-P in either mitochondria or matrix vesicles directly induce calcification of collagen fibrils in no way diminishes the importance of their discovery. The identification of these Ca-P particles and of the membrane-bound matrix vesicles has opened up a new field of investigation into the mineralized tissues that promises to produce significant information on important biologic phenomena in mineralized tissues.

## Other Factors and Components That May Regulate Calcification of Collagen Fibrils

As already mentioned, although the specific stereochemistry and spatial organization of the collagen fibrils of bone, dentin, cementum, and other tissues result in the formation of nucleation sites within the hole zone regions, these factors, although necessary, may not be sufficient in vivo.[10] Even if metastability in the extracellular fluids is adequate for nucleation by the collagen fibrils, there may be other structural and chemical factors along with the collagen fibrils that constitute necessary and biologically sufficient conditions for heterogeneous nucleation of Ca-P crystals. For example, although purified collagen fibrils in dialysis bags[35] or Millipore chambers[60] do calcify in vivo when placed in the peritoneum or subcutaneously, calcification does not occur for several weeks compared with the rapid calcification (hours) of collagen fibrils in the osteoid of bone.

A number of organic components have been postulated to be an integral part of the nucleation site and therefore to be involved directly in the mechanism of nucleation or to regulate collagen calcification, and in support of which experimental data have been obtained.

Organically bound phosphorus rather than $Ca^{2+}$ has been postulated in detailed arguments as the critical ion, which is either an integral part of nucleation or interacts with the nucleation site in the organic matrix.[5,27,34] In brief, (1) unlike ionic $Ca^{2+}$ bound electrostatically to the organic matrix, the organic phosphate residues are not randomly oriented but rather rigidly disposed and sterically organized according to the stereochemistry of the protein(s) with which it is associated. Such organic phosphate groups might therefore be in sterically oriented positions according to the stereochemistry of the protein, and therefore in a three-dimensional array resembling certain planes of the apatite lattice. They would therefore be an integral part of the heterogeneous nucleation site; (2) although covalently bound to the protein, the organic phosphate groups are still able to react strongly with free $Ca^{2+}$ in a way that would permit the bound $Ca^{2+}$ to also react further with additional inorganic phosphate ions, thus building up a cluster of calcium and phosphate ions that could function as nuclei of apatite crystals; (3) the phosphorylation of certain amino acid residues in particular locations in the protein is also possible enzymatically by protein kinases and ATP, thus assuring exquisite biologic control and localization of the process. This precise cellular control and molecular localization of the calcification process make the postulated role of organically bound phosphorus very attractive from both physical chemical and biologic standpoints.

Experimentally, the first step was to determine if phosphoproteins were present in bone and other mineralized tissues. To date, all calcified tissues, both normal and pathologic have been shown to contain phosphoproteins.[61-67] All of the phosphoproteins contain O-phosphoserine [Ser(P)]. Bone, cartilage, and cementum in addition contain significant amounts of O-phosphothreonine [Thr(P)].[65,68-71] Protein kinases have been isolated from several connective tissues that specifically phosphorylate the Ser(P) residues in vitro using ATP as a source for the phosphoryl groups.[27]

Functionally, the phosphoproteins have met a number of criteria necessary to function as facilitators of the nucleation of apatite crystals within the collagen fibrils. For example, the phosphoproteins of dentin strongly bind large amounts of $Ca^{2+}$,[72] and $^{31}P$ NMR studies have in addition shown that the Ser(P) residues are able to form ternary complexes with $Ca^{2+}$ and inorganic phosphate ions,[73] i.e.,

$$\text{protein-O-P} \begin{array}{c} \diagup O \\ \diagdown O \end{array} \text{---} Ca^{2+} \text{---} P_i$$

ternary complex.

Similarly, careful calcium ion binding studies of dentinal collagen by Li and Katz[74] have clearly shown a significant increase in the number of bound $Ca^{2+}$ ions as a function of the number of phosphoprotein molecules complexed with collagen, and consequently the concentration of Ser(P) in the collagen-phosphoprotein complexes.

Although the physical chemical data demonstrate that the physical chemical properties of the phosphoproteins would permit them to participate in the mineralization of the collagen fibrils, at least three important questions had to be answered before any hypothesis could be formulated: (1) Are the phosphoproteins of bone synthesized by bone cells, i.e., are they truly bone proteins or, like albumin and others, are they synthesized elsewhere and bound and concentrated in bone? (2) If synthesized by bone cells, by which cells? (3) Where are they located in the tissue? Are they in the region where initiation of mineralization in vivo occurs? Appropriate answers to all three questions were minimum requisites before phosphoproteins could be considered to have the potential for participating in calcification.

Tissue and then cell culture experiments established that the phosphoproteins were synthesized by bone, and in particular by the osteoblasts.[75,76] Further, when animals were given $^{33}P$,[77,78] light and electron microscopy autoradiography showed that the $^{33}P$ [identified chemically as Ser(P) and Thr(P)] was first located within the osteoblast (and odontoblast in dentin) and then excreted and concentrated at the sites where mineralization was initiated. These findings, demonstrating that the phosphoproteins are synthesized in bone by the appropriate cells and are located where mineralization was first occurring indicate that the phosphoproteins meet the minimum biologic requirements for their consideration as facilitators of the heterogeneous nucleation of apatite crystals by collagen fibrils, or as an integral part of the nucleation site itself.

Analyses of uncalcified and calcifying turkey tendon (before ossification occurs) have shown that there are no detectable phosphoproteins in uncalcified turkey tendon in regions that eventually calcify, or in whole tendons that never calcify. However, once mineralization begins, phosphoproteins are detected and increase in concentration as increasing amounts of mineral are deposited.[69]

Recent experiments measuring the lag time, i.e., time to induce nucleation of Ca-P solid phase during in vitro calcification of bone collagen, supported the role of phosphoproteins in facilitating nucleation of apatite crystals by bone collagen fibrils.[79] In these experiments, decalcified bone collagen fibrils were placed in metastable Ca-P solutions and the time it takes to initiate Ca-P deposition was measured. Collagen preparations complexed with varying amounts of phosphoprotein containing Ser(P) were used. The results clearly demonstrated that a striking correlation existed between the lag time (time to initiate nucleation) and the amount of phosphoprotein complexed to the collagen as measured by the Ser(P) concentration (Fig. 3–9).

In summary, while the role of the phosphoproteins in facilitating calcification remains an hypothesis only, their postulated and experimentally demonstrated physical chemical properties and biologic characteristics provide strong supporting data for their projected role in the initiation of calcification.

Several other components and factors have also been implicated in the initiation, facilitation, or inhibition of mineralization. Proteolipids and complexed acidic phospholipids[80] have been prepared from a variety of sources, and their ability to initiate calcification from metastable solutions of Ca-P in vitro has been examined. These lipid components have been found to be very effective heterogeneous nucleators of apatite in vitro.[81-83] Although these lipid components have not been located ultrastructurally, the most likely source of these components would appear to be cellular membranes. Therefore, they may be present in the membranes of the matrix vesicles, which themselves are derived from the plasma membrane. Thus, they are possibly involved in the calcification of matrix vesicles. Their ability to nucleate apatite crystals in vitro without any additional components suggests that they may be nucleation substrates rather than facilitators.

It seems clear that there must also be a number of factors that delay or tend to inhibit the deposition of Ca-P by influencing the rate of nucleation (lag time) and the number of nucleation sites by diminishing or abolishing secondary nucleation and multiplication; by decreasing the metastability of the extracellular fluids bathing the collagen fibrils of bone; or by decreasing the metastability of structural nucleators in tissues other than bone.[51] The molecules that have received most attention and that have been most intensely studied are the proteoglycans.

Proteoglycans are found in all vertebrate mineralized tissues, especially cartilage. They exemplify the importance of *not* relying solely on calcium-binding as the factor determining whether or not an organic constituent acts as a nucleation agent.[5,13,27,34] Among the factors equally as important as $Ca^{2+}$ binding ability are the configuration of the component, whether it exists in solution or in the solid state, the stereochemistry of the reactive groups, and, most importantly, whether the $Ca^{2+}$ in the reactive groups that form complexes with $Ca^{2+}$ can still react with inorganic phosphate ions. If not, the bound $Ca^{2+}$ will essentially be chelated or clathrated. Unable to react with inorganic phosphate ions, it will be unable to take part in the formation of embryos or nuclei of $Ca^{2+}$ and $P_i$ and thus unable to participate in nucleation or calcification. Indeed, such components would prevent or inhibit nucleation and other steps in calcification, rather than facilitate it.

The state of aggregation is particularly important. Aggregates of a macromolecule packed in a very particular way in the solid state might easily form a highly specific three-dimensional steric and electrical

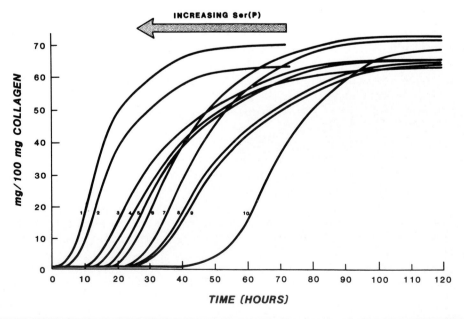

**Fig. 3–9** Lag time in hours of in vitro nucleation of a Ca-P solid phase from a metastable solution of Ca-P as a function of the amount of phosphoprotein complexed to collagen as measured by Ser(P) concentrations. Lag time, viz., time for a collagen phosphoprotein complex to initiate mineralization in vitro, decreases with increasing amounts of phosphoprotein complexed to the collagen. (Reproduced with permission from A Endo and MJ Glimcher, unpublished.)

array of side-chain groups derived from adjacent macromolecules that would constitute a nucleation site.[5,13] The bound $Ca^{2+}$ ions might even be reactive enough to bind $P_i$ ions. However, no further reaction to build up embryos and nuclei occurs because the necessary specific three-dimensional steric array of side chains from adjacent macromolecules is lacking. Thus, it is possible that some components may act to block nucleation when they are in solution, yet facilitate nucleation when in the solid state, and vice versa.

The phosphoproteins are examples of such components: when dissolved in a metastable solution of Ca-P, they essentially delay the onset of spontaneous precipitation,[84] whereas bound to collagen fibrils in the solid state, phosphoproteins in the solid state facilitate the nucleation of Ca-P from solutions of Ca-P in metastable equilibrium.[79]

In early studies of calcification, the observed ability of proteoglycans to bind $Ca^{2+}$ via their carbonyl and sulfate side chain groups led most investigators to postulate that these components somehow directly initiated crystal formation or at least facilitated calcification.[85-87] Later, it was pointed out that calcium binding could also make proteoglycans an inhibitor by preventing the $Ca^{2+}$ concentration in the extracellular fluid from reaching a level sufficient for heterogeneous nucleation by the collagen fibrils.[13,34] The phenomenon was likened to that of tanning skin collagen[34]; tanning was markedly facilitated when the proteoglycans and other noncollagenous substances were removed from the skin.[88] In both the tanning and calcification of collagen, collagen side chains are available for chemical and physical interactions with other chemical components. This was demonstrated when it was shown that the collagen in native skin failed to calcify in vitro when exposed to metastable solutions of Ca-P, whereas skin first treated with hyaluronidase and other enzymes or extracted with salt solutions of high ionic strength did mineralize.[13,34]

The proteoglycans have a number of other physical chemical characteristics that theoretically would tend to inhibit calcification. In addition to binding $Ca^{2+}$ ions, proteoglycan gels inhibit the diffusion of $Ca^{2+}$ and exclude inorganic phosphate ions.[5,27]

Evidence also supports an inhibitory role for the proteoglycans in calcification. During the calcification of cartilage in endochondral ossification, the amount of proteoglycan in the tissue progressively decreases from the completely uncalcified regions to the regions undergoing calcification.[89] Moreover, during this time the proteoglycan macromolecules are degraded and reduced in size.[90] Not only the decrease in size but the decrease in molecular weight and chain length[34] will decrease the number of $Ca^{2+}$ ions that can be bound by the proteoglycans, thus "exposing" the collagen fibrils and permitting them to function

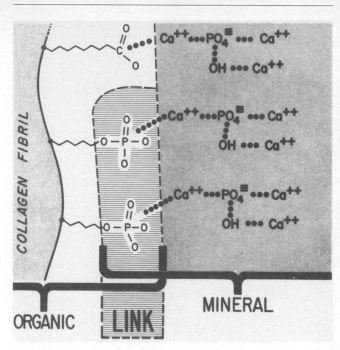

**Fig. 3–10** Schematic diagram illustrating how protein-bound phosphomonoester groups may be constituents of both the organic and the mineral phases and thus serve as a bridge, chemically and physically linking the organic structural molecules of the organic matrix to the inorganic mineral crystals (Reproduced with permission from Glimcher MJ: Recent studies of the mineral phase in bone and its possible linkage to the organic matrix by protein-bound phosphate bonds. *Philos Trans R Soc Lond [Biol Sci]* 1984;304:479–508.)

as heterogeneous nucleators for the formation of apatite crystals. On the basis of analyses from direct puncture of the epiphyseal cartilage fluid, similar conclusions have been reached by Howell and associates,[91-95] Pita and associates,[96,97] Posner and associates,[98] and Chen and Boskey,[99,100] who have conducted extensive experiments on the function of proteoglycans during in vitro calcification. Similarly, electron probe microanalysis of bone has shown more sulfate in the relatively sparsely mineralized osteoid of bone than in the more mineralized mature regions.[101,102] The "protective" function of the proteoglycans in inhibiting the reaction between extracellular fluid components and collagen fibrils by binding and by decreasing diffusion is also illustrated in cartilage by the increased reaction of antibodies to type II collagen after reaction of the tissue with hyaluronidase.

On the other hand, some investigators still believe that the proteoglycans are directly involved in the nucleation and initiation of calcification, based principally on extensive electron micrographic studies.[46,103,104] Included are studies that showed that a particular protein component, the alpha(II) C-terminal propeptide "chondrocalcin" was intimately associated with the mineral crystals in growth plate cartilage, and with proteoglycan in the initial deposits of the mineral phase.[105]

As for other structural factors, Li and Katz[74,106] have demonstrated that the collagen molecules in rat tail tendon are so closely packed that the diffusion of ions such as phosphate must be seriously limited. In contrast, the pathways in bone collagen are much larger, allowing diffusion of the hydrated phosphate ions to and within the collagen fibrils or bone without restriction. These structural factors would therefore have a tendency to inhibit calcification in some normally uncalcified tissues like tendon, while facilitating it in bone.

A large number of other substances are allegedly able to decrease or inhibit mineralization in vitro and in vivo. These include pyrophosphate, fluoride, polypeptides containing phosphorus, and magnesium.[5,27] Presumably, in addition to binding calcium (Fig. 3–10),[27] many of these substances decrease or inhibit calcification by interacting with the Ca-P nuclei to decrease their number or "inactivate" the Ca-P nuclei of the metastable solution phase.[5]

## Summary

From the physical chemical standpoint, the formation of a solid phase of Ca-P in bone represents a phase transformation, a process exemplified by the formation of ice from water. Considering the structural complexity and abundance of highly organized macromolecules in the cells and extracellular tissue spaces of mineralized tissues generally and in bone particularly, it is inconceivable that this phase transformation occurs by homogeneous nucleation, i.e., without the active participation of an organic component acting as a nucleator. This is almost surely true in biologic mineralization in general. Electron micrographs and low-angle neutron and X-ray diffraction studies clearly show that calcification of collagen fibrils occurs in an extremely intimate and highly organized fashion: initiation of crystal formation within the collagen fibrils in the hole zone region, with the long axes (c-axis) of the crystals aligned roughly parallel to the long axis of the fibril within which they are located. Crystals are initially formed in hole zone regions within individual fibrils separated by unmineralized regions. Calcification is initiated in spatially distinct nucleation sites. This indicates that such regions within a single, undirectional fibril represents independent sites for heterogeneous nucleation. Clearly, sites where mineralization is initiated in adjacent collagen fibrils are even further separated, emphasizing even more clearly that the process of progressive calcification of the collagen fibrils and

therefore of the tissue is characterized principally by the presence of increasing numbers of independent nucleation sites within additional hole zone regions of the collagen fibrils. The increase in the mass of Ca-P apatite accrues principally by multiplication of more crystals, mostly by secondary nucleation from the crystals initially deposited in the hole zone region. Very little additional growth of the crystals occurs with time, the additional increase in mineral mass being principally the result of increase in the number of crystals (multiplication), not size of the crystals (crystal growth). The crystals within the collagen fibers grow in number and possibly in size to extend into the overlap zone of the collagen fibrils ("pores") so that all of the available space within the fibrils, which has possibly expanded in volume from its uncalcified level, is eventually occupied by the mineral crystals.

It must be recognized that the calcification of separate tissue components and compartments (collagen, mitochondria, matrix vesicles) must be an independent physical chemical event. The solid phase of Ca-P crystals of one component cannot directly cause or influence the initiation of calcification (nucleation) in another separate component.

## References

1. Levy M: Chemische Untersuchungen uber osteomalacische Knochen. *Hoppe Seylers Z Physiol Chem* 1894;19:239–270.
2. De Jong WF: La substance minerale dans les os. *Recl Trav Chim Pays-Bas Belg* 1926;45:445–448.
3. Roseberry HH, Hastings AB, Morse JK: X-ray analysis of bone and teeth. *J Biol Chem* 1931;90:395–407.
4. Glimcher MJ, Bonar LC, Grynpas MD, et al: Recent studies of bone mineral: Is the ACP theory valid? *J Crystal Growth* 1981;53:100–119.
5. Glimcher MJ: Composition, structure, and organization of bone and other mineralized tissues and the mechanism of calcification, in Greep RO, Astwood EB (eds): *Handbook of Physiology: Endocrinology.* Washington, DC, Am Physiological Soc, 1976, vol 7, pp 25–116.
6. Brown WE, Chow LC: Chemical properties of bone mineral. *Ann Rev Mater Sci* 1976;6:213–236.
7. Wadkins CL, Luben R, Thomas M, et al: Physical biochemistry of calcification. *Clin Orthop* 1974;99:246–266.
8. Termine JD: Mineral chemistry and skeletal biology. *Clin Orthop* 1972;85:207–241.
9. Posner AS: Crystallite chemistry of bone mineral. *Physiol Rev* 1969;49:760.
10. Glimcher MJ: Recent studies of the mineral phase in bone and its possible linkage to the organic matrix by protein-bound phosphate bonds. *Philos Trans R Soc Lond (Biol Sci)* 1984;304:479–508.
11. Elliot JC: The problems of the composition and structure of the mineral components of the hard tissues. *Clin Orthop* 1973;93:313–345.
12. Bonar LC, Roufosse AH, Sabine WK, et al: X-ray diffraction studies of the crystallinity of bone mineral in newly synthe-

sized and density fractionated bone. *Calcif Tissue Int* 1983;35:202–209.

13. Glimcher MJ: Molecular biology of mineralized tissues with particular reference to bone. *Rev Mod Phys* 1959;31:359–393.

14. Landis WJ, Glimcher MJ: Electron diffraction and electron probe microanalysis of the mineral phase of bone tissue prepared by anhydrous techniques. *J Ultrastruc Res* 1978;63:188–223.

15. Woodward HQ: The composition of human cortical bone. *Clin Orthop* 1964;37:187–193.

16. Pellegrino ED, Biltz RM: Mineralization in the chick embryo: I. Monohydrogen phosphate and carbonate relationships during maturation of the bone crystal complex. *Calcif Tissue Res* 1972;10:128–135.

17. Eanes ED, Harper RA, Gillessen IH, et al: An amorphous component in bone mineral, in Gaillard PJ, van der Hoff A, Steendyk R (eds): *Proceedings of the 4th European Symposium on Calcified Tissues*. Amsterdam, Excerpta Med, 1966, pp 24–26.

18. Termine JD: Amorphous Calcium Phosphate: The Second Mineral of Bone, PhD thesis. Cornell University, New York, 1966.

19. Termine JD, Posner AS: Infrared analysis of rat bone: Age dependency of amorphous and crystalline mineral fractions. *Science* 1966;153:1523–1525.

20. Termine JD, Posner AS: Amorphous/crystalline inter-relationships in bone mineral. *Calcif Tissue Res* 1967;1:8–23.

21. Roufosse AH, Landis WJ, Sabine WK, et al: Identification of brushite in newly deposited bone mineral from embryonic chicks. *J Ultrastruct Res* 1979;68:235–255.

22. Grynpas MD, Bonar LC, Glimcher MJ: Failure to detect an amorphous calcium phosphate solid phase in bone mineral. *Calcif Tissue Int* 1984;36:291–301.

23. Fawcett RW: A radial distribution function analysis of an amorphous calcium phosphate with calcium to phosphate molar ratio of 1.42. *Calcif Tissue Res* 1973;13:319–325.

24. Aue WP, Roufosse AH, Roberts JE, et al: Solid state $^{31}$P NMR studies of synthetic solid phases of calcium phosphate: Potential models of bone mineral. *Biochem* 1984;23:6110–6114.

25. Roufosse AH, Aue WP, Glimcher MJ, et al: An investigation of the mineral phases of bone by solid state $^{31}$P magic and sample spinning NMR. *Biochemistry* 1984;23:6115–6120.

26. Roberts JE, Bonar LC, Grynpas MD, et al: Characterization of the youngest mineral phases of bone by solid state phosphorus-31 magic angle sample spinning nuclear magnetic resonance and x-ray diffraction. In press.

27. Glimcher MJ, Krane SM: The organization and structure of bone, and the mechanism of calcification, in Ramachandran GN, Gould BS (eds): *Treatise on Collagen*. New York, Academic Press Inc, 1968, vol 7B, pp 68–251.

28. Glimcher MJ: A basic architectural principle in the organization of mineralized tissues, in Milhaud G, Owen M, Blackwood HJJ (eds): *Proceedings of the 5th European Symposium on Calcified Tissues, 1967*. Paris, Societe d'Edition d'Enseignement Superieur, 1968, pp 3–26.

29. White SW, Hulmes DJS, Miller A, et al: Collagen-mineral axial relationship in calcified turkey leg tendon by X-ray and neutron diffraction. *Nature* 1977;266:421–425.

30. Berthet-Colominas C, Miller A, White SW: Structural study of the calcifying collagen in turkey leg tendons. *J Mol Biol* 1979;134:431–445.

31. Engstrom A: Apatite-collagen organization in calcified tendon. *Exp Cell Res* 1966;43:241–245.

32. Glimcher MJ, Hodge AJ, Schmitt FO: Macromolecular aggregation states in relation to mineralization: The collagen-hydroxyapatite system as studied in vitro. *Proc Natl Acad Sci USA* 1957;43:860–867.

33. Lowenstam HA: Minerals formed by organisms. *Science* 1981;211:1126–1131.

34. Glimcher MJ: Specificity of the molecular structure of organic matrices in mineralization, in Sognnaes RF (ed): *Calcification in Biologic Systems*. Washington, DC, American Association for the Advancement of Science, 1960, pp 421–487.

35. Mergenhagen SE, Martin GR, Rizzo AA, et al: Calcification in vivo of implanted collagen. *Biochim Biophys Acta* 1960;43:563–565.

36. Glimcher MJ, Barr J, Goldhaber P: unpublished data.

37. Lehninger AL: Mitochondria and calcium ion transport. *Biochem J* 1970;119:129–138.

38. Shapiro IM, Greenspan JS: Are mitochondria directly involved in biologic mineralization? *Calcif Tissue Res* 1969;3:100–102.

39. Shapiro IM, Lee NH: Calcium accumulation by chondrocyte mitochondria. *Clin Orthop* 1975;106:323–329.

40. Shapiro IM, Wuthier RE: A study of the phospholipids of bovine dental tissue. II. *Arch Oral Biol* 1966;11:513–519.

41. Shapiro IM, Wuthier RE, Irving JT: A study of the phospholipids of bovine dental tissues. I. *Arch Oral Biol* 1966;11:501–512.

42. Brighton CT, Hunt RM: Mitochondrial calcium and its role in calcification. *Clin Orthop* 1974;100:406–416.

43. Anderson HC: Vesicles associated with calcification in the matrix of epiphyseal cartilage. *J Cell Biol* 1969;41:59–72.

44. Anderson HC: Calcium-accumulating vesicles in the intercellular matrix of bone, in Elliott K, Fitzsimons DW (eds): *Ciba Foundation Symposium, Hard Tissue Growth, Repair and Remineralization*. Amsterdam, Elsevier, 1973, pp 213–246.

45. Morris DC, Vaananen HK, Anderson HC: Matrix vesicle calcification in rat epiphyseal growth plate cartilage prepared anhydrously for electron microscopy. *Metab Bone Dis Relat Res* 1984; 5:131–137.

46. Bonucci F: The locus of initial calcification in cartilage and bone. *Clin Orthop* 1971;78:108–139.

47. Ali SY: Analysis of matrix vesicles and their role in the calcification of epiphyseal cartilage. *Fed Proc* 1976;35:135–142.

48. Ali SY, Craig-Gray J, Wisby A, et al: Preparation of thin cryosections for electron probe analysis of calcifying cartilage. *J Microsc* 1977;111:65–76.

49. Wuthier RE: A review of the primary mechanism of endochondral calcification with special emphasis on the role of cells, mitochondria and matrix vesicles. *Clin Orthop* 1982;169:219–242.

50. Anderson HC: Evolution of cartilage, in Slavkin HC (ed): *The Comparative Molecular Biology of Extracellular Matrices*. New York, Academic Press Inc, 1972, pp 200–205.

51. Glimcher MJ: On the form and function of bone: From molecules to organs. Wolff's law revisited, 1981, in Veis A (ed): *The Chemistry and Biology of Mineralized Connective Tissues*. Amsterdam, Elsevier/North-Holland, 1981, pp 618–673.

52. Landis WJ, Hauschka BT, Rogerson CA, et al: Electron microscopic observations of bone tissue prepared by ultracryomicrotomy. *J Ultrastruct Res* 1977;59:185–206.

53. Landis WJ, Paine MC, Glimcher MJ: Electron microscopic observations of bone tissue prepared anhydrously in organic solvents. *J Ultrastruct Res* 1977;59:1–30.

54. Glimcher MJ, Katz EP, Travis DF: The organization of collagen in bone: The role of noncovalent forces in the physical properties and solubility characteristics of bone collagen, in Comte P (ed): *Symp Int Biochim Physiol Tissu Conjonctif 1966*. Lyon, France, Societe Ormeco et Imprimerie du Sud-Est, 1966, pp 491–503.

55. Landis WJ, Paine M, Hodgens K, et al: unpublished data submitted to *J Ultrastruct Res*.

56. Thyberg J, Friberg U: Ultrastructure and acid phosphatase of

matrix vesicles and cytoplasmic dense bodies in the epiphyseal plate. *J Ultrastruct Res* 1970;33:554–573.

57. Landis WJ: Temporal sequence of mineralization in calcifying turkey leg tendon, in WT Butler (ed): *The Chemistry and Biology of Mineralized Tissues.* Birmingham, AL, EBSCC Media, 1985, pp 360–363.

58. Nylen MU, Scott DB, Mosley VM: Mineralization of turkey leg tendon: II. Collagen-mineral relations revealed by electron and X-ray microscopy, in RF Sognnaes (ed): *Calcification in Biological Systems.* Washington, DC, American Academy for the Advancement of Science, 1960, pp 129–142.

59. Robinson RA, Watson ML: Collagen-crystal relationships in bone as seen in the electron microscope. *Anat Rec* 1952;114:383–409.

60. Glimcher MJ: unpublished data.

61. Glimcher MJ: Phosphopeptides of enamel matrix. *J Dent Res* 1979;58B:790–806.

62. Veis A, Spector AR, Zamoscianyk H: The isolation of an EDTA-soluble phosphoprotein from mineralizing bovine dentin. *Biochim Biophys Acta* 1972;257:404–413.

63. Linde A, Bhown M, Butler WT: Non-collagenous proteins of rat dentin: Evidence that phosphoprotein is not covalently bound to collagen. *Biochim Biophys Acta* 1981;667:341–350.

64. Seyer JM, Glimcher MJ: Isolation, characterization and partial amino acid sequence of a phosphorylated polypeptide (E$_4$) from bovine embryonic dental enamel. *Biochim Biophys Acta* 1977;493:441–451.

65. Glimcher MJ, Kossiva D, Roufosse A: Identification of phosphopeptides and gamma-carboxyglutamic acid-containing peptides in epiphyseal growth plate cartilage; proteins of bone cementum; comparison with dentin, enamel and bone. *Calcif Tissue Int* 1979;27:187–191.

66. Anderson RS, Schwartz ER: Phosphorylation of proteoglycans from human articular cartilage by a cAMP-dependent protein kinase. *Arthritis Rheum* 1984;27:1023–1027.

67. Oegema TR Jr, Brown N, Dziewiakowski D: The link protein in proteoglycan aggregates from the Swarm rat chondrosarcoma. *J Biol Chem* 1977;252:6470–6477.

68. Cohen-Solal L, Lian JB, Kossiva D, et al: The identification of O-phosphothreonine in the soluble noncollagenous phosphoproteins of bone matrix. *FEBS Lett* 1978;89:107–110.

69. Glimcher MJ, Brickley-Parsons D, Kossiva D: Phosphopeptides and carboxyglutamic acid-containing peptides in calcified turkey tendons: Their absence in uncalcified tendon. *Calcif Tissue Int* 1979;27:281–284.

70. Glimcher MJ, Lefteriou B, Kossiva D: Identification of O-phosphoserine, O-phosphothreonine and -carboxyglutamic acid in the noncollagenous proteins of bovine cementum; comparison with dentin, enamel and bone. *Calcif Tissue Int* 1979;28:83–86.

71. Linde A, Bhown M, Butler WT: Non-collagenous proteins of dentin: A re-examination of proteins from rat incisor dentin utilizing techniques to avoid artifacts. *J Biol Chem* 1980;255:5931–5942.

72. Lee SL, Veis A: Studies on the structure and chemistry of dentin collagen-phosphoryn covalent complexes. *Calcif Tissue Int* 1980;31:123–134.

73. Lee SL, Glonek T, Glimcher MJ: $^{31}$P nuclear magnetic resonance spectroscopic evidence for ternary complex formation of fetal phosphoprotein with calcium and inorganic orthophosphate ions. *Calcif Tissue Int* 1983;35:815–818.

74. Li SL, Katz E: On the state of anionic groups of demineralized matrices of bone and dentin. *Calcif Tissue Res* 1977;22:275–284.

75. Glimcher MJ, Kossiva D, Brickley-Parsons D: Phosphoproteins of chicken bone matrix: Proof of synthesis in bone tissue. *J Biol Chem* 1984;259:290–293.

76. Gotoh Y, Sakamoto M, Sakamoto S, et al: Biosynthesis of O-phosphoserine-containing phosphoproteins by isolated bone cells of mouse calvaria. *FEBS Lett* 1983;154:116–120.

77. Weinstock M, Leblond CP: Radioautographic visualization of the deposition of a phosphoprotein at the mineralization front in the dentin of the rat incisor. *J Cell Biol* 1973;56:838–845.

78. Landis WJ, Sanzone CF, Brickley-Parsons D, et al: Radioautographic visualization and biochemical identification of O-phosphoserine and O-phosphothreonine-containing phosphoproteins in mineralizing embryonic chick bone. *J Cell Biol* 1984;98:986–990.

79. Endo A, Glimcher MJ: The potential role of phosphoproteins in the in vitro calcification of bone collagen, in Goldberg VM (ed): *Transactions of the Orthopaedic Research Society.* Park Ridge, The Orthopaedic Research Society, 1986, vol 11, p 221.

80. Raggio CL, Boyan BD, Boskey AL: In vivo induction of hydroxyapatite formation by lipid macromolecules. *J Bone Joint Surg*, in press.

81. Odutuga AA, Prout RES, Hoare J: Hydroxyapatite precipitator in vitro by lipids extracted from mammalian hard and soft tissues. *Arch Oral Biol* 1975;20:311–316.

82. Boskey AL, Posner AS: The role of synthetic and bone-extracted Ca-phospholipid-PO$_4$ complexes in hydroxyapatite formation. *Calcif Tissue Res* 1977;23:251.

83. Boyan BD: Proteolipid-dependent calcification, in Butler WT (ed): *The Chemistry and Biology of Mineralized Tissues.* Birmingham, AL, EBSCO Media, 1985, pp 125–131.

84. Nawrot CT, Campbell DJ, Shroaeder JK, et al: Dental phosphoproteins—Induced formation of hydroxyapatite during in vitro synthesis of amorphous calcium phosphate. *Biochemistry* 1976;15:3445–3449.

85. Sobel AE: Local factors in the mechanism of calcification. *Ann NY Acad Sci* 1955;60:713–732.

86. Sobel AE, Burger M: Calcification: XIV. Investigation of the role of chondroitin sulfate in the calcifying mechanism. *Proc Soc Exp Biol Med* 1954;87:7–13.

87. Sylven B: Cartilage and chondroitin sulfate: II. Chondroitin sulfate and the physiological ossification of cartilage. *J Bone Joint Surg* 1947;29:973–976.

88. Burton D, Reed R: Mucoid material in hides and skins and its significance in tanning and dyeing. *Discuss Faraday Soc* 1954;16:195–201.

89. Lohmander S, Hjerpe A: Proteoglycans of mineralizing rib and epiphyseal cartilage. *Biochim Biophys Acta* 1975;404:93–109.

90. Buckwalter JA: Proteoglycan structure and calcifying cartilage. *Clin Orthop* 1983;172:207–232.

91. Howell DS: Bone formation: biochemistry of calcification. *Isr J Med Sci* 1976;12:91–97.

92. Howell DS, Carlson L: The effect of papain on mineral deposition in the healing of rachitic epiphyses. *Exp Cell Res* 1965;37:582–596.

93. Howell DS, Carlson L: Alterations in the composition of growth cartilage septa during calcification studied by microscopic X-ray elemental analysis. *Exp Cell Res* 1968;51:185–195.

94. Howell DS; Marquez JF, Pita JC: The nature of phospholipids in normal and rachitic costochondral plates. *Arthritis Rheum* 1965;8:1039–1046.

95. Howell DS, Pita J, Marquez J: Phosphate concentration and sodium activity of fluids obtained by micropuncture in epiphyseal cartilage. *Fed Proc* 1965;24:566.

96. Pita JC, Cuervo LA, Madruga JE, et al: Evidence for a role of proteinpolysaccharides in regulation of mineral phase separation in calcifying cartilage. *J Clin Invest* 1970;49:2188–2197.

97. Pita JC, Muller F, Howell DS. Disaggregation of proteoglycan aggregates during endochondral calcification: Physiological role of cartilage lysozyme, in Burleigh M, Poole R (eds): *Dynamics of Connective Tissue Macromolecules.* Amsterdam, Elsevier/North Holland, 1975, pp 247–258.

98. Posner AS, Blumenthal NC, Boskey AL, et al: Formation and transformation of amorphous calcium phosphate to hydroxyapatite, a bone analogue, in calcified tissue, in Czitober M, Eschberger J (eds): *Calcified Tissue.* Vienna, Facta Publications, 1973, pp 1–4.

99. Chen CC, Boskey AL: The effect of proteoglycans on in vitro hydroxyapatite growth. *Calcif Tissue Int* 1984;36:285–290.

100. Chen CC, Boskey AL: Mechanisms of proteoglycan inhibition of hydroxyapatite growth. *Calcif Tissue Int* 1985;37:395–400.

101. Baylink D, Wergedal J, Stauffer M, et al: Effects of fluoride on bone formation, mineralization, and resorption in the rat, in Vischer TL (ed): *Fluoride in Medicine.* Bern, Hans Huber, 1970, pp 37–69.

102. Baylink D, Wergedal J, Thompson E: Loss of proteinpolysaccharides at sites where bone mineralization is initiated. *J Histochem Cytochem* 1972;20:279–292.

103. Bonucci E, Dearden LC, Mosier HD Jr: Effects of gluococorticoid treatment on the ultrastructure of cartilage and bone. *Adv Exp Med Biol* 1984;171:269–278.

104. Poole AR, Pidoux I, Reiner A, et al: An immunoelectron microscopic study of the organization of proteoglycan monomer, link protein, and collagen in the matrix of articular cartilage. *J Cell Biol* 1982;93:921–937.

105. Poole AR, personal communication.

106. Katz EP, Li S: Structure and function of bone collagen fibrils. *J Mol Biol* 1973;80:1–15.

## Acknowledgments

This work was supported in part by the New England Peabody Home for Crippled Children, Inc., National Institutes of Health Grants AM 34078 and AM 34081, and National Science Foundation Grant PCM-8216959.

This chapter was reproduced with permission from Glimcher MJ: The nature of the mineral component of bone and the mechanism of calcification, in Avioli LV (ed): *Metabolic Bone Disease,* ed 2. Orlando, Florida, Grune and Stratton Inc, to be published.

# Osteoporosis: The Structural and Reparative Consequences for the Skeleton

Joseph M. Lane, MD

Charles N. Cornell, MD

John H. Healey, MD

## Introduction

Osteoporosis is a problem of epidemic proportions in the United States. The magnitude of this disorder was studied by Holbrook and associates.[1] Their extensive evaluation of musculoskeletal disorders clearly demonstrated that the incidence of osteoporosis increases dramatically with age and that women are affected more frequently than men. Several studies have reached similar conclusions.[2-5] In a study of a group in Michigan, more than one half of the women 45 years of age and older showed evidence of osteoporosis as defined by osteopenia on spinal radiographs. Osteoporosis was demonstrated in nine of ten women after the age of 75, and was associated with wedge fractures of vertebrae in one of every five women. Perhaps 70% of all fractures occurring in women older than 45 years are related to osteoporosis.[6,7] It has been estimated that osteoporosis accounts for more than $6 billion in economic costs annually.[1]

The three primary fractures most often seen by orthopaedists in patients with osteoporosis are vertebral fractures, hip fractures, and forearm fractures (Colles' fractures) (Fig. 4–1). Although spinal fractures lead primarily to deformity and Colles' fractures produce dysfunction, hip fractures severely

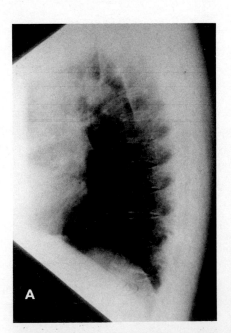
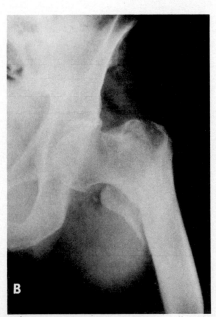
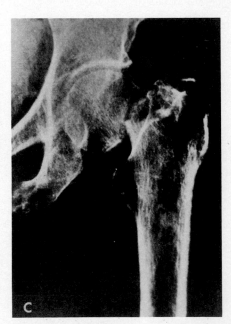
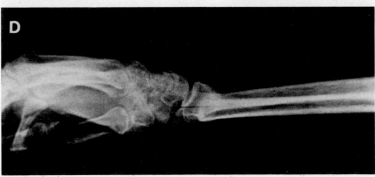

**Fig. 4–1** Radiographs illustrating typical osteopenic fractures. **A:** Lateral view of thoracic spine demonstrating wedge fractures of T9, T10, and T12. **B:** Anteroposterior view of an intertrochanteric fracture of the left hip. **C:** Anteroposterior view of a femoral neck fracture of the left hip. D: Lateral view of a Colles' fracture with dorsal tilt.

affect ultimate quality of life and challenge survival.[1,8] One patient in 20 past the age of 65 years currently occupying a hospital bed is recovering from a hip fracture. Given the best of care, 40% of patients sustaining a hip fracture will not survive for two years after this injury. Of the patients in nursing homes, 70% will not survive for one year.[1,9-12] Only one third of patients suffering hip fractures return to a lifestyle and level of independence comparable to those before the injury.

Appropriate treatment of skeletal injuries secondary to osteoporosis requires an understanding of the effect of osteoporosis on (1) the bone's material and structural properties; (2) the mechanisms of fracture; and (3) the mode of fracture healing.

## Bone Biomechanics

The skeleton serves as a mineral reserve, hemopoietic repository, and structural support. The structural elements have important biomechanical properties.[13] Bone is a composite material consisting of type I collagen (tensile strength) and hydroxyapatite mineral (compressive strength). Bone is anisotropic in structure and consistency. Histologic and microradiographic analyses have shown that bone has well-defined areas of nonmineralized osteoid, partially mineralized osteoid, and fully mineralized osteoid. Nonmineralized osteoid usually constitutes 1% to 2% of the total bone volume. Although all mature bone is essentially lamellar, the cortex is relatively compact with a high volume-to-surface ratio. Interspaced within the cortex are haversian canals with a central blood vessel. Circumferential rings are applied around the vessel to form each osteon. "Cutting cones" of osteoclasts can be identified removing old cortical bone to be remodeled or replaced with a new osteonal system.

Trabecular bone is also largely lamellar but it has a high surface-to-volume ratio. Rather than remodeling by "tunneling resorption" within the trabeculae, there is remodeling on the surface. Osteoclasts initially carve out Howship's lacunae. Within these lacunae, osteoblastic bone formation occurs secondarily.

The material properties of bone are governed by the microdensity of the material. Carter and Hayes[14] demonstrated that, in a homogeneous material, compressive strength is proportional to the square of the

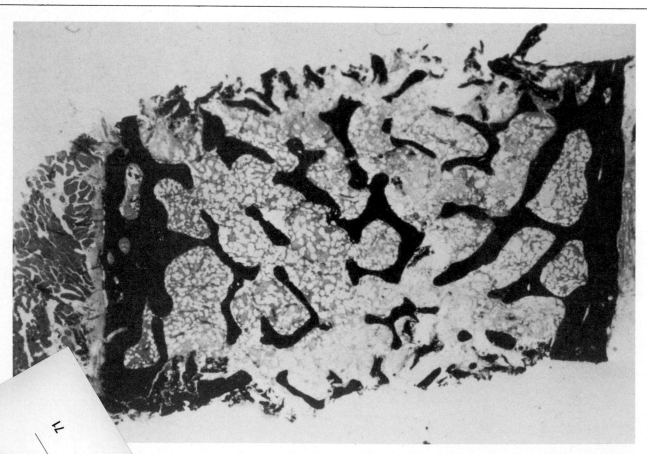

ew of an undecalcified transiliac bone biopsy specimen. The trabeculae show connectivity to cortex in the
inimal connectivity in the midportion of the medullary canal and this area has the least structural

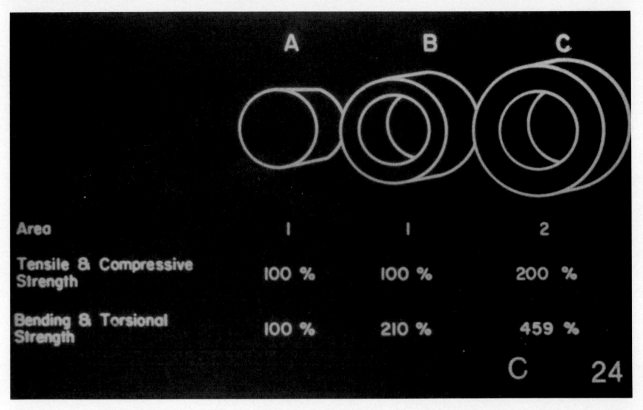

**Fig. 4–3** Biomechanical considerations of structural strength. Solid rod A and tube B have equal cross-sectional areas. The tube's distribution is further from the epicenter. The rod and the tube have equal axial strengths but the tube has 110% more bending and torsional strength than the rod A. Tube C has a mass twice that of the rod, a torsional strength four times greater than that of the rod.

density. When not homogeneous, the material's weakest point is the area of least density. The area between the two cortical end plates of the ilium contains trabecular bone of low density. The central third of the medullary canal frequently has the lowest density of trabeculae and is the site where failure occurs during compressive and shear testing. Failure or fractures occur at the site of the lowest density when there is a nonhomogeneous distribution of bone density (Fig. 4–2). This emphasizes the importance of the structural distribution of the bone mass.

Bone geometry determines bone strength.[15,16] The tensile strength of a solid rod is the same as that of a tube with the same cross-sectional area of material. However, the tube has a greater moment of inertia and is significantly stronger than the rod when withstanding bending or torsional stresses (Fig. 4–3). Consequently, the farther the material is distributed away from the center of the object, the stronger is the structural strength of that material in torsion and bending. An example of this principle is seen in the femoral diaphysis of an aging individual. As one grows older, the outer periosteal diameter and the inner endosteal diameter increase, shifting the bone

mass further from the epicenter of the bone. Theoretically, these changes in bone geometry have the potential to maximize skeletal strength for any given amount of bone mass and could partially compensate for the decreased bone mass that accompanies aging.[17] For instance, a 10% increase in the diameter of a long bone can compensate for a 30% decrease in bone mass. In reality, increases in the diameter of long bones rarely exceed 2% of the original diameter per year.[18,19] Furthermore, although this process has been demonstrated to occur in males,[19-21] some reported data suggest that the female skeleton does not widen with aging. In addition, certain parts of the skeleton, such as the femoral neck, are deficient in periosteum and cannot compensate for loss of endosteal bone mass. These observations partially explain the predilection for fracture of the femoral neck in elderly women.

Careful dissection of the tibia demonstrates another principle of structural distribution and material properties. The anterior and posterior aspects of the diaphysis are respectively under the greatest tensile and compressive stresses caused by the bowing of the tibia and the greater strength of muscles in the posterior compartment of the leg. The medial and lateral·aspects of the tibia are in a more neutral plane and sustain significantly less tensile and compressive loads. Analyses of the tibial cortices show that the osteonal count is greatest in the medial and lateral aspects of the diaphysis in the neutral plane, and lowest in the area of anterior diaphysis under the greatest tension. Symmetric stressing of the tibia in animals has clearly demonstrated the inhibition of osteonal remodeling and the development of bone apposition on the outer diameters of the anterior and posterior tibial cortex.[22] Immobilization of the tibia and calcium deficiency will produce an increase in osteonal remodeling in the unstressed medial and lateral tibia. Two concepts can be generated from these studies: modeling and remodeling (Fig. 4–4).

In modeling, general appositional growth occurs on the surface of the loaded bone at the greatest distance from the epicenter of the bone. It does not follow Frost's[23] metabolic bone unit concept of resorption followed by formation. Modeling is illustrated clinically by periosteal bone formation in stressed bones. It is also seen after aseptic necrosis in which the dead trabeculae provide a lattice upon which new appositional bone growth occurs. Lastly, it is clearly illustrated in the external fracture callus in which bone formation occurs unilaterally, without preliminary bone resorption.

Conversely, remodeling involves an initial process of removing bone from within. This is illustrated by the cutting-cone osteoclastic resorption of cortical bone or Howship's lacunar indentations into trabecular bone. In both instances the bone is temporarily weakened during the remodeling process before it is partially restrengthened by new bone formation. Furthermore, the initial mineralization is incomplete so the new bone is weaker. The new metabolic bone unit is significantly decreased in compressive strength compared to the preexisting highly mineralized bone. Lastly, the production of porosities and subsequent reossification during the remodeling process result in a multicomponent bone rather than a single unit of reinforced collagen in bone. This remodeled bone differs from reinforced concrete which is entirely produced *de novo* at one time. It is similar to the process of boring holes into preexisting concrete, producing microfractures and weakness. Plugging up the hole with new concrete will never return its original strength. Osteonal and remodeled bone is initially significantly weaker than the cortical bone it replaced. The body recognizes skeletal stress, perhaps by a piezoelectric feedback, and will only remodel the least stressed bone. Bone cells respond to the so-called "Wolff's law"[15] and deposit bone appositionally in an effort to increase the structural strength of loaded areas.

The implications of modeling and remodeling are clear in terms of osteoporosis. Bone that has undergone significant remodeling and porosity has a markedly weakened microstructure. Conversely, modeled bone maintains an intact microstructure without faults or stress risers while augmenting lamellar bone mass by appositional growth.

Normal metabolic circumstances avoid rapid bone turnover or production of excess osteoid, and protect the bone's mechanical structure. Enhanced remodeling runs the risk of producing microweaknesses. Patients with hyperparathyroidism, hyperthyroidism, and even Paget's disease, with its enhanced bone mass, all have hypermetabolic remodeling states and are noted for their high incidence of stress fractures. Efforts to strengthen bone by promoting the remodeling process are less likely to succeed than those that augment bone by direct modeling.

Bone consists of both cortical and trabecular material. Each of these two types of bone has a different structural role. Areas suffering large, multidirectional impact stresses do best with the trabecular bone pattern. Cortical bone's primary function is protection against torque and bending loads. Cortical bone forms slowly and its dimensions have been developed in response to a long history of specific recurring stresses. The vertebral body consists of a cortical outer shell and a large trabecular interior bone volume. Carter and Hayes[14] showed that removing the cortex lessened the mechanical strength of the vertebral body during compressive testing by only 7%. Consequently, 93% of the compressive strength of the vertebral body is maintained by the trabecular

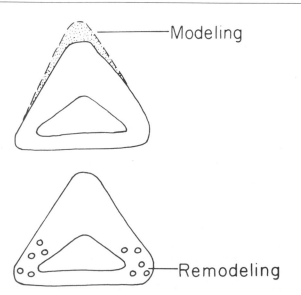

**Fig. 4–4** Modeling represents appositional bone deposition on periphery of a structure. Remodeling is turnover within the original dimensions of the structure. Modeling occurs on the most loaded regions of bone and remodeling on the least loaded areas.

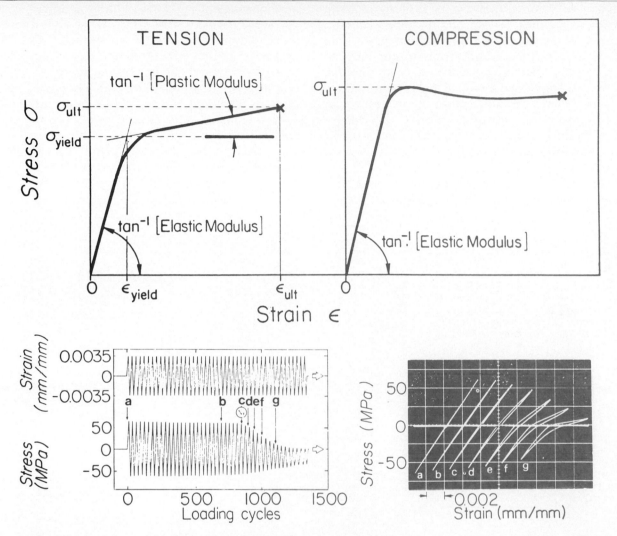

**Fig. 4–5**  Biomechanical considerations of material failure. As demonstrated by stress/strain plots (top), under either tension or compression loads, material undergoes a reversible elastic deformation followed by plastic irreversible deformation until failure occurs (point x on the plots). Under cyclic loading (bottom), failure occurs during each cycle into the plastic region of the stress/strain curve. (Reproduced with permission from Wright TM, Hayes WC: Mechanics of fractures and fracture propagation, in Owen R, Goodfellow J, Bullough P (eds): *Scientific Foundations of Orthopaedics and Traumatology*. London, William Heinemann Medical Books, Ltd, 1980, pp 252–257.)

bone. This has similarly been noted in the subchondral area of the femur and the proximal tibia. The femoral neck has little trabecular bone and depends on cortical bone for its integrity. It fails mainly in torque and bending modes against which trabecular bone offers little protection.

Bones rich in trabecular bone sustain the first ravages of osteoporosis because of their high surface-to-volume ratio. The metaphyses of the distal radius, proximal humerus, and the vertebral bodies lose trabecular bone soon after menopause and these are the sites of early postmenopausal fractures. Cortical bone is slower to dissolve because of its low surface-to-volume ratio. Its loss occurs later, during so-called "senile osteoporosis," and results in cortical bone fractures in areas such as the hip.[24]

## Mechanisms of Fracture

Fractures occur from either repetitive microinjury with propagation of the fracture line (fatigue failure) or from acute trauma.[25] Bone is a viscoelastic substance. A load may deform the bone but, once the load is removed, the bone will regain its original shape (Fig. 4–5). Once the point of elasticity has been passed, permanent plastic deformation does occur. At this point, remodeling or modeling of the bone occurs in an effort to regain structural strength. If this process is deficient, microfractures will coalesce, leading to a weakened cortex and later fracture after mild trauma. The classic example of this process is the stress fracture. These fractures are most frequently seen in the rib, pubic ramus, tibia, and femoral neck. Acute trauma can be superimposed on these microfractures. It is uncertain what initiates hip fractures. Many observers contend that more than 50% of hip fractures result from torque-induced failure of the femoral neck cortex, and that the fracture is completely sustained before the patient strikes the floor. Certainly, most spinal trabecular fractures represent repetitive injuries with microcollapse leading to ultimate deformity. Most patients are unaware of a specific event leading to each spinal fracture.

Unfortunately, noninvasive measures of bone density report only gross mass per unit volume. Bone is

not homogeneous and that volume contains areas of decreased density with microstructural imperfections. Despite this limitation, Melton and Riggs[7] showed that the femoral hip fracture rate clearly depends on gross bone mass. They found 4/1,000 hip fractures per year in patients with a bone mass of 1.0 g/cm$^2$ as identified on the dual-beam absorptiometry instrumentation. A 50% decrease in mass was associated with a fourfold increase of hip fracture rate (16/1,000 patients per year). Thus, a gross loss of bone mass increases the fracture rate exponentially. The incidence of hip fracture is indirectly related to the bone density squared. This clinical evidence cor-

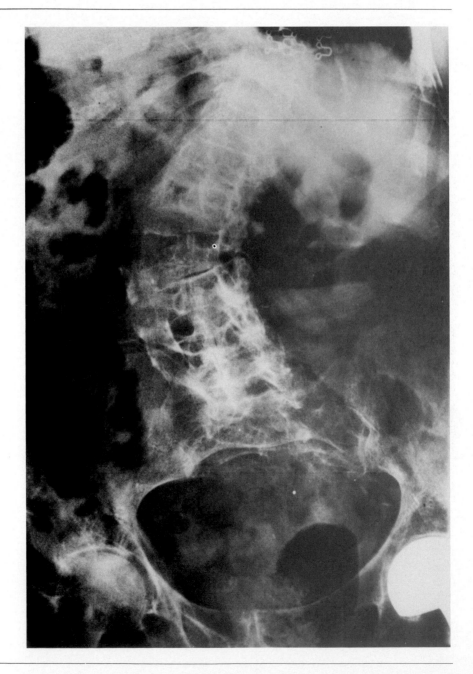

**Fig. 4–6** Anteroposterior view of lumbar scoliosis in a patient who previously underwent hemiarthroplastic replacement for a right hip fracture. The left lumbar scoliosis demonstrates a lateral spondylolisthesis at L3-L4 in an osteopenic skeleton.

roborates laboratory tests in which bone strength is related to the square of the bone density (strength = density$^2$).

Load distribution may accentuate fracture. Healey and Lane[26] have shown that 58% of patients with idiopathic osteoporosis develop scoliosis. Conversely, 76% of patients with adult idiopathic kyphoscoliosis will have osteoporosis (Fig. 4–6). Furthermore, patients with unstable idiopathic scoliosis (>30 degree curves) have a spinal bone density two standard deviations below the age-related mean. The kyphoscoliosis shifts the body weight, increasing a load on the anterior vertebral body trabecular bone. The stress concentration accentuates the fracture risk of select vertebrae. The major sites of fractures are (1) the apex of the kyphos, (2) the transition between the thoracic and the lumbar vertebral bodies, and (3) the apex of the lumbar scoliotic curve. Kyphoscoliosis is a clear risk factor and contributes to specific sites of fracture.

## Fracture Healing

Under normal conditions, fracture healing is accomplished by endochondral bone repair. The six clear stages identified are impact, induction, inflammation, soft callus, hard callus, and remodeling and modeling.[27,28] The stage of impact occurs from the moment of initiation of injury to the dissipation of energy. This leads to both soft-tissue and bony trauma. It is followed by the stage of induction in which a series of inductive factors such as kinins, electronegativity, low pH, and low oxygen tension all initiate the process of tissue repair. Specific agents such as bone morphogenic protein may be important in inducing and modulating repair. During the stage of inflammation which follows there is bone resorption of the necrotic osseous tissue, the initiation and development of vasoformative elements, and the ingrowth of primitive mesenchymal tissue. The stage of soft callus is the conversion of primitive mesenchymal tissue into a soft chondroid element. The stage of hard callus is the calcification of the cartilage bars, deposition of fiber bone upon the cartilage bars, and, ultimately, its conversion into lamellar bone. The last stage of remodeling and modeling reorganizes the microscopic and anatomic structure of the bone, restoring maximal strength to the bone.

Osteoporosis seriously compromises the last two stages of hard callus and remodeling.[13] The synthesis of bone and its mineralization are keenly dependent upon calcium supplied either from diet or calcium reserves (bone). Osteoporotic patients have a low calcium pool, with an inadequate calcium diet and poor structural calcium bank. Callus mineralization is thus slowed. The stage of remodeling and modeling itself is even further prolonged because of the competition for calcium with the rest of the body. Secondary hormonal factors, which are already active in maintaining calcium homeostasis at the expense of the osteoporotic skeleton, may also seriously compromise fracture healing. Consequently, although the first stages of bone repair through the soft callus stage may proceed without interference in osteoporosis, the mineralization and the ultimate remodeling of the callus are prolonged. Hip fractures in the elderly remain positive by bone scan well into the third year and union cannot be fully ascertained until then. Healing itself can be clearly stimulated by physiologic levels of vitamin D, nutritional levels of calcium for that individual (1,500 mg of elemental calcium per day), a normal nitrogen balance (adequate calorie intake), and appropriate exercise stimulation.[29] Exercise aligns collagen in bone deposition, particularly during the stage of remodeling and modeling. Osteoporotic individuals rarely receive appropriate calcium and vitamin therapy after a fracture. Studies at The Hospital for Special Surgery have demonstrated a 10% systemic bone loss in the unaffected skeleton after long-bone fractures despite "adequate" calcium intake.

### Vertebral Fractures

Vertebral fractures are the common result of osteoporosis (Fig. 4–1). Most fractures are unrecognized at the time of onset and are often found in the course of a routine examination. Acute fractures may be quite painful, leading to disability for as long as six weeks. The distribution of fractures is clearly related to the structural alignment of the spine with a majority occurring at the apex of the thoracic kyphos, the transitional zone of the thoracic lumbar spine, and at an apex of any existing lumbar scoliotic curve.[26] The initial treatment consists of conservative bed rest, hot packs, muscle relaxants, and physical activity as soon as possible. Orthotics should be used only to mobilize the patient. Once the patient is ambulatory, the orthotics should be removed because they lead to stress bypass and discourage bone retention within the spine. Long-term treatment should consist of an exercise program to maintain strength and flexibility. Thoracic extension exercises strengthen the upper back muscles supporting the thoracic spine. Abdominal strengthening exercises help to support the lumbar spine. Secondary arthritis associated with malalignment may lead to areas that require specific exercises. Severe secondary scoliosis may require custom-fitted orthoses. Major surgical indications after spinal fractures are related primarily to acute spinal canal impingement. At The Hospital for Special Surgery, 3% of the patients develop sensory level and neuromuscular evidence of cord compression. A computed tomographic (CT) scan, magnetic resonance imaging (MRI), and myelograms may be necessary in any patient with persistent day and night pain and abnormal neurologic findings. These fractures may require anterior decompression akin to the technique used for tuberculosis.[30] The incorporation of bone grafts, usually from the iliac crest, may take some time. Therefore, these patients require protection in a molded polyethylene body jacket starting four vertebral bodies above the level of fusion for as long as nine months.

A dilemma facing the physician is the diagnosis and appropriate treatment of a previously unrecognized compression fracture of the thoracic and lumbar spine. An algorithm created at The Hospital for Special Surgery has been useful in guiding the evaluation of these patients and leading to the correct diagnosis (Fig. 4–7). The initial question is whether the trauma (for example, falling down a flight of stairs) was sufficient to account for the fracture. Conversely, should lifting a window or tripping on the carpeting be considered insufficient trauma? In cases of major trauma the orthopaedist must decide whether the fracture is stable and can be treated conservatively, or unstable requiring surgical intervention and stabilization with instrumentation. In the absence of major trauma it is critical to determine whether in fact there is structural continuity of the fractured vertebral body. If radiographs do not show any lack of continuity or clear structural deficiency, the degree of generalized osteopenia should be determined. Noninvasive techniques, including a quantitative CT scan[31] and dual-beam absorptiometry,[32,33,34] appear to be efficacious. Further studies of the fractured vertebral body, including bone and CT scans, are warranted if structural deficiencies are clearly identified or no osteopenia is evidenced by densitometry analysis of the skeleton. These studies may reveal metastatic or primary malignant tumors. The nontumorous diseases that can lead to localized structural insufficiency include Paget's disease and hemangioma of bone.

In generalized osteopenia the differential diagnosis centers on a bone marrow abnormality, endocrinopathy, osteoporosis, or osteomalacia. An abnormal erythrocyte sedimentation rate, CBC, or serum protein electrophoresis suggests that a bone marrow disorder may exist and a diagnosis of myeloma, leukemia, or other hematologic disorder should be considered. If hematologic screening studies are negative, blood studies should be performed to measure thyroid function, parathyroid function, estrogen and endogenous steroid levels, and glucose level. Increased 24-hour urine hydroxyproline (derived from bone collagen turnover) values should be found in high turnover conditions produced by hormonal imbalances. If endocrinopathy studies are noncontributory, the differential diagnosis of osteopenia rests purely between osteoporosis and osteomalacia. Alkaline phosphatase, calcium, phosphorous, and vitamin D levels may be helpful, but a final diagnosis may require a transiliac bone biopsy to differentiate osteomalacia and osteoporosis. Unfortunately, osteoid mineralization defects are commonly missed by noninvasive procedures. At The Hospital for Special Surgery 25% of patients with compression fractures treated by the orthopaedic service had endocrinopathies, 2% had marrow abnormalities, and 30% demonstrated hyperosteoidosis on bone biopsy. The remainder had osteoporosis or a combination of osteoporosis and one of the above-mentioned disorders.

## Hip Fractures

Hip fractures present a major risk of mortality and permanent morbidity in patients with osteoporosis (Fig. 4–1). The two predominant types of hip fractures are subcapital femoral neck and intertrochanteric fractures. Subcapital fractures are associated with a high risk of nonunion and/or aseptic necrosis of the femoral head. Intertrochanteric fractures have a low risk of nonunion but can lead to malalignment, including retroversion and varus deformities with penetration of the head by the internal fixation device. These fractures all require open reduction and internal fixation or hemiarthroplasty (Fig. 4–8). A study at New York Hospital[6] of 77 patients demonstrated that one third had evidence of hyperosteoidosis (more than 5% trabecular osteoid). Although 40% had marked trabecular bone loss, all patients more than 50 years old had decreased bone mass compared to young individuals. Twenty-five percent had increased metabolic turnover indices, including high osteoclast counts. In that study, bone histomorphometry appeared to be a good predictor of outcome after treatment for femoral neck fracture. Patients who had trabecular bone volumes within 60% of normal had successful union rates of 85% to 90%, whereas patients who had severe trabecular bone loss (<60% of normal) had a union rate of <33% in women and 50% in men. These investigators concluded that significant metabolic bone disease, particularly osteoporosis, leads to a high rate of unsuccessful union after femoral neck fractures. Intertrochanteric fractures have not been comparably studied.

The incidence of hip fracture increases with longevity; approximately 32% of women and 17% of men will sustain a hip fracture by the age of 90 years.[7,35] It is disturbing that the age- and sex-adjusted hip fracture rates have increased significantly since World War II. Hip fracture rates have been affected by several factors. Studies from Finland indicate that

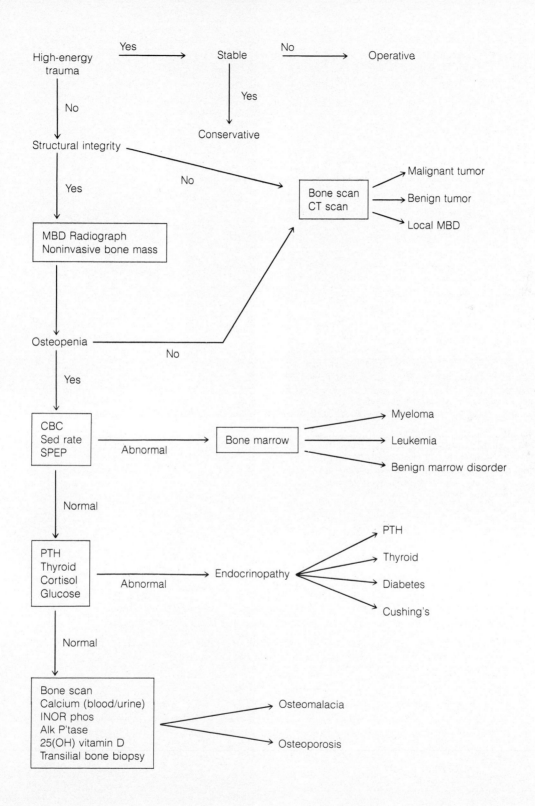

**Fig. 4–7** Algorithm for evaluation of osteopenia.

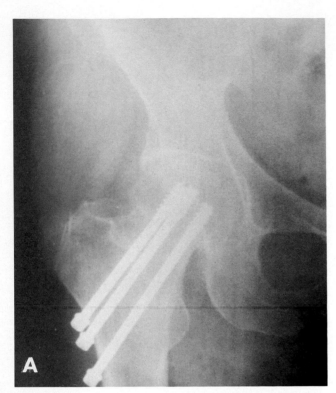

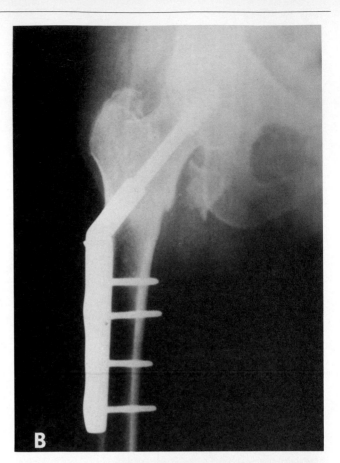

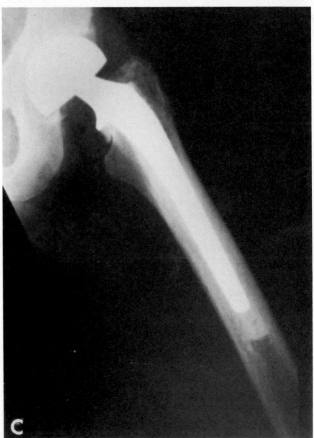

**Fig. 4–8**  Treatment of hip fractures. **A:** Anteroposterior view of a femoral neck hip fracture reduced and stabilized with three Asnis pins. **B:** Anteroposterior view of a femoral intertrochanteric hip fracture reduced and stabilized with a Richards hip compression screw. **C:** Anteroposterior view of a femoral neck hip fracture corrected with a bipolar hemiarthroplasty.

populations using fluoridated water (1 ppm) have one third the fracture rate of patients using nonfluoridated water (corrected per decade).[36] Patients from areas in Yugoslavia[37] with high calcium intakes have a fracture rate one third to one fourth that of patients from areas with low levels of calcium in the diet. This low dietary calcium intake is comparable to the average American intake.

The treatment options for hip fractures include percutaneous pinning or hemiarthroplasty (Fig. 4–8). Pinning has a very low mortality rate (1% excess mortality),[38] but patients with metabolic bone disease have a poor union rate and often require secondary procedures. Long-term mortality may be increased in these patients since they may not regain mobility. Hemiarthroplasties have a higher initial mortality rate, but in the long-run may actually lead to better function and survival. Other studies testing the efficacy of hemiarthroplasty versus pinning in the osteopenic population are now underway in a number of institutions, so this question may be more clearly answered in the future.

The use of sodium fluoride has decreased vertebral fractures but its effect on hip fracture is uncertain.[39,40] One preliminary study in a group of Australian patients treated with sodium fluoride (1 mg/kg/day) suggested higher fracture rates, but a large collaborative study by Riggs and associates[39] suggested that the fracture rate is not actually increased. Long-term studies of patients receiving fluoride therapy at The Hospital for Special Surgery have suggested a 50% decrease in the rate of fractures after two years of fluoride treatment.[40]

## Colles' Fractures

Colles' fractures occur in the distal wrist, most often in postmenopausal women (Fig. 4–1). These fractures frequently lead to foreshortening and malalignment of the wrist. A conservative, nonsurgical approach often results in imperfect reduction but is usually accepted in an effort to regain and retain function. External fixators may permit early function of the hand and the elbow while maintaining alignment, allowing for ultimate healing and preserving the relationship of the radius and ulna. Young individuals have a better potential for healing and must be treated rigorously to maintain alignment. The same conditions could be extended to the elderly if appropriate fixation with low morbidity were developed.

## Pelvic Fractures

Pelvic fractures, particularly in the region of the pubic rami, frequently occur in an osteoporotic population. They may be more common in individuals with underlying hyperosteoidosis. Therapy is directed primarily toward resolving the symptoms rather than restoring skeletal continuity. Healing always occurs even with conservative management. Mobilization, first with a walker and then with crutches, may be sufficient. Pain should be the guide for weight-bearing, and no surgical intervention is warranted.

## Exercise

According to Wolff's law,[15] form follows function. The skeleton, particularly the osteoblasts and osteoclasts, responds to structural demands. A clear distinction must be made between modeling and remodeling. Immobilization leads to bone resorption, particularly in unstressed areas. Conservative levels of exercise maintain bone mass but do not lead to appositional bone growth (modeling). Stringent exercise leads to modeling of the skeletal area that is repetitively stressed. Studies in postmenopausal populations have clearly demonstrated that a reasonable level of exercise (walking 5 miles a week, dancing, and limited forceful activity) can decrease the traditional postmenopausal loss of bone from 2% per year to less than 0.5%[41] per year. Other studies have also found that exercise can limit the tendency for remodeling of stressed bones and thereby prevent loss of bone strength.

In younger groups, Jacobsen and associates[41] demonstrated that high-performance swimmers and typical college women had comparable bone mass whereas tennis players with a high level of "impact loading" had significantly greater amounts of trabecular bone within the spine. Stress loading against impacts leads to augmented bone mass. Exercise has also been shown to protect even patients with anorexia nervosa. Rigotti and associates[42] demonstrated a significant diminution in bone mass in anorexic individuals who did not exercise. However, in anorexic individuals who carried out a general exercise program regularly, bone loss was not statistically different from that of controls. Thus, exercise can partially protect bone mass from loss even during short periods of nutritional deprivation.

Exercise carried to the point of loss of body fat and the development of amenorrhea may ultimately be deleterious. Cann and associates[43] showed that women who jogged 40 miles a week developed amenorrhea, unlike those who jogged 25 miles a week. Quantitative CT scans showed significantly lower spinal mass in the former than in women who ran shorter distances and who continued to menstruate.

Exercise, therefore, can maintain bone mass by inducing modeling and augmented bone formation in impact-loaded bones. If amenorrhea or endocrine dysfunction results from an exercise program, the benefits of exercise may be offset.

It is possible that the physiologic signal of exercise is reproduced through bioelectricity. Tadduni and

**Table 4–1**
**Effects of various substances on bone**

| Substance | Amount | Effect on Bone |
|---|---|---|
| Calcium | 1,000 to 1,500 mg/day | Prevents bone loss/improves bone quality |
| Vitamin D | 400 to 800 units/day | Prevents bone loss/improves bone quality |
| Estrogen | 0.625 mg/day (1 to 25 days/mo) | Prevents bone loss |
| Progesterone | 10 mg/day (15 to 25 days/mo) | Prevents endometrial cancer from estrogen therapy |
| Calcitonin | 50 to 100 units/day (3 to 7 days/wk) | Prevents bone loss |
| Sodium fluoride | 1.0 to 1.3 mg/kg/day | Increases bone mass |

Brighton[44] indicated that capacitive coupling can prevent loss of bone from disuse osteoporosis. Whether bioelectricity can mimic the signal from exercise and actually lead to augmentation of bone mass is uncertain. Although augmented bone production can occur in the young, there are little data to indicate that people past the age of 45 years can markedly increase their bone mass unless they are starting from a state of major deprivation.

## Prevention

The best treatment of osteoporosis is prevention. Reasonable nutrition, including appropriate calcium and vitamin D intakes, preservation of proper hormonal balance (estrogen supplementation), and appropriate exercise are essential in preventing the development of osteoporosis, particularly in the high-risk individual.[45] True osteoporosis requires more than repair of fractures. Re-establishment of exercise programs and adequate nutrition in patients with osteoporosis may protect the remaining bone mass and enhance fracture healing. Specific therapies for osteoporosis, including sodium fluoride, estrogen and progesterone, calcitonin, and bone remodeling programs, have been discussed in greater detail elsewhere in this chapter and in other reviews.[2,11,12,37,39,40,46-51] Calcium, physiologic levels of vitamin D, estrogen and progesterone, and calcitonin halt bone loss while sodium fluoride augments bone mass (Table 4-1).

## Summary

We have discussed the biomechanical and biomaterial properties of bone with emphasis on the micro-environment. The microdensity of bone tissues deter-mines the resistance to compressive forces (strength = density$^2$). The structural orientation of bone determines the ability of bone to withstand torsion and bending forces. Highly remodeled bone is brittle and fractures easily because of the multiple reversal planes within the bone plates. Conversely, augmentation of bone on the periphery by modeling leads to increased material microstrength and structural macrostrength. Consequently, appositional modeling augments whereas remodeling diminishes bone strength.

Hip fractures, spinal fractures, Colles' fractures, and pelvic fractures have been discussed in terms of their pathophysiology and treatment. An algorithm (Fig. 4–7) has been presented for the differential diagnosis of patients with recently discovered spinal compression fractures. Lastly, a discussion of exercise demonstrated its beneficial role, especially in the retention of bone mass.

## References

1. Holbrook TL, Grazier KL, Kelsey JL, et al: *The Frequency of Occurrence, Impact, and Cost of Selected Musculoskeletal Conditions in the United States*. Park Ridge, Illinois, American Academy of Orthopaedic Surgeons, 1984, chap 5, pp 24–72.
2. Lane JM, Vigorita VJ, Falls M: Osteoporosis: Current concepts and treatment. *Geriatrics* 1984;39(4):40–47.
3. Wallach S: Management of osteoporosis. *Hosp Pract* 1978;13(12):91–98.
4. Spencer H: Osteoporosis: Goals of therapy. *Hosp Pract* 1982;17(3):131–138, 143–148.
5. Johnston CC Jr, Norton JA Jr, Khairi RA, et al: Age related bone loss, in Barzel A (ed): *Osteoporosis II*. New York, Grune and Stratton, 1979, pp 91–100.
6. Scileppi KP, Stulberg B, Vigorita VJ, et al: Bone histomorphometry in femoral neck fractures. *Surg Forum* 1981;3:543–545.
7. Melton LJ III, Riggs BL: Epidemiology of age-related fractures, in Avioli LV (ed): *The Osteoporotic Syndrome*. New York, Grune and Stratton, 1983, pp 45–72.
8. Jensen GF, Christiansen C, Boesen J, et al: Epidemiology of post-menopausal spinal and long bone fractures. *Clin Orthop* 1982;166:75–81.
9. Holbrook TL, Grazier KL, Kelsey JL, et al: *The Frequency of Occurrence, Impact, and Cost of Selected Musculoskeletal Conditions in the United States*. Park Ridge, Illinois, American Academy of Orthopaedic Surgeons, 1984, chap 7, pp 136–173.
10. Kenzora JE, McCarthy RE, Lowell JD, et al: Hip fracture mortality. *Clin Orthop* 1984;186:45–56.
11. Lane JM, Vigorita VJ: Osteoporosis. *Univ Pa Orthop J* 1985;1:22–31.
12. Avioli LV: Post-menopausal osteoporosis: Prevention vs cure. *Fed Proc* 1981;40:2418–2422.
13. Lane JM: Metabolic bone disease and fracture healing, in Heppenstall RB (ed): *Fracture Treatment and Healing*. Philadelphia, WB Saunders Co, 1980, chap 32, pp 946–962.
14. Carter DR, Hayes WC: The compressive behavior of bone as a two phase porous structure. *J Bone Joint Surg* 1977;59A:954–962.
15. Wolff J: *Das Gesetz der Transformation de Enochen*. Berlin, Hirschwald, 1892.

16. Moss ML: The design of bones, in Owen R, Goodfellow J, Bullough P (eds): *Scientific Foundations of Orthopaedics and Traumatology*. London, William Heinemann Medical Books, Ltd, 1980, pp 59–66.

17. Smith RW Jr, Walker RB: Femoral expansion in aging women: Implications for osteoporosis and fractures. *Science* 1964;145:156–157.

18. Jowsey J: *Metabolic Diseases of Bone*. Philadelphia, WB Saunders, 1977, chap 8.

19. Trotter M, Peterson RR: Transverse diameter of the femur: On roentgenograms and on bones. *Clin Orthop* 1967;52:233–239.

20. Martin RB: Age and sex-related changes in the structure and strength of the human femoral shaft. *J Biomech* 1977;10:223–231.

21. Martin RB, Pickett JC, Zinaich S: Studies of skeletal remodeling in aging men. *Clin Orthop* 1980;149:268–282.

22. Barr D: *A Multivariate Mechanical Assessment of Sexual Dimorphism in the Human Hip*, thesis. University of West Virginia, Morgantown, VA, 1977.

23. Frost HM: Tetracycline-based histological analysis of bone remodeling. *Calcif Tissue Res* 1969;3:211–237.

24. Riggs BL, Melton LJ III: Evidence for two distinct syndromes of involutional osteoporosis. *Am J Med* 1983;75:899–901.

25. Wright TM, Hayes WC: Mechanics of fractures and fracture propagation, in Owen R, Goodfellow J, Bullough P (eds): *Scientific Foundations of Orthopaedics and Traumatology*. London, William Heinemann Medical Books, Ltd, 1980, pp 252–257.

26. Healey JH, Lane JM: Structural scoliosis in osteoporotic women. *Clin Orthop* 1984;195:216–223.

27. Heppenstall RB: Fracture healing, in Heppenstall RB (ed): *Fracture Treatment and Healing*. Philadelphia, WB Saunders, 1980, chap 2, pp 35–64.

28. Sevitt S: Healing of fractures, in Owen R, Goodfellow J, Bullough P (eds): *Scientific Foundations of Orthopaedics and Traumatology*. London, William Heinemann Medical Books Ltd, 1980, chap 32, pp 258–272.

29. Steier A, Gegadia I, Schwartz A, et al: Effect of vitamin $D_2$ and fluoride upon experimental fracture healing in the rat. *J Dent Res* 1967;46:675–680.

30. Hodgson AR, Stock FE: Anterior spine fusion for the treatment of tuberculosis of the spine: The operative findings and results of treatment in the first one-hundred cases. *J Bone Joint Surg* 1960;42A:295–310.

31. Gennant HK, Cann CE, Ettinger B, et al: Quantitative computed tomography of vertebral spongiosa: A sensitive method of detecting early bone loss after oophorectomy. *Ann Intern Med* 1984;97:699–705.

32. Wahner HW, Dunn WL, Riggs BL: Non-invasive bone mineral measurements. *Semin Nucl Med* 1983;13(3):282–289.

33. Wahner HW: Bone mineral measurements: A new clinical tool, editorial. *J Nucl Med* 1984;25:383–384.

34. Wahner HW, Dunn WL, Riggs BL: Assessment of bone mineral: Parts I and II. *J Nucl Med* 1984;25:1134–1141, 1241–1253.

35. Gallagher JC, Melton LM, Riggs BL, et al: Epidemiology of fractures of the proximal femur in Rochester, Minnesota. *Clin Orthop* 1980;150:163–171.

36. Simonen O, Laitinen O: Does fluoridation of drinking water prevent bone fragility and osteoporosis? *Lancet* 1985;2:432–434.

37. Matkovic V, Kostial K, Simonovic I, et al: Bone status and fracture rates in two regions of Yugoslavia. *Am J Clin Nutr* 1979;32:540–549.

38. Arnold WD, Lyden JP, Minkoff J: Treatment of intracapsular fractures of the femoral neck. *J Bone Joint Surg* 1974;56A:254–262.

39. Riggs BL, Seeman E, Hodgson SF, et al: Effect of the fluoride calcium regimen on vertebral fracture occurrence in postmenopausal osteoporosis. *N Engl J Med* 1984;306:446–450.

40. Lane JM, Healey JH, Schwartz E, et al: Treatment of osteoporosis with sodium fluoride and calcium: Effects on vertebral fracture incidence and bone histomorphometry. *Orthop Clin North Am* 1984;15:729–745.

41. Jacobsen PC, Beaver W, Gruhle SA, et al: Bone density in women: College athletes and older athletic women. *J Orthop Res* 1984;2:328–332.

42. Rigotti NA, Nussbaum SR, Herzog DB, et al: Osteoporosis in women with anorexia nervosa. *N Engl J Med* 1985;311:1601–1606.

43. Cann CE, Genant HK, Ettinger B, et al: Spinal mineral loss in oophorectomized women: Determination by quantitative computed tomography. *JAMA* 1980;224(18):2056–2059.

44. Tadduni GT, Brighton CT: The treatment of disuse osteoporosis in the rat with a capacitively coupled electrical signal. *Orthop Trans* 1985;9:227–228.

45. Lane JM: Osteoporosis as a preventable nutritional disease. *J Clin Med Nutr* 1985;1:23.

46. Aloia JF, Zanzi I, Vaswani A, et al: Combination therapy for osteoporosis with estrogen, fluoride, and calcium. *J Am Geriatr Soc* 1982;30:13–17.

47. Briancon D, Meunier PJ: Treatment of osteoporosis with fluoride, calcium and vitamin D. *Orthop Clin North Am* 1981;12:629–648.

48. Lane JM, Buss DD: Bone metabolism: Normal physiology and disease, in Asher MA (ed): *Orthopaedic Knowledge Update I: Home Study Syllabus*. Park Ridge, Illinois, American Academy of Orthopaedic Surgeons, 1984, pp 21–22.

49. Lindsay R, Dempster DW: Osteoporosis: Current concepts. *Bull NY Acad Med* 1985;61:301–322.

50. Meema S, Bunker ML, Meema HE: Preventive effect of estrogen on post-menopausal bone loss: A follow-up study. *Ann Intern Med* 1975;135:1436–1440.

51. Recker RR, Saville PD, Heaney RP: Effect of estrogen and calcium carbonate on bone loss in post-menopausal women. *Ann Intern Med* 1977;87:649–655.

# Cartilage Tumors

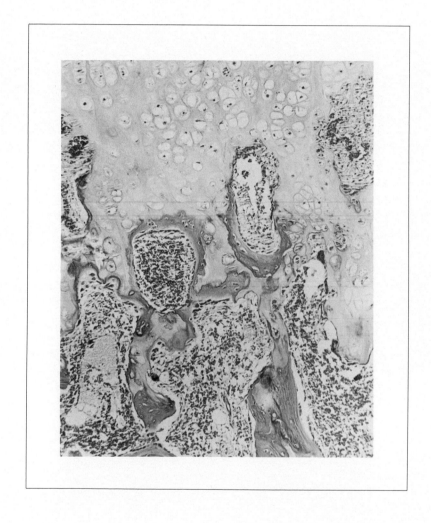

# Benign and Malignant Cartilage Tumors

Michael M. Lewis, MD

Hubert A. Sissons, MD

Alex Norman, MD

Adam Greenspan, MD

## Benign Cartilage Tumors

### Enchondroma (Chondroma)

Enchondroma is a benign tumor characterized by mature cartilage. Lesions located centrally in the bone are customarily called enchondromas whereas those on the outer surface of the cortex are known as periosteal (or juxtacortical) chondromas. Although they may appear at any age, most cases occur in the second to fourth decades of life. There is no sex predilection. The short, tubular bones of the hand (phalanges and metacarpals) are the most common sites (Fig. 5–1). Next in frequency are the femur, humerus, fibula, and ribs. Enchondromas are frequently asymptomatic and pathologic fracture through the tumor often calls attention to the lesion (Fig. 5–2).

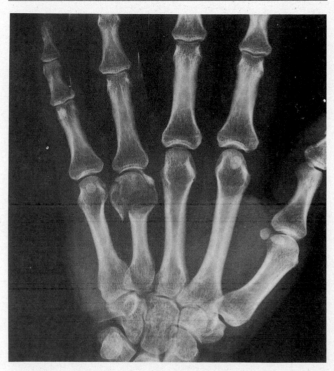

**Fig. 5–2** A 32-year-old woman sustained minor trauma to the right hand. The radiograph demonstrated a pathologic fracture through an enchondroma located at the distal end of fourth metacarpal.

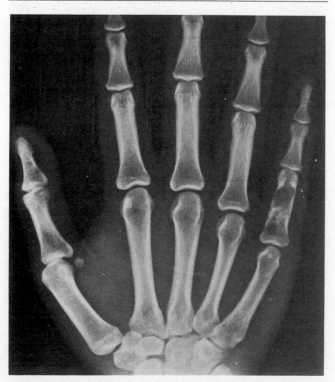

**Fig. 5–1** Enchondroma of the proximal phalanx of the small finger in a 20-year-old woman. The centrally located radiolucent lesion has a well-defined, sclerotic margin.

**Radiographic Findings** General reviews of the radiographic features of cartilage tumors include those of Murray and Jacobson,[1] Sissons and associates,[2] and Wilner.[3] In the short bones, the lesion is frequently radiolucent; in the long bones, annular or comma-shaped calcifications are often seen within the tumor. If the calcifications are extensive, the lesion is called a "calcifying" enchondroma.

Since cartilage grows in a lobular pattern, enchondroma can be recognized radiographically by scalloping of the inner cortical margin. The annular and punctate calcifications are also helpful radiographic hallmarks of a cartilage lesion (Fig. 5–3). The main differential diagnosis, particularly if the lesion is located in the long bone, is medullary bone infarct. At times, it may be difficult to distinguish between these two lesions, particularly when the enchondroma

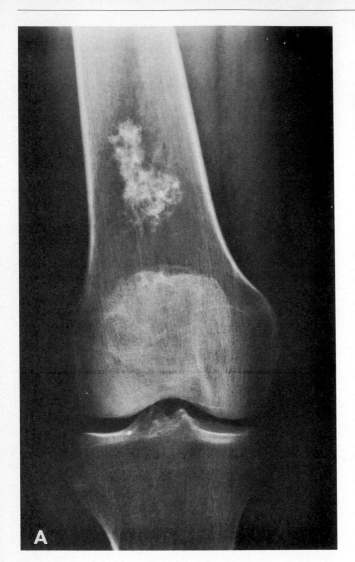

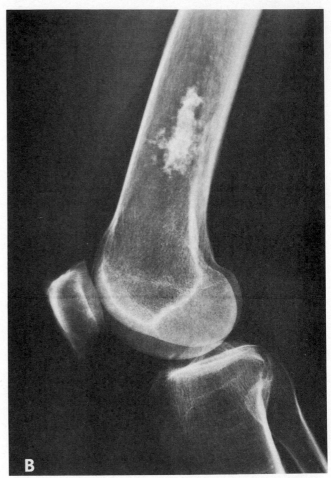

**Fig. 5–3** Anteroposterior **(A)** and lateral **(B)** radiographs demonstrate the typical appearance of enchondroma in a long bone. Note annular and punctate calcifications, the hallmarks of a cartilage lesion.

is small, since both lesions manifest similar calcifications. Helpful radiographic features for diagnosing enchondroma are the lobulation of the tumor, annular, punctate, and comma-shaped calcifications, and a lack of the sclerotic margin usually seen in a bone infarct. If a tumor of the distal phalanx is radiolucent, the enchondroma must be differentiated from an epidermoid inclusion cyst, glomus tumor, or keratoacanthoma. If the lesion reaches the articular end of the bone, a giant-cell tumor should be considered. If a purely radiolucent tumor is in a long bone, another diagnostic possibility is fibrous dysplasia.

**Pathologic Findings** General reviews of the pathologic features of cartilage tumors include those of Sissons and associates[2]; Jaffe[4]; Spjut and associates[5]; Schajowicz and associates[6]; Huvos[7]; Dahlin[8]; Schajowicz[9];

and Steiner.[10] Histologically, cartilage tumors can be recognized by the features of their intercellular matrix. The intercellular matrix has a uniformly translucent appearance, and contains relatively little collagen in comparison with the intercellular matrices of bony tumors such as osteoblastomas and osteosarcomas. The tumor cells themselves are usually located in rounded spaces, or lacunae, as in normal cartilage. In benign cartilage tumors, such as enchondroma, the tissue is sparsely cellular (Fig. 5–4A): the cells, typically with small darkly staining nuclei, fail to show the cytologic features (large nuclei, pleomorphism, double nuclei, mitoses) characteristic of chondrosarcoma. The tumor tissue is usually avascular, and areas of degenerate and calcified matrix are common; calcification is sometimes followed by vascularization and replacement of bone, as in normal endochondral ossification. Because of their slow growth, chondromas erode and expand the overlying cortical bone (Fig. 5–4B) but do not invade it.

Recently, cartilage tumors (chondroma, chondrosarcoma, chondroblastoma, and chondromyxoid fibroma) have been found to give a positive reaction for S-100 protein.[11,12] This is sometimes diagnostically useful, as most other bone tumors do not give this reaction.

**Treatment** A painless enchondroma discovered accidentally in a long bone may be watched without surgical intervention if the radiographic appearance suggests a benign tumor. If the surgeon is concerned about the lesion, biopsy and intralesional curettage can be done. In the more common location in the hand, these lesions are often discovered after pathologic fracture, and surgical treatment in the form of intralesional curettage with bone grafting can have a favorable outcome. The bone graft can be either autogenous or allograft (bank bone).

### Periosteal (Juxtacortical) Chondroma

A periosteal chondroma is a slowly growing benign cartilaginous lesion that arises on the surface of a bone. As the tumor enlarges, it erodes the cortex in a saucer-like fashion, producing a solid buttress of periosteal new bone reaction (Fig. 5–5).

In 1952, Lichtenstein and Hall[13] described periosteal chondroma as a distinct lesion. The lesion is usually small, and occasionally may erode through the cortex into the medullary cavity. These lesions occur in children as well as in adults. There is usually a history of pain and tenderness, often accompanied by swelling at the site of the lesion. The most common location is in the upper humerus. There is no sex predilection.

**Radiographic Findings** The lesion is small and is locat-

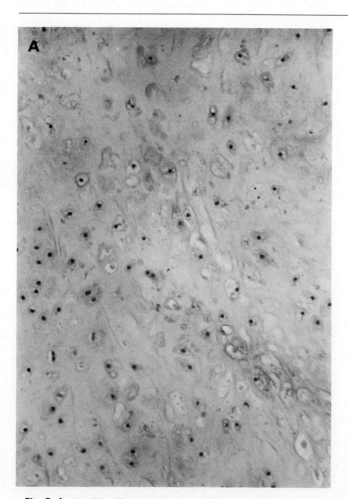
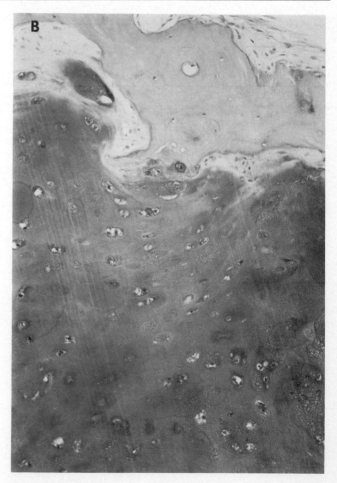

**Fig. 5–4**   **A:** Chondroma. Poorly cellular cartilage (× 235). **B:** Chondroma. Tumor tissue, with expanded but uninvaded cortical bone (× 183).

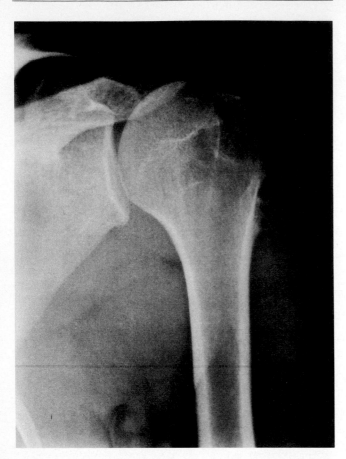

**Fig. 5–5** Periosteal chondroma of the proximal humerus. The lateral cortex is eroded by the tumor and there is a solid buttress of periosteal new bone formation.

ed on the surface of the bone. Characteristically, it erodes the cortex of the bone. A sharp sclerotic inner margin demarcates the lesion and a well-organized buttress of periosteal new bone is often present (Fig. 5–6). Scattered calcifications may be present.

**Pathologic Findings** The histopathologic characteristics of this lesion are identical with those of a conventional enchondroma.

**Treatment** En bloc resection is the treatment of choice for lesions in the long bones. Excision and curettage may be preferred in lesions of the hands and feet. The prognosis is excellent. The lesion occasionally recurs, particularly if it was incompletely resected.

### Enchondromatosis (Ollier's Disease)

Enchondromatosis is characterized by the presence of multiple lesions. Ollier's disease is the term used for enchondromatosis heavily affecting the skeleton, particularly when there is a distinct preference for one side of the body. There is no hereditary or familial tendency in this disorder. Some investigators consider this condition a developmental bone dyspla-

sia rather than a true neoplasm.[1] The clinical manifestations, such as knobby swellings of the digits and disparity in length of the forearm or leg bones, are usually recognized in childhood or adolescence. Enchondromatosis is sometimes a precursor of chondrosarcoma.

**Radiographic Findings** Enchondromas of the hands and feet can be recognized as radiolucent masses of cartilage with the typical foci of calcification noted in chondroid tumors. Linear columns of radiolucent streaks extend from the growth plate into the diaphysis (Fig. 5–7A).

Interference with the growth plate causes shortening and deformity of the bones[14] (Fig. 5–7B). The individual tumors resemble solitary enchondromas. In addition to the intraosseous tumors, some patients show subperiosteal and cortical lesions (Fig. 5–8). Disturbances of growth are common. When enchondromatosis is associated with soft-tissue hemangiomas, the condition is known as Maffucci's syndrome. In the skeleton, the lesions have the same distribution as those in Ollier's disease, that is, a strong predilection for one side of the body.

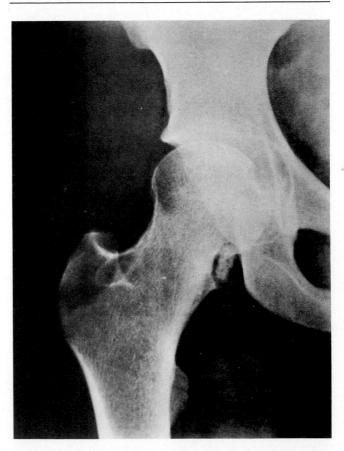

**Fig. 5–6** Periosteal chondroma at the neck of right femur. There is a defect in the cortex at the site of calcified mass and characteristic buttress of periosteal new bone (arrows).

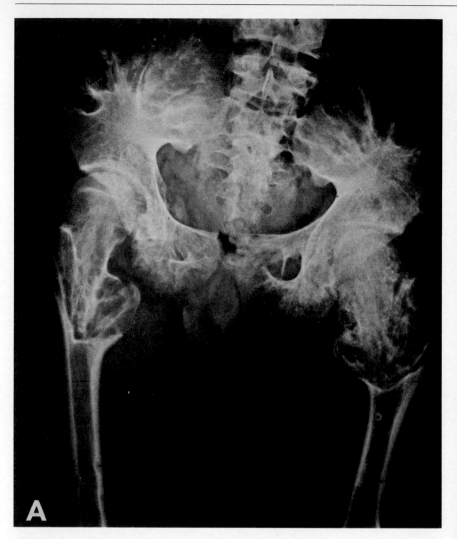

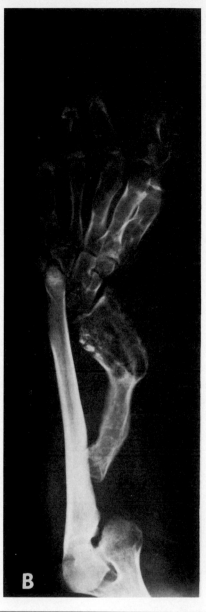

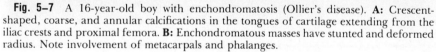

**Fig. 5–7** A 16-year-old boy with enchondromatosis (Ollier's disease). **A:** Crescent-shaped, coarse, and annular calcifications in the tongues of cartilage extending from the iliac crests and proximal femora. **B:** Enchondromatous masses have stunted and deformed radius. Note involvement of metacarpals and phalanges.

**Pathologic Findings** The histologic features of the lesion in enchondromatosis are essentially the same as those of solitary enchondromas, although the multiple lesions tend to be somewhat more cellular. Not all the lesions in enchondromatosis grow progressively, and sometimes the surfaces of inactive cartilage nodules are surrounded by a layer of mature bone (Figs. 5–9 and 5–10). When malignant change occurs, the new tissue shows the usual histologic features of chondrosarcoma. The association between enchondromatosis and chondrosarcoma is sometimes indicated by the presence, in the secondary chondrosarcomas, of areas of benign cartilage tissue corresponding to the pre-existing enchondromatosis.

**Treatment** The treatment of these lesions can be similar to that for solitary enchondroma. Individuality of treatment is the hallmark. However, as there is an increased risk of malignant degeneration, careful follow-up and evaluation are required.

### Solitary Osteochondroma

An osteochondroma (osteocartilaginous exostosis) is a cartilage-capped bony projection on the external surface of the bone. It is the most common benign lesion of bone, and usually occurs in patients in the first two decades of life. Metaphyses of long bones, particularly around the knee and the proximal humerus, are the most common sites of involvement.[10] Growth of an osteochondroma usually stops at the time of skeletal maturity.[4] There are two types of osteochondromas—a pedunculated lesion with a

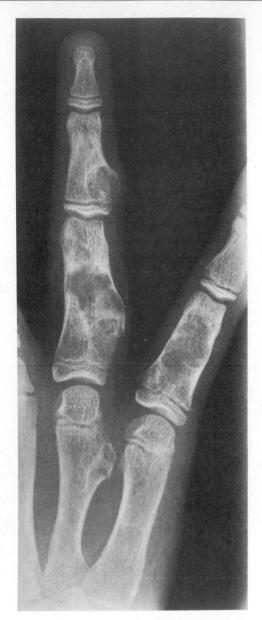

**Fig. 5–8** Subperiosteal and cortical enchondromas involving fourth ray of the left hand of this 12-year-old boy with multiple enchondromatosis.

slender pedicle, usually directed away from the neighboring growth plate, and sessile osteochondroma, which has a broad base.

Osteochondromas can be discovered clinically in several ways. Most commonly, a mass is discovered serendipitously on palpation during physical examination. Less frequently, pain is present, usually caused by pressure of the osteochondroma upon an adjacent vessel or nerve. Pain may also be caused by a pathologic fracture through the stalk.

**Radiographic Findings** The most important radio-

graphic features of osteochondroma are that the continuity of the cortex is interrupted at the base of the lesion and extends onto the stalk and that the medullary cavity of the host bone and the exostosis communicate (Figs. 5–11 and 5–12). This distinguishes an osteochondroma from the similarly located bone masses of juxtacortical osteosarcoma, soft-tissue osteosarcoma, and juxtacortical myositis ossificans. Another radiographic feature of osteochondroma is the presence of calcifications, which are usually in the chondro-osseous zone of the stalk of the lesion. The presence of calcification within the cartilaginous cap is highly suggestive of malignant transformation. This complication is rarely encountered in solitary lesions (less than 1% of cases) but it is more common in multiple cartilaginous exostoses (10% of cases).[4] The chief complications of solitary osteochondroma are pressure on a nerve or vessel, pressure on the adjacent bone with occasional fracture, fracture of the lesion itself, effusion of the bursa exostotica covering the cartilaginous cap, and malignant transformation to chondrosarcoma.

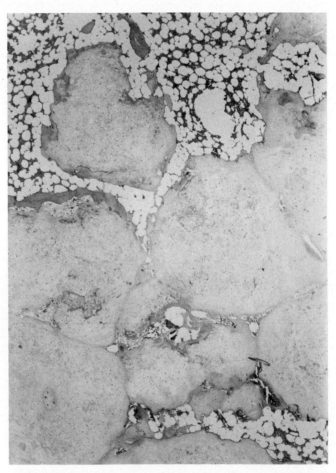

**Fig. 5–9** Enchondromatosis. The multiple nodules of poorly cellular cartilage are rimmed by mature bone (× 36).

**Pathologic Findings** An osteochondroma increases in size by the growth of the cartilage cap, which shows a histologic resemblance to the growing cartilage of the growth plate of a long bone.[10] The proliferating cartilage cells (Fig. 5–11, B and C) become oriented in irregular columns. The cells enlarge, and the tissue is ultimately invaded by vascular connective tissue from the underlying bone and replaced by an extending network of bone trabeculae. The uncalcified cartilage of the cap is not apparent in a conventional radiograph which shows only the outline of the bony part of the lesion (Fig. 5–13).

**Treatment** Many of these lesions can be monitored if they do not cause clinical problems. Surgical removal is indicated if the lesion becomes painful. Surgery may also be required if there is suspected encroachment upon the nerves and/or vessels, if there is a fracture, or if there is concern about the diagnosis. Surgical technique requires, when possible, an extracapsular or marginal type of resection including the entire cartilaginous cap and the overlying periosteum. In cases in which the local anatomy makes this type of resection less desirable, careful intralesional curettage may be the most realistic option. Great care must be taken not to contaminate the soft tissue with the cartilage lesion. After skeletal maturity, any change in the size of the lesion or in the symptoms must be regarded as a possible indication that malignant change is occurring.

### Multiple Osteochondromas (Multiple Cartilaginous Exostoses, Osteochondromatosis, Diaphyseal Aclasis)

This condition is classified as a type of bone dysplasia.[1] The lesion is an autosomal dominant, hereditary disorder. Clinically, osteochondromatosis becomes apparent in childhood as multiple bumps and protuberances, particularly around the knees, ankles, shoulders, and wrists.[4] Pain may be secondary to pressure on a nerve or vessel or result from the development of a bursa exostotica, as described for solitary osteochondroma. Deformities and shortening of bones caused by growth disturbance, particularly in the forearms and legs, are more common than in solitary lesions.

**Radiographic Findings** The radiographic findings are similar to those for a single osteochondroma. Sessile lesions are more frequent in multiple osteochondromatosis (Fig. 5–14). Malignant transformation to chondrosarcoma is more common, and usually the lesions at the shoulder girdle and around the pelvis are at greatest risk.[8,9] The clinical and radiographic signs of this complication are identical to those of malignant transformation of solitary osteochondroma.

Pathologic features of multiple osteochondromas

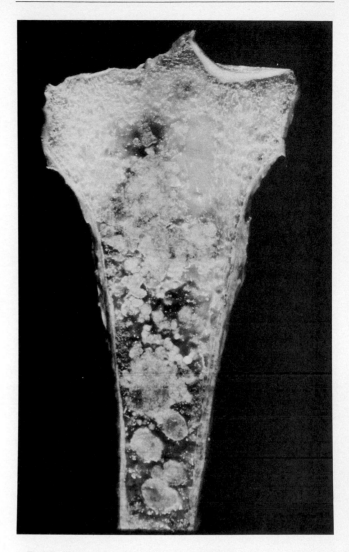

**Fig. 5–10** Enchondromatosis. Longitudinally sectioned tibia demonstrates multiple cartilaginous nodules.

are the same as those of solitary lesions.

**Treatment** Multiple osteochondromas are also treated in an individualized fashion. Like solitary osteochondromas, these lesions are more likely to recur in the younger child and surgery may be deferred, when possible, to a later date. However, the increased risk of malignant degeneration in this condition has to be considered.

### Chondroblastoma

Chondroblastoma is a benign bone tumor of immature cartilage cell derivation with preferential localization in the epiphyses of long bones, such as the humerus, tibia, and femur. It is rare, making up less than 1% of all primary bone tumors.[15] The clinical symptoms, in general, are nonspecific. Pain and swelling, usually present for several months, are the most

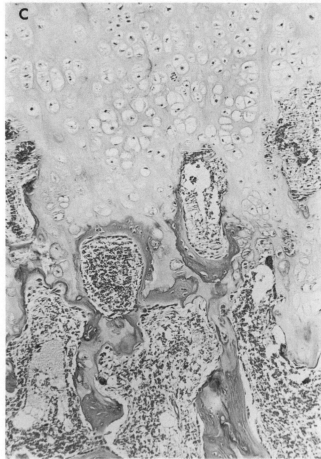

**Fig. 5–11** Pedunculated osteochondroma of distal femur. **A:** The continuity of the cortex of the femur is interrupted at the base of the lesion. The cortex extends on to the stalk of exostosis (arrows). Note that the medullary cavity of the host bone and osteochondroma openly communicate with each other. The calcifications are in the chondro-osseous zone of the stalk (open arrow). **B:** Low-power view of the cartilage cap (× 30). **C:** Higher-power view shows hypertrophic cartilage cells being replaced by endochondral bone (× 100).

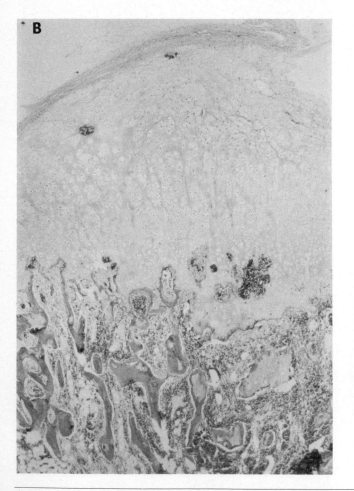

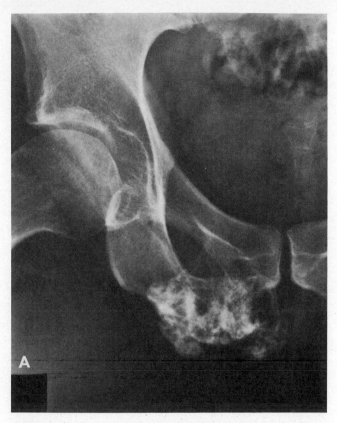

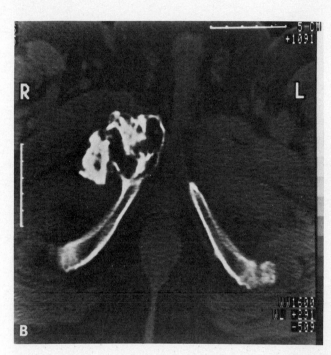

**Fig. 5–12**    Sessile osteochondroma of pelvis. **A:** Conventional radiograph shows a large, calcified, lobulated exostosis attached by the broad base into the right pubic bone. **B:** Computed tomographic scans demonstrate the communication of medullary cavities of the lesion and the host bone.

frequent complaints. Pathologic fracture as a primary manifestation is exceedingly rare.

The lesion occurs before skeletal maturity although some cases have been discovered after obliteration of the growth plate.

**Radiographic Findings**  The lesion arises eccentrically in the bone. The tumor is radiolucent and demarcated by a sclerotic margin. Often, scattered calcifications are present in the lesion (Fig. 5–15). These popcorn-like or punctate calcifications have been noted in 25% of cases.[16] If the calcifications are not apparent, conventional tomograms or a computed tomographic scan can be helpful[17] (Fig. 5–15C).

**Pathologic Findings**  Before the recognition of this entity by Jaffe and Lichtenstein in 1942,[18] it was usually referred to as "epiphyseal chondromatous giant cell tumor."[19] Although the tumor contains giant cells (and it is still sometimes misdiagnosed as giant-cell tumor), Jaffe and Lichtenstein argued that the giant cells were not part of the "primary pattern" of the tumor, and stressed its relationship to cartilage.

These tumors are characterized by highly cellular and relatively undifferentiated tissue made up of round and polygonal cells resembling chondroblasts with distinct outlines, together with multinucleated giant cells of the osteoclast type[18,20,21] (Fig. 5–15D). The presence of small amounts of cartilaginous intercellular matrix and foci of intercellular calcification are typical (Fig. 5–15E).

While the giant cells resemble the same cells in giant-cell tumor, the rounded appearance of the intervening cells contrasts with the spindle-shaped outline of stromal cells in giant-cell tumor. Although relatively little chondroid matrix is present in chondroblastoma, the cells show the same staining reaction for S-100 protein found in other cartilaginous and chondroid tumors.[11,12] The fine pattern of intercellular calcification (Fig. 5–15E) is a typical and diagnostically useful feature.

In a few chondroblastomas, a secondary aneurysmal bone cyst develops, and this can markedly influence the radiographic appearance of the lesion.

In rare cases, pulmonary metastases develop in the absence of any histologic evidence of malignancy either in the primary bone tumor or in the pulmonary metastases.[22-24]

**Treatment**  These lesions can be difficult to eradicate.

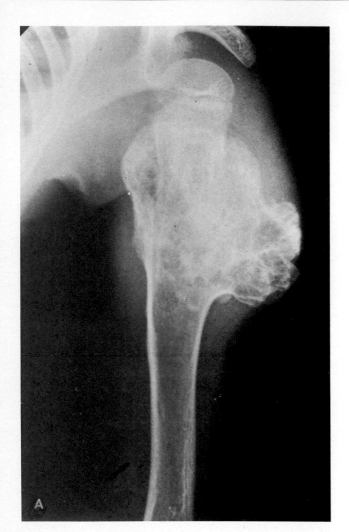

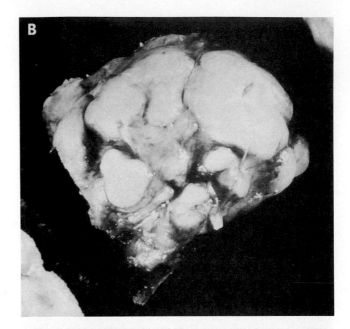

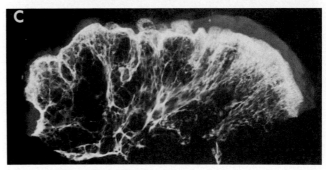

**Fig. 5–13** Sessile osteochondroma of upper humerus. **A:** Large, lobulated lesion with multiple calcifications at the periphery. **B:** Resected tumor, showing lobulated surface. **C:** Slab radiograph. Note the incomplete cap of uncalcified cartilage, deep to which is the network of bone trabeculae making up the bulk of the osteochondroma.

The preferred treatment is extracapsular marginal resection. However, because of their anatomic location in the skeletally immature patient, these lesions are most often treated by intralesional curettage and bone grafting with autogenous bone or allograft bank bone. In the more aggressive local lesion or a recurrent lesion, marginal or wide resection may be considered. Reconstruction may require an autograft, allograft, synthetic replacement, or a combination of these.

### Chondromyxoid Fibroma

This is a rare, benign tumor of cartilage derivation, occurring predominantly in adolescents and young adults, most often in the second or third decades of life.[25,26] It has a predilection for the bones of the lower extremities with the proximal tibia the most frequent site.[7,27] Chondromyxoid fibroma accounts for less than 1% of all primary bone tumors. A male-to-

female ratio of 2:1 has been noted.[10,26] Clinical symptoms include local pain and swelling and the presence of a peripherally located mass.

**Radiographic Findings** Chondromyxoid fibroma presents a characteristic radiographic picture of a radiolucent lesion with a sclerotic, scalloped margin, eccentrically located in the bone, and often eroding or ballooning the cortex (Fig. 5–16A). One characteristic observation is a buttress of periosteal new bone formation. The lesion may be indistinguishable from an aneurysmal bone cyst. Calcifications are not apparent radiologically. The size of the lesion usually ranges from 1 to 10 cm with an average of 3 to 4 cm.

**Pathologic Findings** This tumor is characterized by lobulated areas of spindle-shaped or stellate cells with abundant myxoid or chondroid intercellular material, separated by zones of more cellular tissue with a varying number of multinucleated giant cells.[25,28]

Large pleomorphic cells may be present and can result in confusion with chondrosarcoma. This entity was described by Jaffe and Lichtenstein in 1948.[25] Before their account many examples had probably been regarded as chondrosarcomas; it is now recognized that the tumor is benign. Reported cases of myxomas or myxofibromas of long bones are probably chondromyxoid fibromas. Histologically, the lobulated appearance of the tumor tissue, together with the presence of chondroid matrix and giant cells, is characteristic (Fig. 5–16B).

**Treatment** These lesions are difficult to eradicate fully by means of intralesional curettage and bone grafting with either allograft or autograft bone. However, this may be the initial treatment of choice because of the location of the lesion and the age of the patient. More aggressive or recurrent lesions may require marginal or wide resection.

## Chondrosarcoma

Chondrosarcoma is a malignant tumor characterized by the formation of cartilage by the tumor cells. Several types of chondrosarcoma are recognized, with different clinical, radiographic, and pathologic features.

### Central (Medullary) Chondrosarcoma

This is the most common type of chondrosarcoma. It usually occurs in adults after the third decade of life. The most frequent locations are the pelvis and the long bones, particularly the femur and humerus, but chondrosarcoma may develop in any part of the skeleton.[29] Males are affected twice as frequently as females. Most chondrosarcomas are slowly growing tumors, often discovered accidentally. Occasionally pain and local tenderness may be present.

**Radiographic Findings** The typical chondrosarcoma shows a characteristic expansion of the medullary portion of the bone, with thickening of the cortex and endosteal scalloping often associated with popcorn-like, comma-shaped, or annular calcifications[3] (Fig. 5–17). Occasionally, a soft-tissue mass may be present (Fig. 5–18). In exceptional cases, the tumor can be indistinguishable from an enchondroma, particularly in the early stage. For this reason, all central cartilage tumors in long bones, particularly in adult patients, should be regarded as malignant until proven benign.[30]

**Pathologic Findings** Chondrosarcoma is a malignant tumor characterized by the formation of cartilage, but not bone, by the tumor cells.[2,8] It is distinguished from chondroma by the presence of more cellular and pleomorphic tumor tissue and by appreciable numbers of plump cells with large or double nuclei.

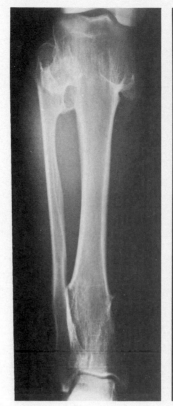
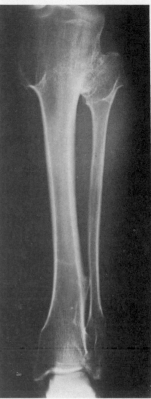

**Fig. 5–14** An 18-year-old boy with multiple, hereditary cartilaginous exostoses. The osteochondromas are predominantly sessile.

Mitotic cells are infrequent.

Chondrosarcoma includes tumors with a wide range of behavior, from slowly growing relatively benign lesions to highly malignant metastasizing tumors. There is a broad parallel between histologic structure and clinical behavior, and it is appropriate to distinguish between low-grade, intermediate, and high-grade chondrosarcomas. This histologic distinction is based on the cellularity of the tumor tissue, the degree of pleomorphism of the cells and nuclei, and the number of mitoses present.[31]

The cartilaginous nature of a well-differentiated (i.e., low-grade) chondrosarcoma is often clear from its gross appearance (Figs. 5–17C, 5–18B, 5–19C, and 5–20C). The tumor tissue is lobulated and has a bluish, translucent appearance. Foci of calcification appear as white, chalky areas. Microscopically, the tissue of a well-differentiated chondrosarcoma differs only slightly from that of an enchondroma (Fig. 5–21A). Intercellular cartilage matrix is abundant in each, but the malignant tumor is more cellular, and the tumor cells are larger and more variable in appearance than those of the benign tumor. Cell nuclei, too, instead of being small and staining darkly,

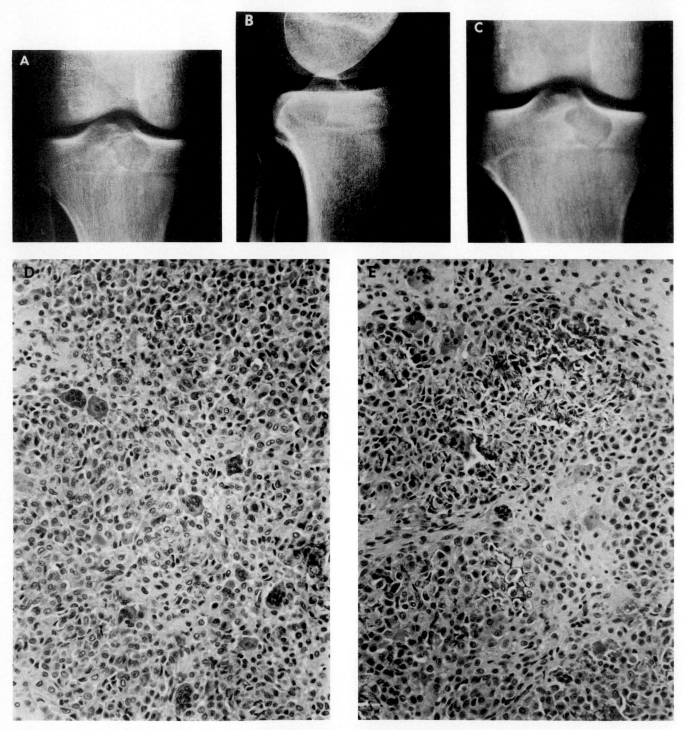

**Fig. 5–15** A 15-year-old girl with chondroblastoma of proximal tibia. Anteroposterior (**A**) and lateral (**B**) radiographs of the knee show an osteolytic, well-defined, eccentrically located lesion in the proximal epiphysis of right tibia. A tomographic scan (**C**) demonstrates small, punctate calcifications within the tumor matrix. **D:** Tumor tissue consisting of rounded cells with scattered giant cells (× 235). **E:** One area shows chondroid matrix, with fine intercellular calcifications (× 235).

are larger and have a more dispersed pattern of chromatin. When present, bizarre cells with pleomorphic nuclei (Fig. 5–21B) are clear evidence of malignancy. A more subtle indication, according to some authorities, is the presence of an appreciable number of binucleate cells.[4,32] Mitoses are not always to be found in low-grade chondrosarcomas. In many of these tumors, only part of the lesion shows histologic

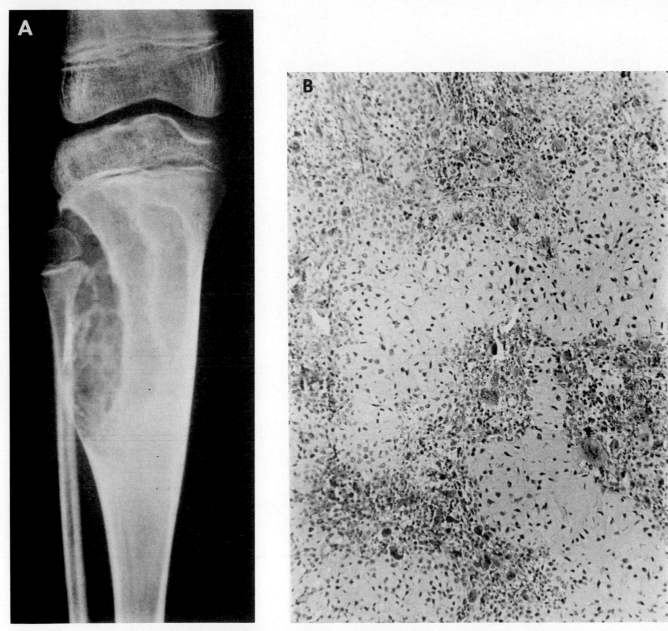

**Fig. 5–16** Chondromyxoid fibroma of tibia. **A:** Large, osteolytic lesion with scalloped, sclerotic border extends from the metaphysis into the diaphysis and balloons the lateral cortex. Well-organized buttress of periosteal new bone is particularly well demonstrated at the distal end of the tumor. **B:** Tumor tissue consisting of lobulated areas of chondroid tissue separated by more cellular tissue containing giant cells (× 72).

evidence of malignancy, and it may be necessary to examine many sections before an unequivocal diagnosis can be made. Because of this, a biopsy report of "chondroma" should not be accepted without the most careful consideration if the clinical and radiologic findings suggest malignancy.

High-grade chondrosarcomas show less resemblance to normal cartilage, both grossly and microscopically. Cellular and nuclear pleomorphism is more pronounced (Fig. 5–21C), and numerous mitot-ic cells may be present. Intercellular cartilage matrix may be less abundant, and the tumor cells, not necessarily enclosed in lacunae, may be spindle-shaped instead of rounded. The tissue of more malignant chondrosarcomas may be highly vascular, in contrast to the tissue of an enchondroma or a low-grade chondrosarcoma.

Chondrosarcomas frequently show evidence of focal calcification (Fig. 5–21D), and this may provide a reliable radiologic indication of the diagnosis.

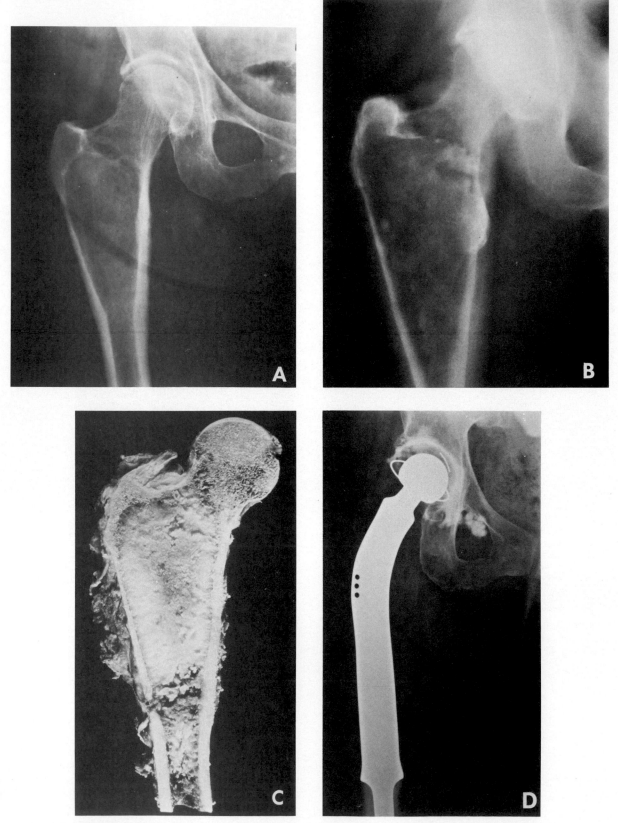

**Fig. 5–17**    Typical central chondrosarcoma of the femur. Conventional radiograph **(A)** and tomogram **(B)** demonstrate an expansile lesion of the medullary portion of bone with annular and punctate calcifications. The medial cortex is thickened. Endosteal scalloping is characteristic of cartilage tumor. In a longitudinally divided femur solid cartilaginous tumor expands the upper part of the shaft **(C)**. The proximal femur has been resected and custom-made prosthesis inserted **(D)**.

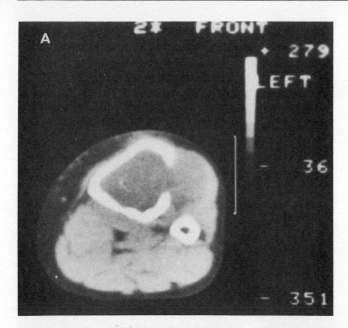

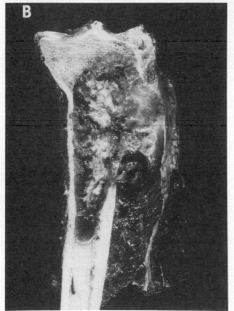

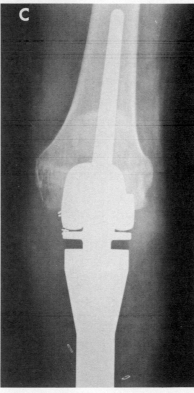

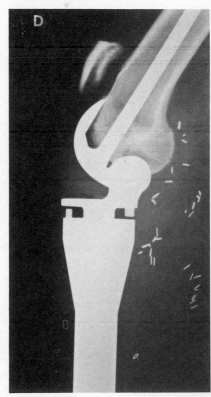

**Fig. 5–18**  Chondrosarcoma of proximal tibia. **A:** Computed tomographic scan demonstrates destruction of the cortex and extension of the tumor into the soft tissue. The latter finding was not well defined on the conventional radiograph. **B:** Longitudinally divided tibia with lobulated cartilaginous tissue in marrow cavity and extending to the adjacent soft tissues. **C and D:** The proximal tibia and distal femur have been resected and replaced by a custom-made, hinge knee prosthesis.

Particularly in well-differentiated, slowly growing tumors, the areas of calcification may undergo replacement by endochondral bone, and this is responsible for the characteristic annular radiographic opacities.

In contrast to benign cartilage tumors, chondrosarcomas show an invasive pattern of growth, extending in the marrow spaces of cancellous bone and in the vascular canals of cortical bone. This pattern of extension, whether apparent grossly or in histologic sections (Fig. 5–21E), is an important diagnostic feature of chondrosarcoma and may indicate this diagnosis when a limited sample of tissue fails to show definite cytologic evidence of malignancy.

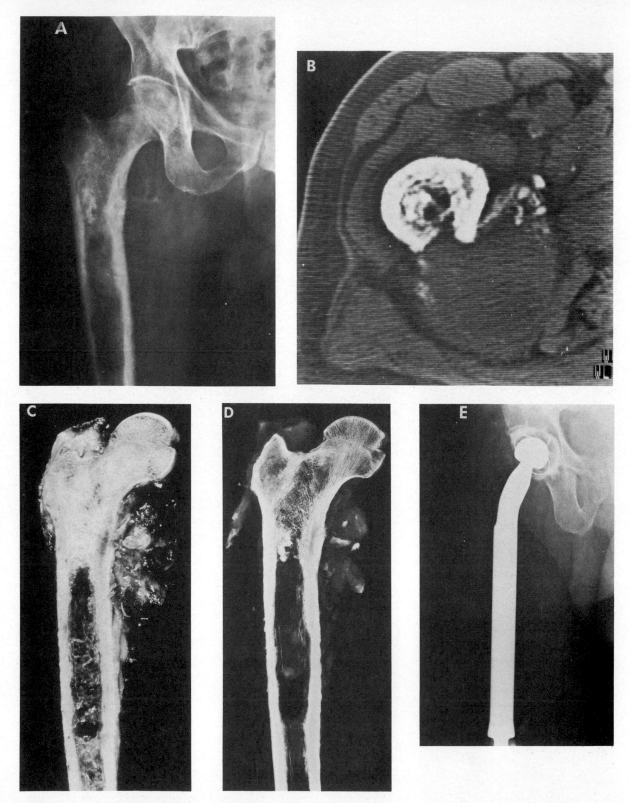

**Fig. 5–19** Chondrosarcoma developing in enchondroma of femur. **A:** Large osteolytic lesion in the medullary portion of right femur. Calcifications in the upper portion represent residue of benign enchondroma. Destructive changes in the distal part of tumor are secondary to chondrosarcoma. **B:** Computed tomographic scan demonstrates a large soft-tissue extension of the tumor with calcifications at the periphery of the mass. Medullary calcifications are also well demonstrated. **C:** Longitudinally divided femur. The marrow cavity is occupied by tumor tissue, some of which has been lost in the preparation of the specimen. **D:** Slab radiograph. The predominantly lytic tumor is eroding the endosteal surface of the cortex; a soft-tissue mass is evident on the medial aspect of the femoral neck. The highly calcified nodule at the upper part of the tumor is a residue of the enchondroma.

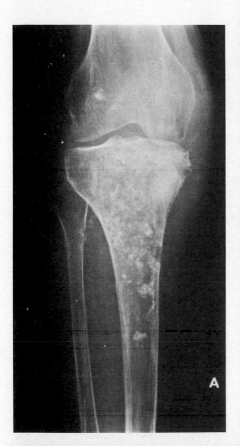
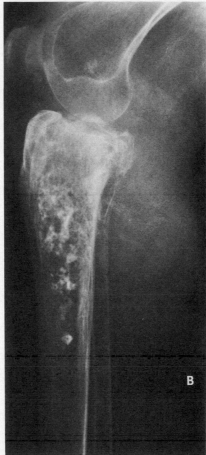
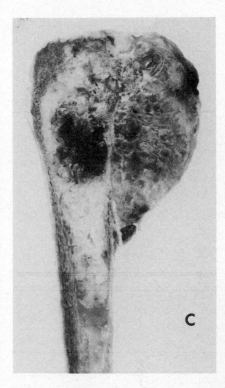
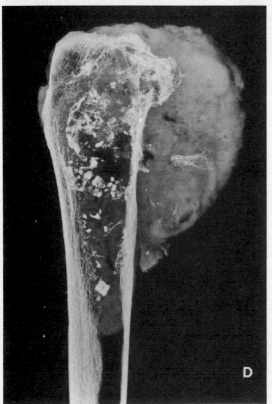

**Fig. 5–20**  Chondrosarcoma developing in enchondromatosis. Anteroposterior (**A**) radiograph shows a large, destructive lesion in the upper tibia with multiple annular and punctate calcifications, characteristic of cartilage tumor. The soft-tissue mass is best demonstrated on the lateral view (**B**). Additional calcific densities are apparent in the enchondromas of the distal femur (arrow). In a longitudinally divided tibia (**C**), the marrow cavity is occupied by lobulated cartilaginous tumor tissue extending through the cortex to form a large subperiosteal mass. Slab radiograph (**D**) shows the heavily calcified opacities within the medullary part of the tumor. These structures, evident in the clinical radiographs, are residues of the preexisting enchondromas.

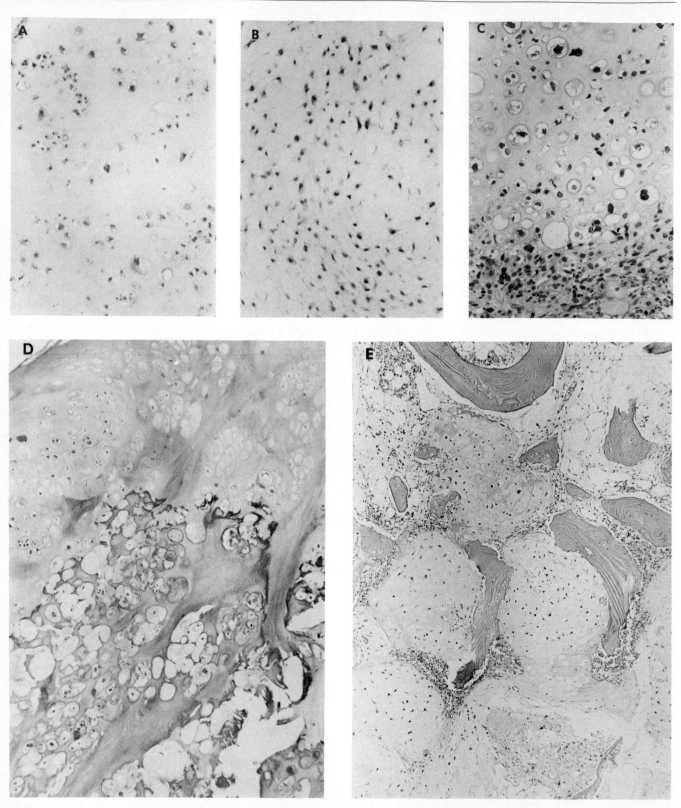

**Fig. 5–21** Histology of chondrosarcoma. **A:** Tissue from a low-grade chondrosarcoma. Abundant cartilage matrix is present and many cells are in round lacunae. A comparison with Fig. 5–4A shows the greater cellularity of the chondrosarcoma and the presence of larger cells with larger and less regular nuclei (× 235). **B:** Tissue from a more malignant chondrosarcoma. In this field the intercellular matrix is less obviously cartilaginous: numerous binucleate and frankly pleomorphic cells are present (× 235). **C:** Tissue from a frankly malignant (high-grade) chondrosarcoma. In this field part of the tissue is recognizable as cartilage, but this merges with pleomorphic spindle-cell tissue (× 235). **D:** An area of calcification, indicated by darker and granular staining of the intercellular matrix, in a low-grade tumor (× 100). **E:** An area where marrow spaces are invaded by tumor tissue. Some bone trabeculae remain (× 100).

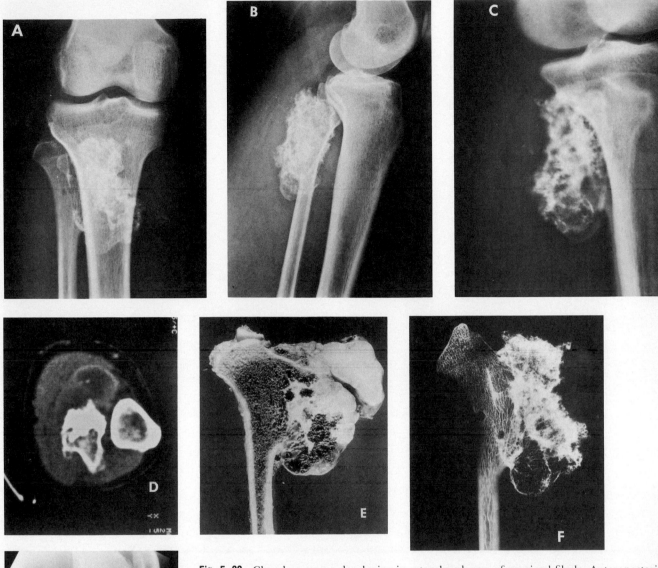

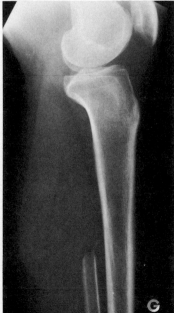

**Fig. 5–22** Chondrosarcoma developing in osteochondroma of proximal fibula. Anteroposterior **(A)** and lateral **(B)** radiographs show a large, lobulated, calcified bony mass attached to the proximal fibula. Lateral tomogram **(C)** demonstrates scattered calcifications within thick cartilaginous cap (arrow), displaced from the main bulk of tumor. Computed tomographic scan **(D)** shows increased thickness of the cartilaginous cap of osteochondroma and dispersed calcifications at the periphery of the mass. Longitudinally divided fibula **(E)** shows large osteochondroma with thick cartilage cap. Slab radiograph **(F)** shows heavy calcification of the deeper part of the lesion. A postoperative radiograph **(G)** with the proximal fibula resected.

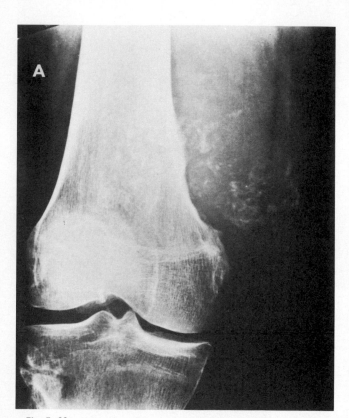
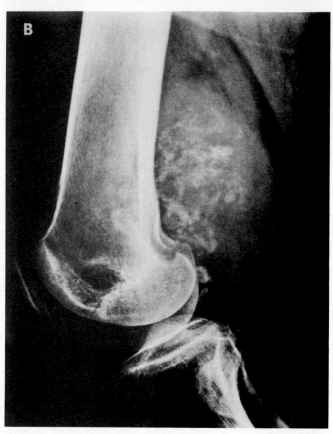

**Fig. 5–23** A 34-year-old man with piosteal chondrosarcoma. Anteroposterior **(A)** and lateral **(B)** radiographs demonstrate a large mass adjacent to the posterolateral cortex of distal femur with scattered punctate and annular opacities.

### Secondary Chondrosarcoma

The term secondary chondrosarcoma is applied to any tumor that arises as a result of malignant change in a benign cartilage lesion, such as an osteochondroma (Fig. 5–22) or enchondroma (Fig. 5–19).[8] Malignant change in solitary enchondroma or osteochondroma is rare. It is more frequent in multiple enchondromatosis or multiple osteochondromatosis. In the latter condition, as many as 10% of cases progress to chondrosarcoma.[4,8]

Secondary chondrosarcomas develop at a somewhat earlier age than primary chondrosarcomas and are of low-grade malignancy, with a relatively benign course and a favorable prognosis.

Clinical features that suggest the possibility of malignant degeneration in an osteochondroma include otherwise unexplained pain and the continued or accelerated growth of the lesion after skeletal maturity. In addition, the rapid growth of a chondrosarcoma can be associated with increased isotopic uptake in a radionuclide bone scan.[33,34] It must be remembered, however, that many benign osteochondromas show increased uptake because of the endochondral ossification occurring at the base of the cartilage cap, and such activity is therefore not always a reliable indication of malignancy.

Additional features that suggest the development of chondrosarcoma include an unusually thick (more than 1 cm) cartilage cap[35,36] and the presence of dispersed calcifications in its tissue.[37] The cytologic features of malignancy include increased cellularity of the tissue, the presence of plump cells with large nuclei, frequent binucleate cells, and pleomorphic and mitotic cells (Fig. 5–21, A to C). When malignant change occurs, cytologic evidence of its existence may be present in only part of the lesion. Thus, it is often necessary to examine many histologic samples of tissue from the cartilaginous cap of an osteochondroma when malignancy is suspected.

### Periosteal (Juxtacortical) Chondrosarcoma

Most primary chondrosarcomas arise centrally in bone, but in rare instances a tumor may originate in the periosteal (juxtacortical) location[38,39] (Fig. 5–23). These neoplasms have the same general radiologic and pathologic features as a central chondrosarcoma. The rare "periosteal osteosarcomas," which also occur on the external surface of long bones, consist largely of cartilage, and can be confused with periosteal chondrosarcoma.[40] Some authorities believe that the two tumors are identical.

## Dedifferentiated Chondrosarcoma

A low-grade chondrosarcoma may occasionally undergo transformation into a rapidly growing aggressive sarcoma in which the tumor tissue no longer retains cartilaginous features. These lesions are termed dedifferentiated chondrosarcomas[41-43] and are the most malignant of all the cartilage tumors. The age and sites of preference are similar to those for conventional chondrosarcoma.

Typically, the patient has had pain for a long time before the onset of rapid swelling and local tenderness. The prolonged pain is probably the result of a slowly growing lesion while the swelling and tenderness may be related to the development of a rapidly growing and more malignant tumor.

**Radiographic Findings** The radiographic features of dedifferentiated chondrosarcoma are variable (Figs. 5–24 and 5–25). One aspect is the radiographic characteristics of a conventional central chondrosarcoma; other features of this tumor are the destructive changes in the bone and the extension of the lesion into the soft tissue to produce a large mass. The focal calcifications in the tumor identify its cartilaginous nature. The hallmark of this lesion is the aggressive portion of the sarcoma engrafted on a benign-appearing chondrosarcoma (Fig. 5–24). The area showing the more long-term nature of the cartilage tumor can usually be distinguished from the aggressive lesion. The large size of the soft-tissue mass and the presence of metastases are also helpful signs in the diagnosis.

**Pathologic Findings** In addition to cartilage, these tumors contain highly cellular sarcomatous tissue which is believed to develop from the cartilaginous component by a process of dedifferentiation. The dedifferentiated tissue may have the appearance of fibrosarcoma, osteosarcoma, or malignant fibrous histiocytoma.[41-44] The histologic diagnosis depends on the identification of the two or more types of tissue, which are often quite distinct from one another. The cartilaginous component is often of low-grade malignancy. In most reported cases, the dedifferentiated component has the histologic structure of malignant fibrous histiocytoma[42] (Fig. 5–24, E and F).

## Mesenchymal Chondrosarcoma

This lesion is exceedingly rare and only 15 (0.24%) cases were noted in the 6,221 tumors reported by Dahlin[8] and Dahlin and Henderson.[45] More than 50% occur in the second and third decades of life.[46] Rarely, these tumors can originate in soft tissues.[47]

**Radiographic Findings** The radiographic characteristics are often nonspecific. However, if two striking features are present, namely, the classic appearance of a chondrosarcoma and a soft-tissue or bony component resembling a round-cell sarcoma, the diagnosis may be proposed[48] (Fig. 5–26A).

**Pathologic Findings** Mesenchymal chondrosarcoma is a highly malignant tumor, characterized by the presence of areas of differentiated cartilage, together with highly vascular spindle-cell or round-cell mesenchymal tissue.[46,48,49]

The microscopic appearances of the two histologic components are strikingly different (Fig. 5–26E). The cellular mesenchymal component, in the absence of recognizable cartilaginous tissue, is sometimes mistaken for Ewing's sarcoma or a malignant vascular tumor (hemangiopericytoma).

## Clear-Cell Chondrosarcoma

A rare and recently recognized variant of chondrosarcoma is the clear-cell chondrosarcoma.[50-52] It is more frequent in males than in females (2:1) and the tumor usually affects patients in the third to fifth decades of life. Many lesions involve the proximal end of the humerus and the proximal or distal end of the femur.

**Radiographic Findings** Clear-cell chondrosarcoma is a predominantly lytic lesion with a sclerotic border and a striking resemblance to chondroblastoma[53] (Fig. 5–27). Occasionally, it may be indistinguishable from the conventional central sarcoma (Fig. 5–28A). It is considered a low-grade malignant neoplasm.

**Pathologic Findings** Histologically, this tumor differs from other chondrosarcomas in that the tumor cells are larger and rounded, with clear or vacuolated cytoplasm (Fig. 5–28B). It may contain areas of calcification (Fig. 5–28C) and these are sometimes sufficiently pronounced to be apparent radiologically.[2] Trabeculae of reactive bone are a rather distinctive feature of this tumor, as is the presence of numerous osteoclast giant cells (Fig. 5–28D). In some cases, the whole tumor shows these distinctive histologic features; in others, areas of conventional chondrosarcoma are present.

Clear-cell chondrosarcomas are of relatively low-grade malignancy, and they have sometimes been confused with chondroblastomas or osteoblastomas.[52] After adequate surgical resection, recurrence is unusual, although metastases have been reported in some cases.

## Treatment of Chondrosarcoma

The treatment of chondrosarcoma is primarily surgical. The objective is to eradicate local disease in such a fashion that the patient's survival is not compromised.[54]

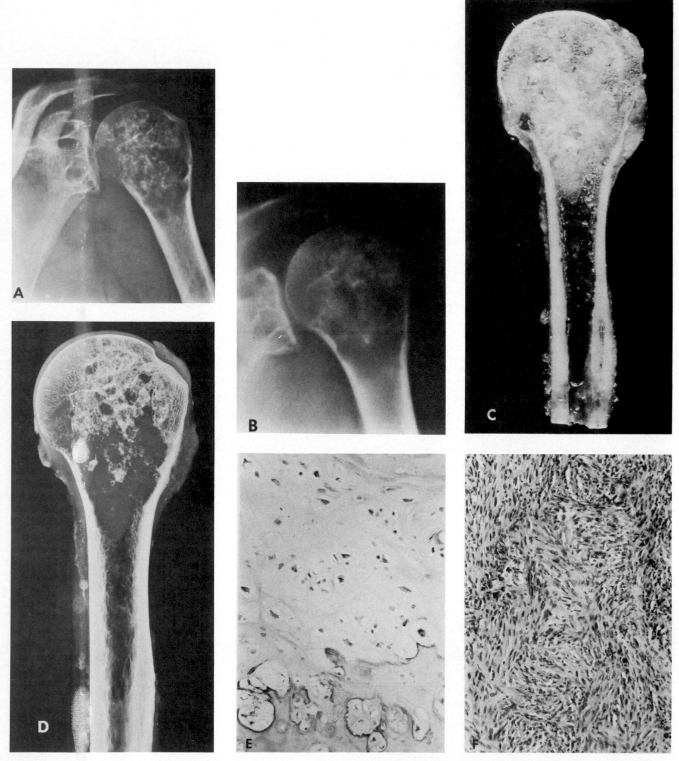

**Fig. 5–24** A 64-year-old man with dedifferentiated chondrosarcoma of the proximal humerus. **A:** Conventional radiograph demonstrates an ill-defined lesion in the humeral head, extending into the neck and shaft. **B:** Trispiral tomogram. The proximal part of the lesion shows typical annular calcifications and scalloping of the endocortex frequent in chondrosarcoma. The distal part of the lesion demonstrates more aggressive features, breaking through the posterolateral cortex and extending into the soft tissues. **C:** Longitudinally divided humerus. The head of the humerus is occupied by loculated cartilaginous tumor tissue that extends through the cortex to the adjacent soft tissue. **D:** Slab radiograph. Note the areas of calcification in the tumor tissue. **E:** Cartilaginous tumor tissue from the central part of the lesion. The darker tissue in the lower part of the field represents an area of calcification. **F:** Dedifferentiated spindle-cell tissue from the subperiosteal mass with the histologic structure of malignant fibrous histiocytoma.

Chondrosarcomas can often be treated by a wide resection, either by means of a wide local resection (limb-sparing)[55] or by wide amputation.[56] There may be selected cases in which chondrosarcoma can be appropriately treated by marginal resection or by radical resection. It is essential that each procedure be individualized for the patient. This includes not only the nature of the surgical procedure, but the different modes of reconstruction, since patients have different life styles and goals. To maximize the chance of success, it is crucial that the initial biopsy be done in a thoughtful and careful fashion, preferably by the surgeon who will be doing the definitive procedure.[57] With this approach adequate tissue for histologic examination will be obtained and potential contamination of normal tissues will be minimized or eliminated. Consequently, the definitive surgical procedure, particularly if limb-sparing is considered, will not be jeopardized. Whether to perform a needle biopsy or an open biopsy depends on the individual situation as well as on the preference and experience of the surgeon and the pathologist. If there is any question of obtaining representative diagnostic tissue it is best to rely on a small open biopsy. An irreversible procedure should not be performed solely on the basis of a frozen-section evaluation, but only after careful review of the definitive sections in relations to the clinical and radiologic information. Preoperative staging is vital.[58] The nature of the surgical procedure and the type of reconstruction, if limb-sparing is chosen, depend on many factors. These include not only the specific bone and the anatomic region of that bone, but also the compartmental status of the lesion, the grade of the lesion, the integrity of the vital neurovascular structures and adjacent soft tissue, and the expectations and goals of the patient. While most chondrosarcomas are of skeletal origin, the same considerations apply to the rarer extraskeletal lesions.

Limb-sparing surgery creates different reconstructive options. These include a synthetic implant, allograft, autograft, vascularized autograft, or a combination of these. The option of performing an arthrodesis or maintaining a mobile joint again depends on the individual situation. Sometimes, in lesions of the clavicle, fibula, or pelvis, wide resection of a limb-sparing type may be achieved without reconstruction[59] (Figs. 5–22G and 5–26E).

Chondrosarcoma of the proximal humerus can often be treated with a modified Tikhoff-Linberg procedure.[60] This is a wide resection of the proximal humerus, including an extra-articular resection of the glenohumeral joint. This procedure is done as an alternative to amputation and can be seriously contemplated if the neurovascular structures in the region of the brachial artery and vein are uninvolved by the tumor.[61] Reconstruction can be done with a

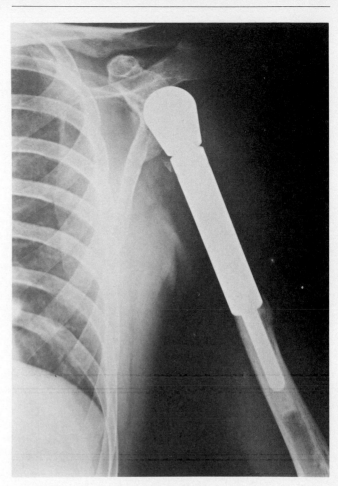

**Fig. 5–25** Postoperative radiograph from another example of dedifferentiated chondrosarcoma of humerus, treated by resection and insertion of metallic prosthesis.

metallic implant spacer (Fig. 5–25), allograft, or autograft. The goal of the surgical procedure is to eradicate the neoplasm and maintain good function of the hand and elbow. Motion at the shoulder region will be passive since the deltoid mechanism and axillary nerve are removed as part of the surgical procedure. However, reconstruction can also be done by means of an arthrodesis with either dual fibular grafts or an allograft. Sometimes a chondrosarcoma involves the scapula in such a fashion that total scapulectomy by itself can be performed, and often no reconstruction is necessary. However, in some recent cases a prosthetic scapula has been used in selected neoplastic resections of this region.

Lesions that involve the proximal femur can often be treated in a limb-sparing fashion if the hip joint is uninvolved.[62] This requires a proximal femur resection of a wide nature; reconstruction can be done with a metallic implant (Fig. 5–17D), allograft, or a combination of these.[63,64] However, there may be

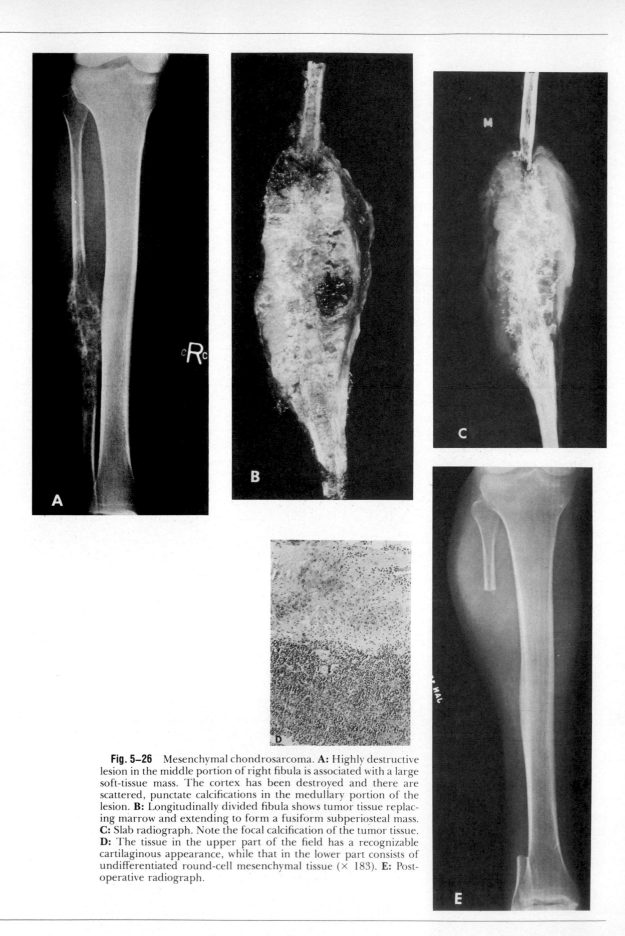

**Fig. 5–26** Mesenchymal chondrosarcoma. **A:** Highly destructive lesion in the middle portion of right fibula is associated with a large soft-tissue mass. The cortex has been destroyed and there are scattered, punctate calcifications in the medullary portion of the lesion. **B:** Longitudinally divided fibula shows tumor tissue replacing marrow and extending to form a fusiform subperiosteal mass. **C:** Slab radiograph. Note the focal calcification of the tumor tissue. **D:** The tissue in the upper part of the field has a recognizable cartilaginous appearance, while that in the lower part consists of undifferentiated round-cell mesenchymal tissue (× 183). **E:** Postoperative radiograph.

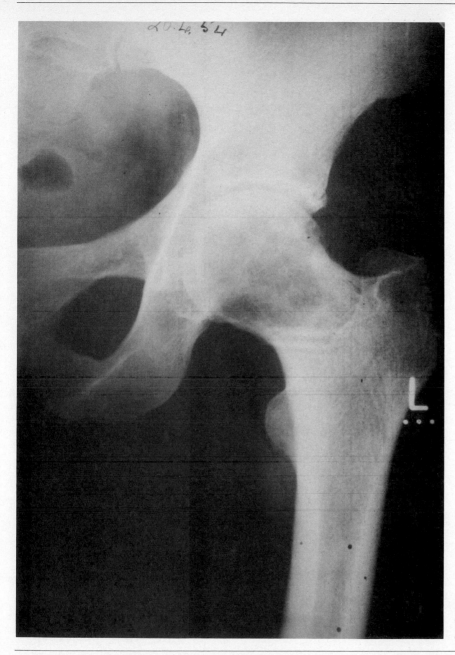

**Fig. 5–27** Osteolytic lesion with sclerotic border in the left femoral head. The resemblance to benign chondroblastoma is striking but the lesion proved to be a clear-cell chondrosarcoma.

some cases in which wide resection in the form of amputation is indicated. This is especially true if there is extensive soft-tissue involvement. With respect to the distal femur and proximal tibia, again wide resection of a limb-sparing type can be done if the posterior tibial nerve and popliteal artery and vein are uninvolved. In these situations, too, the preference of the surgeon and the patient should determine the type of reconstruction, whether it be by metal synthetic implant (Fig. 5–18, C and D), allograft, or arthrodesis.[65-67] However, if the neurovascular bundle is thought to be involved, wide amputation is certainly be the appropriate surgical procedure. The occasional intercalary chondrosarcoma can be treated with wide resection of the limb-sparing type using a metallic implant, allograft, or vascularized autograft.[68]

Finally, it is necessary to consider the rare problem of chondrosarcoma occurring in a long bone of a growing, skeletally immature patient. In this unusual circumstance there may be a role for wide local resection and reconstruction, using the expandable prosthesis as an internal spacer until skeletal maturity is attained.[69]

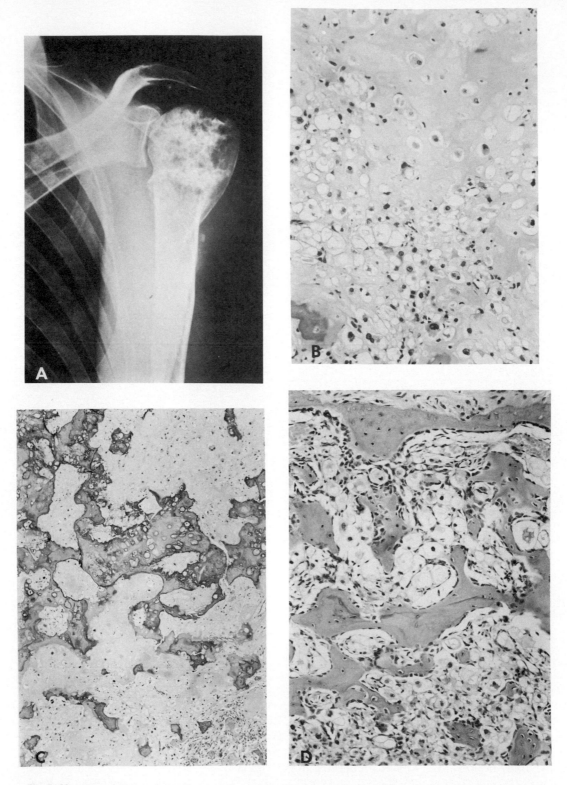

**Fig. 5–28**    Clear-cell chondrosarcoma of the proximal humerus. **A:** Anteroposterior radiograph shows a lytic lesion with multiple calcifications and healed pathologic fracture through the neck of left humerus. The appearance is that of conventional chondrosarcoma. **B:** An area of tumor showing the characteristic large and vacuolated cells. Intercellular cartilage matrix is also present (× 235). **C:** An area with prominent calcification of the cartilage matrix (× 72). **D:** An area with vacuolated cells and reactive bone trabeculae but without cartilage matrix (× 183).

## References

1. Murray RO, Jacobson HG: *The Radiology of Bone Diseases*, ed 2. New York, Churchill Livingstone Inc, 1977.
2. Sissons HA, Murray RO, Kemp HBS: *Orthopaedic Diagnosis*. Berlin, Springer-Verlag, 1984.
3. Wilner D: *Radiology of Bone Tumors and Allied Disorders*. Philadelphia, Lea and Febiger, 1982, vol 1.
4. Jaffe HL: *Tumors and Tumorous Conditions of the Bones and Joints*. Philadelphia, Lea and Febiger, 1968.
5. Spjut HJ, Dorfman HD, Fechner RE, et al: Tumors of bone and cartilage, in *Atlas of Tumor Pathology*, Fascicle 5. Washington, DC, Armed Forces Institute of Pathology, 1971.
6. Schajowicz F, Ackerman LV, Sissons HA: *Histological Typing of Bone Tumors*. Geneva, Switzerland, World Health Organization, 1972.
7. Huvos AG: *Bone Tumors, Diagnosis, Treatment and Prognosis*. Philadelphia, WB Saunders Co, 1979.
8. Dahlin DC: *Bone Tumors: General Aspects and Data on 6221 Cases*, ed 3. Springfield, Illinois, Charles C Thomas, 1981.
9. Schajowicz F: *Tumors and Tumorlike Lesions of Bone and Joints*. Berlin, Springer-Verlag, 1981.
10. Steiner GC: Benign cartilage tumors, in Taveras JM, Ferrucci JT (eds): *Radiology: Diagnosis–Imaging–Intervention*. Philadelphia, JB Lippincott Co, 1986, vol 5, chap 78.
11. Nakamura Y, Becker LE, Marks A: S-100 protein in tumors of cartilage and bone. *Cancer* 1983;52:1820.
12. Monda L, Wick MR: S-100 protein immunostaining in the differential diagnosis of chondroblastoma. *Hum Pathol* 1985;16:287–293.
13. Lichtenstein L, Hall JE: Periosteal chondroma: A distinctive benign cartilage tumor. *J Bone Joint Surg* 1952;34A:691–697.
14. Shapiro F: Ollier's disease–an assessment of angular deformity, shortening, and pathological fracture in 21 patients. *J Bone Joint Surg* 1982;64A:95.
15. Bloem JL, Mulder JD: Chondroblastoma: A clinical and radiological study of 104 cases. *Skeletal Radiol* 1985;14:1–9.
16. McLeod RA, Beabout JW: The roentgenographic features of chondroblastoma. *AJR* 1973;118:464–471.
17. Hudson TM, Hawkins IF Jr: Radiological evaluation of chondroblastoma. *Radiology* 1981;139:1–10.
18. Jaffe HL, Lichtenstein L: Benign chondroblastoma of bone: Reinterpretation of so-called calcifying or chondromatous giant cell tumor. *Am J Pathol* 1942;18:969–991.
19. Codman EA: Epiphyseal chondromatous giant cell tumors of the upper end of the humerus. *Surg Gynecol Obstet* 1931;52:543–548.
20. Dahlin DC, Ivins JC: Benign chondroblastoma. *Cancer* 1972;30:401–413.
21. Schajowicz F, Gallardo H: Epiphyseal chondroblastoma of bone: A clinicopathological study of 69 cases. *J Bone Joint Surg* 1970;42B:205–226.
22. Mirra JM, Ulich TR, Eckardt JJ, et al: "Aggressive" chondroblastoma. *Clin Orthop* 1983;178:276–284.
23. Riddell RJ, Louis CJ, Bromberger NA: Pulmonary metastases from chondroblastoma of the tibia. *J Bone Joint Surg* 1973;55B:848.
24. Huvos AG, Higinbotham NL, Marcove RC, et al: Aggressive chondroblastoma: Review of the literature on aggressive behavior and metastases with a report of one new case. *Clin Orthop* 1977;126:266–272.
25. Jaffe HL, Lichtenstein L: Chondromyxoid fibroma of bone: A distinctive benign tumor likely to be mistaken especially for chondrosarcoma. *Arch Pathol* 1948;45:541–551.
26. Feldman F, Hecht HI, Johnston AD: Chondromyxoid fibroma of bone. *Radiology* 1970;94:249–263.
27. Klein GM: Chondromyxoid fibroma: An unusual location. *Clin Orthop* 1982;164:249.
28. Schajowicz F, Gallardo H: Chondromyxoid fibroma. *J Bone Joint Surg* 1971;53B:198–216.
29. Henderson ED, Dahlin DC: Chondrosarcoma of bone: A study of 280 cases. *J Bone Joint Surg* 1963;45A:1450–1458.
30. Reiter FB, Ackerman LV, Staple TW: Central chondrosarcoma of the appendicular skeleton. *Radiology* 1972;105:525–530.
31. Evans HL, Ayala AG, Romsdahl MM: Prognostic factors in chondrosarcoma of bone. *Cancer* 1977;40:818–883.
32. Lichtenstein L, Jaffe HL: Chondrosarcoma of bone. *Am J Pathol* 1943;19:553–589.
33. Bouvier JF, Chassard JL, Brunat-Mentigny M, et al: Radionuclide bone imaging in diaphyseal aclasis with malignant change. *Cancer* 1986;57:2280–2284.
34. Hudson TM, Chew FS, Manaster BJ: Scintigraphy of benign exostoses and exostotic chondrosarcomas. *AJR* 1983;140:581–586.
35. Lichtenstein L: *Bone Tumors*, ed 5. St Louis, CV Mosby Co.
36. Hudson TM, Springfield DS, Spanier SS, et al: Benign exostoses and exostotic chondrosarcomas: Evaluation of cartilage thickness by CT. *Radiology* 1984;152:595–599.
37. Norman A, Sissons HA: Radiographic hallmarks of peripheral chondrosarcoma. *Radiology* 1984;151:589–596.
38. Schajowicz F: Juxtacortical chondrosarcoma. *J Bone Joint Surg* 1978;59B:473–480.
39. Unni KK, Dahlin DC, Beabout JW: Periosteal osteosarcoma. *Cancer* 1976;37:2476–2485.
40. Bertoni F, Boriani S, Laus M, et al: Periosteal chondrosarcoma and periosteal osteosarcoma. *J Bone Joint Surg* 1982;64B:370–376.
41. Dahlin DC, Beabout JW: Dedifferentiation of low grade chondrosarcomas. *Cancer* 1971;28:461–466.
42. McCarty EF, Dorfman HD: Chondrosarcoma of bone with dedifferentiation: A study of 18 cases. *Hum Pathol* 1982;13:34–36.
43. Johnson S, Tetu B, Ayala AG, et al: Chondrosarcoma with additional mesenchymal component (dedifferentiated chondrosarcoma). *Cancer* 1986;58:278–286.
44. Sanerkin NG, Woods CG: Fibrosarcomata and malignant fibrous histiocytomata arising in relation to enchondromata. *J Bone Joint Surg* 1979;61B:366–372.
45. Dahlin DC, Henderson ED: Mesenchymal chondrosarcoma: Further observations on a new entity. *Cancer* 1962;15:410–417.
46. Henderson ED, Dahlin DC: Mesenchymal chondrosarcoma. *J Bone Joint Surg* 1963;45A:1450–1458.
47. Nakashima Y, Unni KK, Shives TC, et al: Mesenchymal chondrosarcoma of bone and soft tissue. *Cancer* 1986;57:2444–2453.
48. Harwood AR, Kralbich JJ, Fornasier VL: Mesenchymal chondrosarcoma: A report of 17 cases. *Clin Orthop* 1980;158:144.
49. Huvos AG, Rosen G, Dabska M, et al: Mesenchymal chondrosarcoma. *Cancer* 1983;51:1230–1237.
50. Unni KK, Dahlin DC, Beabout JW, et al: Chondrosarcoma: Clear-cell variant: A report of 16 cases. *J Bone Joint Surgery* 1976;58A:676–683.
51. Le Charpentier Y, Forest M, Postel M, et al: Clear-cell chondrosarcoma. *Cancer* 1979;44:633–639.
52. Bjornsson J, Unni KK, Dahlin DC, et al: Clear cell chondrosarcoma of bone: Observations in 47 cases. *Am J Surg Pathol* 1984;8:223–230.
53. Kumar R, David R, Cierney G III: Clear cell chondrosarcoma. *Radiology* 1985;154:45–48.
54. Lewis MM: An approach to the treatment of malignant bone tumors. *Orthopaedics* 1985;8:655–656.
55. Johnston JO: Local resection in primary malignant bone

tumors. *Clin Orthop* 1980;153:73.

56. Gitelis S, Bertoni F, Picci P, et al: Chondrosarcoma of bone. *J Bone Joint Surg* 1981;63A:1248–1256.

57. Lewis MM, Schneider R: Percutaneous needle biopsy of bone, in Taveras JM, Ferrucci JT (eds): *Radiology: Diagnosis–Imaging–Intervention.* Philadelphia, JB Lippincott Co, 1986, vol 5, chap 75.

58. Enneking WF, Spanier S, Goodman MA: A system for the surgical staging of musculoskeletal sarcoma. *Clin Orthop* 1980;153:106.

59. Lewis MM, Ballet F, Kroll P, et al: En bloc clavicular resection operative procedure and postoperative testing of function: Case reports. *Clin Orthop* 1985;133:214–220.

60. Malawer MM, Sugarbaker PH, Lampert M, et al: The Tikhoff-Linberg procedure: Report of 10 patients and presentation of a modified technique for tumors of the proximal humerus. *Surgery* 1985;97:518–528.

61. Marcove R, Lewis MM: Radical en bloc resection of the shoulder girdle: The Tikhoff-Linberg procedure. *Clin Orthop* 1977;124:219–228.

62. Burroughs HJ, Wilson JM, Scales JG: Excision of tumors of the humerus and femur with restoration by internal prosthesis. *J Bone Joint Surg* 1975;57B:148.

63. Lewis MM, Chekofsky K: Proximal femur replacement for neoplastic diseases. *Clin Orthop* 1982;171:72.

64. Sim FH, Chao EYS: Hip salvage for proximal femoral replacement. *J Bone Joint Surg* 1981;63A:1228.

65. Campanacci M: Total resection of the distal femur or proximal tibia for a bone tumor. *J Bone Joint Surg* 1979;61B:445.

66. Marcove R, Lewis MM, Rosen G, et al: Total femur and total knee replacement. *Clin Orthop* 1977;126:147–152.

67. Sim FH, Chao EYS: Prosthetic replacement of the knee and a large segment of the femur or tibia. *J Bone Joint Surg* 1979;61A:887.

68. Mankin HJ, Doppelt SH, Sullivan RT, et al: Osteoarticular and intercalary allograft transplantation in the management of malignant tumors of bone. *Cancer* 1982;50:613–630.

69. Lewis MM: The use of an expandable and adjustable prosthesis in the treatment of childhood malignant bone tumors of the extremity. *Cancer* 1986;57:499–502.

# The Foot and Ankle

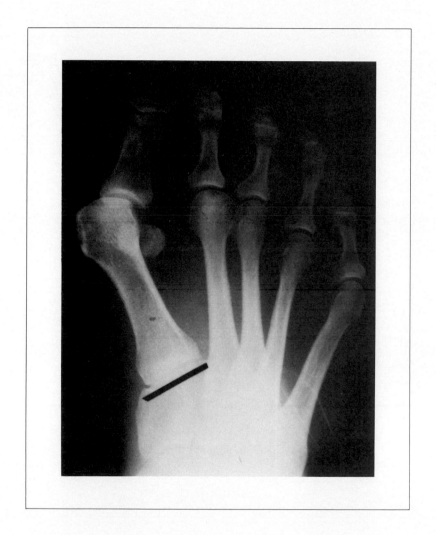

# Congenital Clubfoot: Pathoanatomy and Treatment

Norris C. Carroll, MD

## Pathoanatomy

To better understand the three-dimensional relationships of the ankle mortice, talus, os calcis, navicular, and cuboid, two feet were studied. The first was a left clubfoot from a stillborn baby who was otherwise normal. The second foot was a normal left foot obtained from a 3-week-old term infant who died of congenital heart disease.

The feet were suspended and fixed in 10% neutral-buffered formalin decalcified in 25% formic acid and embedded in paraffin. They were then sliced into 250 sections, stained with safranin O, mounted on glass slides, and projected on a screen for digitization. Each bone was assigned its own individual color. Three reference markers embedded in the paraffin before sectioning ensured accurate stacking of digitized sections. The information was processed and three-dimensional images were reconstructed.

The computer graphic videotape representation of the clubfoot demonstrated posterior positioning of the lateral malleolus (Fig. 6–1). As shown in Fig. 6–2B, it also demonstrated anterior extrusion of the body of the talus with a medial curvature of the neck (as has been reported previously[1-10]) and medial displacement of the navicular, so that it was against the medial malleolus. The os calcis was medially rotated with the posterior part adjacent to the lateral malleolus (Fig. 6–1). The cuboid was displaced medially in relation to the long axis of the os calcis (Fig. 6–3B). The forefoot was adducted and supinated, as was demonstrated by the stacking of the cuneiforms and metatarsals. This was easily visualized in the superior view of the reconstructed foot.

A posterior view of the normal foot (Fig. 6–2C) lets one look through the ankle mortice, whereas in the clubfoot the os calcis was rotated toward the lateral malleolus and, with the anterior extrusion of the body of the talus, little of the body was visible posteriorly. In addition, this view demonstrated the medial displacement of the cuboid in relation to the long axis of the os calcis. The medial view, again, demonstrated the supination and adductus of the forefoot and the medial displacement of the cuboid. Computer technology also enables us to draw vectors that represent the ankle mortice, the axes of the body of the talus and neck of the talus, and the axes of the os calcis, navicular, and cuboid. These axes demonstrate the increased inclination of the neck of the talus

in the clubfoot, the medial displacement of the navicular towards the medial malleolus, the medial displacement of the cuboid in relation to the long axis of the os calcis, and the medial rotation of the os calcis. In addition, the body of the talus was externally rotated in the ankle mortice.

In the past, the pathoanatomy of congenital clubfoot was described differently by different authors because they had viewed the deformity from varying angles.[11-15] With three-dimensional reconstruction, it

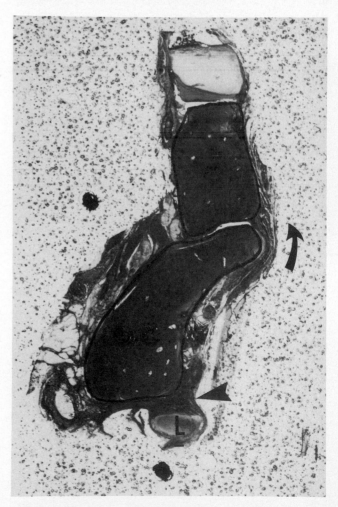

**Fig. 6–1** Section through club foot. Note curved lateral border of foot (long arrow), medial tilting of calcaneocuboid joint, medial displacement of the cuboid (C), posterior displacement of the lateral malleolus (L), thick calcaneofibular ligament (short arrow), and proximity of os calcis (OC) to fibula.

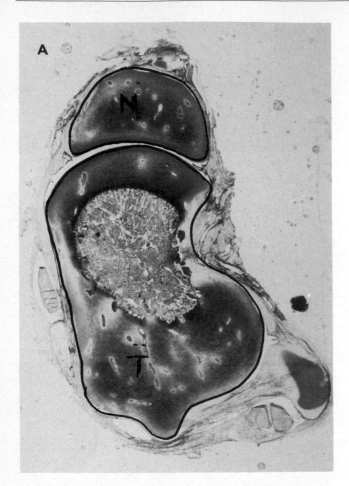

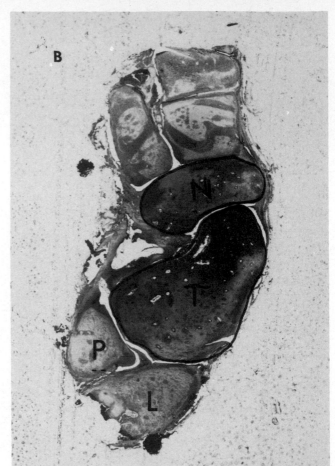

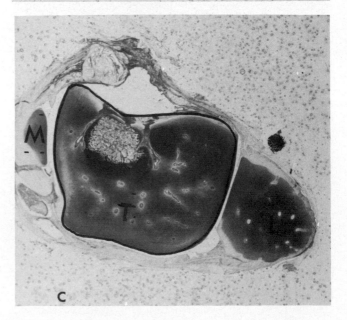

**Fig. 6–2** **A:** Section through normal foot. Note normal alignment of talus (T) and navicular (N). **B:** Section through clubfoot. Note anterior extrusion of body of talus which points laterally, the curve in the neck of the talus, and the medial displacement of the navicular (lateral malleolus [L], tibial plafond [P]). **C:** Section through normal foot. Note normal relationship of body of talus to lateral (L) and medial (M) malleoli.

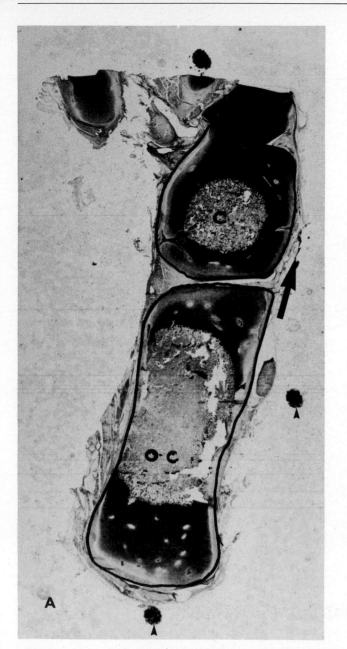

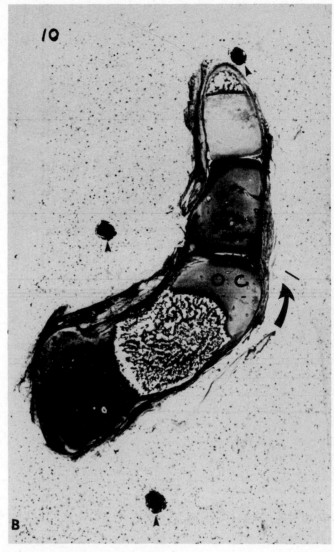

**Fig. 6–3** **A:** Section through normal foot. Note straight lateral border (large arrow) and reference marks (small arrows). **B:** Section through clubfoot. Note curved lateral border (large arrow) and reference marks (small arrows). Note also the medial tilting of the calcaneocuboid joint and the medial displacement of the cuboid (C) and os calcis (OC).

should now be possible to avoid much of this confusion. The author has drawn several conclusions from computed tomographic (CT) examinations, the computer graphics study, dissections of clubfeet, and operative experience.

When the patella points forward, the lateral malleolus is posterior, that is, there is not an internal tibial torsion in congenital clubfoot. This can be proved by a CT scan in which one cut is taken through the femoral condyles and a second through the ankle mortice.

There is a cavus component to a severe clubfoot deformity.[16] This can only be corrected by lengthening the plantar fascia and intrinsic muscles.

There are two columns to the foot, a medial column and a lateral column.[17] The lateral column consists of the os calcis, cuboid, and fourth and fifth metatarsals. The medial column consists of the talus, navicular, three cuneiforms, and the first, second, and third metatarsals. For years, clubfoot surgeons have been talking about medial displacement of the navicular in relation to the head of the talus.[7] Since the medial column and lateral column are joined together, it follows that if the distal portion of the medial column is displaced medially, then the distal portion of the lateral column must be displaced medially. This means that the cuboid is displaced medially. With the cavus and medial displacement of the cuboid, there is a contracture of the long and short plantar ligaments and spring ligament. This displacement is nicely demonstrated in the serial sections from which the computer graphic images were generated.

The long axis of the ossific nuclei of the os calcis and talus are parallel on the anteroposterior and lateral radiographs.[18,19]

The os calcis and the talus are in equinus.

The triceps surae, tibialis posterior, flexor hallucis longus, and flexor digitorum longus muscles are all short.

There is a contracture of the posterior capsule and the collateral ligaments of the ankle. When a z-plasty of the tendo Achillis is performed and the foot is pushed upward, there is no correction of the deformity until the tight capsules of the ankle and subtalar joints are released. This release must include division of the tight posterior lateral structures, namely, the posterior calcaneofibular ligament and the posterior talofibular ligament.[20]

The navicular is subluxated medially against the medial malleolus.

The body of the talus is externally rotated in the ankle mortice.[11] During the correction of a severe clubfoot, the body of the talus should be internally rotated in the ankle mortice and the os calcis must move down and away from the lateral malleolus, that is, the back of the os calcis moves medially. When this is accomplished, the hypoplastic posterior facet of the subtalar joint is easily visualized and it can be seen that the talus does not fit properly against the os calcis once divergence between the long axis of the talus and os calcis has been reestablished.

## Nonsurgical Treatment

The materials needed for nonsurgical treatment are tincture of benzoin, cotton flannelette, plaster, and a pair of scissors.

It helps if the child is hungry during manipulation and reapplication of the cast. A warm bottle of formula is a wonderful distraction. The manipulation begins by palpating the junction between the head and neck of the talus (palpable in the sinus tarsi region). The thumb should be placed against the talus, pushing medially, while the opposite hand applies longitudinal traction to the forefoot to stretch the tibialis posterior and to correct the adductus and supination. With the talus pushed medially and trac-

tion applied to the forefoot, the presence of a correction of the parallelism between the long axis of the talus and os calcis can be determined. If there is a correction, some of the equinus deformity can be corrected by pulling the os calcis away from the lateral malleolus; the back of the os calcis must move medially while the front of the os calcis moves laterally. While the back of the os calcis is being pulled down and away from the lateral malleolus, the front of the os calcis is pushed up to correct the equinus.

The foot should be manipulated for five to ten minutes before the cast is applied. The purpose of the cast is to maintain the position obtained by the manipulation. Once the manipulation is completed, the skin is covered with tincture of benzoin and the foot and leg are then wrapped in a layer of flannelette. Care must be taken to avoid wrinkling the material. The plaster should be dipped in water that is not too hot and left fairly wet so that it can be contoured and molded properly before it sets. The cotton flannelette is not turned down at the top to avoid skin abrasions in the popliteal fossa when the child flexes his knees. The flannelette is, however, turned up to expose the toes. The plaster is molded to correct the forefoot adductus and supination, to correct the external rotation of the body of the talus, the internal rotation of the os calcis, and the equinus of the whole foot. The end of the plaster roll is marked with a little knob. This makes it easier for the parents to remove the plaster by soaking the cast in water and then unwrapping it before the next clinic visit. If the manipulation is done gently, the patient will be more cooperative and a rocker bottom deformity will be avoided.

It is wise to confirm a clinical impression of complete correction by ordering appropriate films such as those recommended by Beatson and Pearson.[18] If the deformity has not been corrected completely, it will worsen if the foot is placed in a splint. It then must be decided whether to continue with manipulations and casting or to arrange a surgical correction. In the author's opinion, a foot that has not been corrected after three months of manipulations and casts should be treated surgically.

## Surgical Treatment

On the basis of the pathoanatomic studies, the author suggests that a severe, resistant clubfoot deformity can be corrected in the following sequence: (1) plantar fascia release; (2) release of Henry's knot; (3) identification of the tibialis anterior, which facilitates the identification of the peroneus longus tendon; (4) protection of the peroneus longus tendon while the calcaneocuboid joint is opened medially; (5) a z-plasty of the tendo Achillis; (6) a z-plasty of the tibialis posterior tendon; (7) a posterior capsulotomy including the posterior calcaneofibular ligament and the posterior talofibular ligament; (8) an open reduction of the talonavicular joint; (9) placement of a K-wire in the body of the talus from behind, correction of the anterior extrusion and external rotation of the body of the talus in the ankle mortice, and advancement of the K-wire across the reduced talonavicular joint; and (10) repair of the lengthened tendons with the foot held in a plantigrade position. In summary, the "bony architecture" must be restored and the muscle forces must be balanced. To avoid overcorrection, part of the deltoid ligament should be preserved and the navicular should not be over displaced in the lateral direction and must not be pinned in a superior position. Tendons must not be overlengthened and the foot must not be cast in an overcorrected position.

## Summary

A better understanding of the pathoanatomy of clubfoot, meticulous attention to detail during surgery, and orthotic maintenance of correction to facilitate remodeling should make it possible to improve the results of treatment.

## References

1. Bechtol CO, Mossman HW: Club-foot: An embryological study of associated muscle abnormalities. *J Bone Joint Surg* 1950;32A:827–838.
2. Hjelmstedt A, Sahlstedt B: Talar deformity in congenital club feet. *Acta Orthop Scand* 1974;45:628–640.
3. Ippolito E, Ponseti IV: Congenital club foot in the human fetus: A histological study. *J Bone Joint Surg* 1980;62A:8–22.
4. Irani RN, Sherman SS: The pathological anatomy of club foot. *J Bone Joint Surg* 1963;45A:45–52.
5. Nichols EH: Anatomy of congenital equino-varus. *Boston Med Surg J* 1897;36:150–153.
6. Parker RW, Shattuck SG: The pathology and etiology of congenital club foot. *Trans Pathol Soc* 1884;35:423–444.
7. Reimann I: *Congenital Idiopathic Club Foot.* PJ Schmidt a/s Vojens, 1967.
8. Scudder CL: Congenital talipes equinovarus. *Boston Med Surg J* 1887;117:397–399.
9. Settle GW: The anatomy of congenital talipes equinovarus: Sixteen dissected specimens. *J Bone Joint Surg* 1963;45A:1341–1354.
10. Shapiro F, Glimcher MJ: Gross and histological abnormalities of the talus in congenital club foot. *J Bone Joint Surg* 1979;61A:522–530.
11. Carroll NC, McMurty R, Leete SF: The pathoanatomy of congenital club foot. *Orthop Clin North Am* 1978;9:225–232.
12. Goldner JL: Congenital talipes equinovarus—fifteen years of surgical treatment. *Curr Pract Orthop Surg* 1969;4:61–123.
13. McKay DW: New concept of and approach to club foot treatment: Section I. Principles and morbid anatomy. *J Pediatr Orthop* 1982;2:347–356.
14. McKay DW: New concept of and approach to club foot treatment: Section II. Correction of the club foot. *J Pediatr Orthop* 1983;3:10–21.
15. McKay DW: New concept of and approach to club foot treatment: Section III. Evaluation and results. *J Pediatr Orthop* 1983;3:141–148.
16. Sherman FC, Westin GW: Plantar release in the correction of deformities of the foot in childhood. *J Bone Joint Surg* 1981;63A:1382–1389.
17. Grant JC: *Boileau Method of Anatomy.* Baltimore, Williams & Wilkins, 1952, p 447.
18. Beatson TR, Pearson JR: A method of assessing correction in club feet. *J Bone Joint Surg* 1966;48B:40–50.
19. Simons G: A standardized method for radiographic evaluation of club feet. *Clin Orthop* 1978;135:107–118.
20. Scott WA, Hosking SW, Catterall A: Club foot: Observations on the surgical anatomy of dorsiflexion. *J Bone Joint Surg* 1984;66B:71–76.

# The Pathophysiology of the Juvenile Bunion

Michael J. Coughlin, MD

Roger A. Mann, MD

## Introduction

The development of a hallux valgus deformity in adolescents or older children is uncommon.[1,2] Deferring an operation until skeletal maturity is reached is a frequent recommendation because of the high recurrence rate in this age group.[1,3–8] Reports of various surgical techniques used to repair the juvenile bunion note inconsistent success. Even series that have employed a similar operative technique report variable success rates. In fact, considerable controversy exists about the indications, timing and choice of operative techniques, and results of treatment.

## Frequency of Occurrence

Piggott[2] noted that in a series of adult patients evaluated for hallux valgus, 57% recalled development of a bunion deformity in adolescence, while only 5% recalled an occurrence after age 20. Hardy and Clapham[9] reported that 40% of hallux valgus deformities in their series occurred prior to age 20. While Scranton[10] observed that a juvenile bunion is "rarely seen before ten years" of age, most series report surgical intervention at an average age of 13, implying early onset of the condition.

While there is no estimate of the frequency of occurrence or of surgical treatment in the United States, Helal[11] estimated that approximately 2,000 adolescents undergo correction for hallux valgus in Great Britain each year. The high incidence of surgical intervention in the female adolescent population[6,7,11–16] may, indeed, correlate with the onset of foot discomfort associated with fashionable footwear.

The juvenile hallux valgus deformity begins in adolescence. Certain adult bunion deformities are significantly more difficult to treat than others and appear to have a higher risk of postoperative recurrence. These, indeed, may have had their onset in the juvenile years.

## Characteristics of Juvenile Hallux Valgus

Understanding the pathophysiology of the hallux valgus deformity forms the basis for treatment. The juvenile bunion deformity differs significantly from the adult bunion (Fig. 7–1).[1,15] Degenerative changes are usually not present at the metatarsophalangeal joint, and bursal thickening is rare. Open proximal phalangeal and proximal metatarsal epiphyses are still present. Frequently, the valgus at the metatarsophalangeal joint and the medial eminence are smaller than in the typical adult deformity.

## Etiology

Various structural factors have been implicated in the development and progression of the juvenile hallux valgus deformity. Pes planus[4,7,10,16–21] and ligament laxity[7,22] have been associated with juvenile hallux valgus. Trott[16] noted that pes planus occurred in 25% of the cases of juvenile bunion, while Scranton and Zuckerman[7] reported a 41% incidence of pes planus in their series. Pronation of the foot changes the axis of the first ray so that with ambulation the first metatarsophalangeal joint has an oblique orientation to the ground. The plantar aspect of the metatarsophalangeal joint is characterized by the sesamoid mechanism, which contains an extension of the double tendon of the flexor hallucis brevis. The plantar medial aspect of the metatarsophalangeal joint is stabilized by the abductor hallucis, and the lateral aspect is stabilized by the adductor hallucis. While these tendons afford significant reinforcement to the plantar medial and lateral metatarsophalangeal joint, the dorsal aspect of the metatarsophalangeal joint is covered by the much thinner extensor hood. As the foot pronates and the metatarsal axis rotates inward, the abductor hallucis assumes a more plantar location and the medial extensor hood, a decidedly weaker structure, is called upon to support the medial metatarsophalangeal joint. In a limited number of patients with pronation of the foot, the metatarsophalangeal joint appears to be less able to withstand the deforming pressures exerted on the soft-tissue supporting structures, leading to hallux valgus deformities.

While a long first metatarsal has been implicated as an increased risk factor for bunion formation,[4,7,21] it appears that the relationship between metatarsal length and development of hallux valgus is fortuitous.[23] Ill-fitting footwear has also been implicated as a cause of bunion progression in the adolescent.[22,24]

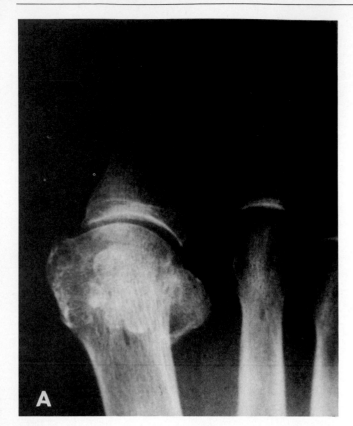 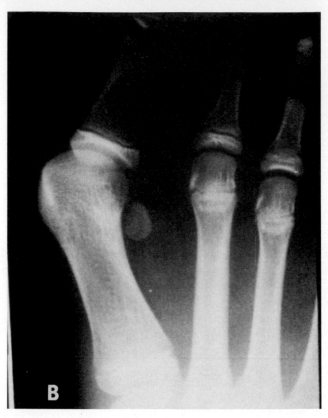

**Fig. 7–1 A:** Medial eminence in adults (note degenerative changes with sagittal sulcus). **B:** Juvenile medial eminence with no obvious degenerative changes.

## Anatomy of Juvenile Hallux Valgus

Anatomic variations in the forefoot may put specific adolescents at risk for hallux valgus development. While the importance of midfoot and hindfoot pathology cannot be overlooked, the shape and orientation of the metatarsophalangeal and metatarsocuneiform joints may be the key to both the development of the adolescent hallux valgus deformity as well as to the correction of this abnormality.

### The Metatarsophalangeal Joint

Variations in the shape of the articular surfaces of the metatarsophalangeal joint may affect the intrinsic stability of the joint and, thus, predispose the hallux to progressive deformity. A round metatarsal head appears to be more prone to the development of hallux valgus,[21,25] while a flattened or chevroned metatarsophalangeal articulation appears to resist deforming forces on the hallux (Fig. 7–2).

In the normal foot, the proximal phalangeal and distal metatarsal articular surfaces are not necessarily oriented at right angles to the long axis of the diaphyses. While hallux valgus of 16 degrees or less is considered normal,[9,23,26] lateral tilting of the articular surfaces of the proximal phalanx and distal metatarsal may be responsible for the static valgus orientation (Fig. 7–3).

The orientation of the metatarsophalangeal joint must be critically evaluated both in assessing a juvenile hallux valgus deformity as well as in choosing the appropriate method of repair. The metatarsal articular orientation (MAO) describes the orientation of the distal metatarsal articular surface in relation to the long axis of the first metatarsal (Fig. 7–4). The phalangeal articular orientation (PAO) defines the orientation of the proximal phalangeal articular surface in relation to the long axis of the proximal phalanx of the hallux (Fig. 7–5). A static structural abnormality resulting in excessive hallux valgus may be secondary either to an abnormally large MAO or PAO, or both.

The presence or absence of joint congruity determines the basis for conservative or surgical treatment of juvenile hallux valgus. A congruous metatarsophalangeal joint is present when the corresponding articular surfaces are aligned in a concentric fashion. A significant amount of valgus can still be present at the metatarsophalangeal joint; however, it is caused by variation in the orientation of either the PAO or

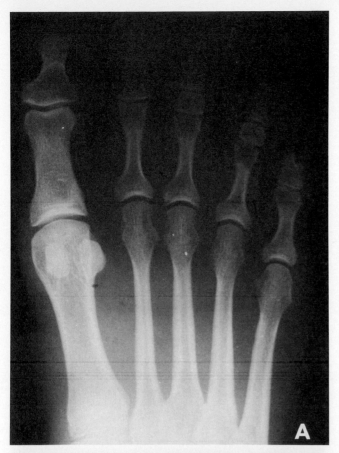

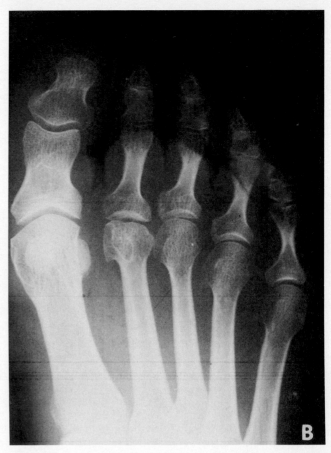

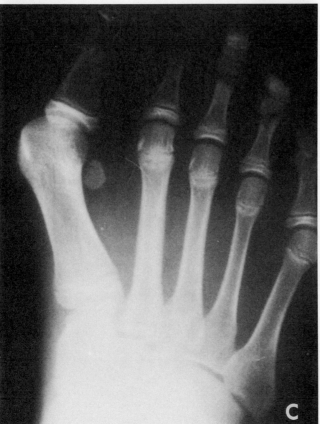

**Fig. 7–2** A flat **(A)** or chevron-type **(B)** metatarsophalangeal articulation is more stable and resists subluxation, while a rounded metatarsal head **(C)** is more prone to subluxation.

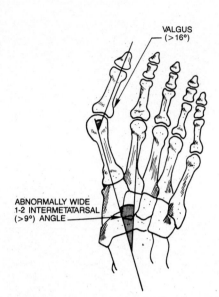

**Fig. 7–3**   A 1–2 intermetatarsal angle greater than 9 degrees is thought to be abnormal; a hallux valgus angle greater than 16 degrees is thought to be abnormal.

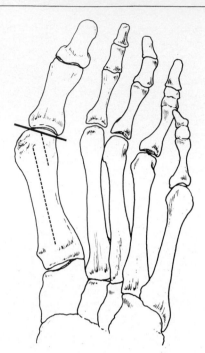

**Fig. 7–4**   The metatarsal articular orientation (MAO) defines the orientation of the articular surface of the metatarsal in relation to the long axis of the metatarsal.

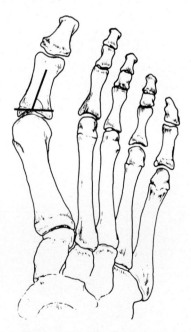

**Fig. 7–5**   The phalangeal articular orientation (PAO) defines the phalangeal articular surface in relation to the long axis of the proximal phalanx.

the MAO (Fig. 7–6). A congruous joint typically is stable; the magnitude of hallux valgus does not appear to increase with time.[2]

With an incongruous metatarsophalangeal joint, the base of the proximal phalanx may deviate or subluxate in relation to the metatarsal articular surface (Fig. 7–7). Early deviation of the metatarsophalangeal joint may progress to significant subluxation, leaving the medial metatarsal head uncovered. Piggott[2] concluded that a congruous metatarsophalangeal joint was a stable joint that would not progress to significant hallux valgus, while the incongruous joint, with slight deviation, was at significant risk for progressive metatarsophalangeal subluxation.

Valgus angulation of the metatarsophalangeal joint can be caused either by tilting of the articular surfaces in relation to the long axis of the metatarsal and phalanx or by joint displacement. It is important to appreciate this distinction, for if a hallux valgus deformity with a congruent metatarsophalangeal joint requires correction, an inappropriate realignment of the metatarsophalangeal joint may place the articular surfaces at significant risk for later degenerative arthritis or recurrent hallux valgus.

### The Metatarsocuneiform Joint

The orientation of the metatarsocuneiform (MC) joint may be the most important factor in the development of an increased intermetatarsal angle. The accepted normal value for the intermetatarsal angle is nine degrees (Fig. 7–3).[9,12,26–29] Variations in the shape and orientation of the metatarsocuneiform joint may

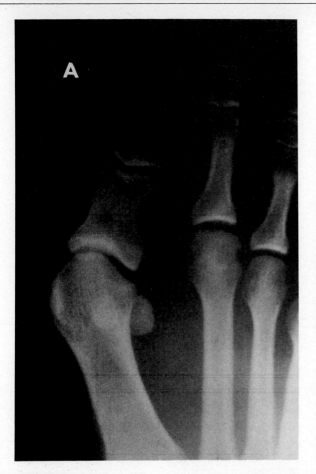

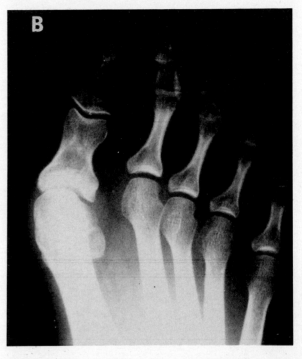

**Fig. 7–6 A:** A congruous joint has concentric apposition of the corresponding metatarsal and phalangeal articular surfaces. Nonetheless, there may be significant valgus at the metatarsophalangeal joint. **B:** A soft-tissue realignment of a congruous joint may put the metatarsophalangeal joint at risk for recurrence or for later degenerative arthritis.

significantly affect stability of the first ray. A horizontal setting tends to resist an increase in the intermetatarsal angle (Fig. 7–8A), while an oblique setting of the MC joint appears to correlate with an increased intermetatarsal angle (Fig. 7–8B). A curved metatarsocuneiform articulation may allow increased mobility and permit medial deviation of the first metatarsal (Fig. 7–8C).[25] A facet present at the lateral base of the proximal first metatarsal may abut so that the first metatarsal base is fixed in varus (Fig. 7–8D).[20,23,25] This facet renders the metatarsocuneiform articulation less flexible, and, thus, the intermetatarsal angle is resistant to change with a distal realignment procedure. Normally, the metatarsocuneiform joint is oriented in a transverse (coronal) axis. The anterior surface of the first cuneiform articulates with the proximal first metatarsal articular surface. The articular surface of the first cuneiform is elliptical, slightly convex, and oriented in a slight plantar-medial direction.[30,31]

Ewald[32] and Berntsen[33] noted that an oblique setting of the metatarsocuneiform joint increased the varus inclination of the first metatarsal, with resultant hallux valgus. The orientation of the metatarsocuneiform joint is not always in alignment on routine radiographs. Simon[34] questioned whether the "apparent orientation" of this joint was merely a radiographic artifact. Haines and McDougall,[30] following numerous metatarsocuneiform dissections, concluded that the orientation of the metatarsocuneiform joint was often oblique with a hallux valgus deformity. While Truslow[35] and Haines and McDougall[30] postulated that, on occasion, an anatomic abnormality in the proximal first metatarsal base was the cause of varus inclination of the first ray, the orientation of the metatarsocuneiform joint appears to exert a profound effect on first metatarsal inclination.[15] Mitchell and associates[15] and others[1,11,28,35,36] concluded that increased varus angulation of the first metatarsal resulted from an abnormal orientation at the metatarsocuneiform joint. McCrea and Lichty[37] and others[30,32,33] noted that in a normal foot, the metatarsocuneiform joint was typically transverse in orientation.

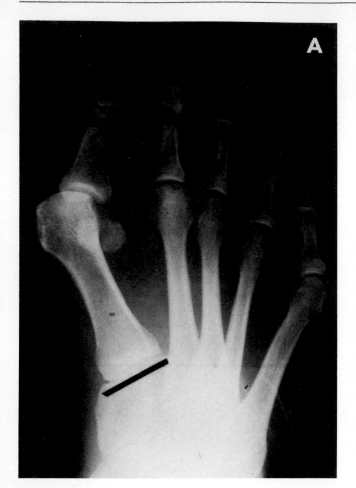
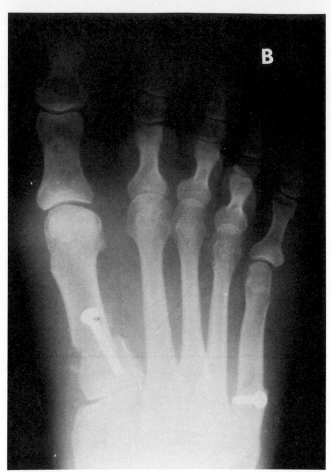

**Fig. 7–7** **A:** With a noncongruous joint, the metatarsophalangeal articulation shows subluxation (note oblique metatarsocuneiform joint orientation). **B:** Postoperative radiographs demonstrating correction with distal soft-tissue repair and proximal metatarsal osteotomy.

### First Metatarsal Orientation

An increased intermetatarsal angle is the abnormality most commonly associated with hallux valgus.[3,8,9,24] Whether it is a primary or a secondary abnormality may be the distinguishing factor between the juvenile and the adult bunion. Piggott[2] and Inman[19] hypothesized that progressive metatarsophalangeal subluxation preceded an increase in the intermetatarsal angle. Antrobus[27] hypothesized that if the intermetatarsal angle returned to a normal range following a distal soft-tissue repair (without metatarsal osteotomy), then the increased intermetatarsal angle deformity was secondary to hallux valgus. DuVries[17] stated that metatarsus primus varus was responsible for the development of hallux valgus in the adolescent, while it was a secondary change in hallux valgus in the adult.

The concept that an increased intermetatarsal angle is the primary deformity in the juvenile, with hallux valgus secondary to it has been frequently postulated (Fig. 7–9).* This distinction may be more than academic. Flexibility at the metatarsocuneiform articulation can have a significant influence, not only on the development of hallux valgus, but also on the type of surgical repair selected and its subsequent success. A fixed, congenitally wide intermetatarsal angle presents a significant risk for postoperative recurrence if only a distal soft-tissue repair is attempted. An equally wide intermetatarsal angle that has developed secondarily to a hallux valgus deformity and retains flexibility at the metatarsocuneiform joint, may be adequately corrected by a distal soft-tissue repair without metatarsal osteotomy.[25] Therefore, the flexibility of the metatarsocuneiform joint plays a key role in any correction.[36]

Often this flexibility can be assessed only at surgery once soft-tissue contractures have been released at the metatarsophalangeal joint. It is interesting, how-

*3,6,12,14,15,17,28,35,36,38,39

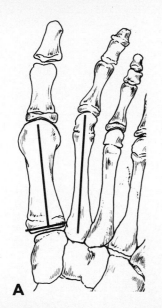
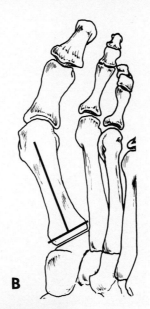
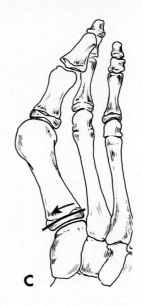

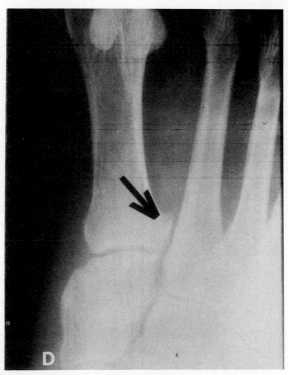

**Fig. 7–8  A:** A horizontal metatarsocuneiform articulation is inherently stable. **B:** An oblique setting to the metatarsocuneiform joint is often nonflexible and may require an osteotomy to correct the varus of the first metatarsal. **C:** A curved metatarsocuneiform articulation may be unstable leading to an increased 1–2 intermetatarsal angle. **D:** An intermetatarsal facet may limit reduction of the intermetatarsal angle at surgery.

ever, that Hawkins and associates[40] noted an average correction of the intermetatarsal angle of 5.2 degrees following distal metatarsal osteotomy and soft-tissue correction. Mann and Coughlin[25] also reported an improvement of 5.2 degrees in the intermetatarsal angle following only a distal soft-tissue repair using the modified McBride procedure. Where flexibility of the metatarsocuneiform joint is present, a distal soft-tissue repair can achieve a significant decrease in the intermetatarsal angle.

When the intermetatarsal angle is evaluated, the value obtained must be assessed in relation to the remaining metatarsals. While nine degrees is the upper normal value for the 1–2 intermetatarsal angle, the orientation of the second metatarsal in relationship to the first metatarsal determines this

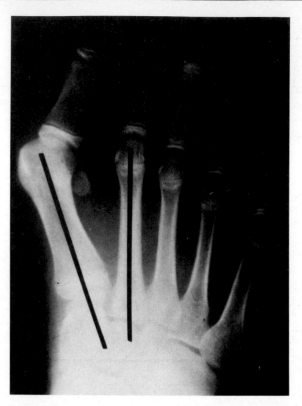 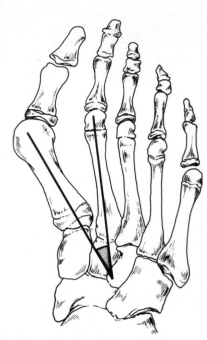

**Fig. 7–9:**  An increased 1–2 intermetatarsal angle is often associated with juvenile hallux valgus.

numerical measurement.[29] If one assumes that the lesser metatarsals are properly oriented, then the 1–2 intermetatarsal angle gives an accurate indication of the amount of first metatarsal varus. Price[29] recommended measuring the angle subtended by the first and fifth metatarsals in order to evaluate metatarsus primus varus and reported that an angle greater than 29 degrees was abnormal. In the absence of valgus of the fifth metatarsal or metatarsus adductus, he found this measurement was a more reliable guide than measurement of the 1–2 intermetatarsal angle.

In the adducted forefoot, the 1–2 intermetatarsal angle does not give a true representation of the amount of varus of the first ray.[4,18] Hallux valgus, associated with metatarsus adductus, has been noted in the juvenile patient[4,6,16,18,21,29] and presents an extremely difficult condition to treat (Fig. 7–10).

Houghton and Dickson[26] postulated that in patients with hallux valgus there was no significant increase in the first metatarsal varus; they concluded that there was an increased valgus of the lateral metatarsals. This conclusion has been challenged by Helal,[11] who reported significant varus of the first metatarsal in 99% of the adolescent patients he evaluated. While the orientation of the second and lesser rays does not influence whether or not the first metatarsal is in true varus, lesser metatarsal orientation does influence the measurement of the intermetatarsal angle. There-

fore, the numerical measurement of the 1–2 intermetatarsal angle does not always give true representation of metatarsal orientation. Furthermore, if significant forefoot adductus is present, the orientation of the lesser metatarsals may make successful repair of a juvenile hallux valgus deformity difficult.

### Open Epiphyses

The belief that surgery should be delayed until skeletal maturity is achieved has been espoused for fear the deformity will progress or that it will recur because of further epiphyseal growth.[3,4,38] Avoidance of epiphyseal injury either to the proximal phalanx or to the proximal metatarsal epiphysis is an important reason for either delaying or avoiding surgery in these regions. Bonney and MacNab[3] noted a recurrence rate of 42% in bunion repairs where there was an open epiphysis, while Scranton and Zuckerman[7] noted a 20% recurrence rate in adolescents with an open epiphysis. An open phalangeal or metatarsal epiphysis does not preclude osteotomy. In fact, in the juvenile population, surgical repair of the hallux valgus deformity routinely requires an osteotomy in order to effect an adequate correction. Avoidance of iatrogenic epiphyseal injury, however, requires precise localization of the epiphysis if a proximal osteotomy is performed. Surgical correction of metatarsus primus varus by means of an osteotomy distal to the

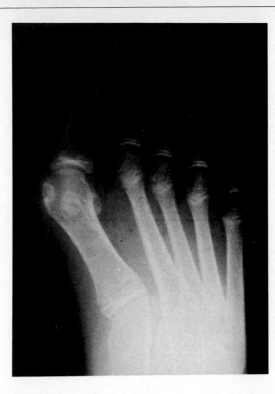

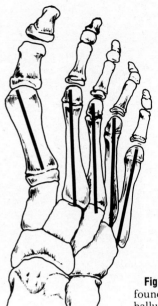

**Fig. 7–10:** Metatarsus adductus is found not uncommonly with juvenile hallux valgus and presents a difficult problem to treat.

epiphysis may, on occasion, result in a progressive postoperative metatarsal angulation into varus.[3] It is for this reason that many reports have cautioned against surgery in the young adolescent.[1,3,4,7,8,11]

Serial measurements of foot growth in adolescents have determined that a girl attains full foot growth usually by 14 years of age.[41,42] However, at age 12 a girl typically has only 0.8 cm of total foot growth remaining. It is highly likely that less than one half of this total growth can be attributed to the proximal metatarsal epiphysis, indicating that growth of this epiphysis is slight after age 12. Boys achieve maturity of foot growth at an average age of 16 years. At age 12, there is approximately 2.7 cm of total growth remaining. Because of the significant amount of growth remaining in the proximal metatarsal epiphysis, postponement of surgery may be considered until the juvenile male patient is closer to skeletal maturity.

Biomechanically, the orientation of the proximal first metatarsal epiphysis may contribute to increased metatarsus primus varus or postoperative recurrence. Luba and Rosman[6] hypothesized that the varus orientation of the proximal first metatarsal epiphysis creates compression forces medially and tension forces laterally, which theoretically stimulate more growth on the lateral aspect of the epiphysis (Fig. 7–11). These forces tend to increase the varus inclination of the first metatarsal. Alteration of the longitu-

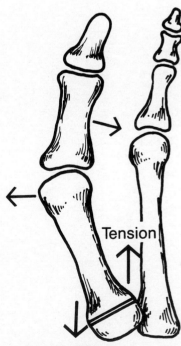

**Fig. 7–11** The orientation of the proximal first metatarsal epiphysis may contribute to increased metatarsus primus varus by tension forces laterally, which stimulate growth of the lateral epiphysis. (Redrawn with permission from Luba R, Rosman M: Bunions in children: Treatment with a modified Mitchell osteotomy. *J Pediatr Orthop* 1984;4:44–47.)

dinal axis of the first ray by surgical correction proximal to the epiphysis may tend to decrease lateral tension forces, thereby decreasing the rate of lateral epiphyseal growth. Osteotomy distal to the epiphysis may also achieve enough correction to slow lateral epiphyseal growth, but may produce the risk of recurrence if lateral overgrowth occurs. Hallux valgus correction distal to the epiphyseal line may put the patient at considerable risk for recurrence if these lateral tensile forces on the epiphysis continue to cause overstimulation of lateral epiphyseal growth. Correction of the varus inclination at the metatarso-cuneiform joint by cuneiform osteotomy may achieve correction at the site of the abnormality and avoid damage to an open epiphysis.

Theoretically, a selective partial lateral epiphyseal arrest at an early age would allow gradual correction of the increased intermetatarsal angle. Although the abnormality is thought to be at the metatarsocunei-form joint, dynamic changes occurring with relative medial overgrowth of the proximal first metatarsal would correct metatarsus primus varus with time. Since it has only limited documentation,[42,43] the efficacy of this technique has yet to be confirmed.

## Conservative Care

Most adolescents with a bunion deformity do not require aggressive surgical treatment.[38] An asymptomatic patient with a mild bunion deformity may be evaluated intermittently for progression of the deformity. Patients who have a flexible pes planus deformity or hyperelasticity with a mild hallux valgus abnormality may benefit from a medial arch support.[1,10,21] Wearing roomy footwear may be the most significant factor in successful conservative care. In contrast, fashionable, constricting footwear plays a role in exacerbating the juvenile bunion. While the asymptomatic adolescent obviously does not require surgery,[10] Chomeley[38] observed that adolescents will rarely, if ever, wear bunion-last shoes, so that efforts at promoting conservative footwear in this age group

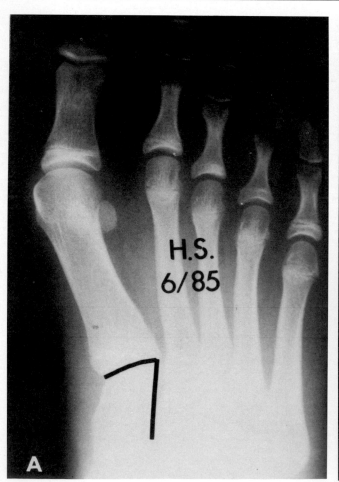
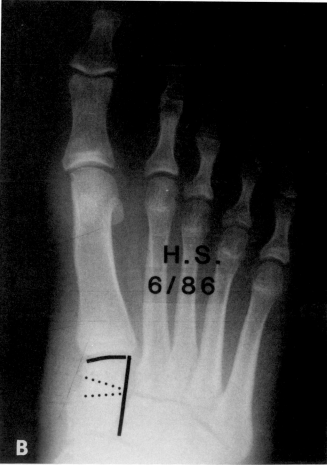

**Fig. 7–12** **A:** Preoperative hallux valgus in juvenile. **B:** Distal soft-tissue realignment combined with opening wedge cuneiform osteotomy.

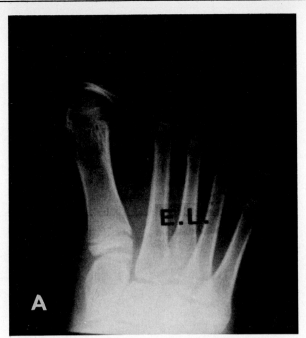
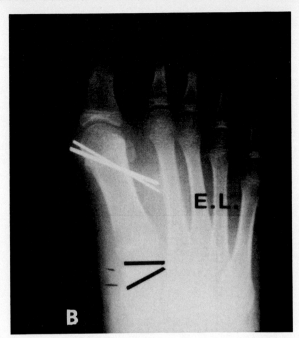

**Fig. 7–13  A:** Preoperative juvenile hallux valgus with increased intermetatarsal angle and incongruous metatarsophalangeal articulation. **B:** Radiograph demonstrating opening wedge cuneiform osteotomy with distal closing wedge metatarsal osteotomy.

are futile. Pain, due to shoe pressure over the medial aspect of the foot, even with conservative footwear, is a common reason for surgical intervention.[1,6,8,10,12-14,39] Progression of the deformity is, as well, a frequent indication for surgical correction[8,10,18] Cosmesis is occasionally mentioned as an indication,[6,12,13,39] but it can be difficult to differentiate from pain and discomfort as an indication.

Even with moderate to severe deformities, conservative care is certainly warranted until the patient is mature enough to cooperate adequately during postoperative care. Conservative care is advised in the juvenile with hyperelasticity or significant pes planus in which postoperative recurrence is common. The decision to correct the juvenile bunion surgically should never be made hurriedly.

### The Rationale for Surgical Correction

In evaluating a patient for surgery, it is important to recognize concurrent abnormalities such as joint hyperelasticity, pes planus, a tight Achilles tendon, or spasticity, as these factors may effect the overall success rate. Analysis of the orientation of the metatarsophalangeal joint establishes whether or not there is a congruous or incongruous articulation.

With a mild hallux valgus deformity with metatarsophalangeal joint subluxation of 25 degrees or less, a distal soft-tissue realignment such as a modified McBride procedure (without excision of the

lateral sesamoid) or a distal metatarsal osteotomy,[12,15,40,44] are acceptable methods of treatment. If the hallux valgus deformity is greater than 25 degrees with concurrent MP subluxation, a distal soft-tissue realignment may be combined with a proximal osteotomy to decrease the intermetatarsal angle (Fig. 7–7). Depending upon the patient's age and the amount of growth remaining at the first metatarsal epiphysis, a metatarsal osteotomy may be placed distal to the epiphysis, or an opening-wedge first cuneiform osteotomy may be performed proximal to the epiphysis if the first ray is not already excessively long (Fig. 7–12).

While a congruous metatarsophalangeal articulation is uncommon in the juvenile with hallux valgus (Piggott reported a 9% incidence[2]), on occasion this deformity requires surgical correction. A realignment of the metatarsophalangeal joint is contraindicated in this situation, as it may result in articular malalignment with subsequent pain, stiffness, and degenerative joint disease.[5] For this structural abnormality, extra-articular repair is indicated. The following procedures may be considered: (1) distal metatarsal osteotomy[15,24,40,44,45]; (2) proximal phalangeal osteotomy[22,23,28]; (3) proximal metatarsal osteotomy[22,23,28]; (4) metatarsocuneiform arthrodesis[20,36]; and (5) cuneiform osteotomy.[3,46] With a congruous metatarsophalangeal articulation, a distal metatarsal osteotomy may be performed without metatarsophalangeal articular realignment (Fig. 7–13). Osteotomies localized to the proximal phalanx and proximal first metatarsal must be either carefully placed or deferred until epiphyseal growth has been completed. The choice of opening wedge, closing wedge, or crescentic osteotomy in the proximal metatarsal region depends upon whether lengthening, shortening, or merely maintenance of metatarsal length is desired.

Frequently, a juvenile bunion is characterized by a metatarsocuneiform joint that is in fixed varus and has little flexibility, even after release of metatarsophalangeal joint soft-tissue contractures. Usually, metatarsophalangeal joint subluxation is present. Assessment of the flexibility of the metatarsocuneiform joint gives an indication of the rigidity of the intermetatarsal angle. While preoperative evaluation of the foot may give some indication of this flexibility, occasionally adequate evaluation can be made only during an operation following the release of the soft-tissue contractures about the metatarsophalangeal joint. Radiographic analysis of the metatarsocuneiform joint for the presence of fixed obliquity or a curvilinear orientation of the joint also gives information about metatarsocuneiform joint flexibility. An increased intermetatarsal angle must be corrected by osteotomy to prevent the probable recurrence of the hallux valgus deformity.[8,13,15,28] A distal soft-tissue release and realignment may repair the distal deformity, but a proximal osteotomy is necessary to realign the first metatarsal. All elements of the deformity must be corrected at the time of surgery[1,3,16,35] to minimize the chance of recurrence.

## Repair of the Juvenile Bunion

Because the metatarsus primus varus deformity must be corrected, osteotomy is frequently necessary. Distal metatarsal osteotomies, while not close to the location of the true deformity, nonetheless, have in certain cases provided an adequate repair.[47] Wilson[47] reported an 88% satisfactory repair rate with a midmetatarsal oblique osteotomy, while Helal[11] reported 100% success with a similar technique.

While many have found the Mitchell repair to be a satisfactory technique,[6,12,13,15] Ball and Sullivan[48] recently reported a 61% recurrence rate with this type of repair. Mitchell and associates[15] reported a 22% postoperative rate of metatarsalgia with the Mitchell repair, and Ball and Sullivan[48] reported a 44% incidence of metatarsalgia following surgery. Displacement of the small distal fragment, rotational instability, dorsiflexion or plantarflexion malunion, nonunion, shortening of an already short first metatarsal, incomplete correction, and avascular necrosis are some of the complications noted following the Mitchell procedure.[1,12,13,18,48]

Proximal osteotomies have been used with varying success. An opening wedge osteotomy has been recommended for repair of the juvenile bunion[3]; however, Scranton and Zuckerman[7] reported a 35% failure rate with this technique, and Goldner and Gaines[18] cautioned that the lengthening of the first ray following an opening wedge osteotomy tightens the extensor mechanism leading to postoperative recurrence. A closing wedge osteotomy was recommended by Scranton and Zuckerman[7] but was noted to have a 25% recurrence rate.

A distal soft-tissue repair alone, such as a modified McBride procedure, has been found to be inadequate for correction of the typical juvenile bunion. Helal and associates[5] reported a 46% failure rate with this technique and noted that, although initially the McBride procedure did well, it did not hold up with time. Scranton and Zuckerman[7] reported a 75% failure rate with this technique. Bonney and MacNab[3] reported that following a distal soft-tissue repair, the intermetatarsal angle returned to its original preoperative angle or experienced an increased metatarsal angle in 63% of the operative cases. A combination of a distal soft-tissue repair with a proximal metatarsal osteotomy has had reported success. Simmonds and Menelaus[8] reported an 80% success rate, while Trott,[16] using a similar technique, reported success in 91% of his patients. Goldner and Gaines[18] combined a metatarsocuneiform fusion with a distal soft-tissue realignment and reported an 88% success rate.

A double osteotomy technique was recommended by Durman,[28] who used an opening wedge proximal phalangeal osteotomy and a closing wedge distal metatarsal osteotomy. Amarnek and associates[22] used a crescentic osteotomy of the proximal phalanx and the proximal metatarsal. While they reported success with this procedure, care must be taken not to disturb an open epiphysis in the juvenile patient.

Cuneiform osteotomy, initially reported by Young,[46] was also used by Bonney and MacNab[3] to realign the metatarsocuneiform joint without disturbing the proximal metatarsal epiphysis.

## Decision Making in the Treatment of the Juvenile Hallux Valgus

The belief that a standard operation is suited for all juvenile patients with hallux valgus is unreasonable. Depending upon the pathophysiology and anatomy of the hallux valgus deformity, various techniques may or may not be appropriate. Furthermore, evaluation of the entire foot may occasionally demonstrate other conditions (such as a contracted Achilles tendon or severe hindfoot valgus) that should be evaluated and possibly treated prior to any hallux valgus repair.

The initial assessment must determine whether the metatarsophalangeal joint is congruous or noncongruous, which will determine whether a metatarsophalangeal joint realignment or an extra-articular repair is necessary. If a noncongruous joint shows significant subluxation at the metatarsophalangeal joint, realignment of the MP joint is acceptable. Using a modified McBride procedure alone, or with a proximal metatarsal osteotomy, or with a cuneiform osteotomy is acceptable. A Chevron or Mitchell osteotomy may also be used in the less severe deformity. Hallux valgus with a congruous joint often requires periarticular osteotomy. A proximal phalangeal osteotomy such as the Akin procedure, and distal metatarsal osteotomies such as the Mitchell, Chevron, Reverdin, and Wilson procedures have all been used.

Further assessment requires evaluation of the intermetatarsal angle. The magnitude of the intermetatarsal angle, the metatarsocuneiform orientation, and the flexibility of the metatarsocuneiform joint must be evaluated. With a significant intermetatarsal angle, a more proximally based osteotomy will achieve greater correction than a distally placed osteotomy. With significant metatarsocuneiform obliquity or an epiphysis that still has considerable growth remaining, a first cuneiform osteotomy may be the treatment of choice.

Finally, the orientation of the lesser metatarsals is considered. Significant forefoot adductus, which is not infrequently associated with the juvenile bunion, is a difficult entity to treat. Correction of the metatarsus primus varus may require a metatarsal osteotomy that produces a negative intermetatarsal angle in order to achieve adequate correction. Rarely, in order to allow adequate realignment of the hallux, multiple metatarsal osteotomies must be performed to correct the forefoot varus.

Postoperative complications are not infrequent with bunion surgery, and care must be taken in treating the juvenile bunion to avoid excessive shortening of the first metatarsal following osteotomy, devascularization of the metatarsal head resulting in avascular necrosis, excessive metatarsal head excision with resection of the medial eminence, and overcorrection with a first metatarsal osteotomy. A procedure should be selected that will correct all the components of the deformity but permit a reasonable means of salvage should the initial procedure fail.

## Summary

While the surgeon may tend to use one procedure in the repair of a hallux valgus deformity, versatility is most important when treating the juvenile bunion. Using a distal soft-tissue repair when subluxation is solely at the metatarsophalangeal joint is an acceptable approach. A metatarsal or cuneiform osteotomy is necessary if the intermetatarsal angle is abnormally large. It is important not to stretch the indications for a bunion technique in order to correct the hallux valgus deformity. If a more severe deformity is present, a more aggressive technique must be used to correct the abnormality. That varying success rates are reported with different techniques testifies to the fact that the juvenile bunion is not suited for a standard hallux valgus repair. The surgical technique used to repair a specific juvenile bunion depends upon the anatomic and physiologic abnormalities present in each patient.

## References

1. Meehan P: Adolescent bunion. American Academy of Orthopaedic Surgeons *Instructional Course Lectures, XXXI.* St Louis, C V Mosby, 1982, pp 262–264.
2. Piggott H: The natural history of hallux valgus in adolescence and early adult life. *J Bone Joint Surg* 1960;42B:749–760.
3. Bonney G, MacNab I: Hallux valgus and hallux rigidus: A critical survey of operative results. *J Bone Joint Surg* 1952;34B:366–385.
4. Halebain J, Gaines S: Juvenile hallux valgus. *J Foot Surg* 1983;22:290–293.
5. Helal B, Gupta S, Gojaseni P: Surgery for adolescent hallux valgus. *Acta Orthop Scand* 1974;45:271–295.
6. Luba R, Rosman M: Bunions in children: Treatment with a modified Mitchell osteotomy. *J Pediatr Orthop* 1984;4:44–47.
7. Scranton P, Zuckerman J: Bunion surgery in adolescents: Results of surgical treatment. *J Pediatr Orthop* 1984;39–43.
8. Simmonds F, Menelaus M: Hallux valgus in adolescents. *J Bone Joint Surg* 1960;42B:761–768.
9. Hardy R, Clapham J: Observations on hallux valgus. *J Bone Joint Surg* 1951;33B:376–391.
10. Scranton P: Adolescent bunions: Diagnosis and management. *Pediatr Ann* 1982;11:518–520.
11. Helal B: Surgery for adolescent hallux valgus. *Clin Orthop* 1981;157:50–63.
12. Carr C, Boyd B: Correctional osteotomy for metatarsus primus varus and hallux valgus. *J Bone Joint Surg* 1968;50A:1353–1367.
13. Das S: Distal metatarsal osteotomy for adolescent hallux valgus. *J Pediatr Orthop* 1984;4:32–38.
14. Jones A: Hallux valgus in the adolescent. *Proc R Soc Med* 1948;41:392–393.
15. Mitchell C, Fleming J, Allen R, et al: Osteotomy-bunionectomy for hallux valgus. *J Bone Joint Surg* 1958;40A:41–59.
16. Trott A: Hallux valgus in the adolescent. American Academy of Orthopaedic Surgeons *Instructional Course Lectures, XXI.* St Louis, C V Mosby, 1972, pp 262–268.
17. DuVries H: *Surgery of the Foot*, ed 2. St Louis, C V Mosby, 1965, pp 436–438.
18. Goldner J, Gaines R: Adult and juvenile hallux valgus: Analysis and treatment. *Orthop Clin North Am* 1976;7:863–887.
19. Inman V: Hallux valgus: A review of etiologic factors. *Orthop Clin North Am* 1974;5:59–66.
20. Lapidus P: Operative correction of the metatarsus varus primus in hallux valgus. *Surg Gynecol Obstet* 1934;58:183–191.
21. McHale KA, McKay DW: Bunions in a child: Conservative versus surgical management. *J Musculoskel Med* 1986;3(1)56–62.

22. Amarnek D, Jacobs A, Oloff L: Adolescent hallux valgus: Its etiology and surgical management. *J Foot Surt* 1985;24:54–61.

23. Mann RA, Coughlin MJ: Hallux valgus and complications of hallux valgus, in *Surgery of the Foot*, ed 5. St Louis, C V Mosby, 1986, pp 66–130.

24. Funk FJ, Wells RE: Bunionectomy with distal osteotomy. *Clin Orthop* 1972;85:71–74.

25. Mann RA, Coughlin MJ: Hallux valgus—etiology, anatomy, treatment, and surgical consideration. *Clin Orthop* 1981; 157:31–41.

26. Houghton G, Dickson R: Hallux valgus in the younger patient: The structural abnormality. *J Bone Joint Surg* 1979;61B:176–177.

27. Antrobus J: The primary deformity in hallux valgus and metatarsus primus varus. *Clin Orthop* 1984;184:251–255.

28. Durman D: Metatarsus primus varus and hallux valgus. *Arch Surg* 1957;74:128–135.

29. Price G: Metatarsus primus varus: including various clinico-radiologic features of the female foot. *Clin Orthop* 1979;145:217–223.

30. Haines R, McDougall A: The anatomy of hallux valgus. *J Bone Joint Surg* 1954;36B:272–293.

31. Sarrafian SK: *Anatomy of the Foot and Ankle*. Philadelphia, J B Lippincott Co, 1983, pp 21–33.

32. Ewald P: Die aetiologie des hallux valgus. *Deutsche Ztsch F Chirurgie* 1912;114:90–103.

33. Berntsen A: De l'hallux valgus, contribution a son etiologie et a son traitement. *Rev Orthop* 1930;17:101–111.

34. Simon WV: Der Hallux Valgus und Seine Chirurgesche Behandlung mit besonderer Berucksichtigung der Ludloff' Schen Operation. *Beitr Klin Chir* 1918;3:467.

35. Truslow W: Metatarsus primus varus or hallux valgus? *J Bone Joint Surg* 1925;7:98–108.

36. Lapidus PW: The author's bunion operation from 1931 to 1959. *Clin Orthop* 1960;16:119–135.

37. McCrea J, Lichty T: The first metatarsocuneiform articulation and its relationship to metatarsus primus adductus. *J Am Podiatry Assoc* 1979;69:700–706.

38. Chomeley J: Hallux valgus in adolescents. *Proc R Soc Med* 1958;51:903–906.

39. Wilson D: Treatment of hallux valgus and bunions. *Br J Hosp Med* 1980;24:548.

40. Hawkins FB, Mitchell CL, Hedrick DW: Correction of hallux valgus by metatarsal osteotomy. *J Bone Joint Surg* 1945;27:387–394.

41. Blais M, Green W, Anderson M: Lengths of the growing foot. *J Bone Joint Surg* 1956;38A:998–1000.

42. Ellis V: A method of correcting metatarsus primus varus. *J Bone Joint Surg* 1951;33B:415–417.

43. Fox I, Smith S: Juvenile bunion correction by epiphysiodesis of the first metatarsal. *J Am Podiatry Assoc* 1983;73:448–455.

44. Zimmer TJ, Johnson KA: The use of the chevron osteotomy for correction of adolescent bunion deformities. Presentation at 1986 American Foot and Ankle Society Annual Meeting, New Orleans, Louisiana, February 19, 1986.

45. Reverdin J: De la deviation en dehors du gros orteil et de son traitement chirurgical. *Trans Int Med Congress* 1881;2:408.

46. Young JD: A new operation for adolescent hallux valgus. *Univ Pa Med Bulletin* 1910;23:459.

47. Wilson J: Oblique displacement osteotomy for hallux valgus. *J Bone Joint Surg* 1963;45B:552–556.

48. Ball J, Sullivan J: Treatment of the juvenile bunion by Mitchell osteotomy. *Orthopedics* 1985;8:1249–1252.

# Lesser Toe Deformities

Roger A. Mann, MD
Michael J. Coughlin, MD

## Introduction

Deformities of the lesser toes usually occur as a result of the long-term use of ill-fitting shoes. This probably accounts for the significantly increased incidence in women (Fig. 8–1). Other causes of lesser toe deformities include anatomic factors, neuromuscular diseases, connective tissue disorders, congenital anomalies, and trauma.

Anatomic factors include (1) a long second ray, resulting in buckling of the toe, which may cause a mallet or hammertoe; (2) an irregularly shaped middle phalanx, which results in a deviated distal phalanx; (3) a long fourth toe, which may result in curling of the fourth toe under the third; and (4) pressure against the second toe by the great toe, resulting in a hammertoe, or a subluxated or dislocated metatarsophalangeal joint.

Neuromuscular diseases such as diskogenic disease, muscular dystrophy, polio, or Charcot-Marie-Tooth disease may lead to deformities of the interphalangeal joints as well as of the metatarsophalangeal joints.

Connective tissue disorders such as rheumatoid arthritis or psoriatic arthritis and nonspecific synovial disorders produce deformities of the lesser toes as well as of the metatarsophalangeal joints.

Trauma may cause deformities of the interphalangeal joints ranging from an isolated hammertoe or mallet toe to a fixed dislocation of an interphalangeal joint.

A congenital anomaly, such as syndactyly, may result in buckling of the toes secondary to differential growth, producing a hammertoe or mallet toe deformity.

A lesser toe deformity may make conventional shoe wear difficult. A soft, laced shoe with an adequate toe box often relieves this problem because it not only provides more room for the toes but also permits padding of the involved toe with lamb's wool, moleskin, foam rubber, and other materials. Padding the foot without providing an adequate toe box area often compounds the patient's problems.

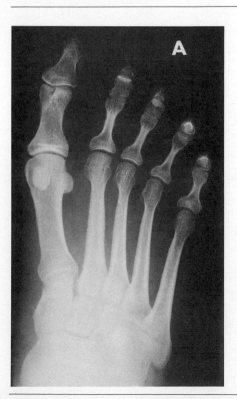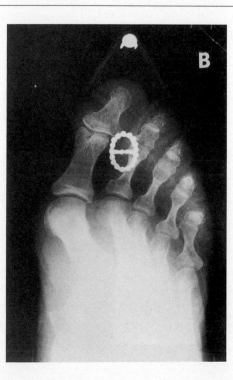

**Fig. 8–1 A:** Anteroposterior radiograph of a normal foot during weight-bearing. **B:** Same foot in a high-heeled, pointed-toe shoe, demonstrating the marked deformities of the toes.

The patient with an insensitive foot presents a more difficult problem. Often an ulceration develops over the bony prominence because there is no discomfort or pain from pressure against the toe. Treatment for this group of patients includes better shoes; however, patients must be taught to inspect their feet carefully each morning and evening. If conservative treatment fails to relieve the problem, surgical intervention should be considered, provided that the patient is a satisfactory surgical candidate and the vascular status is adequate.

Common lesser toe problems include mallet toe, hammertoe, hard corn and soft corn deformities, and claw toe.

## Mallet Toe

A mallet toe is a deformity of a lesser toe, usually the second or third, characterized by a flexion deformity at the level of the distal interphalangeal joint (Fig. 8–2).

### Clinical Complaint

Pressure on the tip of the toe or over the distal interphalangeal joint causes pain.

### Physical Findings

Examination of the toe with the patient standing demonstrates that the distal interphalangeal joint is flexed to almost 90 degrees. This places pressure on the tip of the toe and occasionally on the nail. At times a callus is noted beneath the pad of the toe. The proximal interphalangeal joint may be slightly flexed as well. There is rarely any change at the level of the metatarsophalangeal joint.

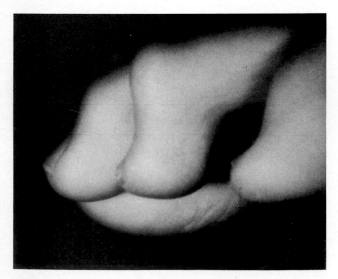

**Fig. 8–2** A mallet toe. (Reproduced with permission from Mann RA (ed): *Surgery of the Foot*, ed 5. St Louis, CV Mosby Co, 1986.)

### Treatment

Conservative treatment consists of wearing a shoe with a roomy toe box to accommodate the patient's forefoot. Although a pad beneath the toe alleviates pressure on the tip of the toe, it may cause pressure on the dorsal aspect of the distal interphalangeal joint as it strikes the top of the shoe.

Surgical treatment is quite successful if conservative management fails.

### Surgical Technique

An arthroplasty is carried out at the level of the distal interphalangeal joint to correct this problem (Fig. 8–3). With the patient under a digital anesthetic block, an elliptical incision is made over the dorsal aspect of the proximal interphalangeal joint. The incision is carried down through the extensor tendon and joint capsule to expose the distal interphalangeal joint. The collateral ligaments are carefully cut, exposing the distal portion of the middle phalanx. The distal portion of the middle phalanx is removed with a rongeur. If a fixed contracture of more than 45 to 50 degrees is present at the distal interphalangeal joint, the flexor digitorum longus tendon should be released to prevent a recurrence. The flexor digitorum longus can be exposed by incising the plantar plate at the bottom of the incision. A tenotomy is then performed. With a deformity of less than 45 degrees, tenotomy usually is not necessary. The arthroplasty site is stabilized with 0.045 K-wire or 3–0 silk incorporating two Telfa bolsters to hold the toe in satisfactory alignment. If the K-wire is used, it is left in place for approximately three to four weeks, after which the toe is taped into correct alignment for another two weeks. If the Telfa bolsters are used, they are removed after one week and the toe is held in correct alignment with adhesive tape for five more weeks. It is important that immobilization be continued long enough for adequate scarring of the soft tissues to occur.

### Results

The expected outcome after an arthroplasty is an ankylosed joint with approximately 10 to 15 degrees of motion. Usually there is no pain at the site of the arthroplasty. There is minimal swelling after a mallet toe procedure.

Complications are rare, although if adequate stabilization of the arthroplasty site is not achieved, a recurrence of the deformity may result.

### Alternative Treatments

Alternative treatments include an arthrodesis of the distal interphalangeal joint. The authors do not prefer fusion because it is difficult to obtain arthrodeses in joints this small.

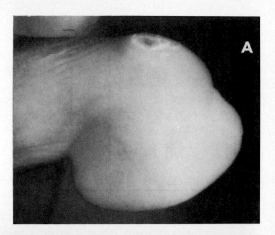

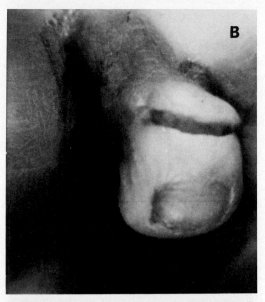

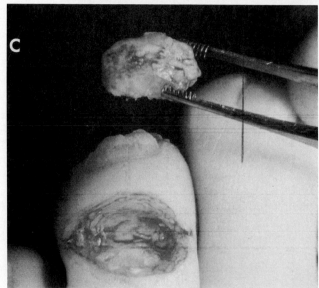

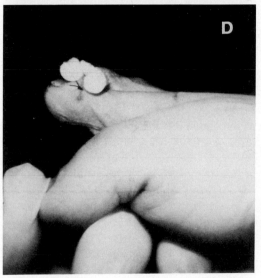

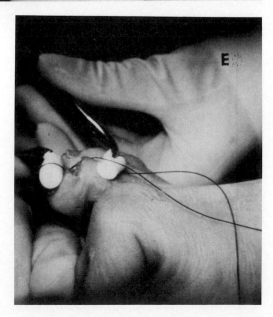

**Fig. 8–3** Technique for correction of mallet toe deformity. **A:** Mallet toe deformity. **B:** Elliptical skin incision centered over the distal interphalangeal joint. **C:** Excision of skin, extensor tendon, and capsule. **D:** Generous excision of the distal portion of the middle phalanx. **E:** Correction of toe with 3–0 silk and two Telfa bolsters. (Fig. 8–3, A and C reproduced with permission from Mann RA (ed): *Surgery of the Foot*, ed 5. St Louis, CV Mosby Co, 1986.)

## Hammertoe

A hammertoe deformity involves a flexion deformity of the proximal interphalangeal joint. A hammertoe may occur as an isolated deformity or in a multiple form involving the second, third, or fourth toes (Fig. 8–4).

### Clinical Complaint

The clinical complaint is pain over the dorsal aspect of the proximal interphalangeal joint. Pressure on the tip of the toes sometimes leads to painful callus formation. A keratotic lesion on the plantar aspect of the corresponding metatarsal head occasionally develops.

### Physical Findings

When the patient stands there is a varying degree of flexion of the proximal interphalangeal joint; at times some mild deformity of the distal interphalangeal joint occurs. Careful evaluation of the metatarsophalangeal joint may determine whether it is involved in the deformity.

When evaluating a hammertoe, it is important to ascertain whether or not it is a fixed deformity or a flexible (dynamic) deformity. In the case of a fixed deformity, only a bony procedure will produce a satisfactory outcome. With flexible or dynamic deformity, a tendon transfer may achieve a satisfactory clinical result. This determination is made at the time of the examination by observing whether or not the hammertoe deformity can be completely corrected by manual pressure on the toe, or whether a fixed deformity is present. As a general rule, if the ankle joint is brought into a plantar flexed position the deformity of the lesser toes straightens. When the ankle is brought into a dorsiflexed position, the involved toes demonstrate the hammertoe deformity.

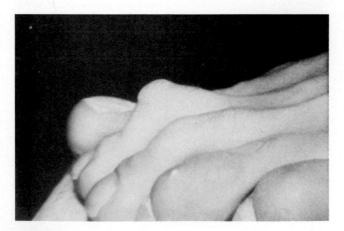

**Fig. 8–4**   A hammertoe.

### Treatment

Conservative management of the hammertoe deformity involves wearing a wide, broad-toed shoe or a shoe with extra depth that provides adequate room for the deformed toes. At times, if the deformity is extremely fixed, some type of toe crest may be used to elevate the tips of the toes off the ground. This, however, does have the disadvantage of elevating the toes slightly, and pressure may develop on the dorsal aspect of the proximal interphalangeal joints as they strike the toe box.

### Surgical Technique

**Fixed Hammertoe**   Surgical management of the fixed hammertoe is carried out with the patient under a digital anesthetic block (Fig. 8–5). An elliptical incision is made over the dorsal aspect of the proximal interphalangeal joint. The callus, extensor tendon, and dorsal capsule are excised. The collateral ligaments are then carefully cut, exposing the distal portion of the proximal phalanx. The distal portion of the proximal phalanx just proximal to the condyles is removed with a rongeur. The toe is then stabilized with 0.045 K-wire drilled distally through the middle phalanx and out through the tip of the toe. It is then advanced in a retrograde fashion into the base of the proximal phalanx but does not cross the metatarsophalangeal joint. An alternative method of fixation is a vertical mattress suture of 3–0 silk incorporating two Telfa bolsters; this also holds the toe in satisfactory alignment. Pin fixation is continued for three to four weeks, after which the pin is removed and the toe is taped in proper alignment for three more weeks. If the Telfa bolsters are used, they are removed after one week and the toe is taped into satisfactory alignment for five weeks.

**Dynamic Hammertoe**   In the case of a dynamic hammertoe, a flexor tendon transfer (Girdlestone procedure) may correct the problem.[1-3] If there is any fixed deformity, this procedure will not produce a satisfactory result.

The flexor tendon transfer is carried out by making a short incision (approximately 5 mm in length) on the plantar aspect of the foot at the level of the proximal flexion crease (Fig. 8–6). After the skin is incised, a mosquito clamp is used to clear away the soft tissues and small venules. The flexor sheath is identified on the plantar aspect of the toe and split longitudinally with a No. 11 blade. A mosquito clamp is then inserted into the flexor sheath and the middle of the three tendons is isolated. This is the flexor digitorum longus tendon, which is characterized by a natural raphe within it. With the tendon under tension, a No. 11 blade is used to release the insertion percutaneously from the base of the distal phalanx.

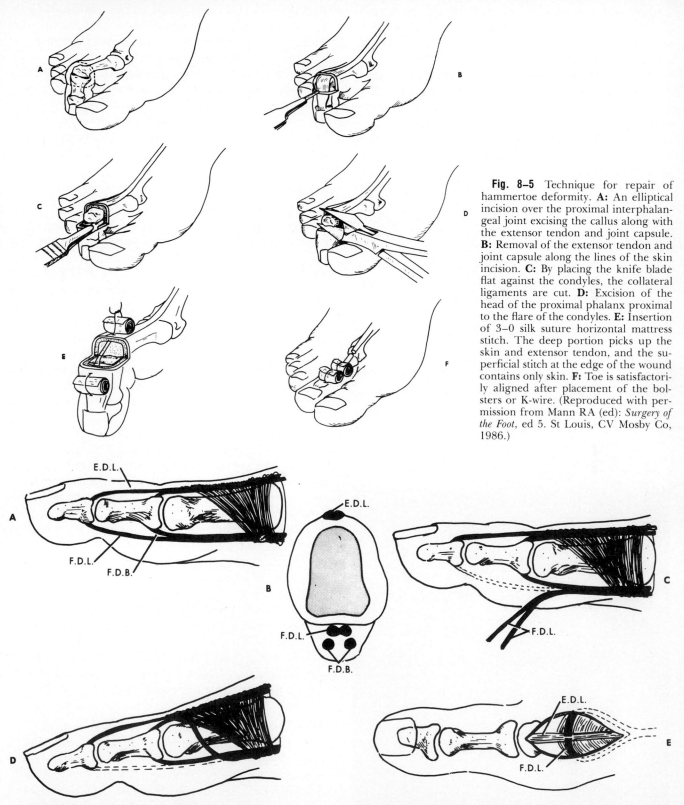

**Fig. 8–5** Technique for repair of hammertoe deformity. **A:** An elliptical incision over the proximal interphalangeal joint excising the callus along with the extensor tendon and joint capsule. **B:** Removal of the extensor tendon and joint capsule along the lines of the skin incision. **C:** By placing the knife blade flat against the condyles, the collateral ligaments are cut. **D:** Excision of the head of the proximal phalanx proximal to the flare of the condyles. **E:** Insertion of 3–0 silk suture horizontal mattress stitch. The deep portion picks up the skin and extensor tendon, and the superficial stitch at the edge of the wound contains only skin. **F:** Toe is satisfactorily aligned after placement of the bolsters or K-wire. (Reproduced with permission from Mann RA (ed): *Surgery of the Foot*, ed 5. St Louis, CV Mosby Co, 1986.)

**Fig. 8–6** Technique for correction of dynamic hammertoe. **A:** Lateral view of a lesser toe demonstrating the anatomy of extensor and flexor tendons. **B:** Cross section of the anatomy through the metatarsal head region. **C:** FDL tendon has been detached from its insertion into the base of the distal phalanx and delivered into the wound at the base of the toe. **D:** The FDL is brought up on each side of the extensor hood through a subcutaneous tunnel. **E:** The FDL is sutured into the extensor digitorum longus tendon under a moderate amount of tension while the metatarsophalangeal joint is held in approximately 20 degrees of plantar flexion. (Reproduced with permission from Mann RA (ed): *Surgery of the Foot*, ed 5. St Louis, CV Mosby Co, 1986.)

Once this is achieved, the tendon is delivered into the wound and two tails are created along the natural cleavage plane. It is important that the tendon halves be separated proximally to the level of the metatarsophalangeal joint.

The next incision is centered over the dorsal aspect of the proximal phalanx, directly over the extensor tendon. The incision is carried down through subcutaneous tissue and fat to expose the extensor tendon. A clamp is then passed on each side of the extensor hood to emerge from the proximal plantar wound. The clamp should stay along the extensor hood without penetrating it or entrapping the digital neurovascular bundle. A mosquito clamp is placed into the slot created on each side of the extensor hood and one tail of the flexor tendon is brought up on each side of the proximal phalanx. The toe is held in approximately 20 degrees of plantar flexion, and the flexor tendon is then sutured into the extensor tendon under a moderate amount of tension. Postoperative care consists of ambulation with the foot in a wooden shoe for a period of about three weeks, after which the foot is progressively mobilized.

### Results

Repair of a fixed hammertoe creates an ankylosis between the cut end of the proximal phalanx and the

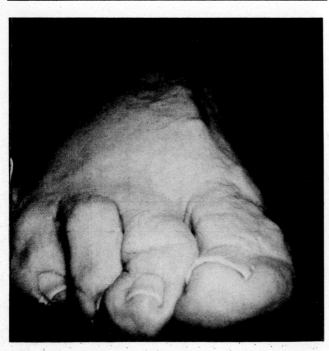

**Fig. 8–7** Postoperative picture after repair of hammertoe involving the second toe. Note the way the second toe has "molded" to the shape of the great toe, resulting in some lateral deviation of the second toe.

remaining articular surface of the middle phalanx. This permits 10 to 15 degrees of motion at this joint. There is rarely pain at the level of the arthroplasty, but if pain persists an injection of steroid preparation into the area usually eliminates the problem.

After the flexor tendon transfer, the toe is usually held quite straight, and little or no voluntary motion of the interphalangeal joints is possible. The patient can extend and flex the toes about the metatarsophalangeal joint, but motion at the interphalangeal joints is sacrificed.

### Complications

Postoperative swelling may persist for two to six months. As a general rule, the swelling is minimal but it may persist. This can annoy the patient. A hammertoe deformity occasionally recurs, but this usually happens because an inadequate amount of bone was removed or because a tight flexor tendon was present and not released at the time of surgery. As a general rule, if the adjacent toes appear to demonstrate tightness of the flexor tendon preoperatively, consideration should be given to release of the flexor tendon at the time of the hammertoe repair. Molding of the hammertoe is the term used to denote the shape of the hammertoe after a repair. If a hallux valgus deformity is present, or if an adjacent toe is crooked when a hammertoe deformity is being corrected, the hammertoe will usually be molded into the same shape as the adjacent toes (Fig. 8–7). This often results in some lateral deviation of the toe at the level of the proximal interphalangeal joint. If this molding did not occur, the toe would have a tendency to overlap the adjacent toe. Preoperative counseling should include a discussion of this possibility.

Complications after flexor tendon transfer are infrequent. Occasionally the patient may have slight residual flexion of the proximal interphalangeal joint, but as a general rule if a complete range of motion is present preoperatively the toe will be held in full extension by the transferred tendon. Occasionally the patient notes some transient numbness after a flexor tendon transfer. This is the result of manipulation of the small cutaneous nerves at the time of surgery.

### Hammertoe and the Metatarsophalangeal Joint

If a hammertoe deformity is associated with a variable degree of dorsiflexion of the metatarsophalangeal joint, treatment of the joint should usually be carried out at the same time as the hammertoe repair. If a mild dorsiflexion contracture is present when the patient stands, then a lengthening of the extensor tendon and a dorsal capsulotomy should be performed at the same time as the hammertoe repair. If a pin is used to stabilize the proximal interphalangeal joint, it can be driven across the metatarsophalangeal joint to stabilize it in a neutral position for about three weeks. If the proximal interphalangeal joint is stabilized with Telfa bolsters, the metatarsophalangeal joint should be kept taped down into a neutral position for approximately three weeks. In either case, the basic principle is that the metatarsophalangeal joint must be held in a corrected position for at least three weeks postoperatively or the deformity will recur.

If there is dorsal subluxation of the metatarsophalangeal joint with the hammertoe, it may be necessary not only to lengthen the extensor tendon and the dorsal joint capsule but also to cut the collateral ligaments to bring the joint down into neutral position. As a general rule, this joint must be pinned for four weeks to prevent a recurrence.

If a complete dislocation of the metatarsophalangeal joint is present along with a hammertoe formation, it is imperative that the dislocation be reduced and the hammertoe repaired.

### Alternative Methods of Treatment

A hammertoe deformity can be treated by an arthrodesis of the proximal interphalangeal joint. This produces a satisfactory result, but it is technically much more demanding and the possibility of obtaining a successful arthrodesis is about 50%. At times the pseudarthrosis created is painful, and for this reason arthrodesis is not the author's procedure of choice.

## Hard Corns

A hard corn is a thickening of the epithelium over a bony prominence, usually involving the fifth toe.

### Clinical Complaint

The patient with a hard corn experiences pain when pressure is applied to the thickened, cornified area of skin.

### Physical Findings

The physical examination demonstrates a thick callus over the dorsolateral aspect of the small toe, which is generally quite sensitive to palpation. There may be a mild flexion deformity at the level of the proximal interphalangeal joint.

### Treatment

Conservative management consists of trimming the corn and protecting the area with some type of a soft cushion over the toe. Patients should be advised to obtain a shoe that provides adequate space for their toes. At times, a small felt pad can relieve the pressure on the involved area.

Surgical management consists of excising the distal portion of the proximal phalanx, as described above for a hammertoe, or possibly removing the lateral condyle of the proximal phalanx of the fifth toe.

### Surgical Technique

With the patient under digital anesthetic block, a longitudinal incision is made over the dorsal aspect of the small toe (Fig. 8–8). It is centered over the proximal interphalangeal joint. The incision is usually placed in this area to prevent a scar from forming over the lateral aspect of the fifth toe where pressure is usually applied by the shoe. If the distal portion of the proximal phalanx is to be removed, this is done in the same manner as described for a hammertoe. If, however, only the condyle is to be removed, then the condyle is exposed and removed with a smaller rongeur. It is important to make a concavity where the previous convexity existed, to ensure that an adequate amount of bone has been removed. On occasion, a portion of the lateral aspect of the middle phalanx needs to be excised as well.

Postoperatively the patient should wear a wooden shoe or a sandal. After the soreness subsides, regular shoes can be worn.

### Results

The usual result is satisfactory. It may take approximately four to six weeks for the hard corn to soften and resolve after the surgical procedure.

### Complications

Complications include prolonged swelling, as occurs after a hammertoe procedure, and, occasionally, recurrence of the corn if an inadequate amount of bone was resected. If too much bone is resected from the phalanx, the small toe may become floppy.

## Soft Corns

A soft corn is the same type of deformity as a hard corn, except that it occurs between two toes. The moisture between the toes produces a soft corn instead of the normal dry hard corn noted on the lateral side of the fifth toe. Two types of soft corns occur, one in the web space between the fourth and fifth toes and the other more distal on the toe, secondary to a small exostosis on the phalanx.

### Clinical Complaint

The patient's main complaint is pain over the corn when the foot is in a shoe. Occasionally, when the soft corn is at the base of the fourth web space there may be a significant degree of maceration and occasionally an infection or sinus tract formation occurs.

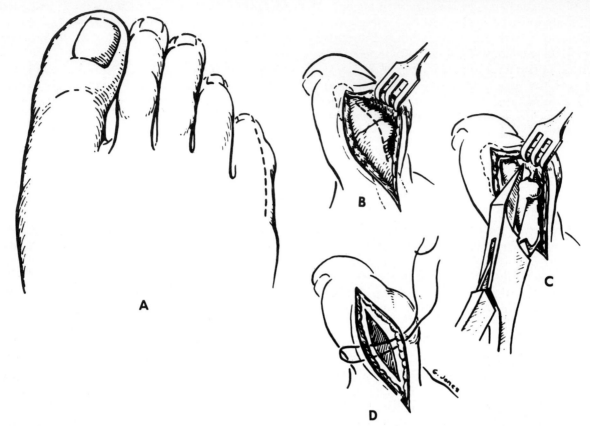

**Fig. 8–8**  DuVries technique for condylectomy for a hard corn on the fifth toe. **A:** Longitudinal incision over the dorsal aspect of the fifth toe. **B:** Skin and capsule retracted. **C:** Fibular condyle or the distal portion of the proximal phalanx is amputated. **D:** Skin and capsule are closed with mattress suture. (Reproduced with permission from Mann RA (ed): *Surgery of the Foot*, ed 5. St Louis, CV Mosby Co, 1986.)

### Physical Findings

On physical examination a distal soft corn is characterized by a small callus, which when carefully palpated reveals an underlying exostosis (Fig. 8–9). Direct pressure on the callus produces pain. The callus is usually no more than 2 to 3 mm in diameter. The soft corn in the fourth web space demonstrates a thickened callus in the web space, which at times is macerated (Fig. 8–10A). Figure 8–10B demonstrates the origin of a soft corn secondary to pressure of the distal portion of the proximal phalanx of the small toe against the lateral base of the proximal phalanx of the fourth toe.

### Treatment

Conservative management consists of adequate padding of the area, either with lamb's wool or by placing a small piece of felt or moleskin between the toes to relieve the pressure on the exostosis. If the patient is comfortable with this padding, no further treatment is necessary.

### Surgical Technique

Surgical treatment of the soft corn located distally on the phalanx begins with a digital anesthetic block. A small incision over the area of the corn is carried down through subcutaneous tissue and fat to expose the underlying exostosis. This is removed with a fine-tipped rongeur to create a concavity. A single suture is usually used to close the capsule and skin. Postoperatively, the patient wears a sandal or a wooden shoe until the swelling subsides. Normal shoe wear can then be resumed.

The treatment of the soft corn in the fourth web space involves resection of the distal portion of the proximal phalanx, since it is the pressure from this against the base of the lateral aspect of the proximal phalanx of the fourth toe that causes the problem. This has been described above in the treatment of hard corns. Postoperatively, the patient wears a sandal or wooden shoe until the wound heals.

### Results

The expected result of an excision of a soft corn involving a distal phalanx is complete resolution of the problem. Rarely is any type of complication noted. The result after excision of the distal portion of the proximal phalanx has been discussed above.

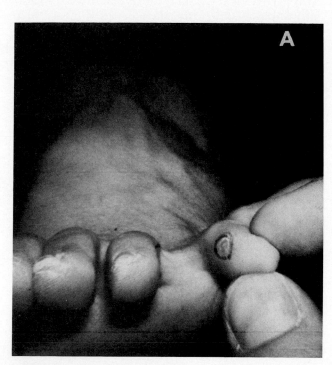

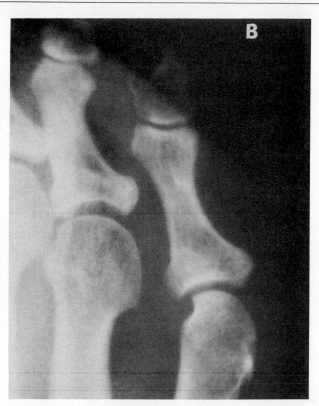

**Fig. 8–9   A:** Soft corn on medial aspect of the tip of the small toe. **B:** Radiograph of the small toe demonstrating a small exostosis on the medial aspect of the distal phalanx producing a soft corn. (Fig. 8-9B reproduced with permission from Mann RA (ed): *Surgery of the Foot*, ed 5. St Louis, CV Mosby Co, 1986.)

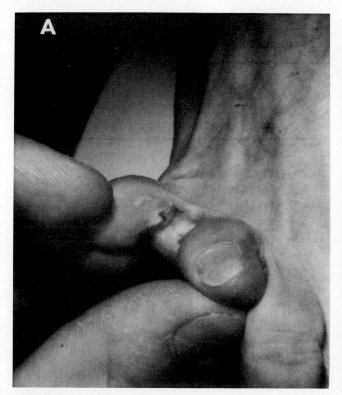

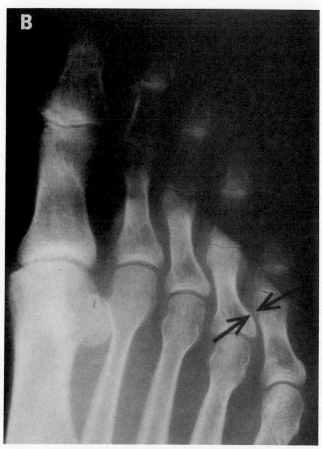

**Fig. 8–10   A:** Soft corn in the fourth web space. **B:** Radiograph demonstrating origin of soft corn.

### Complications

After excision of a soft corn from the distal phalanx, the soft corn occasionally recurs if an inadequate amount of bone was resected. If too much of the distal phalanx was removed during treatment of a soft corn in the fourth web space, the small toe may become floppy. Occasionally, postoperative swelling persists for many months.

### Alternative Methods

There is no way to treat a soft corn of the distal portion of the phalanx except excision of the exostosis.

A soft corn in the fourth web space may be treated by a syndactyly between the fourth and fifth toes, which eliminates the skin between the toes and hence relieves the soft corn. This procedure is certainly satisfactory, although the authors prefer to remove the distal portion of the proximal phalanx since it is much simpler and gives as good a result. Some people also resist having a syndactyly carried out.

Another alternative treatment method is to remove the lateral aspect of the base of the proximal phalanx of the fourth toe. The rationale for this procedure is that it is the pressure from the distal portion of the proximal phalanx of the fifth toe against this lateral flare of the proximal phalanx of the fourth toe that creates the soft corn. Although this alternative appears viable, it is a much more extensive procedure and the loss of the lateral aspect of the base of the proximal phalanx of the fourth toe may result in some instability of the metatarsophalangeal joint with subsequent medial drift of the fourth toe. Our method is simpler and gives a most satisfactory result.

### Overlapping Fifth Toe

An overlapping fifth toe is a congenital anomaly involving the fifth metatarsophalangeal joint in which the small toe deviates medially and rests on top of the fourth toe to a variable degree.

### Clinical Complaint

The patient's main complaint is discomfort over the fifth toe. This can become quite bothersome, particularly for women wearing tight hose. As a general rule men tolerate this problem quite well.

### Physical Findings

The physical examination demonstrates that the fifth toe overrides the fourth toe to a variable degree.

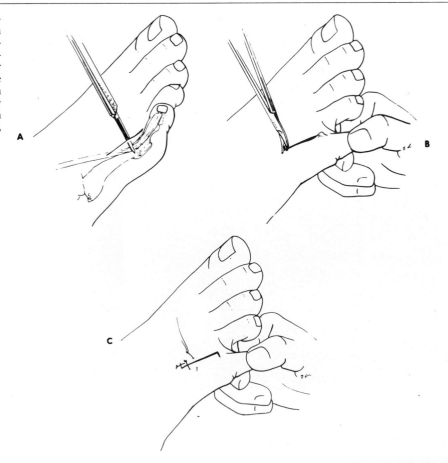

**Fig. 8–11** DuVries technique for correction of overlapping fifth toe with moderate skin contracture. **A:** Longitudinal incision made over the fourth metatarsal interspace. **B:** Fifth toe is plantar flexed to bring the fibular margin of the incision distal and the tibial margin proximal. **C:** Wound sutured in new position. (Reproduced with permission from Mann RA (ed): *Surgery of the Foot,* ed 5. St Louis, CV Mosby Co, 1986.)

There is also some mild dorsiflexion at the metatarsophalangeal joint. In older patients the toe assumes a somewhat flat appearance in the anteroposterior plane, secondary to the pressure exerted against it for many years by the shoe. The toe itself often makes an indentation along the dorsolateral aspect of the fourth toe.

### Treatment

Conservative management consists of a shoe with a toe box broad enough to prevent pressure on the small toe.

If conservative management fails, surgical treatment is fairly successful in alleviating the problem. Women should be advised that when the fifth toe is realigned adjacent to the fourth toe, the foot becomes somewhat wider, making stylish footwear somewhat more difficult to wear.

### Technique

The surgical procedure preferred by the authors is one in which an incision is made in the dorsal aspect of the web space and carried down through subcutaneous tissue (Fig. 8–11). The extensor tendon and dorsal capsule are cut subcutaneously and the toe is pulled down into marked plantar flexion so that any remaining contracted tissue is released. Once this is achieved, the toe usually remains in place. With the toe then held in full plantar flexion, the skin along the lateral side of the incision is displaced distally and the skin incision is closed. This permits the lateral skin to be translated distally in relation to the medial skin margin. The toe is held in a slightly overcorrected (plantar-flexed) alignment for a period of six weeks in a wooden shoe. The patient is then allowed to wear regular shoes.

### Results

The outcome is usually satisfactory (Fig. 8–12). As a rule, adequate alignment of the toe is achieved, although in some cases the toe still assumes a slightly dorsiflexed position because of marked contracture. Usually, however, the crossing over does not recur.

### Complications

The main complication is recurrence of the deformity, which happens in about 5% to 10% of cases. Occasionally there is some mild postoperative swelling, but it is usually of no significance.

### Alternative Methods of Treatment

Resection of all or part of the proximal phalanx with a syndactylization of the fourth web space can produce a satisfactory result. The fifth toe is slightly, but usually not significantly, shortened by this procedure. The advantage of this procedure is that the deformity does not recur if the soft tissues are adequately released.

The Ruiz-Mora[4] procedure has also been used for this deformity (Fig. 8–13). An elliptical plantar incision is made in the long axis of the fifth toe, after which the proximal phalanx is removed. The toe is then reduced and the incision closed in a medial-lateral direction, thereby permitting the small toe to be aligned in mild plantar flexion. This too gives a satisfactory result, although the toe may be somewhat floppy and occasionally tends to dorsiflex slightly.

## Cockup Deformity of the Fifth Toe

The cockup deformity of the fifth toe usually occurs spontaneously although it may be seen with other disease processes such as rheumatoid arthritis. In these cases the proximal phalanx is dislocated onto the neck of the metatarsal and sits at a right angle to the metatarsal shaft (Fig. 8–14).

### Clinical Complaint

The main complaint is chafing of the small toe against the shoe.

### Physical Findings

The physical examination demonstrates a fixed dislocation of the fifth metatarsophalangeal joint. The joint cannot be reduced. Occasionally subluxation or dislocation of the adjacent metatarsophalangeal joint occurs.

### Treatment

Conservative treatment consists of a broad-toed shoe that removes stress from the fifth toe.

Surgical treatment for this condition requires adequate decompression of the joint so that the toe can be brought back into satisfactory alignment. This is achieved with a Ruiz-Mora procedure, as described above. This procedure has the advantage of shortening and decompressing the toe. The dermoplasty on the plantar aspect helps to achieve a satisfactory alignment.

### Result

The outcome is usually satisfactory, although sometimes there is mild dorsiflexion at the metatarsophalangeal joint. The toe itself may be somewhat floppy.

### Complications

There are few or no complications associated with the Ruiz-Mora procedure. The shortness and the floppiness of the toe are usually the patient's main complaints.

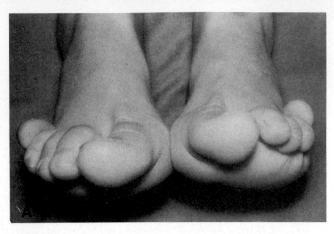
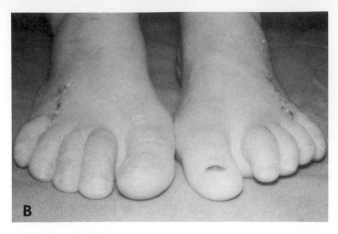

**Fig. 8–12** DuVries technique for repair of overlapping fifth toe. **A:** Preoperatively. **B:** Postoperatively. (Reproduced with permission from Mann RA (ed): *Surgery of the Foot*, ed 5. St Louis, CV Mosby Co, 1986.)

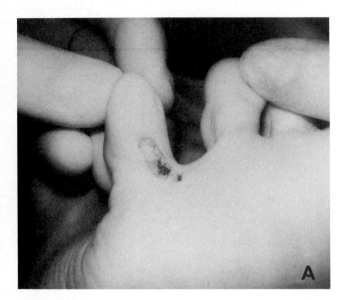
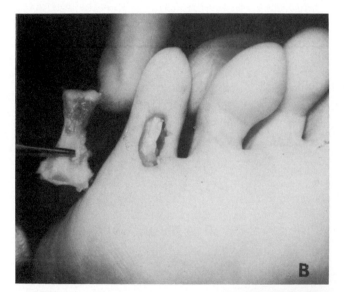
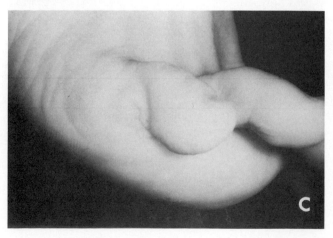

**Fig. 8–13** Technique for the Ruiz-Mora procedure. **A:** An elliptical incision deviating somewhat medially is made on the plantar aspect of the small toe. **B:** The proximal phalanx is removed through this incision. **C:** The incision is closed in a transverse fashion, thereby bringing the small toe into slight plantar flexion and medial deviation. (Reproduced with permission from Mann RA (ed): *Surgery of the Foot*, ed 5. St Louis, CV Mosby Co, 1986.)

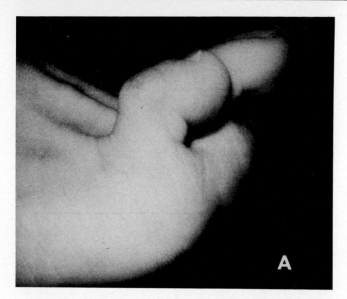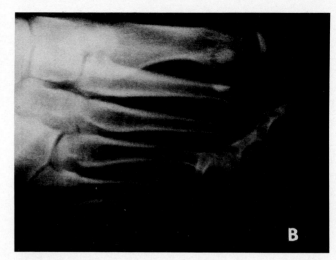

**Fig. 8–14** **A:** Cockup of the fifth toe. **B:** Radiograph demonstrating cockup of fifth toe. Note that the proximal phalanx is subluxated and almost at right angles to the metatarsal shaft. (Reproduced with permission from Mann RA (ed): *Surgery of the Foot*, ed 5. St Louis, CV Mosby Co, 1986.)

### Alternative Methods of Treatment

A partial excision of the base of the proximal phalanx with syndactylization of the fifth toe to the fourth toe can be used. The results cosmetically are about the same as for the Ruiz-Mora procedure, although the toe is usually less floppy. The only objection patients have to this is the syndactyly itself.

### Claw Toes

A claw toe deformity is characterized by dorsiflexion of the metatarsophalangeal joint to a variable degree, associated with hammertoe deformities of the lesser toes. As a general rule, all toes are involved (Fig. 8–15A). The great toe manifests similar findings with dorsiflexion at the metatarsophalangeal joint and flexion of the interphalangeal joint. The deformity itself may be rigid or flexible. Not infrequently it is associated with a cavus-type foot deformity, a neuromuscular disorder such as polio or Charcot-Marie-Tooth disease, or degenerative disk disease. Most frequently, it is idiopathic. The claw toe deformity may be flexible and readily correctable or quite rigid. Claw toes are the result of an imbalance between the intrinsic and extrinsic muscle groups. This deformity can be particularly impressive after a compartment syndrome that results in contractures of the long extensor and flexor tendons associated with a variable degree of weakness or dysfunction of the intrinsic muscles. On occasion, a single ray (toe and metatarsal) may be affected.

### Clinical Complaint

The patient's main complaint is metatarsalgia caused by dorsiflexion at the metatarsophalangeal joints that secondarily forces the metatarsal heads into the plantar aspect of the foot, which not infrequently results in some atrophy of the plantar fat pad. As the deformity progresses, the cockup deformity of the lesser toes becomes more bothersome and there is chafing of these toes against the shoe. There may be concomitant deformities of the hindfoot if the problem is secondary to a cavus foot or a neuromuscular disease such as Charcot-Marie-Tooth disease.

### Treatment

Conservative management of the problem involves redistributing the pressure away from the metatarsal head region and back toward the softer area of the longitudinal arch. This is accomplished with an orthotic device, soft shoes, and a toe box adequate to relieve the stress on the toes. If, however, the deformity is severe, conservative management is usually ineffective.

Surgical management of the problem depends on the degree of the deformity and its rigidity. If a significant deformity of the hindfoot exists, as is common in Charcot-Marie-Tooth disease and/or a cavus foot, reconstruction of the hindfoot usually takes precedence over the forefoot reconstruction. Once the hindfoot is corrected the forefoot realignment can be undertaken.

If the deformity is flexible, a satisfactory result can be achieved with a flexor tendon transfer along with

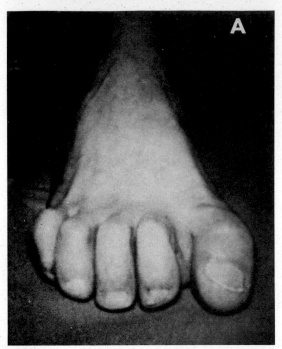

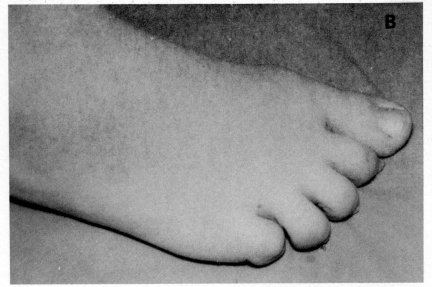

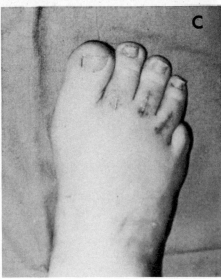

**Fig. 8–15 A:** Claw toe deformity involves a hammertoe associated with dorsiflexion at the metatarsophalangeal joint. **B:** Preoperative picture, before flexor tendon transfer for dynamic claw toes. **C:** Postoperative result. Note the extension of the lesser toes. The fifth toe was not included but should have been. (Fig. 8–15, B and C reproduced with permission from Mann RA (ed): *Surgery of the Foot*, ed 5. St Louis, CV Mosby Co, 1986.)

releases of the extensor tendon and dorsal capsule of the metatarsophalangeal joint (Fig. 8–15, B and C). If the deformity is fixed, it can be repaired with an arthroplasty, as described previously, with resection of the distal portion of the proximal phalanx along with extensor tenotomies and extensive dorsal capsulotomies. In these cases, the proximal interphalangeal joint should be stabilized with a 0.045-inch wire, which is then driven across the metatarsophalangeal joint to hold it in satisfactory alignment until adequate soft-tissue healing occurs around the area. In these cases the pins should be left in place for approximately six weeks. If the contracture is very rigid, release of all the flexor tendons may be necessary.

If the great toe is involved, an arthrodesis of the interphalangeal joint and a transplantation of the extensor hallucis longus into the neck of the first metatarsal (Jones procedure) should be used to realign the first ray.

### Results

The outcome is somewhat variable. If the deformity is not too severe, a satisfactory result can usually be achieved. In cases in which there is marked rigidity of the foot, an adequate reduction may be achieved. However, with time this deformity tends to recur. The recurrence may result from the residual long or short flexor function, if these flexors were not released, or from the constant dorsiflexion force across the metatarsophalangeal joints during walking.

### Complications

The main complication associated with the treatment of multiple claw toes is recurrence. This may result from insufficient release of the soft-tissue and/or tendon contractures.

## Disorders of the Metatarsophalangeal Joints

Disorders of the metatarsophalangeal joints are less common than those involving the lesser toes. However, it is often a problem with the metatarsophalangeal joint that produces the deformity of the lesser toe. Disorders of the metatarsophalangeal joints are more frequent in women because of ill-fitting shoes. The most common disorders include subluxation, dislocation, clawing, synovitis, crossover toe and avascular necrosis.

The most frequent causes of deformity of the metatarsophalangeal joint include anatomic factors, neuromuscular diseases, connective tissue disorders, trauma, avascular necrosis, and congenital anomalies.

The anatomic factors include excessive length of the second metatarsal, which may result in increased stress upon the joint. Stress probably accounts for the fact that this joint is the most frequently dislocated or subluxated. An excessively long ray may buckle at the metatarsophalangeal joint when it is placed in a tight shoe. This buckling places increased stress on the plantar capsule, which may result in deterioration of the plantar plate (joint capsule and plantar aponeurosis), predisposing the metatarsophalangeal joint to subluxation or dislocation. Lateral pressure from the hallux against the second toe, or dorsal pressure when the hallux underlaps the second toe, may lead to subluxation or dislocation of the metatarsophalangeal joint.

Neuromuscular disorders often lead to chronic hypertension of the metatarsophalangeal joints, resulting in clawing of the toes with eventual dorsal subluxation.

Neuromuscular disorders that may affect the metatarsophalangeal joint include diskogenic disease, the muscular dystrophies, neurologic disorders such as Charcot-Marie-Tooth disease, polio, Friedreich's ataxia, and peripheral neuropathies (for example, diabetes, leprosy).

Connective tissues disorders such as rheumatoid arthritis, psoriatic arthritis, and nonspecific synovitis may lead to chronic thickening of the synovial tissue with distention and eventual disruption of the joint capsules and collateral ligaments. Chondrolysis of the articular surfaces may compound the problem.

Trauma may result in an isolated dislocation of the metatarsophalangeal joint or possibly an intra-articular fracture. After trauma to the leg, an unrecognized compartment syndrome may occur, resulting in severe fixed clawing of the metatarsophalangeal joints. Similar findings also occur after a severe crush injury to the foot or leg.

Avascular necrosis of the metatarsal head, such as occurs in Freiberg's infraction, may lead to a painful metatarsophalangeal joint that some times becomes subluxated or painful secondary to a large dorsal osteophyte.

The congenital causes of metatarsophalangeal joint problems are usually those associated with an idiopathic pes cavus, congenital overlapping fifth toe, and a cockup deformity of the fifth metatarsophalangeal joint.

### Subluxation of the Metatarsophalangeal Joint

A subluxation of the metatarsophalangeal joint is the term used when there is a dorsal angulation of the metatarsophalangeal joint of variable degree but when the joint is still intact and not dislocated. A broad range of deformity is associated with a subluxation. The deformity may be a very minor or a rather advanced dorsal angulation. When multiple toes are involved, the term "clawing" is used to describe the metatarsophalangeal joint deformity. Generally speaking, subluxation of the metatarsophalangeal joints is usually associated with a deformity of the lesser toes, namely hammertoe formation of variable degree.

**Clinical Complaint** The main problem associated with subluxation is pressure on the dorsal aspect of the lesser toes as they impinge against the shoe. Secondarily, as the deformity becomes more severe, metatarsalgia may develop secondary to depression of the metatarsal heads.

**Physical Findings** The physical findings in a patient with a subluxation of the metatarsophalangeal joint vary from very minor dorsal angulation to a predislocation state. The deformity may be quite flexible or fixed, depending on the cause. When it involves the second toe as a result of pressure from the great toe, the deformity may not be reduced unless the great toe is moved out of the way and a space is created for the second toe. When it is associated with a connective tissue disorder such as rheumatoid arthritis, there may be joint destruction, with or without advanced synovitis, which may prevent reduction. When it is associated with a chronic neurologic disorder, a rather marked fixed dorsal subluxation may be associated with fixed hammertoes.

**Treatment** The conservative management of subluxation requires that the patient wear a shoe with an adequate toe box. A small sling-type device can be created to help hold the toe in better alignment when a dynamic deformity is present. A soft metatarsal support can be used beneath the metatarsal heads if the subluxation is accompanied by metatarsalgia.

Surgical management is dictated by the severity of the subluxation. Minor dorsal subluxation is treated by lengthening of the extensor digitorum longus and brevis tendons, with or without a dorsal capsulotomy. The toe is then maintained in satisfactory alignment for approximately six weeks to ensure that the correction is lasting.

**Results** The expected result is complete correction of the deformity. At times there is a slight overcorrection.

**Complications** The only complications are those of undercorrection or overcorrection of the metatarsophalangeal joint. If it is undercorrected, the cockup deformity remains; if it is overcorrected, the toe tends to be in a slightly plantar flexed position, which can be bothersome. Neither complication is significant.

### Severe Subluxation of the Metatarsophalangeal Joint

When severe subluxation of the metatarsophalangeal joint is associated with rheumatoid arthritis, an arthroplasty of the metatarsophalangeal joint involves removal of all or part of the metatarsal head. If more than two joints are involved, we believe that a formal rheumatoid procedure consisting of resection of all of the metatarsal heads with an arthrodesis of the first metatarsophalangeal joint should be performed.

When the advanced subluxation involves the second metatarsophalangeal joint secondary to an advanced hallux valgus deformity, the hallux valgus deformity must be corrected at the same time to create a space for the second toe. If there is no physical space for the toe, any form of treatment on the second toe will fail.

Not infrequently the patient with severe subluxation also has an associated hammertoe. In more advanced cases of subluxation, the deformity is usually quite fixed and realignment is difficult.

**Technique** Surgical treatment consists of release of the extensor tendons and performance of a complete dorsal capsulotomy along with release of the collateral ligaments. Once release is achieved, the toe is sharply plantar flexed to lyse the remaining adhesions. If an associated hammertoe exists, it must be treated at the same time. If plantar flexion power at the metatarsophalangeal joint is not adequate, adding a flexor tendon transfer to the procedure provides a form of active flexion to the metatarsophalangeal joint and helps achieve stability.

The surgical approach to this problem is through a dorsal incision, starting over the middle phalanx and extending proximal to the metatarsophalangeal joint. The flexor digitorum longus tendon is harvested from the plantar aspect of the foot, as described previously. The extensor tendons are released, as are the joint capsules and the collateral ligaments. This release usually permits reduction of the metatarsophalangeal joint. The distal portion (condyles) of the proximal phalanx is then removed to reduce the hammertoe deformity. Next, a 0.045-inch Kirschner wire is drilled out through the middle phalanx and the tip of the toe. It is driven in a retrograde fashion across the proximal interphalangeal joint. The two tails of the flexor digitorum longus tendon are brought up on each side of the extensor hood and sutured to it, holding the metatarsophalangeal joint in 10 to 20 degrees of plantar flexion in relation to the long axis of the metatarsal. After the toe is adequately aligned, the K-wire is advanced across the metatarsophalangeal joint to stabilize the repair (Fig. 8–16, A to C).

Postoperatively, the foot is placed in a wooden shoe and the pins are left in place for three weeks. After pins are removed, the toes are taped for another three weeks to ensure satisfactory alignment of the joints.

**Results** The degree of correction usually depends on the severity of the deformity. As a general rule, if the metatarsophalangeal joint can be adequately mobilized and the proximal interphalangeal joint reduced, a satisfactory result can be achieved. There may be some mild residual cocking up and flexion of the toe.

**Complications** Complications are related to the severity of the deformity. As mentioned above, a complete correction cannot be achieved in all patients. The vascular status of the toe must be carefully monitored after this type of procedure because arterial compromise may occur if the toe is stretched out over the pin; if the toe is compressed too much along the pin, venous compromise may occur. In either of these cases, if the vascular status is still marginal two to three hours after surgery, the pin should be removed and the toe supported with soft-tissue dressings.

**Alternative Methods of Treatment** There are a number of ways to treat this condition. The main principle involved is that the metatarsal head should be retained if possible, except in patients with connective tissue disorders. The authors prefer to leave the base of the proximal phalanx intact whenever possible. Some authors believe that the base of the proximal phalanx can be resected and a syndactyly created between adjacent toes to create satisfactory positioning. It has been our experience, however, that when this procedure is used the deformity tends to recur. Because of

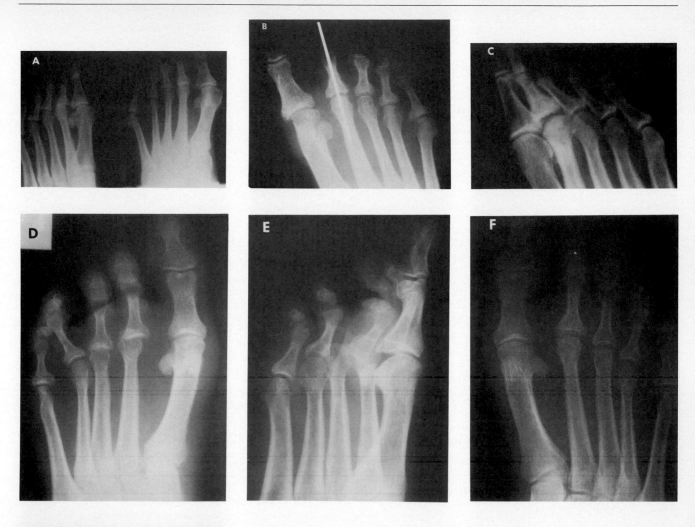

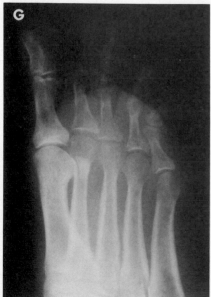

**Fig. 8–16** **A:** Dislocation of the second metatarsophalangeal joint associated with a hallux valgus deformity. **B:** Reduction of the metatarsophalangeal joint with pin fixation and correction of hallux valgus deformity. **C:** Postoperative radiograph demonstrating satisfactory reduction one year after surgery. **D:** Radiograph with dislocation of the second and third metatarsophalangeal joints. **E:** Oblique radiograph demonstrating dislocation of the second and third metatarsophalangeal joints. **F:** Postoperative radiograph after reduction of the second and third metatarsophalangeal joints by arthroplasty and flexor tendon transfer. **G:** Oblique postoperative radiograph. (Fig. 8–16, A to C reproduced with permission from Mann RA (ed): *Surgery of the Foot*, ed 5. St Louis, CV Mosby Co, 1986.)

the syndactylization the involved toe and the adjacent toe subluxate dorsally. The toe also has a tendency to shorten, which can be unsightly.

Resection of the proximal phalanx in its entirety, or the proximal half of the proximal phalanx, should also be avoided. Resection tends to result in a cockup deformity of the remaining "nubbin" of toe, along with unsightly shortening.

Resection of the metatarsal head usually results in a transfer lesion, and generally this procedure is not indicated for subluxation of the metatarsophalangeal joint.

### Dislocation of the Second Metatarsophalangeal Joint

A dislocation of the metatarsophalangeal joint[5] involves the second ray most often but may involve others as well. In a dislocation the proximal phalanx sits on the dorsal aspect of the metatarsal head, which results in plantar flexion of the metatarsal head. Metatarsalgia is almost invariably associated with this condition. When only a single metatarsophalangeal joint is dislocated, it usually involves the second ray, since it is the longest and probably is subjected to the greatest degree of stress against the shoe. It is also subjected to extrinsic pressure from the great toe pressing against it and not infrequently it overlaps the great toe, which can also help bring about the dislocation. The dislocation is occasionally secondary to trauma. Dislocation of multiple metatarsophalangeal joints is almost invariably associated with some type of connective tissue disorder such as rheumatoid arthritis or psoriatic arthritis.

**Clinical Complaint** The primary complaints are pressure from the toe striking the top of the shoe and pain that develops under the metatarsal head.

**Physical Findings** The physical examination usually demonstrates a moderate degree of dorsal angulation of the metatarsophalangeal joint and an accompanying hammertoe deformity. These deformities are usually quite fixed in nature and cannot be reduced. Occasionally a patient can spontaneously dislocate and reduce the metatarsophalangeal joint. Moderately advanced synovial reaction is often present in patients with dislocated metatarsophalangeal joints. There may be ulceration under the second metatarsal head associated with the dislocation.

**Treatment** Conservative management involves the use of a shoe with extra depth that provides sufficient room for the toes. Not infrequently, a metatarsal support is needed to relieve the stress on the metatarsal heads. Wearing conventional shoes is extremely difficult for the individual with dislocated metatarsophalangeal joints.

The surgical treatment involves reduction of the metatarsophalangeal joint. Unfortunately, reducing the joint while maintaining normal motion is, in our experience, almost impossible. The main principle of treatment is the creation of an arthrofibrosis of the joint. This provides joint stability and, usually, lasting benefit at the expense of loss of joint motion.

**Technique** The surgical procedure we favor is an arthroplasty of the metatarsophalangeal joint. A longitudinal dorsal incision begins over the middle phalanx, as in the treatment of a subluxated metatarsophalangeal joint, and is carried to a level just proximal to the metatarsophalangeal joint. The extensor tendons, dorsal capsule, and collateral ligaments are cut. Any proliferative synovium is removed. Longitudinal pressure is then placed on the toe to determine how much traction is needed to carry out a reduction. The traction is then slowly reduced to determine how much the proximal phalanx overlaps the metatarsal head region. As a general rule, the overlaps measure 3 to 4 mm; at this point the distal portion of the metatarsal head is removed. The edges are then smoothed off so that the proximal phalanx sits laterally at the end of the metatarsal and remains there as the ankle is dorsiflexed and plantar flexed. If the joint continues to dislocate dorsally, more metatarsal head should be removed. It is rarely necessary to remove more than one half of the metatarsal head. The metatarsal head is beveled to create a smooth new articulating surface. Almost invariably a hammertoe is present, and the distal portion of the proximal phalanx is removed. Once again, a 0.045-inch Kirschner wire is passed out through the middle phalanx to the tip of the toe and then advanced through the proximal phalanx and into the metatarsal head. Once this is achieved, alignment of the toe should be satisfactory. Several toes may be treated in this manner (Fig. 8–16, D to G).

Postoperatively, the pin is left in place for approximately three weeks. It is then removed and the patient is allowed to walk while wearing a wooden shoe. Gentle, passive range-of-motion exercises are instituted as well. The wooden shoe is discontinued after six weeks, at which time the patient can wear any comfortable shoe.

**Results** Approximately 30% to 40% of the motion of the metatarsophalangeal joint is lost after this type of procedure because of the arthrofibrosis that develops. This loss is compatible with satisfactory foot function. It is important to encourage the patient to work on range of motion after the pin is removed at three weeks. Rarely does the metatarsophalangeal joint redislocate.

**Complications** The main complication is excessive stiffness of the metatarsophalangeal joint. Generally, however, if the pin is removed at three weeks and first passive and then active range-of-motion exercises are begun, stiffness is not a problem. Swelling occasionally persists for various periods secondary to the extensive nature of the procedure. The vascular status of the toe must be carefully monitored postoperatively to avoid venous or arterial compromise. Occasionally a transfer lesion occurs adjacent to the metatarsophalangeal joint if an excessive amount of metatarsal head was removed. This, however, is seldom of much concern to the patient.

**Alternative Methods of Treatment** Although the authors believe arthroplasty is currently the best method of handling this difficult problem, it is by no means the only one. Other authors prefer to do a partial phalangectomy associated with a syndactylization for this condition. It has been our experience that although an initial satisfactory result is achieved, long-term findings not infrequently include cocking up of the involved toes and recurrence of the deformity. Resection of the proximal phalanx usually creates a short, stubby, unsightly toe. The toe also becomes floppy, making it difficult for the patient to put on socks and shoes.

Although some surgeons prefer to use an implant for this condition, it does not produce results equal to or superior to ours.

## Crossover Toe

A crossover toe is a deformity usually involving the second metatarsophalangeal joint, in which the second toe overlaps the great toe. This is most often caused by disruption of the medial or lateral collateral ligament along with degeneration of the plantar plate on the same side as the collateral ligament degeneration.

**Clinical Complaint** The main problem associated with a crossover toe is, again, pressure of the toe against the shoe. The toe sits on top of the great toe or a lesser toe and makes wearing shoes extremely difficult. If the toes are merely deviated, as a general rule the main complaint is a cosmetic one.

**Physical Findings** The physical examination demonstrates that when the patient stands, the involved toe, which is usually the second, sits on top of the great toe or the third toe. The deformity is sometimes fixed and cannot be brought back into alignment. At other times the toe can easily be brought into alignment. In the case of deviating toes, the deformity is readily correctable, but as soon as the pressure is removed from the toes the deformity once again recurs (Fig. 8–17A).

**Treatment** Conservative management of the cross-

over toe requires wearing a shoe large enough to accommodate the toes. Occasionally a sling can be created to pull the second toe back into alignment, which works if the deformity is not too rigid.

**Technique** Surgical treatment for a crossover toe involves the same basic steps as treatment for a subluxated metatarsophalangeal joint. The surgical principle involves releasing the contracted dorsal structures, releasing the contracted collateral ligament, plication if possible of the degenerated collateral ligament, and the use of a flexor tendon transfer to provide some plantar flexion force against the proximal phalanx. Occasionally bony decompression of the metatarsophalangeal joint is necessary, as described for dislocation of the metatarsophalangeal joint.

The surgical approach is through an incision starting over the middle dorsal aspect of the proximal phalanx and carried proximal to the metatarsophalangeal joint. The extensor tendon and dorsal capsule are released if necessary. The collateral ligament on the side to which the toe has deviated is severed to relieve any contracture. The collateral ligament on the side away from the deviation is then inspected. Not infrequently this tissue is completely degenerated and an actual hole is present. If some tissue is present, attempts can be made to place one or two sutures in this tissue and reef it to reapproximate the collateral ligament.

If hyperextension of the metatarsophalangeal joint has occurred, the flexor tendon may be transferred to the extensor hood to provide some plantar flexion pull on the proximal phalanx. The slip of flexor tendon on the side where the collateral ligament has been disrupted is tightened more than on the opposite side to hold the toe in satisfactory alignment.

Postoperatively, the toe is taped in a corrected position and held this way for approximately six weeks while the patient wears a wooden shoe. As a general rule, pin fixation is not used (Fig. 8–17, B and C).

**Results** The alignment of the crossover toe can be significantly improved and at times completely corrected. At other times, however, varying degrees of deformity persist. Voluntary control of the toe is usually lost after surgery.

**Complications** The major complication is usually recurrence of the deformity. Vascular compromise is rarely a problem.

**Alternative Methods of Treatment** Some surgeons prefer to perform a partial proximal phalangectomy along with syndactyly for this problem. Again, for the reasons mentioned above, the authors do not favor

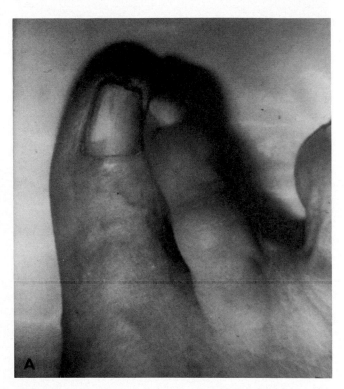

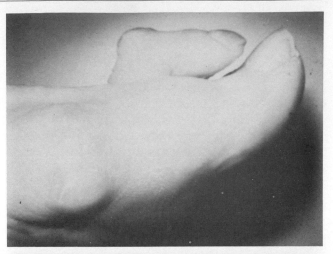

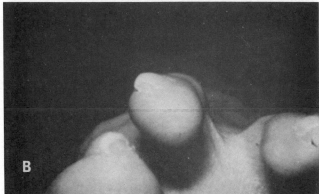

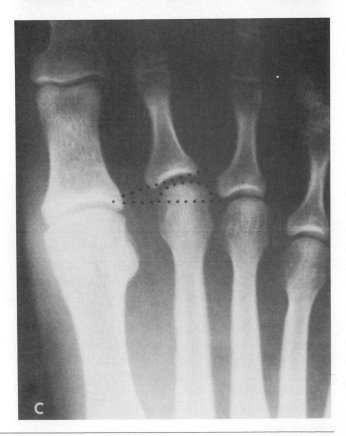

**Fig. 8–17 A** and **B:** Crossover second toe. **C:** Radiograph demonstrating crossover second toe.

this procedure. We believe that a proximal phalangectomy in and of itself does not produce a satisfactory outcome because of the marked shortening and destabilization of the toe.

Treatment for deviated toes is essentially the same; however, if no dorsal angulation is present at the metatarsophalangeal joint, it is not necessary to carry out a flexor tendon transfer.

### Synovitis of the Metatarsophalangeal Joint

Nonspecific synovitis usually affects the second and third metatarsophalangeal joints. It is associated with spontaneous thickening of the synovial tissue within the joint, and has no apparent cause. All tests for rheumatoid disease or other types of known connective tissue disorders are negative. The condition, which usually starts as swelling of the metatarsophalangeal joint, can lead to subluxation and eventual dislocation of the joint, with or without an associated hammertoe.

**Clinical Complaint** The main complaint is usually pain on the plantar aspect of the foot beneath the involved metatarsal head. Patients often state that they feel as though they are walking on a painful lump on the bottom of the foot. At times the involved toe is swollen and demonstrates a variable degree of hammertoe formation.

**Physical Findings** The physical examination demonstrates generalized thickening about the involved metatarsophalangeal joint. Squeezing the metatarsophalangeal joint causes a moderate amount of discomfort. When the joint is grasped by two fingers of each hand, the marked thickening of the involved joint contrasts sharply to the adjacent metatarsophalangeal joints. This condition is often confused with an interdigital neuroma. As a general rule, only a single metatarsophalangeal joint is involved in this condition, unlike rheumatoid arthritis or other forms of generalized arthritides.

**Treatment** The conservative method of treatment is the use of anti-inflammatory medications along with a soft metatarsal support to remove stress from the involved joint. If this treatment fails, injection of a steroid preparation into the joint may be indicated.

If conservative management fails, a synovectomy of the metatarsophalangeal joint is performed. If an associated subluxation is present, flexor tendon transfer is added to the procedure to produce some plantar flexion of the metatarsophalangeal joint. If a hammertoe is also present, it too is corrected.

Postoperatively, the patient wears a wooden shoe for a period of four weeks to allow the soft-tissue reaction to subside and to permit the joint to become stabilized.

**Results** The results after synovectomy are usually good since the natural course of the condition is development of a fixed subluxated or dislocated metatarsophalangeal joint, with or without a fixed hammertoe deformity.

**Complications** Almost invariably swelling of the toe is a problem for many months after surgery. Even if a hammertoe procedure is not done, there is often significant swelling of the toe secondary to the reaction brought about by the synovitis. Not infrequently a certain degree of stiffness of the metatarsophalangeal joint ensues. A long-term complication is hammertoe formation if none was present initially.

### Freiberg's Infraction

Freiberg's infraction is a collapse of the metatarsal head because of avascular necrosis. It may take many forms, from minimal physical findings to complete collapse (Fig. 8–18).

**Clinical Complaint** Most patients complain of pain about the metatarsophalangeal joint. In longstanding cases, the main complaint is pain with dorsiflexion of the joint.

**Physical Findings** The physical examination usually demonstrates some thickening about the metatarsophalangeal joint, although the synovial reaction is not as severe as that noted with nonspecific synovitis. Not infrequently a dorsal ridge is noted on the metatarsal head, and dorsiflexion of the metatarsophalangeal joint causes discomfort.

**Treatment** Conservative management of the problem consists of wearing a low-heeled shoe with an adequate toe box. Occasionally taping the toe into a plantar flexed position helps to alleviate the problem.

If conservative management fails, surgical intervention is often successful. A cheilectomy is performed to debride the joint and remove the dorsal spurring.

**Technique** Through a hockey-stick incision starting in the web space and curving over the metatarsal head, the extensor tendons are swept aside and the joint capsule opened. Generally, a moderate degree of synovial tissue is encountered, and is removed. The metatarsal head is identified and the loose articular cartilage is removed. The metatarsal head is beveled to create a smooth articular surface upon which fibrocartilage may form.

Postoperatively, the patient wears a wooden shoe for approximately three weeks and is then encouraged to work on active and passive range of motion of the joint. The patient then wears a sandal and gradually progresses to regular shoes.

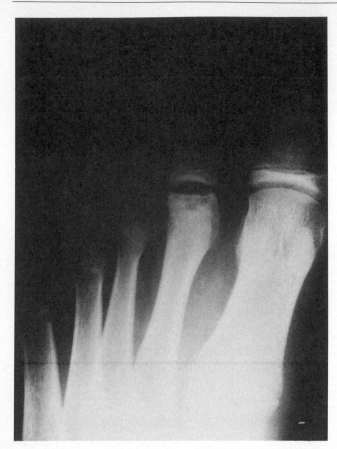

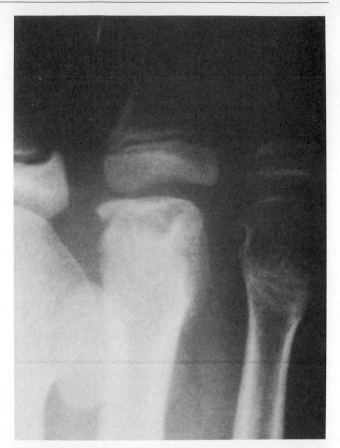

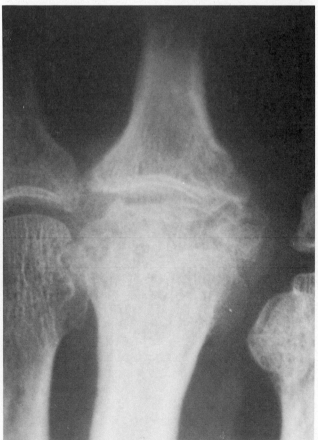

**Fig. 8–18** Examples of Freiberg's infraction involving the second metatarsophalangeal joint.

**Results**  Debridement and cheilectomy of the metatarsal head produce a satisfactory result. Often some stiffness persists at the level of the joint, but the pain is usually relieved.

**Complications**  Occasionally swelling of the involved toe persists, but it is not common. The main complication is persistent pain, which is also unusual.

**Alternative Methods of Treatment**  Some surgeons advocate the removal of the metatarsal head if it is severely involved or removal of part of the proximal phalanx. The authors do not believe that a single metatarsal head should be removed, since a transfer lesion invariably occurs. Resection of the proximal phalanx

usually does not bring about a satisfactory long-term result.

## References

1. Girdlestone GR: Physiotherapy for hand and foot. *J Chartered Soc Physiother* 1947;32:167.
2. Parrish TF: Dynamic correction of claw toes. *Orthop Clin North Am* 1973;4:97.
3. Taylor RG: The treatment of claw toes by multiple transfers of flexor into extensor tendons. *J Bone Joint Surg* 1951;33B:539.
4. Ruiz-Mora J: Plastic correction of over-riding 5th toe. *Orthop Letters Club* 1954;6.
5. DuVries HL: Dislocation of toe. *JAMA* 1956;160:728.

# Functional Anatomy of the Ankle Joint Ligaments

Roger A. Mann, MD

The configuration of the ligamentous structures about the ankle joint is related to the functional axes of the ankle and subtalar joints. This functional relationship is not fully recognized at times by clinicians evaluating the stability of the ankle joint and considering surgical reconstruction of the ligaments about the ankle joint. This review discusses the basic biomechanical relationships of the ankle joint ligaments to the subtalar and ankle joint axes and relates them to clinical problems in the ankle region.

Inman's monograph[1] presents the anatomic relationships that exist between the ankle and subtalar joints in relation to the ligamentous structures crossing these joints. Most of the biomechanical data for this review were obtained from his classic work and correlated with clinical data.

The axis of the ankle joint passes below the tip of the medial and lateral malleoli when it is viewed in the frontal plane and externally rotated approximately 20 to 30 degrees in relation to the knee joint axis[2] (Fig. 9–1). The motions occurring at the ankle are dorsiflexion and plantar flexion. At initial contact with the ground, rapid plantar flexion occurs, followed by progressive dorsiflexion, which lasts until approximately 40% of the walking cycle has been completed, when plantar flexion once again begins, reaching a maximum at the time of lift-off, at which point dorsiflexion begins and continues through the swing phase (Fig. 9–2). The muscle control of the ankle joint is provided by the anterior compartment muscles, which through an eccentric (lengthening) contraction permit controlled plantar flexion to occur at the time of initial contact with the ground, after which the posterior calf musculature becomes active (Fig. 9–3).

The posterior calf muscles function by undergoing an eccentric (lengthening) contraction during the midstance phase. This controls the forward move-

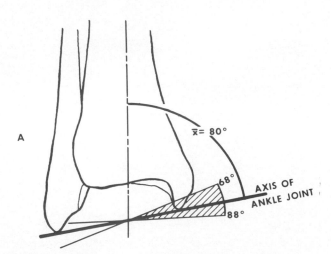

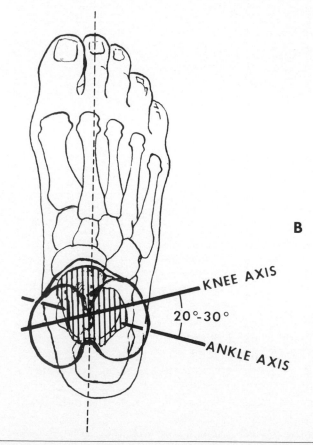

**Fig. 9–1  A:** Angle between the axis of the ankle joint and the long axis of the tibia. **B:** Relationship of the knee, ankle and foot axes. (Reproduced with permission from Mann RA: Biomechanics of the foot, in American Academy of Orthopaedic Surgeons *Atlas of Orthotics*. St Louis, CV Mosby Co, 1975.

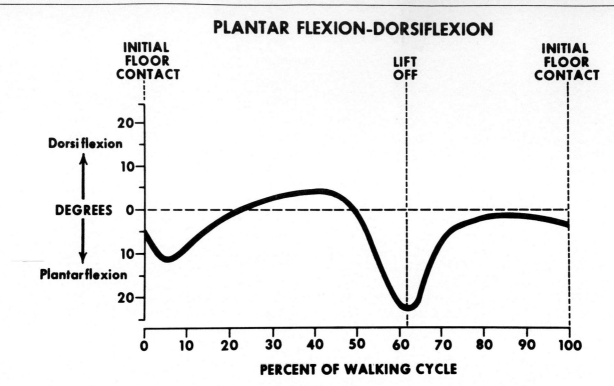

**Fig. 9–2** Range of motion of the ankle joint. (Reproduced with permission from Mann RA: Biomechanics of the foot, in American Academy of Orthopaedic Surgeons *Atlas of Orthotics*. St Louis, CV Mosby Co, 1975).

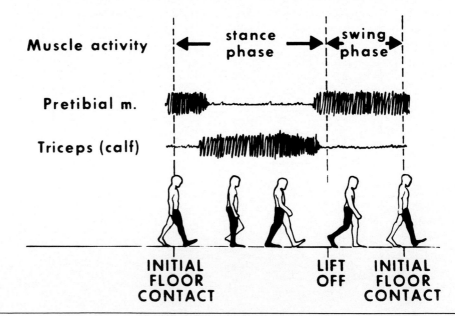

**Fig. 9–3** A schematic representation of the phasic activity of the leg muscles during normal gait. (Reproduced with permission from Mann RA: Biomechanics of the foot, in American Academy of Orthopaedic Surgeons *Atlas of Orthotics*. St Louis, CV Mosby Co, 1975.

ment of the tibia over the fixed foot. Next, they undergo a concentric (shortening) contraction initiating plantar flexion of the ankle joint. At approximately 50% of the walking cycle, prior to full plantar flexion, their electrical activity ceases. The anterior compartment muscles become active again at the time of lift-off to provide dorsiflexion of the ankle joint through the swing phase.

In the transverse plane, internal and external rota-

tion of the lower limb, which includes the pelvis, femur, and tibia, occurs with each step (Fig. 9–4). At the time of initial contact with the ground, internal rotation occurs in the lower extremity. This internal rotation is secondary to the loading response of the subtalar joint. As weight is applied to the subtalar joint, it assumes a position of eversion within the constraints of the shape of its articular surfaces and the surrounding ligament and muscle supports. As a result, there is internal rotation in the tibia and femur above. The internal rotation reaches a maximum at the time of foot-flat, at which time progressive external rotation of the foot begins. The external rotation is initiated in the contralateral pelvis and is transmitted distally. As the contralateral (swing) leg is moving forward, the pelvis acts as a "crank," providing the force that causes the external rotation of the femur and tibia. This force crosses the ankle joint, and is then translated by the subtalar joint to invert the calcaneus. The internal rotation reaches a maximum at the time of lift-off, when external rotation resumes. The external rotation is a rather dynamic event, whereas the internal rotation at the time of initial contact with the ground is a rather passive event. Since little or no transverse plane motion occurs within the ankle joint, the subtalar joint acts as an oblique hinge beneath the ankle joint, converting the transverse plane motion of the tibia to rotation of the calcaneus, which then passes it distally to the foot. The axis of the subtalar joint passes obliquely across the foot at an angle of about 16 degrees and in the horizontal plane at about 42 degrees, although there is a moderate degree of variation (Fig. 9–5). Subtalar joint rotation is greater in a person with a flat foot and less in a person with a cavus foot configuration

(Fig. 9–6). The subtalar joint motion directly affects the function of the transverse tarsal joint, which consists of the talonavicular and calcaneocuboid joint. When the subtalar joint is everted, the transverse tarsal joint is "unlocked," producing a supple forefoot; whereas at toe-off, the subtalar joint is in maximum inversion, the transverse tarsal joint is "locked," and the forefoot is rigid (Fig. 9–7).

The next anatomic consideration is the shape of the trochlear surface of the talus. This surface, from an anatomic standpoint, is not a section of a cylinder but rather a section of a cone (Fig. 9–8). The apex of the cone is directed toward the medial malleolus and the base is directed toward the lateral malleolus. The ligamentous structures around the medial and lateral sides of the joint must be different to accommodate this conical configuration.

Rotation occurs about a small area at the apex of the cone on the medial side of the ankle joint during dorsiflexion and plantar flexion. The deltoid ligament is constructed to accommodate this apical rotation as it fans out from the medial malleolus and attaches into the talus. On the lateral side of the ankle joint, which is the open end of the cone, there is motion over a larger area. Instead of a single ligamentous attachment, the lateral ankle ligament con-

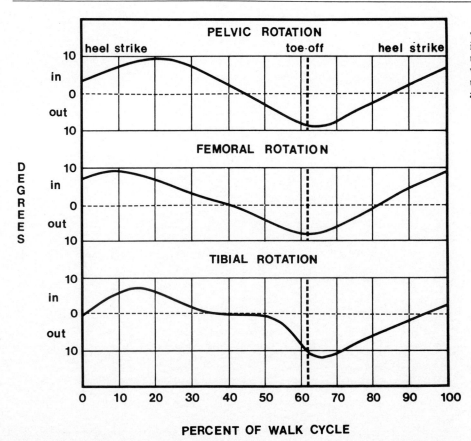

**Fig. 9–4** Transverse rotation of the pelvis, femur, and tibia during a normal walking cycle. Note that there is inward rotation until foot-flat at 15% of the cycle, after which there is progressive outward rotation until toe-off, when inward rotation once again begins.

PERCENT OF WALK CYCLE

sists of three distinct ligament bands—the anterior and posterior talofibular ligaments and the obliquely placed calcaneofibular ligament.

Because it crosses two joints (the ankle and subtalar joint), the calcaneofibular ligament is the most complex of the lateral collateral ligaments. It arises from the tip of the fibular malleolus and passes obliquely downward and posteriorly to insert into the calcaneus. Since this ligament crosses both the ankle and subtalar joints, it must permit simultaneous motion in both. The direction that the calcaneofibular ligament assumes as it passes to insert into the calcaneus is such that it parallels the horizontal axis of the subtalar joint. The anterior talofibular ligament passes from the distal aspect of the fibula and inserts into the neck of the talus. The posterior talofibular ligament arises from the medial aspect of the distal fibula and passes almost horizontally to insert along the posterior aspect of the talus.

If the anatomic position of the ligament and its

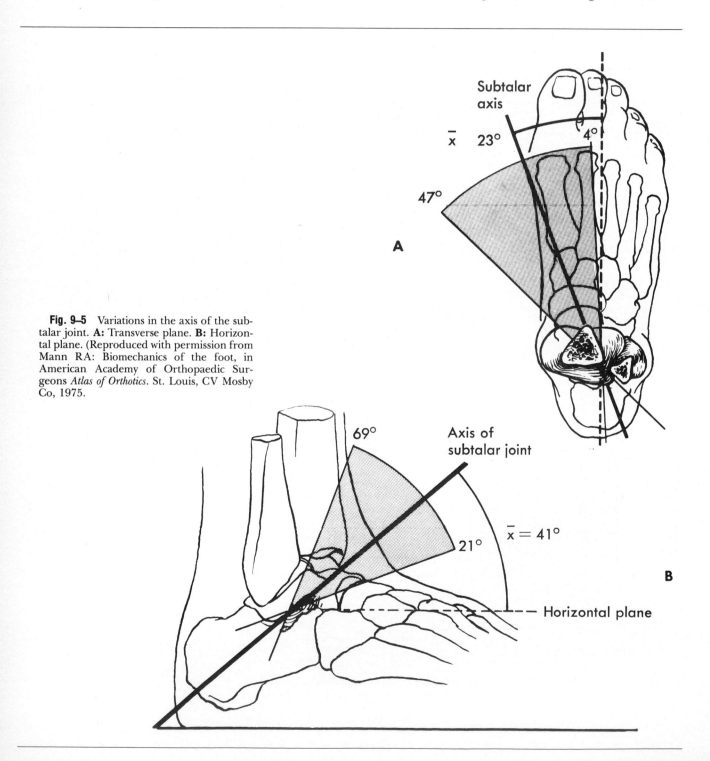

**Fig. 9–5** Variations in the axis of the subtalar joint. **A:** Transverse plane. **B:** Horizontal plane. (Reproduced with permission from Mann RA: Biomechanics of the foot, in American Academy of Orthopaedic Surgeons *Atlas of Orthotics*. St. Louis, CV Mosby Co, 1975.

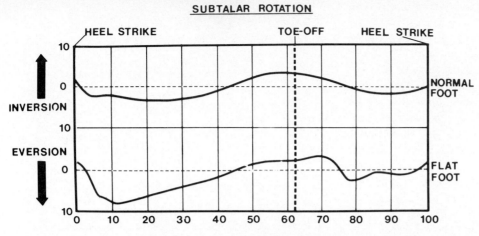

**Fig. 9–6** Subtalar joint motion in a normal individual and a flat-footed individual.

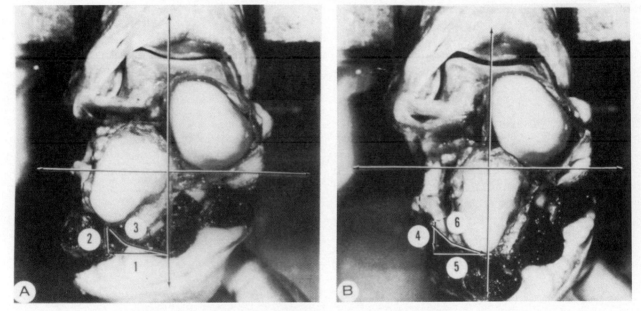

**Fig. 9–7** Anatomic model of the hindfoot demonstrating the effect of valgus of the calcaneus and varus of the calcaneus in relationship to the talus. **A:** When the calcaneus is in valgus, the transverse tarsal joint, which consists of the talonavicular and calcaneocuboid joints, is unlocked, giving rise to a flexible forefoot. **B:** When the calcaneus is in varus, the transverse tarsal joint is locked and the forefoot is rigid. (Reproduced with permission from Sarrafian SK: *Functional Anatomy of the Foot and Ankle.* Philadelphia, JB Lippincott Co, 1983.)

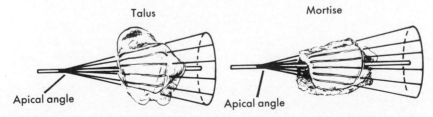

**Fig. 9–8** Curvature of the trochlear surface of the talus creates a cone whose apex is based medially. From this configuration one can observe that the deltoid ligament is well suited to function along the medial side of the ankle joint, whereas laterally, where more rotation is occurring, three separate ligaments are necessary. (Reproduced with permission from Inman VT: *The Joints of the Ankle.* Baltimore, Williams & Wilkins Co, 1976.)

relationship to the position of the ankle joint are taken into account, the calcaneofibular ligament is in line with the fibula and acts as a collateral ligament during dorsiflexion, whereas the anterior talofibular ligament is in line with the fibula and acts as a collateral ligament in plantar flexion (Fig. 9–9).

When Inman[1] measured the angle between the calcaneofibular and anterior talofibular ligaments (Fig. 9–10), he found an average angle in the sagittal plane of about 105 degrees (range, 70 to 140 degrees). This wide variation may shed some light on the lateral stability of the ankle joint itself. If the angle between the calcaneofibular and talofibular ligaments becomes too great (that is, more than 120 to 125 degrees), the stability provided by these collateral ligaments may not be adequate since neither is in line with the fibula. This may be the anatomic configuration in an individual who has chronic lateral ankle instability without a history of significant trauma. The divergence of the two ligaments is such that each ligament provides stability only at the extremes of dorsiflexion or plantar flexion and little or no stability when the ankle joint is in its midrange of motion.

As inversion and eversion of the subtalar joint occurs, the calcaneofibular ligament rotates around the posterolateral aspect of the ankle and calcaneus. As demonstrated in Fig. 9–11, the relationship between the calcaneofibular ligament and the subtalar axis produces a cone-shaped configuration. As inversion of the subtalar joint occurs, the calcaneofibular ligament rotates anteriorly along the surface of the cone; as the subtalar joint everts, the ligament moves posteriorly. It is this movement of the calcaneofibular

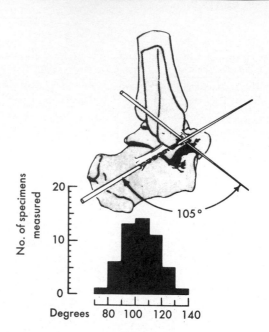

**Fig. 9–10** Average angle between calcaneofibular and talofibular ligaments is sagittal plane. Although average angle is 105 degrees, there is considerable variation, from 70 degrees to 140 degrees. (Reproduced with permission from Inman VT: *The Joints of the Ankle.* Baltimore, Williams & Wilkins Co, 1976.)

ligament about the posterolateral aspect of the ankle and calcaneus that permits unrestricted motion in the subtalar joint. This fact must be carefully considered when a ligament repair of the ankle joint is being contemplated, since failure to reestablish the cal-

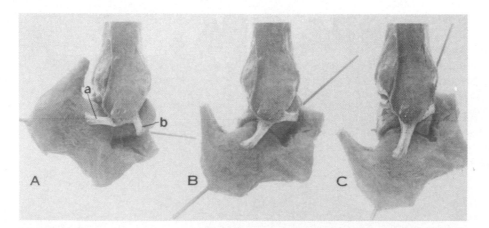

**Fig. 9–9** Calcaneofibular ligament (a) and anterior talofibular ligament (b) are shown. **A:** In plantar flexion, anterior talofibular ligament is in line with fibula and provides most of support to lateral aspect of ankle joint. **B:** In neutral position of ankle joint, both anterior talofibular and calcaneofibular ligaments provide support to joint. Relationship of calcaneofibular ligament to subtalar axis, which is depicted in the background, is noted. Note that this ligament and axis are parallel to each other. **C:** In dorsiflexion, calcaneofibular ligament is in line with fibula and provides support to lateral aspect of ankle joint. (Reproduced with permission from Inman VT: *The Joints of the Ankle.* Baltimore, Williams & Wilkins Co, 1976.)

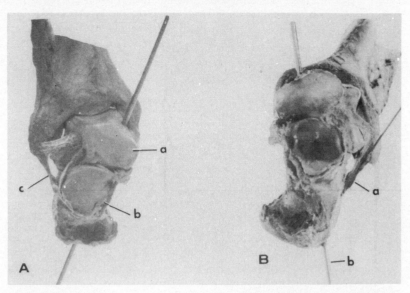

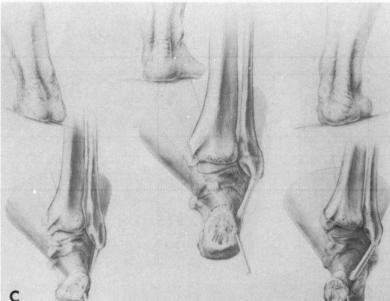

**Fig. 9–11  A:** Anterior view of transverse tarsal joint. Head of talus (a). Head of calcaneus (b). Calcaneofibular ligament (c). Rod passing through head of talus and exiting on lateral aspect of calcaneus demonstrates axis of subtalar joint. **B:** Same specimen viewed from below. Kirschner wire has now been placed through fibers of calcaneofibular ligament (a). Note direction of ligament extending from malleolus to lateral side of calcaneus. **C:** Functional arrangement of calcaneofibular ligament. This drawing explains the mechanism in which free motion is permitted in the subtalar joint without restriction by calcaneofibular ligament. Imaginary cone has been drawn around axis of subtalar joint. The calcaneofibular ligament is shown converging from its fibular attachment to calcaneus. Since the ligament lies on surface of cone the apex of which is the point of intersection of functional extensions of ligament and axis of subtalar joint, motion of calcaneus under talus is allowed without undue restriction from ligament, which is merely displaced over surface of cone. (Reproduced with permission from Inman VT: *The Joints of the Ankle.* Baltimore, Williams & Wilkins Co, 1976.)

**Fig. 9–12**  Example of forefoot valgus. This anatomic alignment of the forefoot will impart an inversion or varus torque to the ankle joint, which may cause or aggravate chronic lateral ankle joint instability.

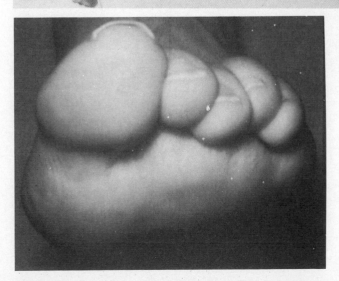

caneofibular ligament anatomically may result in decreased motion in the ankle and/or subtalar joint.

Another factor affecting the stability of the ankle joint is the anatomic alignment of the forefoot. If the forefoot is in a position of valgus, so that there is significant plantar flexion of the first metatarsal, inversion torque must be applied to the hindfoot before the foot can be placed flat on the ground. If the degree of forefoot valgus is severe, the result may be chronic ankle sprains. This must be carefully looked for when examining a patient with chronic lateral ligament instability (Fig. 9–12).

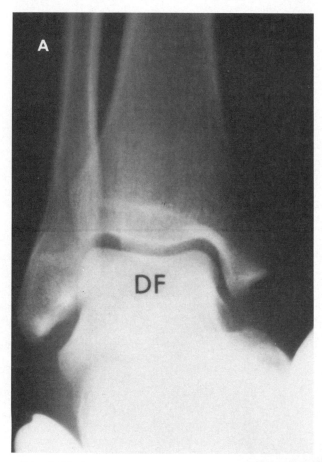

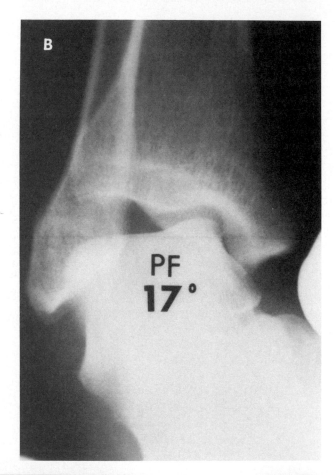

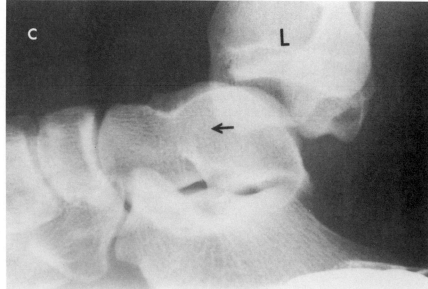

**Fig. 9–13** Stress radiographs of ankle in dorsiflexion demonstrating no instability in the calcaneofibular ligament. Same ankle stressed in plantar flexion demonstrates loss of stability caused by disruption of anterior talofibular ligament. Note anterior subluxation that is present when this ligament is torn. (Reproduced with permission from Mann RA: Biomechanics of the foot and ankle, in Mann RA (ed): *Surgery of the Foot*, ed 5. St Louis, CV Mosby Co, 1986.)

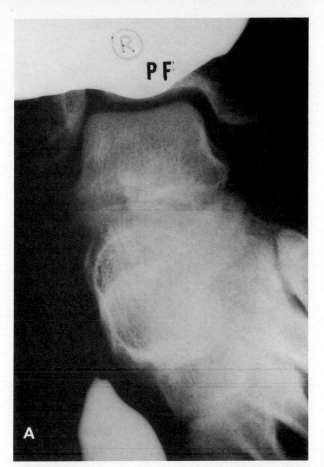 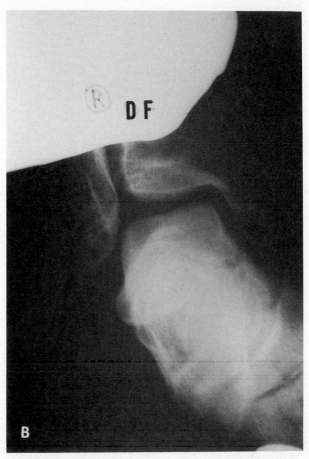

**Fig. 9–14 A:** Stress radiographs of ankle in plantar flexion, demonstrating no ligament instability. **B:** Same ankle stressed in dorsiflexion demonstrates laxity of calcaneofibular ligament. (Reproduced with permission from Mann RA: Biomechanics of the foot and ankle, in Mann RA (ed): *Surgery of the Foot*, ed 5. St Louis, CV Mosby Co, 1986.)

Correlating the biomechanics of the ankle ligaments with their anatomic alignment makes reasonable the assumption that when an injury occurs with the ankle joint in plantar flexion the anterior talofibular ligament is stressed and injured. In plantar flexion, the calcaneofibular ligament is displaced somewhat posteriorly and is horizontal to the ground, providing little or no lateral ankle joint stability. Conversely, if the injury occurs with the foot in dorsiflexion, the calcaneofibular ligament is stressed because it is in line with the fibula and the anterior talofibular ligament is displaced anteriorly in a more horizontal plane and may not be injured. With this in mind, one should attempt to elicit the mechanism of injury by obtaining a careful history from the patient in order to assess which ligament is injured. Palpation of each ligament also gives the clinician insight as to which ligament or ligaments are injured. Finally, when stress radiographs are contemplated, it is important to stress the ankle so that both the anterior talofibular and calcaneofibular ligaments can be evaluated. It is usually the anterior talofibular ligament that is disrupted, because most injuries occur with the foot in a plantar flexed position; in certain instances, however, only the calcaneofibular ligament is involved, as when the patient steps in a hole and sustains an inversion stress. On some occasions, both the anterior talofibular ligament and the calcaneofibular ligament are torn.

When stress radiographs of the ankle are done, the foot should be in plantar flexion to establish the competency of the anterior talofibular ligament and in neutral to slight dorsiflexion to establish the competency of the calcaneofibular ligament; the anterior drawer test should also be used to evaluate the competency of the anterior talofibular ligament. Stress radiographs of the uninvolved ankle should also be taken for comparison. Testing the ankle ligaments in this manner makes possible a more accurate diagnosis of the injured ligament or ligaments (Figs. 9–13 to 9–15).

If a ligament reconstruction is done, the normal

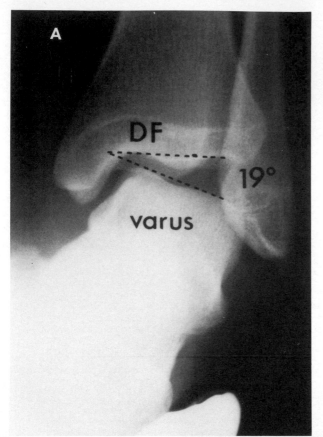
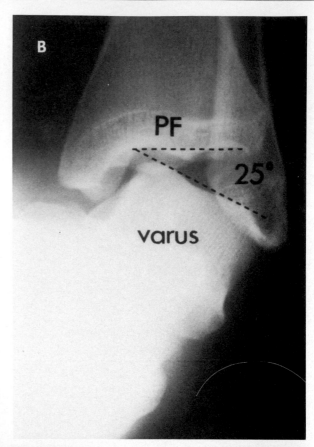
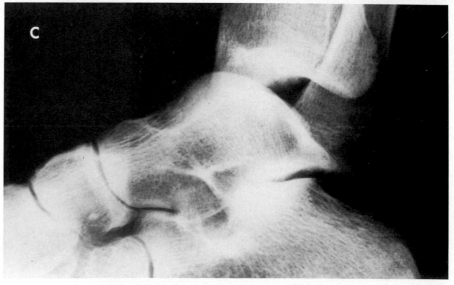

**Fig. 9–15** Stress radiographs of ankle joint in dorsiflexion, plantar flexion, and anteriorly, all demonstrating evidence of ligament disruption. This indicates complete tear of lateral collateral ligament structure. (Reproduced with permission from Mann RA: Biomechanics of the foot and ankle, in Mann RA (ed): *Surgery of the Foot*, ed 5. St Louis, CV Mosby Co, 1986.)

anatomic alignment should be restored as much as possible, so as to minimize restricting motion of the subtalar joint. If a tenodesis is carried out, as is so often done, a band of tendon passes from the area of the fifth metatarsal to the fibula, which from an anatomic standpoint is at right angles to the calcaneofibular ligament. Under these circumstances, a tenodesis produces adequate stabilization of the subtalar joint but unfortunately also restricts its motion. This may impede the performance of an active individual, such as a dancer or a professional athlete, who places severe demands upon the ankle and subtalar joint, but who also requires a full range of motion.

### References

1. Inman VT: *The Joints of the Ankle*. Baltimore, Williams & Wilkins Co, 1976.
2. Isman RE, Inman VT: Anthropometric studies of the human foot and ankle. *Bull Prosthet Res* 1969;10–11:97.

# The Knee

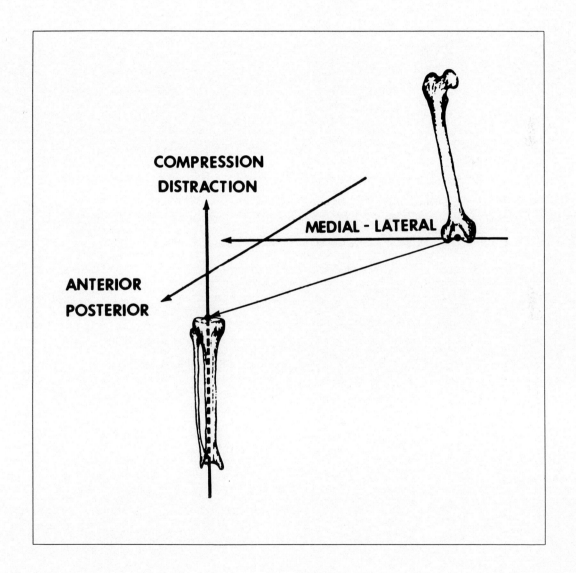

# Evaluation of Fixation Methods
# in Cruciate Ligament Replacement

David L. Butler, PhD

## Introduction

Many orthopaedic surgeons perform ligament replacements because the anterior cruciate ligament (ACL) is frequently injured but difficult to repair. Among the many ACL grafts used clinically are the iliotibial tract and band,[1] semitendinosus[2] and gracilis tendons,[3] central and medial portions of the patellar tendon,[4,5] quadriceps and prepatellar retinaculum[6] and meniscus.[7] Despite many reported clinical successes, no one replacement has gained wide acceptance.

The variable success of these procedures can be attributed to many factors, including initial graft selection,[8] surgical placement of the graft with the proper pretensioning force and knee flexion angle,[9] the rehabilitation program[10] and the patient's willingness to comply with it, and obtaining rigid fixation of the graft ends. Rigid fixation includes proper attachment of graft bone to underlying bone with staples, screws, and sutures and attachment of soft tissue to bone with sutures and staples. Rigid fixation is probably the most important factor in the success of these procedures during the initial stages of healing.

Several clinical goals are associated with attainment of rigid fixation. The first is joint stability under repetitive forces. Joint stability is important to the patient whose knee is subjected to the often large cyclic forces of walking and running. Stability is just as important, however, to the patient undergoing a lower-force, postinjury rehabilitation program such as continuous passive motion (CPM). In both loading regimens, achieving stability requires the graft tissue and its attachments to possess adequate strength and fatigue resistance.

The second clinical goal is the ability to resist sudden traumatic loads. These are usually larger forces not unlike those that produced the original injury. A graft is especially vulnerable to these forces soon after surgery when revascularization and cellular proliferation weaken the tissue and when soft tissue-to-bone or bone-to-bone healing has not yet occurred. In this situation, a single episode of overloading can compromise the reconstruction.

The third clinical goal is eventual transfer of forces from the fixation device to the biologic graft. Unless the attachment of soft tissue or bone end to underlying bone heals, the graft remains at risk and fails when the staple or screw loosens, breaks, or is removed by the surgeon.

Ligament graft fixation has been evaluated in several laboratory studies[11-13] using cadaveric specimens to test the effectiveness of different tissue types and fixation methods in resisting simulated in vivo cyclic and traumatic loads. Three important factors—donor age, tissue types and fixation techniques, and testing methods employed—can affect the results and, thus, the conclusions drawn by the investigators. Therefore, after examining these three factors to determine their influence on mechanical fixation of tissue grafts, the author will evaluate these studies[11-13] in light of these factors.

## Factors in Graft Fixation

### Donor Age

It is important to use young cadaveric donors when evaluating graft-fixation methods. Donors in the second and third decades most closely match the age range of patients who receive ligament reconstructions.[14] Using soft tissue and bone from older donors is less desirable because bone can become weak and osteoporotic, providing poor bone ends for a patellar tendon-bone (PT-bone) graft and inadequate fixation beds on the femur and tibia. Furthermore, Noyes and Grood[15] showed that ACL-bone units undergo significant, twofold to threefold reductions in stiffness and strength between 20 and 50 years of age and that ligament failures predominate in this age range, whereas bone avulsion failures and further reduction in mechanical properties occur thereafter. Therefore, it is likely that the soft-tissue component of the graft also loses strength and stiffness with age and the graft bone ends, if present, and the underlying bony bed become osteoporotic as well. Should these changes have occurred in a donor, the resulting data would underestimate true graft and fixation mechanical properties.

### Tissue Types and Fixation Techniques

Numerous cadaveric tissues and fixation methods have been employed in laboratory studies.[11-13] These include prepatellar retinaculum with quadriceps and patellar tendon ends, secured over the top with staples or screws; PT-bone units fixed with staples, screws, or buttons; semitendinosus and gracilis tendons and fascia lata held with staples; iliotibial band and distal bone fixed with staples or screws; and meniscus held with sutures. The mechanical behavior of these replacements depends on the ability of the fixation device to anchor the graft to bone. However, the results are also greatly affected by the inherent strength and stiffness of graft tissues, which can vary significantly.[8,16] An example of this variation is shown in Table 10–1 where the initial strengths of different graft tissues from young donors (mean age, 26 years) are expressed as percentages of ACL maximum force from an earlier study.[15] Note that only the PT-bone unit exceeds the strength of the ACL-bone unit while the semitendinosus and gracilis tendons are 70% and 49% of the ligament value, respectively. In light of these differences, it is important that investigators compare fixation methods using the same tissue types, preferably contralateral specimens from the same donor. In these left-right comparisons it is also important that the investigators place the devices in the same locations in the graft and bone by means of reproducible installation procedures.

## Testing Methods

Two types of tests are commonly employed to evaluate the mechanical response of different fixation methods: the cyclic test and the failure test. The cyclic test tries to simulate repetitive loading on implanted grafts. It is typically performed at slow rates to simulate either CPM or walking speeds and at force levels comparable to those the graft might experience in vivo. The cyclic test can be performed in two ways.

One method is to control the maximum elongation placed on the substitute during each cycle and to measure the unloading that occurs over time. This is called the cyclic relaxation test. Examples of the elongation vs time and load vs time plots for such a test are shown in Fig. 10–1A. The unloading can be caused by the loss of fixation strength over time, the goal of the experiment, but can also result from the viscoelastic or time-dependent behavior of the tissue. Separating these two variables requires performing another set of cycles after a waiting period to see if the tissue has "recovered" from the viscoelastic changes. The post-test to pretest difference in peak force represents this recovery and can be subtracted from the total force to give the restraining action of the fixation device alone.

The second type of cyclic test is the cyclic creep test in which maximum force is controlled during each

**Table 10–1**
**Maximum loads for nine common ligament replacements**[*†]

| Values | No. | Maximum Load (N) | Percent of Anterior Cruciate | Maximum Load/Unit Width (N/mm) | Maximum Stress (MPa) |
|---|---|---|---|---|---|
| Measured values | | | | | |
| Anterior cruciate ligament-bone | 6 | 1725 ± 269 | 100 | Width measures not done | 37.8 ± 3.8 |
| Bone-patellar tendon-bone | | | | | |
|   Central third | 7 | 2900 ± 260[‡] | 168 | 208 ± 24 | 58.3 ± 6.1[‡] |
|   Medial third | 7 | 2734 ± 298[‡] | 159 | 162 ± 13 | 56.7 ± 4.4[‡] |
| Semitendinosus | 11 | 1216 ± 50 | 70 | Width measures not done | 88.5 ± 5.0[¶] |
| Gracilis | 17 | 838 ± 30[§] | 49 | Width measures not done | 111.5 ± 4.0[¶] |
| Distal iliotibial tract (18 mm wide) | 10 | 769 ± 99[§] | 44 | 44 ± 6 | 19.1 ± 2.9[#] |
| Fascia lata (16 mm wide) | 18 | 628 ± 35[#] | 36 | 39 ± 2 | 78.7 ± 4.6[¶] |
| Quadriceps-patellar retinaculum- | | | | | |
| patellar tendon | | | | | |
|   Medial | 7 | 371 ± 46[¶] | 21 | 24 ± 4 | 15.4 ± 3.4[#] |
|   Central | 6 | 266 ± 74[¶] | 15 | 17 ± 3 | 16.1 ± 1.8[¶] |
|   Lateral | 7 | 249 ± 54[¶] | 14 | 19 ± 4 | 9.7 ± 1.5[¶] |
| Calculated values[**] | | | | | |
| Distal iliotibial tract | | | | | |
|   25 mm wide | — | 1068 | 62 | | |
|   Plus adjacent 10 mm of fascia | — | 1468 | 85 | | |
|   Plus adjacent 20 mm of fascia | — | 1868 | 108 | | |
| Fascia lata (45 mm wide) | — | 1800 | 104 | | |

[*]Adapted with permission from Noyes FR, Butler DL, Grood ES, et al: Biomechanical analysis of human ligament grafts used in knee ligament repairs and reconstructions. *J Bone Joint Surg* 1984;66A:344–352. Initial strengths are compared to the results for the anterior cruciate ligament from an earlier study.[15]
[†]Data are given as means and standard errors of the mean.
[‡]Statistically different from the maximum value for the anterior cruciate ligament: P<.05.
[§]P<.01.
[#]P<.005.
[¶]P<.001.
[**]Calculated by adjusting test values to new specimen widths.

cycle and the increase in elongation or "stretching out" is measured over time (Fig. 10–1B). Viscoelastic effects must also be measured and eliminated from these calculations. The creep experiment probably better resembles in vivo loading of grafts, but it is more difficult to perform in the laboratory.

The second kind of experiment is the failure test. This test is designed to determine the mechanical properties of a graft subjected to a single overload event typical of the forces that might have caused the injury. These tests are performed at high rates to simulate trauma and to test the bone and soft tissue together.[17] Force and elongation are measured simultaneously and are plotted in a curve like the one shown in Fig. 10–2. Important structural mechanical properties obtained from this curve are stiffness, maximum force, elongation to maximum force, and energy to failure. Stiffness represents the change in force caused by a change in the elongation, that is, a resistance to elongation, and is measured as the maximum slope of the force-elongation curve. The maximum force, the highest point on the curve, is the ultimate strength produced by the graft tissue and fixation device. The maximum elongation (not labeled) is the amount the graft-bone unit must be stretched to achieve maximum force. The energy to failure is measured as the area under the entire force-elongation curve.

## Recent Fixation Studies

Three recent studies have examined fixation methods under different loading conditions. These studies will be evaluated using the factors just discussed.

### Study 1

Burks and associates[11] evaluated three fixation procedures and three tissue types. They used a CPM apparatus and a knee arthrometer to determine laxity in cadaveric knees at 20 degrees of flexion and 20 lb of anterior drawer. The laxities of the intact knee and ACL-cut knee were first determined to provide baselines for evaluating the different fixation methods. Each knee was then reconstructed to reproduce intact knee laxity by one of three methods: the Marshall-MacIntosh procedure,[6] which uses prepatellar retinaculum and quadriceps and patellar tendon run over the top and secured with staples and screws; the Lambert procedure,[18] which uses the central one-third PT-bone unit placed in 9-mm drill holes in the femur and tibia and secured with 6.5-mm A-O cancellous screws; or the technique described by Mott[2] in which a free semitendinosus tendon is looped over a bony bridge proximally and the two ends are secured distally with an A-O screw and washer. The knees were then subjected to CPM in a

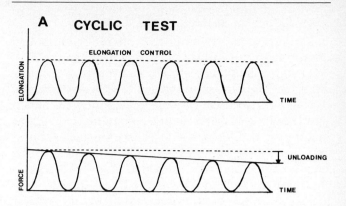

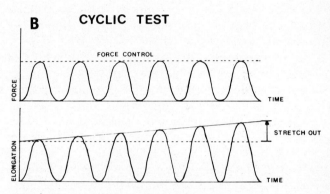

**Fig. 10–1** Two methods for performing cyclic testing on installed grafts. **A:** In cyclic relaxation tests, the elongations applied to the tissue are controlled and the drop in peak force or relaxation is measured. **B:** In cyclic creep tests, the forces are controlled and the increase in elongation or stretching out is measured.

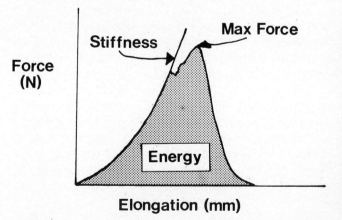

**Fig. 10–2** Force-elongation curve produced during the failure test. Stiffness, maximum force, elongation to maximum force (not shown), and energy to failure are values taken from this test.

commercial unit between 20 and 70 degrees of flexion. CPM tests were performed on the knee at 10 c/min for three days in a cooler to permit the desired number of cycles (at ten times the normal rate) without producing decomposition of the specimens. The post-test CPM laxity was then measured and any graft failures recorded. Stability before and after

CPM was defined as maintaining anterior laxity within 2 mm of that of the intact knee.

The investigators found that the intact knees had an average anterior laxity of 5.8 mm. When the ACL was cut, the laxity increased by an average of 6.4 mm. All three PT-bone units failed at the tibial attachment during CPM. In each case the tibial bone plug pulled past the screw. Five of eight semitendinosus tendons failed near the femoral end. Three of these failures occurred where the tendon entered the hole in the femoral condyle. The proximal bony bridge was moved proximally in the last two knees, producing a less acute angle at the entry point on the femur. Failure then occurred proximally to the bridge, however. The best results were found with the prepatellar retinacular tissues: only one of nine specimens became "unstable" during CPM.

To interpret these results properly, the factors of donor age and testing methods must be examined. The average age of the donors was not specified. However, one of the investigators (D. Daniel, personal communication), indicated that these were older donors. The bony beds available for fixing the tissues may, therefore, have been osteoporotic, and the bone ends of the patellar tendon may have been weak as well. If bone strength was reduced because of aging, the ability of any fixation method to secure the graft must be questioned. Aging could have been the cause for the PT-bone unit failures, in which the cancellous screws cut through the bone. The testing method, performing CPM in an actual system, was reasonable since it duplicated the types of loads the graft should experience. However, the fact that tests were performed at ten times the conventional rate raises questions about the possibility of fatigue in these grafts at their attachment points. The separate studies using semitendinosus tendons to examine the effects of different proximal attachment points provided worthwhile data. Although the sample size was small, the studies suggested that acute graft angles in the over-the-top region place the soft tissue at risk for abrasion and failure. Additional tests of this kind are warranted.

### Study 2

Kurosaka and associates[12] conducted an interesting study that involved two separate but related projects. The first was designed to evaluate different fixation methods in four tissue types. These included (1) PT-bone units placed through drill holes and secured by sutures over buttons, staples, or a 6.5-mm A-O screw[18]; (2) iliotibial tract and semitendinosus tendon, the former by stapling at both ends and the latter by stapling proximally and leaving the distal end attached; and (3) meniscus tied over bone by the method of Tillberg.[7] Tests were conducted on seven

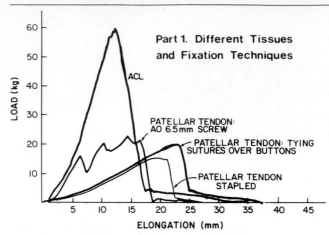

**Fig. 10–3** Typical force-elongation failure curves for the ACL-bone unit and for PT-bone units fixed with screws, buttons, and staples. (Reproduced with permission from Kurosaka M, Yoshiya S, Andrish JT: A biomechanical comparison of different surgical fixation techniques of graft fixation in anterior cruciate ligament reconstruction. Read before the Interim Meeting of the American Orthopaedic Society for Sports Medicine, Las Vegas, Nevada, January 23, 1985.)

cadaveric donor knees with a mean age of 59 years. Axial failure tests were performed on the grafts with the knees at 45 degrees of flexion.

The second project was designed to evaluate the effect of screw diameter on the strength of medial and lateral PT-bone units. Both ends of each graft were held with either A-O 6.5-mm or custom 9.0-mm screws using the Lambert procedure.[18] Tissues from three young (mean age, 20 years) donors were used. The testing methods were identical to those in the first project.

Typical curves from the first project are displayed in Fig. 10–3. Load-elongation curves for PT-bone units secured with screws, with buttons, and with staples are contrasted with a failure curve for the ACL-bone unit. When data for each tissue were averaged, the ACL-bone unit generated a maximum load of 61.1 kg whereas the stapled PT-bone unit produced only 13.1 kg of force. The PT-bone units held with staples and with screws failed at 25.3 and 21.9 kg, respectively. The iliotibial band, semitendinosus tendon, and meniscus produced 11.2 to 14.6 kg of force. In the second project, the intact, 10-mm-wide PT-bone units developed an average maximum force of 104.3 kg. The graft with the 9.0-mm screw produced about 46% of this load, significantly more than the graft with the 6.5-mm screw (20%).

Several conclusions can be drawn from both projects. First, ACL maximum load in the first project was only one third of the value (1,730 N or 175 kg) for ACL from young donors.[15] The low force level was probably the result of using tissue taken from older donors. Kennedy and associates[19] also found low ACL values when using older donors. Therefore, the relative strengths of these PT-bone units secured with staples or tied over buttons (Fig. 10–3) were really only 12% and 14% of ACL maximum load from young donors.[15] (The potential strengths of these fixation methods are difficult to estimate, however, since better fixation and higher loads would probably be obtained with young cadaveric soft tissue and bone.)

The second project, which used younger donors, provided more meaningful data. The PT-bone unit maximum force of 104.3 kg was more characteristic of patellar tendon but still only about one half of the 2,000 N PT-bone strength obtained with comparably aged donors (found by adjusting the 2,800 N average force in Table 10-1 from 14 mm to 10 mm of tissue width). It is appropriate, then, to compare the graft strengths with the original ACL maximum force baseline of 1,730 N.[15] The results were disappointing, however, since the 6.5-mm screw provided only 12% of ACL strength and the 9.0-mm screw only 28%. These values for installed grafts were low, given that the inherent strength of the PT-bone unit is 160% of the ACL.[8]

The conclusions drawn by Kurosaka and associates seem appropriate. First, an interference fit should be sought for the graft bone in each tunnel to provide additional resistance to loading. Second, these fixation methods should also be examined by cyclic creep loading to determine how they would perform during simulated in vivo loading. Finally, the low strength values measured make it imperative that the grafts and fixation methods be adequately protected from large forces during the early remodeling phase after surgery.

### Study 3

VanKampen and associates[13] evaluated augmented ACL reconstructions in five limbs from five older donors. Each composite graft consisted of a flat strip of polyurethane braid or augmentation device sutured to one of five biologic substitutes: PT-bone, prepatellar retinaculum, semitendinosus tendon, gracilis tendon, and iliotibial band. The biologic tissue was fixed distally with an A-O screw and washer. The augmentation device was then sutured to the tissue in midsubstance and secured proximally to a hook attached to the load frame. Testing conditions consisted of preconditioning the grafts to 10 lb, 20 lb, and then 10 lb (each a single cycle) and then cycling the composites either 40 or 480 times at 8

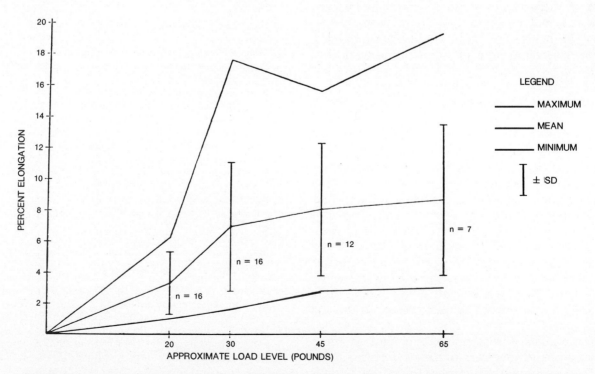

**Fig. 10–4**  Increasing residual elongation at higher peak cyclic loads. The mean value is shown at each load as well as the range. (Reproduced with permission from VanKampen C, May S, Flood C, et al. Comparison of reconstructions in cadavers. Read before the Synthetic Ligament Workshop, Carmel, California, 1984.)

c/min to increasing peak loads of 20, 30, 45, and 65 lb. The motor of the commercial CPM unit was used to apply the load. Those grafts that did not break during cycling were then tested to failure. The elongations were measured at peak loads and the failure cycle number and failure site were recorded.

VanKampen and associates[13] found that preconditioning the composite grafts produced a 0% to 4% residual elongation. Forty cycles of loading to 20 lb produced another 1% to 6% increase in elongation. As shown in Fig. 10-4, loading to higher peak forces produced further increases in elongation. The investigators also determined that the peak load level was more important in determining the percent elongation than was the number of cycles applied at each load level. The maximum loads that the grafts could tolerate were about 89 lb for the PT-bone unit and about 60 to 65 lb for the other grafts.

How should this study be interpreted? First, while a composite graft was tested, only the augmentation device was gripped proximally; the biologic tissue was gripped distally. This means that the device-suture-graft interface was actually tested. Thus, the true strength of the graft and device remains unknown. In fact, the investigators recommended that in future studies both components be gripped proximally. Their attempts to perform a cyclic creep test to control forces on the grafts seem plausible and worthy of additional study. However, for more careful control of these forces, these tests should be performed in a materials testing machine. Nonetheless, these experiments were important because they used repetitive loading to simulate in vivo conditions.

## Summary

Laboratory studies designed to simulate in vivo loading of a ligament graft and fixation method are affected by the age of the cadaveric donor, the types of tissue and fixation device employed, and the testing methods used. The use of older donors compromises the graft bone, underlying bone bed, and soft tissue. Staples, sutures, and screws all provide different fixation strengths depending on the tissue to be held. Cyclic testing of the graft better evaluates the performance of the composite during the activities of daily living, while high-speed failure tests indicate the replacement's ability to resist a traumatic injury.

Several studies were examined in light of these factors. Each study had certain merits but also limitations. Further studies are required for careful evaluation of the cyclic response of cancellous screws of different sizes, barbed staples, and other methods of graft fixation. Only then can recommendations be made as to the best device to use for achieving the clinical goals of joint stability, adequate resistance to traumatic loads, and proper graft attachment healing.

## References

1. Insall J, Joseph D, Aglietti HP, et al: Bone block iliotibial-band transfer for anterior cruciate insufficiency. *J Bone Joint Surg* 1981;63A:560–569.
2. Mott HW: Semitendinosus anatomical reconstruction for cruciate ligament insufficiency. *Clin Orthop* 1983;172:90–92.
3. McMaster JH, Weinert CR Jr, Scranton P: The diagnosis and management of isolated anterior cruciate ligament tears: A preliminary report on reconstruction with the gracilis tendon. *J Trauma* 1974;14:230–235.
4. Jones KG: Reconstruction of the anterior cruciate ligament: A technique using the central one-third of the patellar ligament. *J Bone Joint Surg* 1970;52A:1302–1308.
5. Noyes FR, Butler DL, Paulos LE, et al: Intraarticular cruciate reconstruction: I. Perspectives on graft strength, vascularization, and immediate motion after replacement. *Clin Orthop* 1983; 172:71–77.
6. Marshall JL, Warren RF, Wickiewicz TL, et al: The anterior cruciate ligament: A technique of repair and reconstruction. *Clin Orthop* 1979;143:98–106.
7. Tillberg B: The late repair of torn cruciate ligaments using menisci. *J Bone Joint Surg* 1977;59B:15–19.
8. Noyes FR, Butler DL, Grood ES, et al: Biomechanical analysis of human ligament grafts used in knee ligament repairs and reconstructions. *J Bone Joint Surg* 1984;66A:344–352.
9. Grood ES, Hefzy MS, Butler DL, et al: On the placement and the initial tension of anterior cruciate ligament substitutes. *Transactions of the 29th Orthopaedic Research Society Meeting.* Park Ridge, Illinois, Orthopaedic Research Society, vol 8, 1983, p 92.
10. Grood ES, Suntay WJ, Noyes FR, et al: Biomechanics of the knee-extension exercise. *J Bone Joint Surg* 1984;66A:725–734.
11. Burks R, Daniel D, Losse G: The effect of continuous passive motion on anterior cruciate ligament reconstruction stability. *Am J Sports Med* 1984;12:323–326.
12. Kurosaka M, Yoshiya S, Andrish JT: A biomechanical comparison of different surgical fixation techniques of graft fixation in anterior cruciate ligament reconstruction. Read before the Interim Meeting of the American Orthopaedic Society for Sports Medicine, Las Vegas, Nevada, January 23, 1985.
13. VanKampen C, May S, Flood C, et al: Comparison of reconstructions in cadavers. Read before the Synthetic Ligament Workshop, Carmel, California, 1984.
14. Butler DL, Grood ES, Noyes FR, et al: On the interpretation of our anterior cruciate ligament data. *Clin Orthop* 1985;186:26–34.
15. Noyes FR, Grood ES: The strength of the anterior cruciate ligament in humans and rhesus monkeys: Age-related and species-related changes. *J Bone Joint Surg* 1976;58A:1074–1082.
16. Butler DL, Grood ES, Noyes FR, et al: Effects of structure and strain measurement technique on the material properties of young human tendons and fascia. *J Biomech* 1984;17:590–596.
17. Noyes FR, DeLucas JL, Torvik PJ: Biomechanics of anterior cruciate ligament failure: An analysis of strain-rate sensitivity and mechanisms of failure in primates. *J Bone Joint Surg* 1974;56A:236–253.
18. Lambert KL: Vascularized patellar tendon graft with rigid internal fixation for anterior cruciate ligament insufficiency. *Clin Orthop* 1983; 172:85–89.
19. Kennedy JC, Hawkins RJ, Willis RB, et al: Tension studies of human knee ligaments. *J Bone Joint Surg* 1976;58A:350–355.

# Preoperative Planning for High Tibial Osteotomy

Joseph R. Cass, MD

This chapter will review important aspects of preoperative planning for high tibial osteotomy. Included is a brief review of historical developments as well as current traditional concepts in patient selection. Procedures used in high tibial osteotomy will be outlined. The importance of the angular correction and its attainability will be discussed in more detail.

The initial procedure is commonly credited to J. P. Jackson, who reported on eight high tibial osteotomies in 1958.[1] Coventry published his early results in 71 patients in 1965[2] and 1973.[3] Bauer and associates[4] and Harris and Kostuik[5] added their reports in 1969 and 1970. The operation, with variations, converted a varus knee to a valgus knee by resecting an appropriate wedge of bone. Short-term results, as reported by the various investigators, were satisfactory in 80% to 90% of the patients. With longer follow-up, reports indicate that continued satisfaction can be expected in 60% of the patients seven to ten years after osteotomy.[6-8]

The incidence of reported complications following this procedure varied from 10% to nearly 60%. The types of complications (Table 11–1) and their frequency depend on the technique and fixation used for osteotomy.[9]

The classic indications for the procedure have been outlined by Coventry.[10] Important considerations are the age, weight, and activity level of the patient. The pain should be localized to the medial side of the joint, although Coventry does not believe that the presence of patellofemoral pain is an absolute contraindication. The range of motion should be nearly 90 degrees with less than 20 degrees of flexion contracture.[9]

Traditionally, lateral instability has been a contraindication to high tibial osteotomy. Currently this contraindication is being reassessed. The closer study of patients less than 40 years old and those with instability and early degenerative changes may alter this perception.

Prodromos and associates[11] have begun to elucidate the dynamics of the varus knee deformity and have classified some patients as high medial loaders. It must be emphasized that the clinical assessment of "varus thrust" does not correlate with the presence or absence of a high medial load. Thus, the clinician presently has no way of determining whether a patient is a high or low medial loader. Technetium-99

bone scanning has been advocated for preoperative assessment in those patients with poorly localized pain. If the increased uptake of $^{99m}$Tc is not confined to the medial compartment, upper tibial osteotomy may not be successful. The efficacy of this particular procedure has not been critically assessed, however.[10]

Interest in using associated procedures with the high tibial osteotomy varies. In their study of 60 knees, Keene and Dyreby[12] found that arthroscopic findings, including exposed subchondral bone in the lateral or patellofemoral compartments, were of no value in predicting the outcome of osteotomy. In this particular study, the arthroscopic procedure was used for diagnostic assessment and not for treatment of any intra-articular problem. Therefore, it cannot be stated categorically that arthroscopy is of no assistance in the treatment of patients with medial compartment gonarthrosis. The Keene and Dyreby study stated only that arthroscopic findings cannot be utilized to predict the results of high tibial osteotomy.[12] These data have recently been updated and confirmed.[13]

The use of tibial tubercle elevation (Maquet procedure) in addition to high tibial osteotomy must be seriously questioned. Of three studies available, two[14,15] reported very disappointing results, and one by Putnam and associates reported a 68% satisfaction rating.[16] With such minimal support from the literature and the proven success of total knee arthroplas-

---

**Table 11–1**
**Complications of high tibial osteotomy**

Complications

Infection
Neurologic
  Peroneal nerve
  Posterior tibial nerve
Vascular
  Compartment syndrome
Bone healing
  Delayed union
  Nonunion
  Loss of correction
Malalignment
Intra-articular fracture
Instability
Thromboembolism
Sympathetic dystrophy

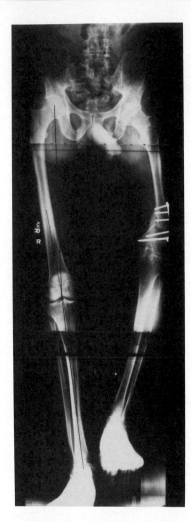

**Fig. 11–1** Anatomic axis (dotted line), the angle formed by lines drawn along the femoral and tibial diaphysis. Mechanical axis (solid line), the angle formed by lines drawn from the center of the femoral head through the center of the knee joint, and from the center of the knee joint to the center of the ankle joint. Ideally, a straight line from the center of the femoral head to the ankle joint should pass through the center of the knee joint.

ty, the use of this combined procedure for bicompartmental disease is of less than certain efficacy.

Abrasion chondroplasty is currently popular. Its use could be considered at the time of osteotomy. Alternatively, if the patient's pain recurs after a period of time without the loss of alignment, abrasion chondroplasty is an option. The results in either setting await critical scrutiny.

More recently, data have begun to appear on the use of high tibial osteotomy in younger patients with or without concomitant ligament instability. Its efficacy has been reported in the treatment of medial

compartment arthrosis in the patient under 50 years of age.[17] Some investigators are using realignment as a way of protecting ligament reconstructions. Again, these procedures have not undergone critical review.

A great deal of emphasis has been placed on the anatomic axis, the mechanical axis, and medial compartment load. These concepts can be a source of confusion. If a bowed leg is changed to a knock knee, the forces will be lateralized. The question of how much angulation changes the force by what magnitude, however, can be answered differently.

Before examining the data from a clinical and biomechanical standpoint, a brief definition of the various axis systems is in order. The anatomic axis is that angle formed by lines drawn from the center of the femoral and tibial diaphyses across the knee joint on the anteroposterior radiograph. Five to 7 degrees of valgus is considered normal (Fig. 11–1). The normal mechanical axis is considered to be a straight line from the center of the femoral head to the center of the ankle joint. On the anteroposterior radiograph, this line should pass through the center of the knee joint. A full-length standing radiograph is required for this assessment (Fig. 11–1).

Using the clinical data derived from five major investigators, Bauer and associates[4] recommended alignment in 3 to 16 degrees of valgus, a relatively broad range. Coventry[3] recommended 5 degrees of overcorrection as compared with a normal of 5 to 8 degrees of valgus. Kettelkamp and associates[18] recommended 8 to 11 degrees of valgus. These recommendations define valgus with respect to the anatomic alignment. Maquet recommended 2 to 4 degrees of valgus with respect to the mechanical axis.[19,20] These above recommendations were all based on an analysis of patient result.

The correction to 7 to 10 degrees of valgus in the anatomic axis system should give a satisfactory result 80% to 90% of the time. Excessive valgus angulation was not found to be as much a mechanical as a cosmetic problem.

Three long-term studies report follow-ups of longer than seven years. Based on these data, Vainionpaa and associates[8] recommended 5 to 8 degrees and Coventry 7 to 9 degrees of anatomic valgus.[6] Insall and associates,[7] however, found that in the long-term the degree of correction did not correlate with the outcome, that the basic disease process seemed to continue in spite of "satisfactory" realignment.

As mentioned earlier, the effect of recurrence of deformity on the decline in quality of results remains unknown. Although 25% of the patients in Insall and associates' study[7] and 8% (17 of 213) in Coventry and Bowman's study[6] had a measurable decrease in their valgus angulation with time, no study has as yet addressed this question specifically, saying only that it can occur if not adequately corrected initially.

Reports providing biomechanical data give conflicting information. The investigations are either static force assessments based on radiographic measurements or dynamic force assessments based on gait assessment of motion, transducer-measured force, electromyographically measured muscle activity, or dimensions measured in cadavers. In all cases, the calculations are complex.

The static evaluations are based on standard anteroposterior radiographs such as used by Kettelkamp and associates in their assessment,[18,21] or on full length standing radiographs used by Maquet and others.[19,20] The distinction is again made between the anatomic axis of 5 to 7 degrees of valgus and the mechanical axis drawn from the center of the femoral head, ideally through the center of the knee joint and then through the center of the ankle.

Based on Kettelkamp's and associates' measurements, there is normally a force of 0.25 times body weight (BW) on the medial plateau. The goal of an osteotomy is to decrease the elevated medial plateau force to less than 0.5 BW. Those patients who had a force less than 0.5 BW on the medial plateau had a satisfactory result in all but one case.[18]

Maquet made his calculations using a full-length radiograph and imparted a much stronger role to the iliotibial band, calling it the "pelvic deltoid" that helps balance the knee in a varus deformity. Accordingly, however, this approach increases the load on the knee much as the abductors increase the load on the hip. Again, he believed that 2 to 4 degrees of valgus with respect to the mechanical axis was most appropriate.[19,20]

These studies were done at a relatively primitive phase in the history of joint force calculations. Just as with the radiographic method of force estimation, certain assumptions are made with the gait-related assessment of knee forces. In 1980, Nissan reviewed the basic assumptions made in knee biomechanical studies and varied certain parameters.[22] He found that varying the estimated point of application of the intercondylar force (vertical force) by less than 1 cm markedly varied the result. Also, varying the geometric center of the knee by less than 1 cm greatly changed the result. The results in both the preceding as well as the following studies, then, must be looked at in the light of these findings.

In 1980, Johnson and associates demonstrated that because the body's center of gravity remained medially displaced with respect to the knee during normal gait, there remained an adductor moment.[23] The radiographic calculations did not take this fact into account. As represented in Figure 11–2, when static assessments are used, the forces on the knee are relatively small as the magnitude of the adductor moment is quite small. However, if dynamic force estimations are used, there is a much greater load on

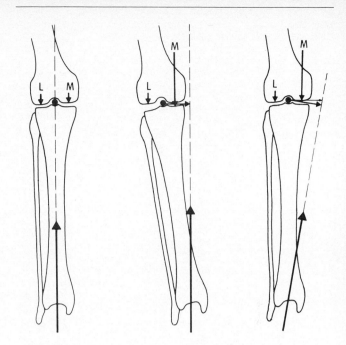

**Fig. 11–2**   This figure demonstrates the adductor moment arm. On the left, there is no adductor moment arm when only the static force assessment is used. When the static force assessment for a varus knee is used (center), there is a small moment arm. When a dynamic force assessment is used for a normally aligned knee, the moment arm is even larger. Johnson and associates[23] used this information to support his hypothesis of a continued adductor moment about the knee. (Reproduced with permission from Johnson F, Leitl S, and Waugh W: The distribution of load across the knee. *J Bone Joint Surg* 1980;62B:346–349.)

the medial compartment. Harrington[24] demonstrated this fact in a more quantitative fashion. As seen in Table 11–2, the amount of angulation measured radiographically did not predict well the type of loading. For example, with a varus deformity of 9 degrees measured on a static system, there seemed to be no lateral loading. Lateral loading was predicted to be present dynamically. Similarly, valgus of 8 degrees resulted in a discrepancy between the two methods; statically, in 8 degrees of valgus the forces were primarily lateral. The opposite was true dynamically. Even with a valgus deformity of 20 degrees, a medial plateau force existed. See Table 11–2.

Recently, the effect of adductor moment on the medial load has been quantified by Prodromos and associates.[11] Again, the tendency to equate varus thrust, a clinical impression, with high medial loading, a mechanical assessment, must be avoided. It seems that even the most sophisticated radiographic measurements are crude estimates of forces, and that gait techniques may give us more accurate information. The applicability of this information to practicing orthopaedists is limited at this time, however.

Assuming that the surgeon has carefully calculated

**Table 11–2**
**Static and dynamic loading patterns***

| Case | Age | Sex | Height (m) | Weight (kg) | Deformity (degrees) | Gait | | | Joint Force | | Location of Center of Pressure[†] | |
|---|---|---|---|---|---|---|---|---|---|---|---|---|
| | | | | | | Velocity (m/sec) | Cadence (steps/min) | Stride Length (m) | Static | Dynamic | Static | Dynamic |
| 1 | 75 | F | 1.57 | 61.2 | Varus, 2 | 1.02 | 96 | 1.32 | 650 | 941 | M, 1P | M, 2P |
| 2 | 69 | F | 1.68 | 63.4 | Varus, 5 | 0.43 | 60 | 0.81 | 851 | 1008 | M, 1P | M, 2P |
| 3 | 62 | F | 1.55 | 58.9 | Varus, 3 | 0.74 | 145 | 0.81 | 851 | 1075 | M, 1P | M, 2P |
| 4 | 64 | F | 1.57 | 62.1 | Varus, 9 | 1.33 | 136 | 1.12 | 1165 | 1658 | M, 1P | M, 2P |
| 5 | 58 | F | 1.63 | 61.7 | Varus, 12 | 1.38 | 131 | 1.42 | 1120 | 1299 | M, 1P | M, 1P |
| 6 | 72 | F | 1.57 | 61.2 | Varus, 17 | 0.51 | 111 | 1.02 | 1277 | 1546 | M, 1P | M, 1P |
| 7 | 68 | F | 1.67 | 61.6 | Varus, 31 | 1.42 | 140 | 1.17 | 1030 | 1792 | M, 1P | M, 1P |
| 8 | 64 | F | 1.57 | 62.1 | Valgus, 8 | 1.19 | 128 | 1.02 | 582 | 941 | L, 2P | M, 2P |
| 9 | 62 | F | 1.63 | 63.5 | Valgus, 8 | 0.91 | 107 | 1.07 | 582 | 1434 | L, 2P | M, 2P |
| 10 | 71 | F | 1.60 | 72.6 | Valgus, 20 | 0.46 | 120 | 0.51 | 941 | 1210 | L, 1P | L, 2P |
| 11 | 60 | F | 1.57 | 56.7 | Valgus, 20 | 0.56 | 100 | 0.81 | 874 | 1254 | L, 1P | L, 1P |
| 12 | 55 | M | 1.55 | 41.0 | Valgus, 30 | 1.79 | 116 | 1.42 | 941 | 1837 | L, 1P | L, 1P |
| 13 | 59 | F | 1.70 | 63.5 | Flexion, 23 | 0.55 | 81 | 0.79 | 627 | 1034 | M, 2P | M, 2P |
| 14 | 15 | M | 1.52 | 41.0 | Flexion, 40 | 1.70 | 125 | 1.62 | 650 | 1434 | M, 2P | M, 2P |
| 15 | 60 | F | 1.70 | 63.5 | Flexion, 40 | 0.53 | 79 | 0.81 | 784 | 1434 | M, 2P | M, 2P |
| 16 | 70 | F | 1.55 | 63.5 | Flexion, 41 | 0.81 | 140 | 1.12 | 987 | 2016 | M, 2P | M, 2P |
| 17 | 39 | M | 1.82 | 74.8 | Normal | 2.22 | 150 | 1.72 | 739 | 2334 | M, 2P | M, 1P |
| 18 | 63 | F | 1.75 | 65.8 | Normal | 1.71 | 104 | 1.98 | 597 | 1595 | M, 2P | M, 1P |
| 19 | 61 | M | 1.78 | 74.8 | Normal | 1.38 | 170 | 1.78 | 687 | 2079 | M, 2P | M, 1P |

*The anatomic alignment of varus or valgus gives different predictions of location of the center of pressure depending on whether static or dynamic force measurements are used. (Reproduced with permission from Harrington IJ: Static and dynamic loading patterns in knee joints with deformities. *J Bone Joint Surg* 1983;65A:247–259.)
[†]M = medial; L = lateral; 1P = one-point bearing contact; 2P = two-point bearing contact.

# HIGH TIBIAL OSTEOTOMY
## Preoperative Planning
### 1 mm=1° (56 mm)

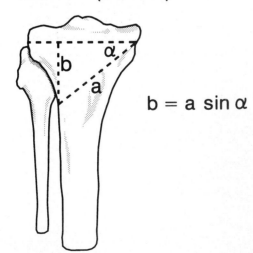

$$b = a \sin \alpha$$

**Fig. 11–3** This is the geometric way to ascertain the width of the tibial wedge. Magnification secondary to the radiograph must also be taken into account. Thus, if this procedure is done under fluoroscopic guidance, the angle between two Kirschner wires can be measured, assuring that the appropriate wedge will be taken.

the appropriate alignment based on these diverse data, the critical wedge must be attained. The attainability is related to three factors: (1) the adequacy of preoperative planning; (2) the accuracy of intraoperative estimation; and (3) the incidence of postoperative recurrence. Preoperative planning can take any one of three approaches. Measurements of the anatomic or preferably mechanical axis can be utilized to estimate the amount of wedge necessary. Quantitative gait measurement facilities can be used. Computer software programs can be used to estimate the force redistribution given the angular correction. For most, careful radiographic measurements are the cornerstone. These measurements must be done keeping geometric concepts in mind. The commonly accepted estimation that 1 mm = 1 degree is true only if the tibia is 56 mm wide, which is a relatively narrow tibial width. The measurement can be individualized as demonstrated in Figure 11–3.

Even when the size of the required wedge is known, its attainment is by no means certain. Looking at the clinical studies noted previously, appropriate correction was not obtained in 36% of Bauer and associates' patients,[4] 9% of Coventry's patients,[3] 48% of Kettelkamp and associates' patients,[18] and 10% of Maquet's patients.[19] Other studies report that up to 60% of patients were incorrectly aligned. In Hagstedt and associates' study specifically examining attainability, 82% of the time the desired wedge was attained to within ± 3 degrees.[25]

Various methods are available to ensure satisfactory alignment. The height of the wedge in the lateral tibial cortex can be measured and then the wedge can be removed. A technique that many have found very helpful is to perform the procedure under fluoroscopic guidance. Occasionally, jig systems are available.

As mentioned earlier, although postoperative recurrence is known to occur, the recurrence is unpredictable, and changes in the alignment in the early postoperative period can be caused by inadequate immobilization or delayed union. Late recurrence is probably secondary to continued high medial forces and secondary degenerative changes.

To summarize, traditional criteria for patient selection still apply. With the use of associated procedures and the problem of the younger patient with medial compartment gonarthrosis, the indications may be expanding, but the data are incomplete. Certainly in the short-term and probably in the long-term, appropriate angular correction is important, aiming for 8 to 10 degrees of anatomic axis and 2 to 4 degrees of mechanical axis valgus. It must be remembered, however, that static radiographic assessments markedly underestimate medial compartment forces. Furthermore, there may be a clinically indistinguishable group of patients known as high medial loaders who would not obtain satisfactory relief of symptoms in spite of appropriate realignment. Finally, a careful surgical technique to ensure that the appropriate wedge is taken must be used. If not, the preoperative assessment will be futile.

## References

1. Jackson JP: Osteotomy for osteoarthritis of the knee, in Proceedings of the Sheffield Regional Orthopaedic Club. *J Bone Joint Surg* 1958;40B:826.
2. Coventry MB: Osteotomy of the upper portion of the tibia for degenerative arthritis of the knee: A preliminary report. *J Bone Joint Surg* 1965;47A:984–990.
3. Coventry M: Osteotomy about the knee for degenerative and rheumatoid arthritis. *J Bone and Joint Surg* 1973;55A:23–48.
4. Bauer GCH, Insall J, Koshino T: Tibial osteotomy in gonarthrosis (osteoarthritis of the knee). *J Bone Joint Surg* 1969;51A:1545–1563.
5. Harris WR, Kostuik JP: High tibial osteotomy for osteoarthritis of the knee. *J Bone Joint Surg* 1970;52A:330–343.
6. Coventry MB, Bowman PW: Long-term results of upper tibial osteotomy for degenerative arthritis of the knee. *Acta Orthop Belg* 1982;48:139–156.
7. Insall JN, Joseph DM, Msika C: High tibial osteotomy for varus gonarthrosis: A long-term follow-up study. *J Bone Joint Surg* 1984;66A:1040–1048.
8. Vainionpaa S, Laike E, Kirves P, et al: Tibial osteotomy for osteoarthritis of the knee: A five-to ten-year follow-up study. *J Bone Joint Surg* 1981;63A:938–945.
9. Morrey BF: Upper tibial esteotomy: Analysis of prognostic features: A review. *Adv Orthop Surg* 1986;9(5):213–222.
10. Coventry MB: Current concepts review—upper tibial osteotomy for osteoarthritis. *J Bone Joint Surg* 1985;67A:1136–1140.
11. Prodromos CC, Andriacchi TP, Galante JO: A relationship between and clinical changes following high tibial osteotomy. *J Bone Joint Surg* 1985;67A:1188–1194.
12. Keene JS, Dyreby JR: High tibial osteotomy in the treatment of osteoarthritis of the knee. *J Bone Joint Surg* 1983;65A:36–42.
13. Keene JS, Monson DK, Roberts JM, et al: Arthroscopic evaluation of patients for high tibial osteotomy. Read before the 53rd Annual Meeting of the American Academy of Orthopaedic Surgeons, New Orleans, Feb, 1986.
14. Bourguignon RL: Combined Coventry-Maquet tibial osteotomy. *Clin Orthop* 1981;160:144–148.
15. Hoffmann AA, Wyatt RW, Jones RE: Combined Coventry-Maquet procedure for two compartment degenerative arthritis. *Clin Orthop* 1984;190:186–191.
16. Putnam MD, Mears DC, Fu FH: Combined Maquet and proximal tibial valgus osteotomy. *Clin Orthop* 1985;197:217–223.
17. Holden DL, James SL, Slocum DB, et al: Long-term results of high tibial osteotomy in patients under 50. Read before the 53rd Annual Meeting of the American Academy of Orthopaedic Surgeons, New Orleans, Feb, 1986.
18. Kettelkamp DB, Wenger DR, Chao EYS, et al: Results of proximal tibial osteotomy. *J Bone Joint Surg* 1976;58A:952–960.
19. Maquet P: Valgus osteotomy for osteoarthritis of the knee. *Clin Orthop* 1976;120:143–147.
20. Maquet P: *Biomechanics of the Knee*, ed 2. Berlin, New York, Springer-Verlag, 1984.
21. Kettelkamp DB, Chao EY: A method for quantitative analysis of medial and lateral compression forces at the knee during standing. *Clin Orthop* 1972;83:202–213.
22. Nissan M: Review of some basic assumptions in knee biomechanics. *J Biomech* 1980;13:375–381.
23. Johnson F, Leitl S, Waugh W: The distribution of load across the knee. *J Bone Joint Surg* 1980;62B:346–349.
24. Harrington IJ: Static and dynamic loading patterns in knee joints with deformities. *J Bone Joint Surg* 1983;65A:247–259.
25. Hagstedt B, Norman O, Olsson TH: Technical accuracy in high tibial osteotomy for gonarthrosis. *Acta Orthop Scand* 1980;51:963–970.

# Classification of Ligament Injuries:
# Why an Anterolateral Laxity or Anteromedial Laxity Is Not a Diagnostic Entity

Frank R. Noyes, MD

Edward S. Grood, PhD

## Introduction

Significant disagreement exists in the literature about the diagnosis and classification of ligament laxities, and many different classification schemes have been proposed.[1-7] New concepts about knee motions and ligament function have evolved over the past five years.[7-12] The concepts presented in this discussion are based, in part, on the previous work of the authors and others, as well as on new information gathered in our laboratory and clinic. This brief discussion, then, is a synopsis of important new concepts that we have presented in greater detail elsewhere.[6,7,11] Our intention is to present, to the clinician interested in knee ligament disorders, kinematic and biomechanical concepts that we believe provide a basis for a rational and valid scheme for the diagnosis and classification of knee ligament injuries.

The major purpose of a classification system is two-fold: (1) to make accurate distinctions between discrete pathologic conditions; and (2) to provide a common descriptive tool for physicians who wish to present clinical cases and to describe the results of their treatment programs. A classification system that permits two distinct types of injuries to be grouped as a single entity prevents the association of a unique natural history or surgical outcome with the injury classification. The existence of several possible natural histories or treatment outcomes interferes with attempts to develop improved treatment methods. Further, using such a classification scheme to report clinical results creates confusion about the actual pathologic condition being treated.

While existing classification systems for knee ligament injuries have advanced the understanding of knee ligament injury and treatment, we believe that modifications are required. The American Orthopaedic Society for Sports Medicine classification system[13] illustrates this point. This system identifies four "rotatory instabilities": anterolateral, anteromedial, posterolateral, and posteromedial. For each type of rotatory instability, a list of ligaments that may be involved is presented. For example, the list for anterolateral instability includes the anterior cruciate ligament, the iliotibial band, the midlateral capsule, and portions of the posterolateral capsule. Because this list involves so many structures, we believe that it does not represent a single diagnostic pathology with a unique natural history. Therefore, we present three

different types of anterior subluxations that may occur after anterior cruciate injury. Additionally, we describe the individual components of a "rotatory instability" in terms of the abnormalities that occur, such as changes in anterior translation, internal tibial rotation, and the center of tibial rotation. We use kinematic and biomechanical principles to explain ligament "instabilities." Our classification scheme is based on four concepts: (1) Ligament injuries must be diagnosed according to the specific anatomic defect, not abnormal motion or laxity. (2) The clinical laxity examination must be analyzed by a six degrees-of-freedom system (three-dimensional motion) to detect abnormalities. (3) Rotatory subluxations can be characterized by the separate translations that occur to the medial and lateral tibial plateaus. (4) The functional disruption of each ligament and capsular structure is diagnosed using select laxity tests in which the primary and secondary ligamentous restraints have been experimentally determined.

## Concept 1: Ligament Injuries Must Be Diagnosed According to Specific Anatomic Defect, Not Abnormal Motion or Laxity

The term "instability" has been used to describe both an abnormal looseness caused by ligament injury and the giving-way of the knee joint during activity. In the latter case, instability is a symptom of ligament injury, inadequate muscular control of the joint, altered neurologic function and control mechanisms, or mechanical blocks such as torn meniscus and loose bodies that interfere with knee joint motion. Because more than one factor is usually responsible for the giving-way event, "instability" does not indicate the precise cause of the giving-way episode.

"Laxity" is a general term meaning "looseness" and is not a diagnostic term for an abnormality. Actually, the knee joint requires looseness to function normally. The knee has a normal laxity or may have an abnormal laxity as a result of a ligament injury. The knee laxity examination is performed to detect an increased amount of motion (translation or rotation) or an abnormal position (subluxation). These findings are clinical signs. Although a clinical sign may be diagnostic of a specific ligament defect, it does not represent the diagnosis. This is true for other aspects of physical diagnosis as well. For example, a cardiologist after detecting the clinical sign of a grade III systolic ejection murmur would record the sign as a finding observed during examination. The diagnosis, however, would be separately recorded. A diagnosis, such as aortic valvular stenosis, indicates the affected anatomic part. In a similar way, the sign of an abnormal laxity must not be considered the diagnosis. It would be incorrect to record anterolateral laxity of the knee as a diagnosis. Rather, the specific anatomic defect of the anterior cruciate ligament and any other associated ligamentous or capsular structures should be recorded as the diagnosis. In the past, abnormal laxities (signs) have been labeled as the diagnosis, causing confusion as to the exact ligamentous and capsular defect present.

### Concept 2: The Clinical Laxity Examination Must Be Analyzed by a Six Degrees-of-Freedom System (Three-Dimensional Motion) To Detect Abnormalities

The terms "anterolateral instability" or "anteromedial instability" are imprecise and do not represent a specific definable motion or set of motions. Some classification systems use only one degree of freedom, internal-external tibial rotation, to describe the "rotatory laxities." In other classification systems, the terms anteromedial or anterolateral laxity imply a combination of two motions: anterior tibial translation and internal-external tibial rotation. The AOSSM classification[13] defines anteromedial instability as representing three motions: tibial abduction, external tibial rotation, and anterior tibial translation. An almost infinite number of combinations of joint motions actually exist that could occur in anteromedial instabilities, depending on the abnormalities in any one, two, or three of the degrees of freedom. The same is true for anterolateral instability or posterolateral instability. Because these terms are imprecise and do not define the specific change in each degree of freedom of motion involved, communicating the results of treatment often presents a significant problem.

#### Six Joint Motions (Degrees-of-Freedom)

Since the major function of the knee ligaments is to limit motion between the tibia and femur, the physician who understands all of the possible motions is

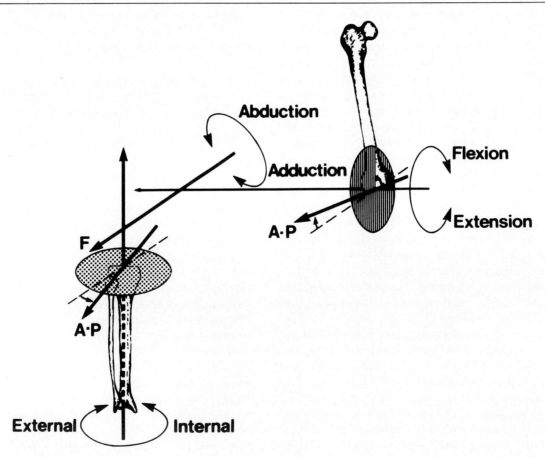

**Fig. 12–1** The three joint rotations in the knee joint. Flexion/extension occurs about the medially and laterally oriented axis in the femur. Internal and external tibial rotation occurs about an axis parallel to the shaft of the tibia. Abduction occurs about a third axis parallel to the femoral sagittal plane and also through the tibial transverse plane.

better able to perform manual stress tests and to determine the specific abnormality that exists. But a diagnosis cannot be based on knowledge of the motion abnormality alone. Rather, an accurate diagnosis requires that knowledge of the precise abnormalities be combined with biomechanical data on which ligaments limit each of the motions. We will discuss the function of individual ligaments after we have classified the possible motions that can occur.

The field of science that describes the motions between objects is known as kinematics. Fundamental to this science is the recognition that six possible motions can occur in three dimensions. Each of the six motions is distinct and independent of the other five motions. The six motions are often referred to as "degrees of freedom," and they form the basis of engineering descriptions of joints.

Figure 12–1 illustrates the three rotational degrees of freedom for the knee joint. Each rotation occurs about one axis. The first of the three axes is the flexion-extension axis, which is located in the femur and oriented in a pure medial-lateral direction, perpendicular to the femoral sagittal plane. Rotation of the tibia about the axis is pure flexion-extension without any associated internal-external rotation or abduction-adduction motions.[10] Since these motions do occur during flexion of a normal knee, the flexion-extension axis of Figure 12–1 does not correspond to the functional flexion axis. The functional flexion axis is skewed in the knee, and even changes its orientation as the knee is flexed.[11] The skewed orientation of the functional axis accounts for the combined motions of flexion, abduction, and tibial rotation.

The second axis shown in Figure 12–1 is located in the tibia and is parallel to the tibial shaft and perpendicular to the tibial transverse plane. Rotations about this axis are pure internal and external tibial rotation motions without any associated abduction-adduction or flexion-extension.[10]

The third axis is for abduction-adduction rotations. It is slightly more difficult to visualize this axis because it is not located in either bone and its orientation can change relative to both. The abduction-adduction axis is always parallel to the femoral sagittal plane.[10] When the knee is flexed, the orientation of the abduction axis changes relative to the femur as it rotates in the sagittal plane. Similarly, the abduction axis is perpendicular to the tibial rotation axis and parallel to the tibial transverse plane.

In addition to the three rotations, there are three linear degrees-of-freedom called translations. While the translations can be described in numerous ways, one simple approach is to visualize relative sliding between the bones along each of the three rotational axes.[10] These sliding motions are illustrated in Figure 12–2. The sliding motion along the flexion-extension

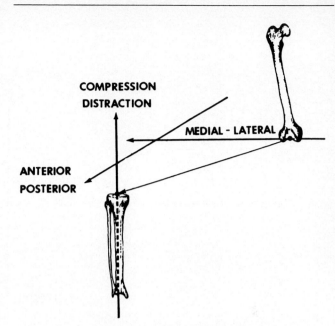

**Fig. 12–2** The three translations of the knee are motions of a point on the tibia parallel to each of the three axes. The point of the tibia we use is located midway between the spines of the tibial plateau and is indicated by the arrow originating from the center point of the femur. Medial/lateral translation is motion of the point parallel to the flexion/extension axis. Anterior/posterior translation is motion of the tibial point parallel to the abduction axis, and compression/distraction translation is motion of the point along the internal and external rotation axis.

axis is the medial-lateral translation between the tibia and femur. The sliding motion along the tibial rotation axis results in joint compression and distraction translation. Finally, sliding motions along the abduction-adduction rotation axis produce anterior-posterior translations, or "drawer" motions, as they are more commonly known.

In summary, there are six possible motions that can occur in the knee; three are rotations and three are translations. To explain these six motions requires describing three axes, one fixed in each "bone," as illustrated in Figure 12–2, and one that moves relative to both. Each axis represents two degrees of freedom, one being a rotation occurring about the axis and the other being a translation, or sliding motion, occurring along the axis.

Three related points must be emphasized. First, the physician must determine the specific increase in motion (amount and direction) of each clinically relevant degree of freedom. In many instances, the knee joint functions with coupled motions, such as the anterior translation that is combined with internal tibial rotation during the Lachman anterior translation test. For proper diagnosis, the physician must understand the effect that ligament defects have upon each of these motions, since one or both may be increased. Second, both the amount of increased motion and the resulting subluxation of the tibial

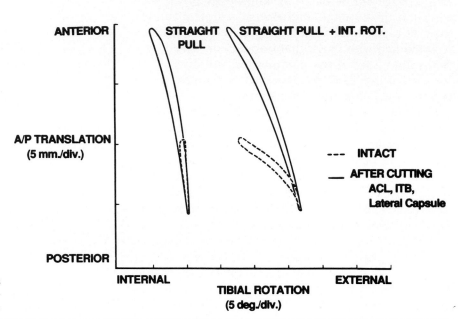

**Fig. 12–3**   Anterior translation versus tibial rotation is shown during the anterior drawer test at 15 degrees of flexion.

plateaus strongly depend on the position of the knee joint, which is also defined in terms of six degrees of freedom. Third, after ligament injury, an abnormal position commonly exists in the axis of internal-external tibial rotation. This abnormal position, which can be clinically detected, is helpful in diagnosing the ligament defect.

In order to interpret the results of the clinical laxity test, a clear separation must be made between abnormalities in joint motion and abnormalities in joint position (subluxation) which occur at the limit of the test. An abnormality in one or more motion limits can cause a subluxation of the knee joint. The precise subluxation depends on the direction and magnitude of the loads applied. Clinical laxity tests are used to detect both abnormal looseness and the final abnormal joint position. The laxity examination usually detects a subluxation rather than complete dislocation (in which contact between the articulating surface of both tibiofemoral compartments is lost).

These motion concepts can be applied to understand what often occurs after an anterior cruciate ligament tear. In cadaver knees, after the anterior cruciate ligament was cut we found an abnormal increase in both anterior tibial translation and internal tibial rotation. However, the increase in anterior tibial translation was the primary abnormality. It increased approximately 100% while the total amount of internal-external rotation increased 15%.

Figure 12–3 shows the data for a Lachman-type anterior translation test conducted at 15 degrees of knee flexion. The amount of anterior tibial transla-

tion that occurred during the test is shown vertically; the position of tibial rotation is shown horizontally. Tibial translation was measured at a point mid-way between the spines. As shown in Figure 12–4, a six degrees-of-freedom electrogoniometer was used to measure knee motion in whole lower limbs obtained from cadavers. The actual motions that occurred during the laxity test were displayed on a monitor.[1,11,12] Note, in Figure 12–3, that an anterior pull produced a few degrees of internal tibial rotation in addition to the anterior tibial translation (coupled motions of anterior translation and internal rotation). Coupled motions also occurred following the cutting of the anterior cruciate ligament and lateral extra-articular structures, but the increase in anterior tibial translation was the predominant abnormality (Fig. 12–3). Such coupled motions can be caused by factors intrinsic to the knee or by the manner in which the clinical test is performed. We found that the amount of internal tibial rotation depended primarily on the testing method, since the clinician was able to apply differing amounts of internal rotation. This explains why it is so difficult to obtain reproducible results. Thus, the Lachman test, like other clinical laxity tests, is variable in terms of the different ways it may be performed and the subsequent clinical findings.

The physician must also understand the phenomenon illustrated in Figure 12–5. The amount of anterior translation occurring in anterior cruciate injuries depends on the position of internal or external tibial rotation at the beginning of the test because the rotation tightens the extra-articular restraints. In

Figure 12–5, only the anterior cruciate ligament was cut. The greatest amount of anterior translation occurred when the neutral rotation position of the tibia was maintained. When the tibia was rotated prior to the start of the test, the amount of tibial translation markedly decreased. Small amounts of additional internal rotation during the test further reduced the amount of tibial translation. The position of external tibial rotation before the anterior drawer test produced a similar but opposite effect.

These results show that the examiner controls the amount of translation by (a) the initial rotational position of the tibia and (b) the amount of rotation imposed during the test. Thus, the clinician must perform the clinical examinations in as reproducible a position as possible to minimize the technique-related differences seen from test to test or between right and left limbs.

The pivot shift and the flexion-rotation drawer tests[14-16] involve a rather complex set of tibial rotations and anterior-posterior translations. Figure 12–6 shows the technique for the flexion-rotation drawer test. In Figure 12–7, the sequence of motions during the test is shown. The results presented in Figure

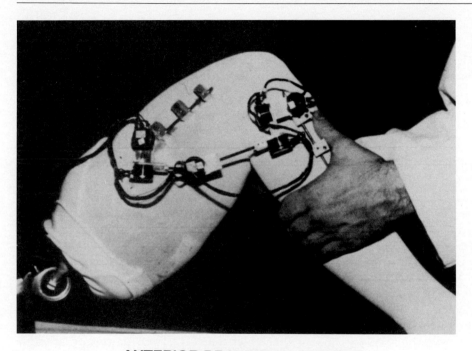

**Fig. 12–4** The six degrees-of-freedom electrogoniometer provides the clinician with immediate feedback on the motions induced during the laxity tests.

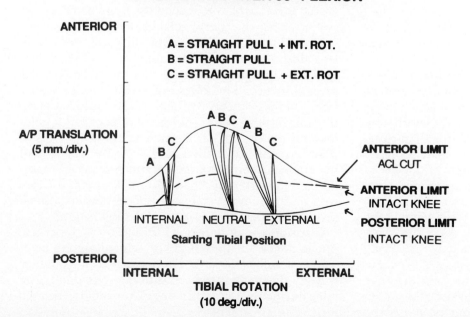

**Fig. 12–5** The amount of anteroposterior laxity depends on the rotational position of the tibia at the beginning of the anterior drawer test.

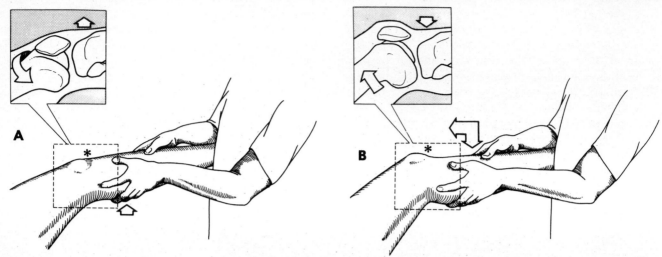

**Fig. 12–6** **A:** Flexion–rotation drawer test, subluxated position. With the leg held in neutral rotation, the weight of the thigh causes the femur to drop back posteriorly and, more importantly, to rotate externally, producing anterior subluxation of the lateral tibial plateau. **B:** Flexion-rotation drawer test, reduced position. Gentle flexion and a downward push on the leg (as in a posterior drawer test) reduces the subluxation. This test assesses the function of the anterior cruciate ligament in the control of both translation and rotation. (Reproduced with permission from Noyes FR, Bassett RW, Grood ES, et al: Arthroscopy in acute traumatic hemarthrosis of the knee. *J Bone Joint Surg* 1980;62A:687–695.)

12–7 are based upon prior studies using whole lower limbs and a three-dimensional (six degrees-of-freedom) electrogoniometer to measure total knee motion.[6] At the beginning of the test (position A), the lower extremity is simply supported against gravity. After ligament sectioning, both anterior tibial translation and internal rotation increase as the femur drops back and externally rotates into a subluxated position. This position is accentuated as the tibia is lifted anteriorly (position B). At approximately 30 degrees of knee flexion, the tibia is pushed posteriorly, reducing the tibia into a normal relationship with the femur (position C). This is the limit of posterior translation of the knee resisted primarily by the posterior cruciate ligament. From position C to position A, the knee is extended to produce the subluxated position again.

The examiner can purposely accentuate the rotational component of the test by inducing a rolling motion of the femur. It is not necessary to produce joint compression or to add a lateral abduction force, as in the pivot shift test. Inducing a rolling motion avoids the sometimes painful aspect of the thud/clunk phenomenon in the pivot shift test. The examiner places a finger along the anterior aspect of the lateral and medial plateau, palpates the tibiofemoral step-off, and estimates the millimeters of anterior subluxation. This test enables the examiner to see easily the translation and rotation movements. As in the Lachman test, tibial translation is detected by observing the forward motion of the tibial plateaus. The examiner observes rotation by watching the patella rotate externally with the femur in the subluxated position, and internally in the reduced position.

The pivot shift and flexion-rotation drawer tests are graded as positive only in qualitative terms, since it is difficult to estimate with any degree of accuracy the actual amount of internal tibial rotation or anterior translation present.

Table 12–1 presents the subjective difference in the pivot shift phenomenon used to grade qualitatively the different types of anterior subluxation. A fully positive pivot shift test grade IV (type III) indicates a gross subluxation of the lateral tibiofemoral articulation and also an increased anterior displacement of the medial tibial plateau. The amount of anterior subluxation indicates laxity of both the anterior cruciate ligament and the secondary extra-articular restraints. Since the lateral tibial plateau has the greater subluxation in a positive pivot shift test, the lateral restraints (iliotibial band, lateral capsule) are not functionally tight; otherwise, they would block the pivot shift test. This does not mean that associated injury to these lateral restraints has occurred, since a physiological slackness of the iliotibial band tibiofemoral attachments is normal at the knee flexion position used in the pivot shift test. We have found the iliotibial band tibiofemoral attachments are tightest past 45 degrees of knee flexion. Thus, most knees with an anterior cruciate tear alone have a positive pivot shift phenomenon (type III subluxation).

Occasionally, in anterior cruciate tears the classic phenomenon of the "thud" or "clunk" of the pivot shift test will be absent. The experienced examiner will still detect an increased slipping sensation in the knee during the pivot shift or flexion-rotation drawer test (type II subluxation). This slipping sensation

## FLEXION ROTATION DRAWER

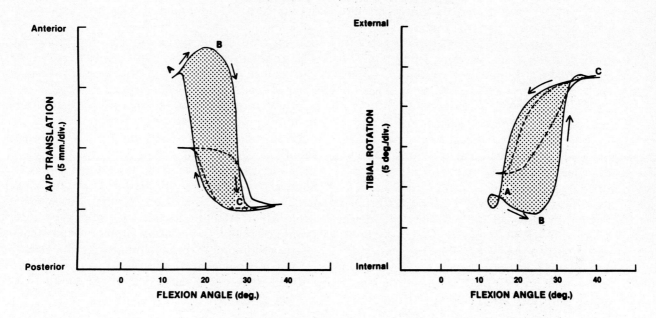

**Fig. 12–7**   The knee motions during the flexion–rotation drawer test are shown for tibial drawer versus knee flexion, and for tibial rotation versus knee flexion. The laxity test is shown for the normal knee (open circle) and after ligament sectioning (dotted circle). The ligaments sectioned were the anterior cruciate ligament, iliotibial band, and lateral capsule. Position A equals the starting position of the test, B is the maximum subluxated position, and C indicates the reduced position.

**Table 12–1**
**Classification of pivot shift tests**

| Laxity Grade | Structures Involved | | | Positive Tests | Comments |
|---|---|---|---|---|---|
| | Anterior Cruciate | Iliotibial Band, Lateral Capsule | Medial Ligaments, Capsule | | |
| Normal | Not loose | Not loose | Not loose | | Physiologic laxity normally present. |
| Moderate (Grade I) | Loose | Not loose | Not loose | Lachman, flexion-rotation drawer, ALRI, pivot shift "slip" but not "jerk" | Subtle subluxation-reduction phenomena. Secondary ligament restraints limit the amount of joint subluxation but may stretch out later with repeat injury. Pivot shift and jerk tests do not show obvious jump, thud, or jerk, although the subluxation may be detected as a "slip" with experience. |
| Severe (Grade II) | Loose | Loose | Not loose | All tests | Hallmark is an obvious jump, thud, or jerk with the gross subluxation-reduction during the test. This indicates laxity of other ligament restraints, either a normal physiologic laxity, (lateral capsule, iliotibial band), or injured secondary restraints. |
| Gross (Grade III) | Loose | Very loose | Very loose | All tests | Hallmark is a gross subluxation with impingement of the posterior aspect of the lateral tibial plateau against the femoral condyle. The examiner must effect reduction to allow further knee flexion. |

indicates an abnormal laxity in which tight extra-articular secondary restraints limit the amount of anterior tibial subluxation after the anterior cruciate ligament is torn. We have found the Lachman and flexion-rotation drawer tests to be the most sensitive in picking up the subtle type II anterior subluxation.

The type IV subluxation, characterized by a loss of the medial and lateral secondary ligament restraints, occurs when the amount of anterior subluxation of the tibia is so large that the posterior margin of the lateral tibial plateau impinges against the femoral condyle and blocks knee flexion during the test. It is important to add both a maximal anterior force and forcible internal tibial rotation of the tibia to see if this maximum subluxation position can be reached. It is easy to hypothesize that the type IV subluxated knee has the worst prognosis, and we have discussed various treatments and their implications elsewhere.[16] In type IV subluxations we recommend acute augmented repairs for acute knee injuries and discussed the possibility of a combined intra-articular and extra-articular surgical approach in chronic cases. Since the qualitative grading of the pivot shift tests does not provide a measurable amount of anterior tibial translation. More objective measurements of anteroposterior translation should be used in reporting clinical results.

### Concept 3: Rotatory Subluxations Can Be Characterized by the Separate Translations That Occur to the Medial and Lateral Tibial Plateaus

Earlier, we described abnormalities in anterior tibial translation and internal tibial rotation that occur in knees with anterior cruciate ligament disruption. We noted that the clinician must be aware of both motions when performing laxity tests in order to interpret properly which limits of motion are abnormal. A simple unifying concept helps to explain the abnormal motions which occur after anterior cruciate disruption: rotatory subluxations can be classified according to the amount of anterior and posterior translation of each tibiofemoral compartment.

Figure 12-8 illustrates a Lachman test performed on a knee in which the combined motions of tibial translation and internal tibial rotation occur about a medially located rotation axis. In this ideal test, only planar motion occurs, and the anterior cruciate rupture doubles anterior translation and slightly increases the internal tibial rotation, as previously presented. The rotation axis then shifts medially. The ratio of tibial translation to degrees of internal tibial rotation determines how far medially the axis of rotation shifts.

The abnormalities in tibial rotation and translation are easily expressed in terms of the different amounts of anterior translation that occur to the medial and lateral compartments. During the laxity tests, the clinician can palpate and observe the anterior translation of each tibial plateau. It is simpler to characterize the anteroposterior translations of the medial and lateral plateaus than to define specifically the individual components of translation, rotation, and rotation axis location that lead to the anterior subluxation. The rotations and translations combine to amplify and reduce the motions of the medial and lateral tibial plateaus, and this phenomenon determines the different translations of the medial and lateral tibiofemoral compartments.

We previously determined that the type of rotatory subluxations that can occur depends on both the ligamentous injury, and the knee flexion position. Some classification systems record the rotational subluxations at only one knee position (90 degrees), while other systems do not state the knee flexion position. However, the subluxation of the medial and lateral tibiofemoral compartment must be recorded at least at two knee flexion positions, and we chose 20 and 90 degrees of knee flexion, as we discuss in greater detail below.

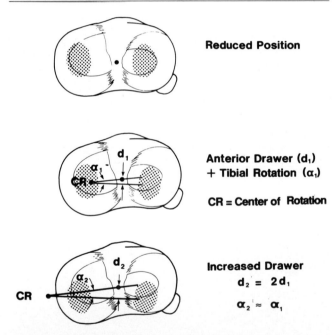

**Reduced Position**

**Anterior Drawer ($d_1$)**
**+ Tibial Rotation ($\alpha_1$)**

**CR = Center of Rotation**

**Increased Drawer**
$d_2 = 2d_1$
$\alpha_2 \approx \alpha_1$

**Fig. 12-8** A simplification of the pathologic knee motions after anterior cruciate ligament sectioning. An understanding of rotatory subluxations requires specifying changes in (1) position of the vertical axis of rotation and (2) displacement of the medial and lateral tibiofemoral compartments. The normal or subluxated position of the joint is determined by the degrees of rotation and the amount of translation. In the figure, an anterior pull is applied to the knee, which has an intact anterior cruciate ligament. There is a normal anterior translation ($d_1$) and internal tibial rotation ($a_1$) about the center of rotation (CR). After anterior cruciate sectioning there is a 100% increase on tibial translation ($d_2$) along with only a slight (15%) increase in internal tibial rotation ($a_2$). This shifts the axis of rotation medially and produces the subluxation of the lateral compartment and medial compartment as demonstrated. Loss of the medial extra-articular restraints would result in a further medial shift in the axis of rotation. This would increase the anterior subluxation of the medial tibial plateau and lateral tibial plateau.

Name _____  Date _____

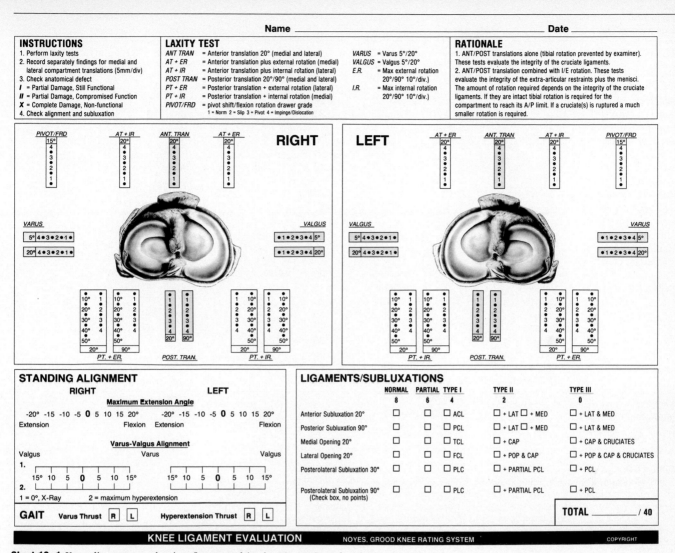

**Chart 12–1** Knee ligament evaluation form used in the Noyes-Grood rating system

## Concept 4: The Functional Disruption of Each Ligament and Capsular Structure Is Diagnosed Using Select Laxity Tests in Which the Primary and Secondary Ligamentous Restraints Have Been Experimentally Determined

Anterior cruciate ligament tears and injury to the extra-articular ligamentous and capsular structures can be diagnosed by using the anterior drawer, pivot shift, and flexion-rotation drawer tests (Chart 12–1). They provide the basic signs that enable the clinician to determine which ligament and capsular structures are injured, based on abnormal motion limits and resultant joint subluxations. The diagnosis, then, is made after the clinician determines which ligaments resist these laxity tests. We perform compartmental anteroposterior and rotation tests, selecting knee flexion positions in which the secondary restraints are "out of the way." This allows for the maximum excursion of the joint to test individual ligaments. It is not possible to "guess" which ligaments are acting as functional restraints, and further, major discrepancies exist in ligament-cutting studies because of meth-

odological differences which we have described elsewhere.[8,17–19]

Chart 12–1 and Table 12–2 present the scheme we use for recording the findings of the ligament laxity tests and the resultant diagnosis. Table 12–2 provides for the first time a comprehensive listing of the primary and secondary restraints for a variety of joint positions and represents our best estimate of ligament function in certain situations since biomechanical studies are still in progress. Brief instructions for using the knee ligament evaluation form are given in the upper left-hand column. The clinician first selects a laxity test for which the primary and secondary resisting ligament restraints have been experimentally determined. Table 12–2 lists the major tests used, along with the primary and secondary ligamentous restraints that resist each test. All knees are tested for (1) anteroposterior translation (drawer test performed without allowing any added tibial rotation); (2) pivot shift and flexion rotation drawer motions; (3) abduction-adduction rotation (amount of medial

**Table 12–2**
**Ligamentous restraints**

| Laxity Test | Primary Restraint* | | | Degrees | Secondary Restraint* | | |
| --- | --- | --- | --- | --- | --- | --- | --- |
| | Medial | Central | Lateral | | Medial | Central | Lateral |
| Anterior drawer | — | ACL | — | 20/90 | TCL + MM | — | ALS |
| Anterior drawer + internal rotation | — | ACL | ALS | 20/90 | — | — | FCL +PLS |
| Anterior drawer + external rotation | TCL + MM | ACL | — | 20/90 | PMS | — | — |
| Flexion-rotation drawer, pivot shift | — | ACL | — | 15 | MM + TCL + PMS | — | ALS + FCL |
| Posterior drawer | — | PCL | — | 20/90 | PMS + TCL | — | FCL + PLS |
| Posterior drawer + external rotation | — | — | FCL + PLS | 30 | — | PCL | — |
| | — | PCL | FCL + PLS | 90 | — | — | — |
| Posterior drawer + internal rotation | TCL + PMS | — | — | 20 | — | ACL + PCL | — |
| | TCL + POL | PCL | — | 90 | — | ACL | — |
| Valgus | TCL + PMS | — | Bone | 5 | — | PCL + ACL | — |
| | TCL | — | Bone | 20 | PMS | PCL | — |
| Varus | Bone | — | FCL + PLS | 5 | — | ACL + PCL | — |
| | Bone | — | FCL | 20 | — | ACL | PLS |
| External rotation | PMS + TCL | — | FCL + PLS | 30 | MM | PCL | — |
| | MM + TCL | PCL | FCL + PLS | 90 | PMS | — | — |
| Internal rotation | TCL + PMS | ACL | ALS | 20 | — | PCL | FCL |
| | TCL + POL | ACL + PCL | ALS | 90 | — | — | FCL |

*ACL = anterior cruciate ligament; ALS = iliotibial band + anterior +mid lateral capsule; FCL = fibular collateral ligament; MM = medial meniscus; PCL = posterior cruciate ligament; PLS = popliteus, posterolateral capsule; PMS = posterior oblique ligament + posteromedial capsule; POL = posterior oblique ligament; TCL = tibial collateral ligament.

**Table 12–3**
**Types of anterior knee subluxations following rupture of the anterior cruciate ligament**

| Type | Medial Ligaments and Capsule | Anterior Translation* | Lateral Ligaments and Capsule | Anterior Translation | Rotation Axis† |
| --- | --- | --- | --- | --- | --- |
| Type I, normal, ACL intact | — | Medial tibial plateau | — | Lateral tibial plateau | Central |
| Type II | Tight‡ | — | Intact | ↑ | Medial compartment |
| | Intact‡ | ↑ | Tight‡ | — | Lateral compartment |
| | Tight‡ | — | Tight‡ | — | Central |
| Type III | Intact | ↑ ↑ | Intact | ↑ ↑ ↑ | Outside knee medially |
| Type IV | Lax§ | ↑ ↑ ↑ | Lax§ | ↑ ↑ ↑ ↑ | Outside knee medially |

*Refers to anterior translation of the medial or lateral tibial plateau during laxity test.
†During Lachman-type anterior drawer test or flexion-rotation drawer test.
‡Physiologic tightness of structure or result of operative treatment.
§Abnormal laxity due to injury or physiologic laxity.

and lateral joint opening without allowing any added internal or external rotation); and (4) the external rotation test at 20 and 90 degrees of flexion (to test the posterolateral complex). This forms the basic minimum set of tests to determine function of the primary ligamentous restraints. Additional drawer tests with internal or external rotation are performed in the more complex rotatory subluxations and grading columns are provided in Chart 12–1 for these supplemental tests. The clinician then marks the test findings on the anatomic drawing of each knee (Chart 12–1). A scale is provided in which each major division equals 5 mm of translation and each minor division equals 2.5 mm. The clinician records the maximum translation for the center of the tibia and for each tibial plateau if the supplemental tests are used. A second scale is provided to record the maximal amount of internal and external tibial rotation.

For most acutely injured knees, a varus-valgus test that reveals a one-grade increase in joint opening indicates a third-degree, or complete, injury to the primary restraint.[18,20] Each subsequent grade indicates damage to the secondary restraints.

The clinician uses the following symbols to record the extent of damage to each structure: I, partial damage, still functional; II, partial damage, compromised function; and X, complete damage, nonfunc-

tional. Biomechanical information on the functional capacity of ligaments and their mechanisms of failure enables the clinician to approximate the injury classification.[18,20,21] However, the assessment of the functional capacity of the damaged ligament and capsular structures is only an approximation. A quantitative measurement of joint stiffness or compliance would provide more precise information.[22–24] Ultimately, it will be necessary to measure the stiffness of each one of the ligament systems (or functional "bumpers")[11] to determine the approximate extent to which the individual structures have been damaged.

The type of subluxation is checked in the lower right-hand corner of the evaluation form. (This will be discussed below using the bumper models.) The form also includes the evaluation of the standing alignment of the knee joint as to degrees of varus-valgus angulation and degrees of hyperextension.

The form is designed so that both clinical signs and diagnosis can be recorded on one page. Note that surgical treatment results must be reported in quantitative terms. All of the concepts presented here can be applied either in a qualitative or quantitative manner.

At least three clinically identifiable types of anterior knee subluxations can occur following a rupture of the anterior cruciate ligament (Table 12–3). These

| Characteristics | Laxity Test | Treatment Considerations |
| --- | --- | --- |
| Normal pattern ACL maintains central restraint | Normal A-P translation | — |
| One or both extra-articular restraints limit compartment translation (<10% of knees with ACL disruption) | Postive Lachman and FRD; grade amount of translation separately for medial and lateral compartments; grade II pivot shift (slipping sensation) | Secondary restraints provide stability if protected from repeat injury. Generally best prognosis; consider nonoperative approach in less athletic individual. Still warrants acute augmented repair in fully competitive athlete since primary restraint is disrupted |
| Typical pattern after ACL disruption | Postive Lachman and FRD; grade III pivot shift (thud, clunk, jerk phenomena) Obvious anterior subluxation, both compartments; grade IV pivot shift (impingement) | Avoid repeat giving-way injuries to protect secondary restraints; acute augmented repair in active athlete; extra-articular procedure may convert to type II but does not restore stability |
| Gross anterior subluxation to due involvement of one or both extra-articular restraints (approximately 20% to 30% of ACL-deficient knees); commonly has associated increased varus or valgus opening or posterolateral subluxation | | Severe functional disability for any kind of athletics; often produces giving-way with activities of daily living; extra-articular procedure alone not warranted; would affect only lateral tibiofemoral compartment translation; in acute and chronic cases, consider need to restore lateral extra-articular restraints |

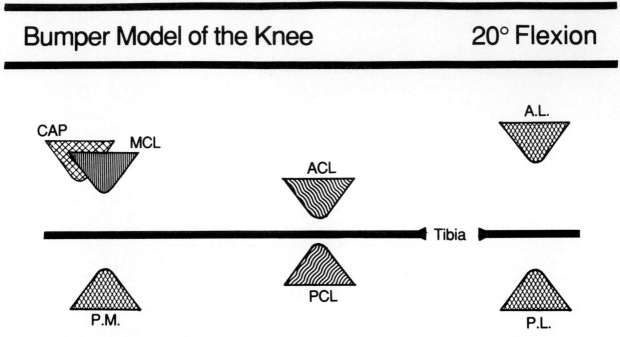

**Fig. 12–9**   The bumper model is used to show how the various structures about the knee limit internal and external rotation and anterior-posterior translation, both at the joint center and at the medial and lateral joint margins. The tibia is represented by the horizontal line the motion of which is limited by the bumpers. Six bumpers, which replace the limiting action of the ligaments, capsular structures, and menisci, are shown. The two central bumpers account for the limiting action of the anterior cruciate ligament (above) and the posterior cruciate ligament (below). The bumpers in the four quadrants are designated MCL and CAP (anteromedial restraints), AL (anterolateral restraints), PM (posteromedial restraints), and PL (posterolateral restraints). These bumpers include the combined effects of several ligamentous, capsular structures and are not meant to designate a single anatomic entity.

types are illustrated in Figures 12–9 through 12–12. The "bumper models" present an analogy, or explanation, of how ligamentous structures resist tibiofemoral motions. The cruciate ligaments are replaced by a set of central bumpers that limit the amount of anteroposterior translation. There are also medial and lateral sets of bumpers that resist medial and lateral tibiofemoral compartment translations. For the medial and lateral bumpers, different ligament structures commonly work together as systems to provide the resistance. The bumpers do not represent exact ligament structures; rather, the bumpers represent the final restraints to tibial motion summating the effect of the ligaments, menisci and capsular structures. For simplicity, we have replaced the tension-restraining, or spring-like effect, of ligaments by an opposite mechanism, namely a compressive bumper. In fact, the stiffness of the spring is replaced by the compressibility of the bumper. The bumper models allow for a clearer understanding of the complex changes in the medial, lateral and central compartments of the knee that occur with ligament injuries. The data for the bumper models are based on experiments conducted on cadaveric lower limbs in which the three-dimensional motions and resultant

joint subluxations were measured before and after ligament sectioning.

Figure 12–9 shows a type I motion pattern of the normal knee. An anterior drawer test may be performed to provide an anterior translation alone or combined with internal or external tibial rotation which would also be resisted by the lateral or medial bumpers respectively. In diagnosing abnormal knee laxities (Chart 12–1), we first perform an anterior drawer (Lachman) without rotation to test the central bumper represented by the anterior cruciate ligament. We then repeat the anterior drawer test first with internal and then with external tibial rotation to test for the maximum excursion of the lateral and medial tibiofemoral compartments. This provides added information on the laxity of the extra-articular ligamentous restraints.

In Figure 12–10, the anterior cruciate ligament was the only structure removed. This figure represents a knee with very tight medial and lateral extra-articular restraints that limit the amount of anterior translation of both tibiofemoral compartments (type II subluxations). The tight medial extra-articular restraints hold the center of rotation close to the medial aspect of the knee joint. The amount of central and lateral tibial

# TYPE II SUBLUXATION                    20° Flexion
## Tight Medial and Lateral Ligaments

### ACL TEAR

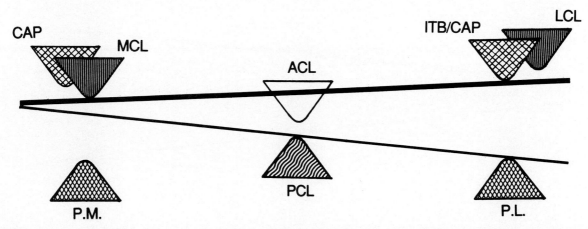

**Fig. 12–10**   In a type II subluxation there is an abnormal tightness (restraining function) of one or both compartments. This can be detected by palpating the amount of anterior excursion of the medial and lateral tibial plateau during the Lachman and flexion-rotation drawer tests. As indicated, the lesion involves the anterior cruciate ligament alone. The lower line represents the posterior limit of tibial excursion with a posterior drawer and external rotation; it is used as a reference line throughout (Figs. 12–9 and 12–11). The upper line represents the anterior limit of tibial excursion resisted by the appropriate ligament bumpers.

# TYPE III SUBLUXATION                   20° Flexion
## Average Looseness

### ACL TEAR

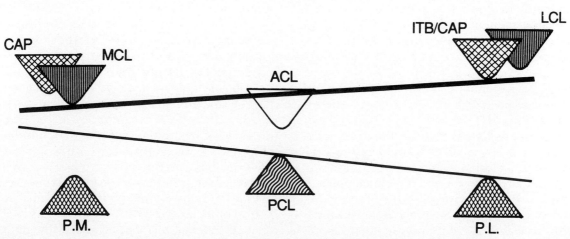

**Fig. 12–11**   Type III anterior subluxation. This is the usual finding after anterior cruciate disruption. The lateral extra-articular structures are physiologically lax between zero and 45 degrees of knee flexion, allowing for increased anterior translation of the lateral tibiofemoral compartment. The lesion involves laxity of both the anterior cruciate and lateral structures (iliotibial band, lateral capsule). The bumper model shows that the relative increase in medial compartment translation is actually greater than in the lateral compartment because the normal position for the medial tibial plateau is actually posteriorly positioned, resting on the posteromedial bumper.

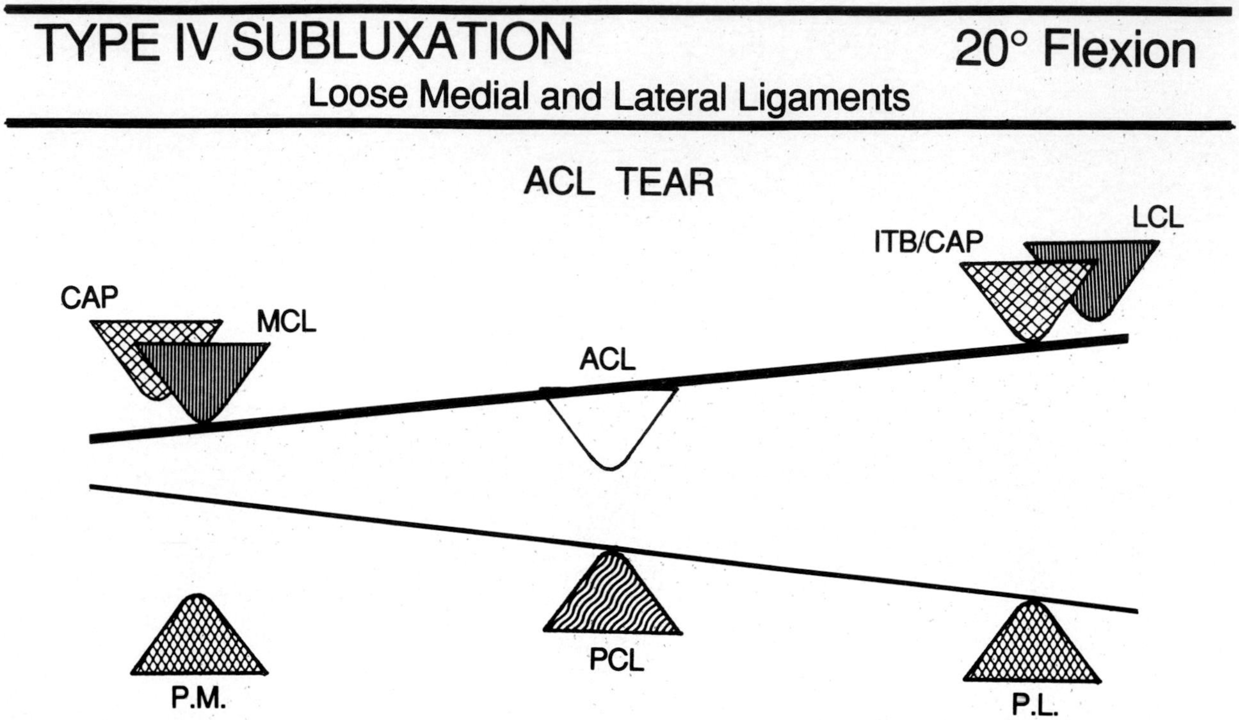

# TYPE IV SUBLUXATION
## Loose Medial and Lateral Ligaments
### 20° Flexion

**Fig. 12–12** Type IV anterior subluxation. There is associated laxity of both the medial and lateral extra-articular restraints. This allows for a gross subluxation of both the medial and lateral tibial plateaus easily palpable during the Lachman and flexion-rotation drawer tests.

translation is only slightly increased. The "bumper model" illustrates how the anterior restraints limit motion during the flexion-rotation drawer test, which allows the maximal anterior excursion of the medial and lateral tibiofemoral compartments. The results of the laxity tests are indicated on the diagnostic map (Chart 12–1) by first recording the amount of central subluxation and, secondly, the amount of the medial and lateral compartment subluxation when tibial rotation is added. The qualitative estimate for the pivot shift phenomenon is listed as a grade II. (See Table 12–1.)

Figure 12–10 presents the most common type of anterior subluxation which occurs after an anterior cruciate injury (type III subluxation). The center of rotation shifts medially far outside the knee joint, with a resultant increase in translation to both the medial and lateral compartments. The anterior subluxation of the lateral tibiofemoral compartment is the greatest. The qualitative estimate of the pivot shift test is grade III. The anatomic lesion includes the anterior cruciate ligament and the lateral extra-articular restraints, which are functionally loose since they do not limit the anterior subluxation of the lateral compartment. A qualification is in order. As previously discussed, the lateral extra-articular structures are physiologically loose at this knee flexion position.

The gross type of anterior subluxation (type IV) is shown in Figure 12–12. In this case, there is an increased translation and resultant subluxation to both the medial and lateral compartments; subsequently, the rotation axis shifts medially even farther outside the knee joint. The qualitative estimate of the pivot shift test is a grade IV, which indicates gross subluxation with impingement of the posterior aspect of the tibia against the femoral condyle. On the diagnostic map, we would record the associated functional damage of the medial extra-articular restraints, accounting for the amount of anterior subluxation of the medial compartment. A second-degree partial damage of the medial ligamentous structures is diagnosed. If there were a significant increase in medial tibiofemoral joint opening (one grade) under valgus stress testing, we would record a third-degree lesion of the medial structures.

The clinical significance of identifying these three types of anterior subluxations rests in their different natural histories and treatment programs.[13,16,25-27] The type II subluxation, characterized by tight extra-articular structures, has a better prognosis; the abnormal motion limits may not progress if no further giving-way episodes occur that damage the secondary restraints. The type III subluxation, which is the most common, has an anterior subluxation to the medial and lateral tibial compartments (greater to the lateral compartment because of associated increases in the internal rotation limits). For those patients with a functional disability, we recommend anterior cruciate reconstruction; we do not recommend a lateral extra-articular reconstruction alone or in combination with an intra-articular procedure. Although a lateral extra-articular procedure may limit anterior subluxation of the lateral compartment, it would not have any significant effect on the medial compartment.

In our clinical experience, a patient with a type IV anterior subluxation may experience frequent giving way with normal activities of daily living. The natural history in these knees is rather poor, as the patient has limited ability to compensate for this magnitude of anterior subluxation. Therefore, we advise patients that the knee joint is significantly at risk for future giving-way episodes, and we recommend, in acute knee injuries, that the patient consider an acute augmented repair of the anterior cruciate ligament. As well, we direct our attention to restoring associated damaged ligamentous structures, particularly the lateral extra-articular tissues. In the chronically unstable knee with similar anatomic defects, we commonly advise both an intra-articular and lateral extra-articular procedure given the gross anterior subluxation that exists. We believe this treatment approach is appropriate for these types of subluxations; however, careful long-term analysis is required. The point we wish to make is that reports of surgical results should define the types of anterior subluxation that were treated.

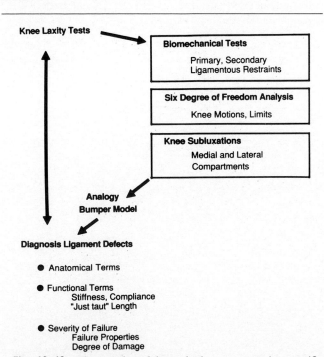

**Fig. 12–13** The results of knee laxity tests require specific biomechanical and kinematic principles (illustrated by the bumper model) for correct diagnosis of ligament defects. Ligament defects are further defined by anatomic, functional and severity categories.

## Summary

To interpret clinical laxity tests, the clinician must apply the kinematic and biomechanical concepts listed in Figure 12–13. These concepts have been briefly introduced here and are discussed in greater detail elsewhere.[7,11]

Figure 12–13 illustrates the importance of first selecting a laxity test to diagnose a specific ligament structure abnormality. The test selected, and the diagnostic information gained, is based on an understanding of the primary and secondary ligamentous restraints which are being tested. It is difficult to guess which ligaments are resisting specific joint displacements; therefore, biomechanical tests must first experimentally determine the restraints. Performing these tests obviates the first level of disagreement that existed when interpretations of clinical laxity tests were based only on "clinical impressions."

The results of the laxity tests must be understood and communicated in terms of the six degrees-of-freedom system that determines abnormalities in motion.

Resultant joint subluxations are readily understood by examining the medial and lateral tibiofemoral compartments separately. Our bumper model illustrates the different types of anterior subluxations that occur after anterior cruciate disruption.

The final diagnosis of a ligament defect must be made in precise anatomic terms. In cases of partial disruption, or after healing occurs, the clinician must analyze the remaining functional capacity of the ligaments. In the future, newer diagnostic machines will provide even more detailed information enabling clinicians to determine the different types of compartmental subluxations under defined loading conditions. These machines will also provide measurements of ligament and joint stiffness. In this way, the functional deficits of the individual ligaments, and the joint as a whole, can be more readily characterized. The concepts that we have presented here can be applied qualitatively by the clinician, and in the future, they can be quantitatively applied. Our goal is to provide the basic scientific and clinical principles upon which the diagnosis and classification of ligament injuries should be based.

## References

1. Hughston JC, Andrews JR, Cross MJ, et al: Classification of knee ligament instabilities: Part I. The medial compartment and cruciate ligaments. *J Bone Joint Surg* 1976;58A:159–172.
2. Hughston JC, Andrews JR, Cross MJ, et al: Classification of knee ligament instabilities: Part III. The medial compartment and cruciate ligaments. *J Bone Joint Surg* 1976;58A:173–179.
3. Muller W: *The Knee: Form, Function, and Ligament Reconstruction.* Berlin, Heidelberg, Springer–Verlag, 1982.
4. Nicholas JA: Lateral instability of the knee. *Orthop Rev* 1977;6:33–44.

5. Nicholas JA: Report of the committee on research and education. *Am J Sports Med* 1978;6:295–304.

6. Noyes FR, Grood ES, Suntay WJ, et al: The three dimensional laxity of the anterior cruciate deficient knee as determined by clinical laxity tests. *Iowa Orthop J* 1983;3:32–44.

7. Feagin JA (ed): *The Crucial Ligaments.* New York, Churchill Livingstone, 1986, chap 10.

8. Grood ES, Noyes FR, Butler DL, et al: Ligamentous and capsular restraints preventing straight medial and lateral laxity in intact human cadaver knees. *J Bone Joint Surg* 1981;63A:1257–1269.

9. Grood ES, Suntay WJ, Noyes FR, et al: Total motion measurement during knee laxity tests. *Transactions of the 25th Annual Meeting of the Orthopaedic Research Society.* Park Ridge, IL., Orthopaedic Research Society, 1979, p 80.

10. Grood ES, Suntay WJ: A joint coordinate system for the clinical description of three dimensional motions: Application to the knee. ASME Trans. *J Biomech Eng* 1983;105:136–144.

11. Feagin JA (ed): *The Crucial Ligaments.* New York, Churchill Livingstone, 1986, chap 9.

12. Suntay WJ, Grood ES, Hefzy MS, et al: Error analysis of a system for measuring three–dimensional motion. ASME Trans. *J Biomech Eng* 1983;105:127–135.

13. Noyes FR, McGinniss GH: Controversy about treatment of the knee with anterior cruciate laxity. *Clin Orthop* 1985;198:61–76.

14. Galway RD, Beaupre A, MacIntosh DL: Pivot shift: A clinical sign of anterior cruciate ligament insufficiency. *Clin Orthop* 1980;147:45–50.

15. Galway HR, MacIntosh DL: The lateral pivot shift: A symptom and sign of anterior cruciate ligament insufficiency. *J Bone Joint Surg* 1972;54B:763.

16. Noyes FR, Mooar PA, Matthews DS, et al: The symptomatic anterior cruciate deficient knee: Part I. The long–term functional disability in athletically active individuals. *J Bone Joint Surg* 1983;65A:154–162.

17. Butler DL, Noyes FR, Grood ES: Ligamentous restraints to anterior-posterior drawer in the human knee: A biomechanical study. *J Bone Joint Surg* 1980;62A:259–270.

18. Noyes FR, Grood ES, Butler DL, et al: Clinical biomechanics of the knee-ligament restraints and functional stability, in Funk FJ (ed): American Academy of Orthopaedic Surgeons *Symposium on the Athlete's Knee: Surgical Repair and Reconstruction.* St Louis, CV Mosby Co, 1980.

19. Torzilli PA, Greenberg RL, Insall J: An in-vivo biomechanical evaluation of anterior-posterior motion of the knee, roentgenographic measurement technique, stress machine, and stable population. *J Bone Joint Surg* 1981;63A:960–968.

20. Ellison A (ed): *Athletic Training and Sports Medicine.* Park Ridge, IL, American Academy of Orthopaedic Surgeons, 1984.

21. Noyes FR, Grood ES, Butler DL, et al: Clinical laxity tests and functional stability of the knee: Biomechanical concepts. *Clin Orthop* 1980;146:84–89.

22. Daniel DM, Malcom LL, Losse G, et al: Instrumented measurement of anterior laxity of the knee. *J Bone Joint Surg* 1985;67A:720–726.

23. Markolf KL, Mensch JS, Amstutz HC: Stiffness and laxity of the knee—the contributions of the supporting structures. *J Bone Joint Surg* 1976;58A:583–594.

24. Markolf KL, Graff–Radfor A, Amstutz HC: In vivo knee stability: A quantitative assessment using an instrumented clinical testing apparatus. *J Bone Joint Surg* 1978;60A:664–674.

25. Noyes FR, McGinniss GH, Mooar LA: Functional disability in the anterior cruciate insufficient knee syndrome: Review of knee rating systems and projected risk factors in determining treatment. *Sports Med* 1984;1:278–302.

26. Noyes FR, Butler DL, Paulos LE, et al: Intra-articular cruciate reconstruction: Part I. Perspectives on graft strength, vascularization and immediate motion after replacement. *Clin Orthop* 1983;712:71–77.

27. Noyes FR, Matthews DS, Mooar PA, et al: Symptomatic anterior cruciate deficient knee: Part II. The success of rehabilitation, activity modification and counseling in functional disability. *J Bone Joint Surg* 1983;65A:163–174.

## Acknowledgment

This work is supported in part by Grant AM 21172 from the National Institute of Arthritis, Diabetes, Digestive and Kidney Diseases and the Cincinnati Sportsmedicine and Orthopaedic Research and Educational Foundation.

# Decision-Making in Acute Anterior Cruciate Ligament Injury

Kenneth E. DeHaven, MD

## Introduction

Acute anterior cruciate ligament (ACL) tear should be suspected when a significant injury (usually a noncontact, cutting mechanism) is followed by immediate disability and the early onset of hemarthrosis. Physical examination will show hemarthrosis, usually a slight lack of full extension, and frequently posteromedial and/or posterolateral joint line tenderness. Of the clinical laxity tests for ACL integrity, the Lachman test is the most reliable in a conscious patient. The classic anterior drawer sign is not reliable under these circumstances, and the lateral pivot shift test requires relaxation that is seldom possible with acute pain and muscle guarding. If the injured extremity was bearing weight at the time of injury, significant associated lesions are also frequently present (meniscus tears in approximately 50% and chondral damage in 20%).

Examination with the patient under anesthesia and arthroscopy are needed to define the ACL laxity profile accurately, to determine whether the ACL tear is complete or partial, and to define significant associated lesions. Depending on the findings, some or all of the surgical treatment may also be carried out under arthroscopic control.

## Examination With the Patient Under Anesthesia

The author tabulated the laxity findings by anterior drawer, anteromedial rotatory instability, lateral pivot shift, and Lachman testing with and without anesthesia in 25 consecutive patients with complete acute ACL disruption[1] (Table 13–1). The anterior drawer sign was not helpful, being negative in 75% of the patients without anesthesia and in 40% with anesthesia. Anteromedial rotatory instability testing was negative in approximately 75% of the patients while awake and while anesthetized. The lateral pivot shift test was quite accurate in patients under anesthesia (although the results were negative in a few), but in 80% of the conscious patients, evaluation was not possible because of muscular guarding. The Lachman test was by far the most helpful, being 84% positive without anesthesia and 100% reliable with anesthesia. The author later encountered two cases in which the Lachman test remained negative under anesthesia despite complete ACL disruption. It

should also be emphasized that the Lachman test is frequently positive with partial ACL tears that do not require surgical treatment.

## Arthroscopy

Whether or not to perform arthroscopy in the presence of acute hemarthrosis requires careful deliberation. Arthroscopy is particularly hazardous for knees with major acute disruption of either collateral ligament along with cruciate disruption. Irrigation fluid will extravasate, causing the collateral ligament tissues to become edematous and difficult to dissect and repair. Massive extravasation causing neurovascular compression syndromes is also possible. If damage to the collateral ligament is sufficient to warrant surgical repair, it is the author's opinion that arthroscopy should not be performed, especially since adequate visualization of interior structures can be obtained through the surgical exposure for repair.

Hemarthrosis without collateral ligament disruption is an excellent indication for arthroscopy, however, and should be carried out with the patient under general or spinal anesthesia to permit adequate ligamentous examination. The use of a tourniquet should be avoided if at all possible because of the likelihood of subsequent open surgery. The hemarthrosis is initially washed out through the telescope

**Table 13–1**
**Clinical tests of ACL laxity in 25 consecutive patients with acute ACL tear**

| Test | Patient | | | |
|------|---------|---|---|---|
| | Conscious | | Anesthetized | |
| | No. | % | No. | % |
| Anterior drawer | | | | |
| Positive | 6 | 24 | 15 | 60 |
| Negative | 19 | 76 | 10 | 40 |
| Anteromedial rotary | | | | |
| Positive | 7 | 28 | 7 | 28 |
| Negative | 18 | 72 | 18 | 72 |
| Lateral pivot-shift | | | | |
| Positive | 4 | 16 | 21 | 84 |
| Negative | 21 | 84 | 4 | 16 |
| Lachman | | | | |
| Positive | 21 | 84 | 25 | 100 |
| Negative | 4 | 16 | 0 | 0 |

sleeve, and a 4- to 5-mm diagnostic telescope utilized. The best view is usually obtained by a constant-flow irrigation system with inflow through the arthroscope sleeve and outflow in the suprapatellar pouch. Arthroscopic pumps are useful to allow a constant distention pressure while maintaining the necessary constant-flow irrigation. Routine probing of the menisci and cruciate ligaments is important, as well as posterior visualization (usually advisable for the medial compartment, but rarely necessary for the lateral compartment).

Several series have documented the lesions encountered in acute knee injury with hemarthrosis.[1-5] The author found that of 145 consecutive patients 105 (73%) had anterior cruciate ligament tears. Two thirds of the complete ACL tears were associated with meniscus tears while an additional 17 patients (12%) had partial ACL tears with more than 50% of the ligament remaining intact. In the remaining 40 cases (27%) of acute hemarthrosis without ACL injury, the author found bucket-handle meniscus tears in 14%, osteochondral fractures in 6%, posterior cruciate ligament tears in 2%, and no significant internal derangement in 5%.

This series also documented a relatively high incidence of lateral compared with medial meniscus tears in conjunction with acute ACL injury (57% lateral and 43% medial). These meniscus lesions are frequently peripheral and amenable to repair. Noyes and associates[5] found an incidence of associated chondral damage of approximately 20% in acute ACL disruption.

## Selection Factors

The key to management of acute ACL injury is deciding whether to use surgical or nonsurgical treatment. Some have advocated initial nonsurgical treatment of all acute ACL tears, citing the widely quoted work of McDaniel and Dameron,[6] which indicated that 75% of patients do well without surgical intervention. They advocated letting patients "experience their disability" and operating only when subsequent functional instability proves it necessary. Theirs was an unselected series, however, and high-risk populations can be identified who do not routinely do well with nonsurgical treatment. More recent studies by Mariani and associates,[7] Hawkins and associates,[8] and Clancy and associates[9] have documented 60% to 85% fair or poor results with nonsurgical management of such high-risk patients. Further, instability episodes while the patients are "experiencing their disability" can cause additional damage to menisci, secondary restraints, and articular surfaces, all of which can compromise the result of delayed surgical treatment. In addition, any opportunity for primary ACL repair (with augmentation) would be lost. Thus, it is just as wrong to say that none of these patients need immediate surgical treatment as it is to say that they all do.

The major factors to be considered before recommending surgical or nonsurgical treatment are age, level of demand, type and extent of associated lesions, degree of laxity, and various individual patient factors. None of these factors, taken by itself, should dictate whether surgical or nonsurgical treatment is more appropriate. Even when all factors are considered together, the relative importance of each has not been definitively established.

In general, the younger the patient (teens to early 20s) the greater the tendency for surgical treatment since these patients tend to be physically active, whereas persons more than 40 years old tend to put less stress on their knees and should do well with nonsurgical treatment. But age is a relative factor and not all teenagers need surgery (some place low demands on their knees), and some individuals more than 40 years old should be considered for surgical treatment if they regularly place high demands on their knees. The approach to those in their 20s and 30s must also be individualized.

Jackson[10] showed that "isolated" ACL tears (especially partial lesions) have a better prognosis than those with associated meniscal and/or chondral lesions. In this author's opinion high-risk patients with complete ACL disruption should be considered surgical candidates even if the acute laxity is minimal. An older patient with low demands but severe laxity is also high-risk. Important individual factors to consider include the patient's motivation and commitment to do what is necessary to obtain a good result from surgical treatment. In addition, the economic realities of family and occupational commitments may make surgical treatment unfeasible for some high-risk patients. Other psychosocial factors can also be of pivotal importance in electing surgical or nonsurgical treatment in individual cases.

The typical high-risk profile shows a younger patient who intends to place high demands on the knee, who has associated meniscal tears, regardless of the degree of laxity, and favorable psychosocial factors. The typical lower-risk profile is that of an older patient who puts low to modest demands on the knee, has minimal associated lesions, mild to moderate laxity, or unfavorable psychosocial factors. It should be emphasized, however, that severe laxity and/or multiple associated lesions can change an otherwise lower-risk patient to a high-risk one.

## General Approach

The general principles are to recommend immediate surgical treatment of the ACL for high-risk patients and nonsurgical treatment of the ACL in lower-risk individuals. Nonsurgical treatment is also recommended for partial ACL tears with more than 50% of the ligament intact in both high-risk and lower-risk individuals. Although most would agree that the patient and family should participate in the decision-making process, meaningful discussion is difficult if not impossible when the diagnosis remains in doubt until after arthroscopy and examination with the patient under anesthesia. Fortunately, the reliability of the Lachman test without anesthesia makes it possible in most instances to arrive at an appropriate treatment decision before operating.

When treating a patient who has an acute hemarthrosis and a positive Lachman test, the important points to remember are that the ACL is torn (but that it is not known whether the tear is complete or partial) and that a meniscus tear is also probable. In a patient who has an acute hemarthrosis but a negative Lachman test, an ACL tear is still possible (in approximately 15% the Lachman test is negative until the patient is examined under anesthesia). Other possibilities include a meniscus tear without ACL tear, osteochondral fracture, or even a posterior cruciate ligament tear.

If the patient has a high-risk profile, the recommended initial approach is examination with the patient under anesthesia, arthroscopy, and surgical treatment whether or not the Lachman test is positive or negative without anesthesia, whether or not the pivot shift test is positive or negative under anesthesia, and whether or not there is an associated meniscal tear.

If the patient has a lower-risk profile, there are two basic approaches. The first is to proceed with examination under anesthesia, arthroscopy, and any necessary meniscus surgery followed by nonsurgical treatment of the ACL. The alternative approach is to begin initial nonsurgical treatment for the ACL injury, followed by possible delayed arthroscopy and meniscus surgery if warranted by continuing problems. Good arguments can be made for each of these approaches and the author uses both. Both approaches may require delayed stabilization if functional instability proves to be a problem.

## Nonsurgical Treatment

If the acute ACL injury is being treated nonsurgically, the knee must function on the basis of the integrity of the secondary ligamentous restraints and dynamic compensation provided by the thigh musculature. Accordingly, the principles of nonsurgical management are to protect the healing secondary restraints and then to carry out a rehabilitation program to maximize dynamic compensation. The author applies a hinged splint with limited motion from 30 to 90 degrees for six weeks, followed by a rehabilitation program similar in concept to that for surgical patients. Quadriceps progressive resistance exercises (PRE) are limited to the arc from 90 degrees to 45 degrees for the first three to four months, while hamstring and hip abductor PRE are also stressed. Quadriceps PRE are performed into full extension (after four months) before the knee is considered to be completely rehabilitated. A protective brace is advised for strenuous activities to help prevent reinjury. Adherence to these selection and treatment guidelines will produce good to excellent results from nonsurgical treatment in 80% to 90% of patients in the lower-risk group. It must be emphasized that nonsurgical treatment does not mean no treatment.

## Summary

Acute surgical treatment is generally recommended for patients in the high-risk category. The relative frequency of surgical compared with nonsurgical treatment in any individual practice setting depends on the patient population and can vary widely from one practice to another even though overall indications may be quite similar.

## References

1. DeHaven KE: Evaluation of the acutely injured knee, in Casscells SW (ed): *Arthroscopy: Diagnostic and Surgical Practice.* Philadelphia, Lea and Febiger, 1984, pp 64–71.
2. DeHaven KE: Diagnosis of acute knee injuries with hemarthrosis. *Am J Sports Med* 1980;8:9.
3. Eriksson E: Sports injuries of the knee ligaments: Their diagnosis, treatment, rehabilitation and prevention. *Med Sci Sports* 1976;8:133.
4. Gillquist J, Hagberg G, Oretorp N: Arthroscopy in acute injuries of the knee joint. *Acta Orthop Scand* 1977;48:190.
5. Noyes FR, Bassett RW, Grood ES, et al: Arthroscopy in acute traumatic hemarthrosis of the knee. *J Bone Joint Surg* 1980;62A:687–695.
6. McDaniel WJ Jr, Dameron TB Jr: Untreated ruptures of the anterior cruciate ligament: A follow-up study. *J Bone Joint Surg* 1980;62A:696–705.
7. Mariani PP, Puddu G, Ferretti A: Hemarthrosis treated by aspiration and casting: How to condemn the knee. *Am J Sports Med* 1982;10:343–345.
8. Hawkins R, Misamore G, Merritt T: Acute nonoperated isolated anterior cruciate ligament tear. *Am J Sports Med* 1986;14:205–210.
9. Clancy W, Ray J, Zoltan D: Acute third degree anterior cruciate ligament injury: A prospective study of conservative nonoperative treatment and operative treatment with repair and patellar tendon augmentation. Presented at the Fourth Congress of the International Society of the Knee, Salzburg, Austria, 1985.
10. Jackson R: Anterior cruciate ligament injuries, in Casscells SW (ed): *Arthroscopy: Diagnostic and Surgical Practice.* Philadelphia, Lea and Febiger, 1984, pp 52–63.

# Neuromuscular Disease and Deformities

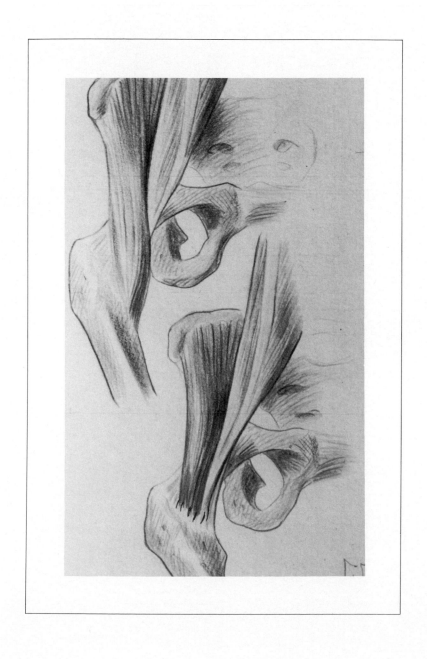

# Surgical Reconstruction of the Upper Extremity in Cerebral Palsy

J. Leonard Goldner, MD

## Introduction

The brain lesion causing alterations of the upper extremity in patients with cerebral palsy is part of a static encephalopathy. The extremity deformity may become more severe during epiphyseal development and extremity growth. Also, aging has the same effect on the primary brain lesion as it has on any nervous tissue.

The goal in managing a patient with neuromuscular dysfunction is to identify the extent and site of the cerebral lesion, establish a baseline of muscle strength and coordination, determine the sensibility pattern of the hand, and attempt to prevent progressive deformity by early night splinting and subsequent surgical treatment. Functional activity is encouraged as the child grows and daytime splinting is avoided if it interferes with sensibility and function.[1-3]

Surgical treatment should assist in maintaining the strength of the muscle-tendon unit, elongate it sufficiently to prevent contracture but maintain function, obtain a balanced grasp and release, and provide reasonable pronation and supination of the forearm. Adequate elbow and shoulder function should be either maintained or obtained.[4-7]

## Anatomic-Pathologic-Neurophysiologic Changes

The brain lesion may result from hypoxia associated with prematurity, trauma during the delivery process, or other conditions causing ischemia. As infant mortality decreases, the incidence of cerebral palsy may increase. The surviving premature infant with a developmental genetic brain syndrome may have permanently altered brain function and extremity deformity.

### Clinical Signs of a Brain Lesion

The clinical signs include (1) hyperreflexia of the biceps, triceps, and brachioradialis muscles; (2) a stretch reflex, which is initiated by rapid flexion and extension movement of the fingers, hand, or forearm; and (3) clonus, which is stimulated by limited stretch of the muscle-tendon unit, resulting in repetitive persistent involuntary movement. The severity of clonus ranges from minimal to continuous or maximal involuntary activity.

## Classification of Cerebral Palsy

The patient's brain lesion and extremity movement provide the basis for classifying the pattern of abnormal neuromuscular function as spastic; athetoid; ataxic; or mixed. Each of these major abnormal functional patterns may be mild, moderate, or severe, and the number of extremities involved is also specified.

Other conditions referred to as tension athetoid, tremor, dystonia, and shudder are manifestations of brain lesions of different locations and severity.[8-10]

The abnormal functional pattern displayed by the patient determines the ultimate prognosis, and particularly surgical decisions. For example, an extremity with pure spasticity will respond after surgical treatment in a more predictable and reliable way than will an extremity affected by spasticity and tension athetosis. In the latter, the preliminary assessment is more difficult, and the results of tendon lengthening and tendon transfers are less reliable.[10]

## Extremity Evaluation (Joint, Muscle, Sensibility)

### General Examination

Initially, the examiner should gain the patient's confidence. The child is encouraged to handle blocks, pick up play objects, manipulate plastic containers or items of clothing, and to perform activities of daily living while the examiner casually observes. If the involvement is primarily one-sided, then the examiner gives play objects to the patient's good hand and requests that the object be placed in the involved hand. In this way, the speed of manipulation of objects, the effectiveness of grasp and release of the involved extremity, and voluntary muscle control are observed.[9,10]

### Contracture Determination

A dynamic or static deformity is detected by the examiner manipulating the extremity. In a dynamic deformity the contracture is caused by spasticity rather than by muscle shortening or joint alteration.

A static contracture is detected by extending or flexing the affected segment of the extremity and determining contracture of the joint capsule or the muscle-tendon unit, which does not correct either with local or general anesthesia. The deformity is fixed. The different kinds of contracture are described as flexion or extension or a combination of both.

**Flexion Contracture**  A dynamic contracture of the flexor digitorum superficialis is detected by the examiner, who holds the patient's hand in maximum extension, the metacarpophalangeal joint in extension, and then extends the proximal interphalangeal joint as much as possible. This position is recorded, the wrist is then placed in neutral position, the metacarpophalangeal joint in neutral position and the interphalangeal joints are extended as much as possible. A dynamic contracture allows complete correction of the interphalangeal joint, whereas a static contracture results in an uncorrectable degree of flexion deformity. The examiner must change the position of the joints of the extremity in order to perform an accurate test.[7,10]

**Extension Contracture**  Muscles and tendons on the extensor surface of the forearm, hand, arm, and shoulder are occasionally contracted. The examiner can determine the difference between static and dynamic deformity by manipulating the involved joints of the extremity and by testing the tension of the muscle-tendon unit of the extensor muscles involved. For example, if the wrist is in full flexion position, the examiner applies tension to the digits and attempts to flex the digits at the metacarpophalangeal joints. If flexion will not occur, then the extensor muscles are contracted. If flexion occurs to 90 degrees, there is little or no contracture.

### Sensory Assessment

The brain lesion causing a pathologic state in cerebral palsy frequently spares epicritic sensation (sharp point determination, and recognition of heat and cold). Recognition of size and shape (stereognosis) is usually diminished and sometimes absent. Adequate stereognosis provides a better prognosis following surgical reconstruction, than if there is diminished stereognosis. However, the latter is not a contraindication to reconstructive surgery. As the patient becomes older, eye-hand coordination is recognized as a valuable means of improving function.[2]

### Patterns of Upper Extremity Deformity

Prior to instituting a surgical program, the surgeon must analyze the existing pattern of the involved upper extremity and formulate a plan. Specific subgroups of patterns have been arbitrarily designated, based on the author's experience. A review of the deformity in 100 consecutive patients showed the following patterns:

In the flexion-pronation pattern (70%), the wrist is flexed, the forearm is pronated, and the thumb is in the palm. The fingers are partially flexed. The degree of deformity varies according to the severity of the spasticity, the age of the patient, and the degree of fixed contractures. The elbow is usually flexed when the patient is walking and moving but may be in a neutral position when the patient is at rest. The shoulder is usually internally rotated and slightly abducted.

A pattern of dorsiflexion of the hand, thumb-in-palm, and pronation of the forearm occurred in 10% of the patients. The wrist extensor muscles are more active than the wrist flexor muscles. Fingers are flexed and the thumb is in the palm. Forearm pronation occurs more frequently than supination. Grasp is performed more quickly than release. The dorsiflexed position slows release.

Forearm supination, hand dorsiflexion, and ulnar deviation occurred in 5% of the patients.

The wrist in neutral position, thumb in the palm intermittently, and moderate dynamic tightness of the finger flexors occurred in 10% of the patients. Grasp and release are performed without difficulty. The wrist is elevated most effectively by a combination of wrist muscle extension and active finger flexion.

In severe flexion deformity of the wrist, flexion of the fingers, and thumb-in-palm (5%), there is digit extension only when the wrist is in full flexion. When the wrist is entended, the fingers are acutely flexed in the palm. There is no active extension of the wrist or of the fingers or thumb.

### Summary of Hand Patterns Correlated With Voluntary Grasp and Release

When the wrist is in acute flexion, the fingers are moderately flexed and the thumb is in the palm. Because of the acute flexion of the wrist, the tension on the finger and thumb extensors is sufficient to diminish the degree of flexion of the digits. As the fingers are actively flexed, the hand automatically elevates, and the subtle strength of the extensor muscles of the wrist and fingers becomes evident.

When there is wrist extension, finger flexion, and thumb-in-palm, the patient's ability to release the digits is limited because of the inherent tension of the flexor muscles on the fingers. The greater the degree of wrist extension, the slower is the speed and range of finger extension.

With the wrist in extension, the forearm in supination, and ulnar deviation of the hand, the fingers are flexed and the thumb is in the palm. In this position, the action of gravity aggravates the dorsiflexed position of the hand which, in turn, leads to a flexed position of all of the digits.

These different positions associated with particular hand patterns influenced significantly the decisions concerning surgical reconstruction.[7,9,10]

## Operative and Nonoperative Goals of Correction of the Hand, Wrist, and Forearm

The thumb is brought out of the palm by releasing the contractures. Also, extension of the metacarpal is improved, the digit is stabilized at the metacarpophalangeal joint, and active flexion of the intrinsics and the flexor pollicis longus, as well as extension of the extensor pollicis longus and abductor muscles is maintained.

Thumb extension is improved by transferring an additional motor to the extensor pollicis longus, plicating and strengthening the abductor pollicis longus, and by diminishing overflow or contracture of the wrist or finger flexors.

Wrist extension is best augmented by a tendon transfer to the extensor carpi radialis brevis. However, excessive transfers will cause a fixed dorsiflexion contracture because of the subtle unrecognized strength of the stretched wrist extensor muscles that automatically become more active as the flexors are weakened and the tendon transfer is performed.[4,8]

An equilibrium of flexion and extension depends on preoperative assessment of the potential strength of the wrist extensors and avoidance of excessive transfers to the extensors. Also, the persistent capability of wrist flexion requires voluntary strength of the wrist and finger flexors and the benefit of gravity when the hand is in the pronated position.

Active forearm supination is usually improved by either release or transfer of the pronator radii teres muscle, and by reinforcement of supination with an active transfer of a flexor muscle to a wrist extensor. If the pronation deformity is severe enough to warrant release of the pronator, then transfer of the pronator through the interosseous space, transfer of a wrist flexor around the ulnar border to the extensor carpi radialis brevis, and release of the pronator quadratus muscle are also indicated. This muscle may be spastic or contracted and active supination will be improved if the pronator quadratus is weakened.

Occasionally, a rotational osteotomy of the radius or the ulna or both may be necessary to stabilize the forearm and hand in a position of maximum function. The position of pronation should not be sacrificed completely, because it is essential for grasp and release, and in the activities of daily living is consistently more important than is supination.

## Goals of Treatment of the Elbow and Shoulder

### Elbow

A flexion deformity of the elbow may be either dynamic or static. The method of surgical treatment depends on the principal category of the patient's deformity and on muscle strength. A dynamic flexed position of the elbow joint can be diminished by tendon lengthening and muscle belly recession. The operation is performed during or prior to rapid growth spurts or when a mild deformity has progressed to one that is moderate or severe.

A static deformity can be corrected at any age, and the earlier the correction the less severe the deformity. The extent of the correction should be limited so that strong active forearm flexion is possible even after this treatment.[10]

### Shoulder

An internal rotation-adduction deformity of the humerus is treated by diminishing the deformity and improving active external rotation of the humerus and glenohumeral abduction and flexion. Soft-tissue releases and limited tendon transfers are usually sufficient to allow this improvement.

Traumatic arthritis of the shoulder joint occasionally develops after long periods of contracture and involuntary glenohumeral motion. A total joint replacement has been used infrequently to diminish pain and maintain reasonable range of motion.

## Major Neuropathologic Concepts That Affect Surgical Procedures

### Stretch Reflex

A stretch reflex will occur if the extremity is moved repetitively by the examiner and if the flexor or extensor muscles have inherent spasticity. This dynamic spasticity is classified as minimal, mild, moderate, or severe. It correlates with hyperactive reflexes and clonus. These characteristics affect the tension on a muscle-tendon transfer and also limit voluntary control. Tendon lengthening will diminish overflow and improve voluntary muscle function.

### Athetosis

Athetosis influences surgical decisions and results. If primary athetosis exists, tendon lengthening alone will produce a less predictable result than if spasticity alone is the major pathologic characteristic. Tendon transfers are less reliable if the muscles are affected by moderate or severe athetosis. When athetosis is mild, however, tendon transfers are reasonably reliable to reinforce demonstrable weakness. For example, a fixed dorsiflexion contracture of the hand is more likely to occur if a strong wrist flexor is transferred to a presumed weak wrist extensor affected by moderate to severe athetoid movement. Muscle testing is important prior to tendon transfers in the athetoid patient, but the result of testing is less reliable than in the patient with spasticity alone. The testing, however, is important for decision-making.

### Ataxia and Its Effect on Surgical Decisions

Grasp and release are potentially possible but

manipulation may be difficult if the extremity is affected by ataxic movements. Reconstructive procedures are of limited success but may be helpful to provide an assistive hand or a hand into which objects can be passed voluntarily. Also, osteotomies and arthrodesis may provide stability and improved grasp and release.[7,10]

## Manual Muscle Testing

The surgeon must have information about individual muscles and groups of muscles prior to making plans for surgical reconstruction of the upper extremity. Although manual muscle testing is not as accurate for cerebral palsy patients as it is for those with peripheral nerve or spinal cord anterior horn lesions, it does provide important information about the individual muscle-tendon unit and gives the surgeon data helpful in predicting the probable results of tendon lengthening, muscle recession, or tendon transfer.

The surgeon who understands the concepts of muscle testing should perform the test regularly, recording the results, and then reaffirming the results at another time. Furthermore, the surgeon should cooperate with the therapist involved so that both can become expert in determining voluntary and involuntary activity and in assessing muscle function without depending on electromyography. Electromyography is most helpful in determining out-of-phase activity but not necessarily in determining muscle strength.

## Information Essential for Planning a Surgical Reconstruction of the Upper Extremity

The age of the patient and pattern of coordination, cooperation, and ability to communicate are useful data. Certain procedures, such as tendon lengthening, can be done at any age and do not require any specific postoperative cooperation other than reasonable discipline.

How well the patient can voluntarily or involuntarily manage a particular muscle or group of muscles is also important.

The surgeon must recognize the effect of joint movement, such as movement of the wrist and finger joints, and extremity position such as that of the shoulder and elbow on muscle-tendon excursion and contracture.

The surgeon must determine whether or not there are voluntary or involuntary contractions of a muscle belly as the digits or wrist are flexed or extended. These muscle stretch responses are described as tenodesis effects, but they may be accompanied by involuntary contraction of a spastic muscle or voluntary contraction of a wrist extensor as the fingers are flexed.

The surgeon should attempt to estimate the strength and resistance of active muscles during a voluntary contraction of an individual muscle or group of muscles and rate these strength maneuvers as normal (5/100%); good (4/80%); fair (3/50%); poor (2/20%), and zero.

The severity of a stretch reflex or an overflow from a particular muscle group should be graded as minimal (1), mild (2), moderate (3), severe (4), or very severe (5).[7,9,10]

## Muscle Physiology and Function Before and After Tendon Lengthening or Transfer

### Phase Activity

Individual muscles contract during their major activity and relax after performing their designated action. Action potentials are not present during the resting phase. However, if a muscle belly fires both during active phase and resting phase, it is not ideal for transfer. This information is obtained by clinical examination and by electromyographic study if the clinical information is not clear. A muscle belly anesthetic block may be helpful in providing this information.

A stretch reflex is determined by repetitive passive extension or flexion of the arm, forearm, and hand. The stretch reflex is classified, as it does affect the accuracy of muscle testing. Muscle testing for strength and assessment of a stretch reflex are tests performed prior to tendon transfers. A muscle with a mild stretch reflex may be transferred safely, whereas one with a severe stretch reflex may cause a reverse deformity. Tendon lengthening, however, is safely performed even in the muscle with a severe stretch reflex, whereas muscle-tendon transfer is not as accurate if the stretch reflex is severe.

### Synergism Associated With Tendon Transfer

The wrist extensors and finger flexors act synergistically to strengthen grasp. The wrist flexors and finger extensors contract simultaneously to improve release. Surgical reconstruction should maintain active wrist motion in both flexion and extension if this is possible, so that synergism will be enhanced. Overactive dorsal extensor tendon transfers will diminish finger release and overactive wrist flexors with weak extensors of the wrist will diminish finger closure. A balanced degree of wrist motion and the appropriate tendon transfers to the extensor tendons of the fingers and flexor tendons of the hand will enhance grasp and release.

### Antagonistic Muscles

Antagonistic muscles affect the decision to perform tendon transfers. Weak hand extension, for example, may be due to weakness of the wrist extensors because of a cortical pathologic lesion; or absent or limited response of the extensor muscles caused by overactivity of the wrist or finger flexors. A muscle belly local anesthetic injection aids in making a differential diagnosis of the cause of an apparent weak muscle action. If the extensors appear to be weak, then the anesthetic is injected into the flexor muscle mass. This is more accurate from a functional standpoint than is peripheral nerve block.

### Combined Muscle Action Pathology and Its Management

Isometric contracture, muscle spasticity, and muscle weakness caused by a cerebral cortical lesion may all co-exist. All three elements are treated by (1) precise lengthening of the flexor pollicis longus tendon at the wrist, if that particular muscle belly is involved; and (2) tendon transfer to the lengthened flexor pollicis longus by the brachioradialis or the flexor digitorum superficialis directly after the lengthening. This concept of tendon lengthening and muscle-tendon reinforcement provides a successful muscle-tendon excursion and function and makes the difference between success and failure after treating an apparent flexion contracture of the flexor pollicis longus.

### How To Determine Contractures of the Upper-Extremity Muscles and Joints

The examiner slowly moves the involved joint and its muscle-tendon unit to a position of maximum extension and flexion in order to determine if a static contracture is present. If a static contracture exists, the affected part of the extremity cannot be moved through a full range of motion when the joint is in the position of maximum extension or flexion. The difference between static and dynamic contracture depends on the ultimate range of joint motion in the positions of maximum flexion or extension.[7,10]

### Sensibility of the Hand

Most patients with cerebral palsy usually recognize the sensations of sharp, dull, heat, and cold. Stereognosis, however, is usually not physiologic. If the patient does have good recognition of the size and shape of objects while not looking at these objects, then the prognosis for final functional improvement is better than if there is astereognosis. A rapid test is performed when the examiner asks the patient to place the arms overhead, to close the eyes, and to describe individual objects that the examiner places initially in the involved hand and then, for comparison, in the uninvolved hand. Both large and small objects are used and the patient's response to the characteristics of these objects is recorded.[2]

### Analysis of the Examination and Formation of a Surgical Plan

Patient deficiencies in performing activities of daily living and in doing specific functions are determined by the patient and the family and are recorded. Also, the desired goals of both the patient and the family, and the expectations of both are recorded. The surgeon must impress the family with the realization that the end result will not necessarily approach normal, although it may improve function of the extremity. A description should be given relative to benefits that occur if the thumb is out of the palm, if the finger flexors are less tight, and if grasp and release are performed more rapidly and wrist extension is improved once the overactive flexors are lengthened and the weak extensors are reinforced.

The surgeon should describe to the patient and the family the changes that will follow if pronation and supination are altered, and if flexion deformity of the elbow is diminished. Emphasis is placed on undercorrection rather than overcorrection, and on the fact that the situation will not be worsened and that the pattern of function will likely be improved.

The surgeon must emphasize the following: (1) a normal extremity will not be obtained; (2) fine coordination is usually not improved; (3) sensibility will not be altered in any way; (4) some aspects of overactivity will continue, although the absolute degree may be diminished; and (5) the degree of athetosis will not necessarily be altered, nor will dystonia be eliminated, although the parts affected by the central lesions will be less deformed.

### Timing and Selection of Surgical Procedures

#### Age of the Patient

The severity of a static contracture or a persistent overflow deformity in a 3-year-old becomes worse as the child becomes older. Bone growth aggravates deformity. Static contractures and dynamic overflow require surgical treatment in the younger patient if there is evidence of progression. Stretching does not benefit either of these conditions, but night splinting is helpful in maintaining a state of equilibrium.

An old static contracture may be diminished by tendon lengthening, and function may be improved by both tendon lengthening and tendon transfer.

These concepts apply not only to children but also to adults.

Longitudinal growth of the extremity aggravates existing deformities and may require a second operation if the original procedure is performed when the patient is about 4 years old. That particular age is reasonable for tendon lengthening or tendon transfers if the other prerequisites have been defined and analyzed. The severity of deformity does increase during childhood, and, for this reason, relatively early correction of static contracture or dynamic overflow is desirable.

Night splinting and active assistive play therapy are helpful in conditioning the patient to two-handed activity. Night splinting with plaster, acrylic, or Orthoplast splints does result in elongation of collagen and diminishes the rapidity of recurrent contracture or the development of a primary contracture.

### Timing of Surgical Treatment

Early surgical treatment is desirable. Age 4 is an appropriate age for treatment of a static deformity. Delayed surgical treatment may also be successful. Surgical treatment should not be delayed, however, because of concern about the child's ability to cooperate or to perform a specific exercise program. In patients this age, muscle strengthening and coordination occur during play, with parental supervision, and with occasional guidance from the surgeon and reinforcement from the therapist. Long periods of therapy and stretching have not proven to be beneficial.

### Effectiveness of Tendon Lengthening

Surgical tendon lengthening followed by night splinting until growth is completed may prevent recurrence of deformity or at least minimize recurrence. In lieu of tendon lengthening, active stretching alone during waking hours is usually ineffective in providing elongation of collagen or in changing dynamic overflow.

### Tendon Transfers Performed in Early Childhood

A tendon transfer of the extensor carpi ulnaris to the extensor carpi radialis brevis or to the extensor digitorum communis is usually satisfactory for strengthening the digits or the entire hand and seldom causes a secondary deformity.

Tendon transfer of the extensor carpi ulnaris from the base of the fifth metacarpal to the base of the fourth or to the tendon insertion of the extensor carpi radialis brevis at the base of the third improves elevation of the wrist, diminishes ulnar deviation, and usually causes no secondary deformities.

### Transfer of a Major Wrist Flexor Tendon to Extensor Tendons

The risk involved in transferring a major flexor tendon to an extensor tendon is relatively great. The result of transferring the flexor carpi ulnaris tendon, for example, to a wrist extensor is less predictable than if a flexor digitorum superficialis is transferred. An extension deformity may result if the potential strength of the extensor muscles is greater than expected once the flexion deformity has been diminished. Thus, overcorrection should be avoided if possible, and slight undercorrection accepted, as grasp and release are easier with undercorrection than with overcorrection.

### Tendon Lengthening Versus Tendon Transfer

The decision to transfer a flexor tendon to an extensor muscle, or an extensor tendon to a flexor muscle of the forearm, depends on the original pattern of deformity. A voluntarily strong, moderately spastic flexor muscle, which fires only in the flexion phase of action, may be safely transferred to a weak extensor tendon-muscle unit. This alteration in muscle balance will improve both grasp and release by diminishing the flexion power and by increasing wrist extension and finger flexion.

An alternative to tendon transfer is tendon lengthening of an overactive wrist flexor muscle-tendon unit. This alternative is adopted if, as the patient grips an object, the wrist extensor tendons are palpable and react voluntarily in that position, even though the patient is not easily able to contract the extensors when the wrist is in flexion. The extensors are not controlled voluntarily because of overactivity of the flexors. Flexor tendon lengthening results in stronger extensor muscle action if the potential for increased strength of the extensors exists.

The overactive spastic flexor muscle, if lengthened, usually requires reinforcement by an adjacent active motor muscle. This combination of procedures is most frequently performed on the flexor pollicis longus. The tendon is lengthened a controlled amount at the wrist, and it is then reinforced with the adjacent brachioradialis, which was transferred to the musculotendinous junction of the flexor pollicis longus.

Extensor muscle strength has an effect on balancing the flexor muscles of the wrist and fingers. If extensor muscles are weak (20%, or 1/5), and either voluntary or involuntary action is present, the extensor muscles are either lengthened or shortened, but in either instance reinforcement is performed.

If the extensor muscles are fair (50%, or 2.5/5), the options are to reinforce the extensor muscles by transferring an extensor motor to the fair extensor muscle; or to transfer strong flexor muscles to the weaker extensor muscles.

Specific flexor muscles can be lengthened in order to strengthen indirectly the weaker extensor muscles.

Once the flexors are weakened by lengthening, the potential strength of the extensors becomes evident.

The extensor muscles can be shortened and reinforced with either a strong flexor or extensor muscle.

If the extensor muscles are of normal strength, then a strong extensor muscle can be transferred to a weakened flexor muscle.[6–8,10]

## Multiple Consecutive Surgical Procedures Performed Under One Anesthetic

Performing multiple consecutive surgical procedures under one anesthetic aims to diminish or eliminate flexion deformity of the wrist, thumb, and fingers in a uniform way that treats both deformities simultaneously; and to enhance strength and excursion of potentially strong extensor muscles and maintain wrist mobility in order to enhance a tenodesis action while improving voluntary strength of both the flexor and the extensor muscles.

The goal is to produce a balanced, voluntary grasp and release with the thumb out of the palm and with sufficient strength in the digits to grasp an object with the hand in dorsiflexion. In this position, the hand should function voluntarily so that the patient is able to release an object relatively quickly.

The set of contracted muscles affecting the thumb should be corrected simultaneously in order to obtain a reasonable balance between thumb flexion and extension and thereby maintain the thumb out of the palm. Weak extensors should be reinforced; strong flexors should be lengthened or transferred; the thumb should be maintained out of the palm, and finger flexors and extensors should function uniformly.

All deformities should be altered at the first surgical operation. Secondary procedures may be necessary, but these occur because of incomplete correction at the time of the primary operation; or as planned second procedures. For example, joint stabilization, additional untreated soft-tissue problems, or problems developed after the first group of procedures are managed during the subsequent surgical effort at balancing the hand and attempting to obtain a reasonable grasp and release.[10]

## Muscle Tension: Strength After Tendon Transfer or Lengthening

The length of a muscle-tendon unit after tendon lengthening or transfer affects the final strength of the individual muscle, because the muscle fibers are stretched which, in turn, increases the contracting force of the muscle (Blix's curve). Excessive muscle fiber tension will diminish excursion and decrease both strength and function. Insufficient muscle ten-

sion will not only limit excursion, but will also weaken muscle contractions. Thus, if muscle fibers are either overstretched or overlengthened, they are weakened.

### Transfer of the Flexor Carpi Ulnaris Tendon to the Extensor Carpi Radialis Brevis

This transfer is indicated if the wrist extensor muscles are weak and if the flexor muscles are strong and active during their contracting phase. Excursion of the flexor carpi ulnaris is tested by gentle traction, measured, and recorded; this information determines the placement of the flexor tendon into the extensor carpi radialis brevis tendon under the proper tension, proper point of attachment, and appropriate direction. For example, an excursion of 4.0 cm in the flexor carpi ulnaris is reduced to 2.4 cm (60% of the original excursion), with the wrist held at neutral position. This increased tension on the transferred tendon is maintained while the tendon is attached to the recipient tendon, which is held in a taut condition by applying proximal traction on the tendon. Excessive tension (4.0 cm—100% of original excursion) on the transferred flexor carpi ulnaris and attachment of the flexor carpi ulnaris to the recipient extensor tendon with the wrist held in dorsiflexion will result in excessive tension on both the recipient and the donor tendons and a subsequent wrist extension deformity.

The amount of spasticity of the flexor carpi ulnaris and its action during both the contracting and the resting phase are important. If the flexor carpi ulnaris is firing frequently and excessively in both the contracting and resting phases, adjustment of the tension on the muscle-tendon unit in its new position is critical, so that excessive stress on the extensor carpi radialis brevis will be avoided after the transfer. If the transferred muscle is contracting both during the resting and the active phase, overcorrection will tend to occur if the strength of the original recipient muscle is greater than was evident preoperatively. Release of the flexor carpi ulnaris may allow increased strength to occur in the recipient extensor carpi radialis brevis. This factor should be determined preoperatively by palpation and by testing flexion grasp. If the extensor carpi radialis longus and brevis muscles are palpated and observed during strong flexion grasp, their inherent strength will become apparent.

There are three factors which, if considered, will usually prevent extension contracture after transfer of the flexor carpi ulnaris to the extensor carpi radialis brevis.

First, the surgeon must recognize the double phase activity of the muscle to be transferred and avoid placing this muscle too tightly in its new position.

The inherent strength of the presumably weak extensor carpi radialis brevis must also be recognized.

This muscle may actually be stronger than suspected and, if that is the case, then the transferred flexor carpi ulnaris should not be inserted into the extensor carpi radialis brevis but, rather, into the extensor digitorum communis if that muscle is weak; or the weaker muscles, such as the flexor digitorum superficialis or one half of the extensor carpi ulnaris, should be used for reinforcement.

Finally, one active muscle should remain on the volar aspect of the wrist. Thus, the flexor carpi radialis and the flexor carpi ulnaris should not both be transferred.

The flexor carpi ulnaris should be considered as the last transfer to the wrist extensor muscles, rather than as the initial transfer. Preoperative muscle belly Xylocaine injections, careful testing of grasp and release, and detection of subtle unrecognized strength in the wrist extensor muscles are critical steps in making these decisions.

### Transfer of the Flexor Digitorum Superficialis Muscle-Tendon Unit to the Extensor Pollicis Longus

The flexor digitorum superficialis of the ring finger is tested and found to have normal strength. The tendon is detached through a palmar wrist-lower forearm incision after tension is applied, so that adequate length is obtained. Release of the tendon from the proximal crease of the involved digit is unnecessary. Sixty percent of the excursion of the flexor digitorum superficialis is then measured by manual traction and documented with a millimeter rule. The extensor pollicis longus is isolated through a separate incision on the dorsum of the hand, and the flexor digitorum superficialis is passed subcutaneously under the dorsal veins and cutaneous nerves and is inserted into the extensor pollicis longus by a buttonhole technique. With the wrist in neutral position, the thumb should be held in abduction 2 cm away from the second metacarpal, extension at 1 cm below the second metacarpal head, and the distal phalanx of the thumb extended 10 degrees. When the hand is extended passively, the thumb will deviate toward the radial aspect of the tip of the index finger; or, to a position where the thumb is opposite the side of the index finger for key pinch. When the hand is flexed, the thumb moves away from the index finger about 4 cm, so that an object can be placed between thumb and hand, or thumb and index by slight flexion of the wrist.

### Other Factors Affecting Muscle-Tendon Tension During and After Transfer

After the tourniquet is released, blood volume in the muscles increases and muscle tension increases moderately.

Skin closure compresses the muscle-tendon unit and increases tension on the transferred muscle-tendon.

The resting tension of the thumb, in its new position after tendon transfer has been completed, should be 20% greater than it is when the digit is in the anatomic position. This modest increase of tension should be present after each tendon transfer.

### Reliability and Predictability of Upper-Extremity Reconstructive Procedures

At the present time there is no consensus concerning the success of tendon transfers in the upper extremity affected by cerebral palsy. However, in over 100 patients with documented static encephalopathy who have been treated and followed for at least ten years by the author, the evidence documents that tendon transfers are generally successful; that tendon lengthenings are valid; and that combining several procedures during the same anesthetic session has produced reliable and predictable results.

Other items that have been observed and documented as useful are as follows:

Manual muscle testing of the upper and lower extremities, which is relatively accurate. The preoperative strength of particular muscles prior to transfer can be assessed and the strength of those muscles postoperatively can be predicted.

Electromyography, which is helpful in certain instances, but not essential. Electromyography is a teaching device. It does provide information about in-phase and out-of-phase muscle activity that may be difficult to detect by clinical examination alone. However, the deficiencies of electromyography require that all aspects of clinical examination be used prior to determining muscles to be transferred, those to be lengthened, and the combinations of each of these procedures.

Simultaneous consecutive multiple operative procedures, which have been questioned and challenged because end results have been difficult to assess. However, if the procedures are coordinated, and if the goal is directed toward improving grasp, release, maintaining wrist motion, and keeping the thumb out of the palm, then simultaneous consecutive procedures performed during one operative session are justified and usually successful.

Elongation of the muscle-tendon unit, which may be performed distally through the tendon or proximally at the muscle belly. The efficacy and accuracy of muscle origin release compared with distal tendon lengthening is cause for disagreement. Preoperative accurate assessment of the individual muscles, degree of stretch reflex, the severity of contracture, the proprioceptive and protopathic status, and the patient's willingness to participate in developing grasp and release are all important in obtaining improvement after multiple tendon transfers.

## Special Considerations

### Wrist Mobility

Wrist mobility should be maintained. The mobile wrist augments thumb and finger extension while wrist flexion is occurring, and the movable wrist also strengthens thumb and finger flexion as wrist extension is performed. Arthrodesis of the radial, carpal, and second and third metacarpal joints is avoided until tendon transfers have been completed and the effort has been made to maintain wrist mobility so that grasp and release are augmented by wrist motion. Arthrodesis is indicated if these attempts to strengthen the extensor muscles with tendon transfers and to maintain adequate strength in grasp are insufficient to allow the patient to hold objects of moderate weight in either a neutral or dorsiflexed position of the hand. If grasp and release are possible, but wrist extensor strength is weak, and if no other muscles are available to strengthen wrist extension, then wrist arthrodesis is considered.

### Selection of Muscle Motors for Transfer

Individual muscles with minimal strength are reinforced if their action is essential in providing function of the entire hand or individual digits. Flexor muscles, if transferred, will function as extensors of the hand or fingers; extensor muscles after transfer will contract voluntarily as flexor motors. Also, the extensor muscles will actively reinforce adjacent weakened extensors, and strong flexor muscles will reinforce adjacent weakened wrist or finger flexors.

A tenodesis action is useful to provide thumb or finger extension or to prevent complete wrist flexion. Extensor tenodesis is more commonly used than flexor tenodesis in stabilizing the cerebral palsy hand.

The brachioradialis or the pronator radii teres muscles may be transferred to either the extensor muscles or to the flexor muscles, depending on the area of greatest need. These muscles function in-phase for both the flexors or extensors, just as do the other muscles of the forearm and hand. However, the most useful and most successful combinations are those of flexors to extensors or extensors to flexors.

### Tenodesis as an Adjunct to Tendon Transfers

A tenodesis action is inherent in all tendon transfers whether the primary motor is active or passive. The myostatic contraction of an active motor is active or passive. The myostatic contraction of an active motor persists after its tendon is transferred, but a passive motor or one that is paralyzed and trans-

ferred will always stretch. For this reason, only the tendon and not the muscle of a passive or paralyzed muscle should be used for tenodesis. The muscle is separated at the junction with the tendon, and the proximal cut end of the tendon is inserted into bone through two drill holes and sutured to itself under maximum tension.

This technique is useful in order to anchor the distal tendon of the extensor carpi radialis longus into the radius to prevent or limit wrist flexion; also, the extensor pollicis longus tendon is anchored into the radius through two drill holes to decrease the thumb-in-palm deformity. Another tenodesis helpful in maintaining finger extension is to anchor the extensor digitorum communis tendons into the distal radius to diminish active or passive flexion of the metacarpophalangeal joints. In each of these instances, the insertion is not disturbed but the tendon at the level of the musculotendinous junction is identified, isolated, and inserted into bone with the digit or hand in the appropriate tight position.

### Elbow Flexor Muscle Belly or Aponeurosis Release Compared With Tendon Lengthening Distal to the Musculotendinous Junction

The proximal muscle belly is released from both the humerus and ulna in order to diminish elbow contracture. Release of the origin of these wrist muscles and the pronator radii teres will allow additional straightening of the elbow joint. However, contracted thumb and/or finger flexor muscles are best lengthened in a controlled way by performing tendon lengthening at the wrist. In this way, over-lengthening is avoided.

**Technique** The suture lines are staggered at the wrist and lower forearm; the guideline for lengthening these muscle-tendon units is 0.5 mm per degree of desired correction. The estimate of proposed correction is made preoperatively and includes a static contracture determination as well as the observed dynamic overflow.

The elbow flexor muscle origins are released if flexion contracture has increased at the elbow joint as extremity growth has occurred. Also, the origin of the pronator radii teres is elevated from the humerus and the ulna if a combined pronation deformity and elbow contracture co-exists. Pronation deformity alone is usually managed by detaching the insertion of the pronator radii teres after which this insertion is either transferred into the extensor carpi radialis longus or brevis tendon or recessed to the periosteum of the radius. The tendon is either attached directly to the radius or to the dorsum of the radius after the tendon has been passed through the interosseous space. In the latter position, the pronator will function as a partial supinator.

### Selection of Patients for Surgical Reconstruction

Those patients with progressive deformity of the elbow, forearm, or hand, regardless of their age, mental status, or number of extremities involved, should be considered for selective surgical procedures. A preoperative trial of splinting and strengthening will usually indicate the limited benefit to be expected from this kind of treatment, and surgical procedures are then more readily considered. The patient should be reasonably cooperative, with evidence of positive motivation. The expectations regarding end results are limited.

Patients with satisfactory protopathic sensibility have a better prognosis than those with astereognosis, proprioceptive deficiency, and a general limitation of sensitivity. Most patients respond to a pinpoint stimulation and thermal changes, but a large number of these patients have limited ability to recognize size and shape of objects. Furthermore, low intellectual function or less than average ability to cooperate in performing activities of daily living are *not* contraindications to surgical reconstruction. However, the prognosis for gross and fine coordination does diminish as the quality of communication and intelligence is lessened, and if motivation is low.

### Muscle Belly Injection

**Peripheral Nerve Blockade** A peripheral nerve blockade paralyzes the entire muscle and provides information about strength of the overactive muscles if they are functioning against a paralyzed muscle. The entire muscle action may be weakened and give spurious data concerning the effect of the muscle weakening that will occur by tendon lengthening. The muscle belly injection with local anesthetic, however, weakens the muscle strength moderately and provides more appropriate information about the action and balance than might be expected by elongating one muscle or group of muscles and thereby allowing stronger action of the opposite muscle group or the antagonist muscles. Injection of these spastic flexor muscles provides information about potential strength of the extensor muscles after the flexors are weakened. The anesthetic injection also gives quantitative information about the unopposed action of the antagonistic extensor muscles, and the effect of the less active agonist flexor muscles on the original deformity. This alteration of muscle activity provides a temporary model but resembles a postoperative situation after the flexor tendons are lengthened.

**Myoneural Junction Injection With 45% Alcohol** This myoneural block weakens the muscle belly for approximately eight weeks after the injection. During this time, the antagonistic muscles affected by the injection demonstrate their strength. For example, if the forearm flexor muscle mass (agonist) is injected with 45% alcohol as described, a baseline of strength of the partially opposed extensor muscles (antagonist) is defined so that management of the flexor muscles and tendons is then planned by either tendon lengthening or transfer or a combination of both procedures.[10]

### Communication Among Physician, Patient, and Family

The patient's ability to learn, perceptual deficiencies, visual defects, and basic intelligence all affect prognosis. Therefore, these factors should be discussed by the physician, family, patient (if possible), and other members of the health care team. Also, the patient's social development, degree of cooperation, and extent of motivation are important in establishing the postoperative program.

Long hours of occupational and physical therapy away from home are not necessary either before or after surgery. A program is established for home exercise, and activity is planned and worked out with a therapist preoperatively. Postoperatively, the emphasis is on grasp and release and on play therapy supervised by the physician and the therapist on a monthly basis after the initial program is planned and accepted by the patient and the family.

Parental expectations should be verbalized preoperatively; the surgeon should modify these, if necessary, before the operation. This requires a detailed explanation of the surgical procedures, a description of the possible preoperative results, and the functional changes that may occur as time passes.

The surgeon must emphasize that the extremity will never be normal, that comparison with the opposite uninvolved extremity is not a guideline for success of the surgical procedures, and that secondary operations are frequently needed in order to complete what was attempted during the first multiple-stage procedure. Cosmetic alterations, the size and length of the incisions, the location of the incisions, and the time necessary for wearing splints are important items that should be explained on more than one occasion to alleviate anxiety of both the patient and the family.

### Recurrent Deformity or Incomplete Correction

These situations are dependent on the age of the patient at the time of the operation, the rate of bone growth after the operation, the use of night splints, and the severity of the original static and spastic deformities. For example, if there is a strong element of athetosis, then predictability of soft-tissue transfers is limited and the accuracy of the prediction is very low.

There is no logical reason to delay surgical procedures until the patient reaches maturity once the indications for these procedures are evident. Deformities worsen as rapid growth occurs, and contractures become more rigid in childhood and adolescence.

### Delay of Surgical Reconstruction

Delaying surgery until maturity is not desirable, but is not necessarily detrimental to relearning or to coordination. Surgical reconstruction of the upper extremity performed at age 16 will improve function in most instances. However, the extent and magnitude of the procedure will be considerably greater when the patient is older than if the initial operations were performed when the patient was 5 years old. If the hand and forearm are balanced when the child is young, this adjustment will provide increased performance, will improve the child's awareness of the extremity, and will improve the usefulness of the extremity during childhood and adulthood.

### Useful and Predictable Surgical Procedures for Upper Extremity Reconstruction

The choice of operative procedures selected for reconstruction of an upper extremity affected by cerebral palsy depends on the pattern of hand and forearm deformities, on muscle strength, on static and dynamic contractures, and on the anatomic balance of the hand and forearm.

The anatomic considerations to be included in any analysis of an upper extremity problem are (1) the strength, voluntary control, and spasticity of the extensor and flexor muscles of the forearm and hand. This consideration includes range of motion and strength of the digit/finger extension and flexion; forearm pronation and supination (active or passive positions); wrist extension and wrist flexion (voluntary or involuntary). (2) Elbow flexion and extension and severity of the deformity. (3) Shoulder abduction-adduction-rotation-overhead elevation.

### Categories of Surgical Procedures

The various surgical procedures selected to realign and correct deformity of the upper extremity in cerebral palsy include tendon lengthening, tendon transfer in order to reinforce weak muscles, release of joint contracture, realignment of muscle tendon direction, capsulodesis, and joint arthrodesis.

Multiple simultaneous procedures are planned according to the anatomic region involved, the topographic area of either flexor or extensor surfaces, and the individual digits or anatomic parts affected. Simultaneous multiple surgical procedures are reliable, predictable, biomechanically sound, and will improve function.

### General Concepts of Management

The general concepts of management of the upper extremity are included in Tables 14–1 through 14–3. These tables summarize information as it relates to indications for certain surgical procedures; the grading of different deformities of the thumb, fingers, wrist, and elbow; and the expected results of specific surgical procedures. Techniques are arranged with individual surgical procedures, but these procedures usually overlap and are done during the same anesthetic session. Results, therefore, require special information and both functional and clinical analysis in order to determine which procedure resulted not only in anatomic improvement but also improvement in clinical function.

### Clinical Cases

To illustrate some of the general concepts presented in Tables 14–1 through 14–3, several clinical cases will be presented.

Figure 14–1 shows the upper extremity of a 16-year-old patient with hemiplegia who has been managed successfully by splinting and stretching in attempts to control the spastic deformities involving the elbow, wrist, fingers, and thumb. Spasticity, however, did not and will not respond to stretching. Attempts at voluntary strengthening of extensor muscles overstretched by spastic flexor muscles usually result in a continuous imbalance. Weak or paralyzed extensor muscles require reinforcement or else agonist flexor muscles will continue to cause overaction and flexion deformity.

The plan of treatment for this patient included the following multiple simultaneous procedures: release of elbow contracture; lengthening of spastic wrist and digit flexors; reinforcement of muscles to the thumb,

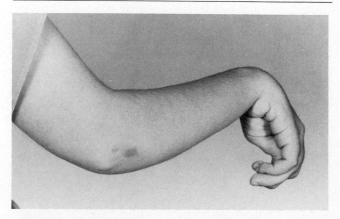

**Fig. 14–1** Upper extremity of a 16-year-old patient with hemiplegia.

**Table 14–1**
**Classification and treatment of muscles with pathologic actions in the upper extremity**

| Abnormal Muscle Characteristics | Treatment |
| --- | --- |
| Class 1a: flexor muscles | Local anesthetic block; tendon lengthening; tendon transfer to extensors or to reinforce flexors |
| Wrist | Lengthen specific flexor muscles (flexor carpi ulnaris, flexor carpi radialis, palmaris longus) |
| Thumb | Controlled lengthening; or lengthening and transfer reinforcement (brachioradialis, flexor digitorum superficialis |
| Finger | Lengthen and/or reinforce flexor digitorum superficialis and/or flexor digitorum profundus) |
| Class 1b: extensor muscles (weak) | Reinforce muscles by transfer or strengthen the extensor muscles indirectly by lengthening the overactive flexors |
| Wrist | Lengthen wrist flexor tendons if contracted or if muscle is hyperactive (palmaris longus, flexor carpi ulnaris, flexor carpi radialis) |
| Fingers/thumb | Reinforce the elongated weakened muscles (extensor digitorum communis, extensor indicis proprius, extensor digiti quinti, extensor pollicis longus, abductor pollicis longus; as indicated, transfer flexor digitorum superficialis, flexor carpi radialis, flexor carpi ulnaris, pronator radii teres |
| Class 2a: flexor muscles (overactive) | Lengthen specific flexor muscles |
| Wrist | Lengthen flexor carpi radialis, flexor carpi ulnaris, palmaris longus |
| Thumb | Lengthen flexor pollicis longus and reinforce with brachioradialis or flexor digitorum superficialis; plicate and/or reinforce abductor pollicis longus |
| Fingers | Lengthen and/or transfer if contracted or if there is overactive dynamic function; transfer specific flexor muscles (e.g., flexor digitorum superficialis) and/or lengthen flexor digitorum profundus) |
| Class 2b: extensor muscles with fair (50%) strength | Reinforce extensor muscles with flexors; lengthen flexor muscles of wrist or digits to strengthen extensor muscles indirectly |
| Thumb | Extensor pollicis longus reinforced with flexor digitorum superficialis, brachioradialis, or palmaris longus |
| Abductor pollicis longus | Plicate and reinforce with brachioradialis, flexor digitorum superficialis, or extensor indicis proprius |
| Class 3a: flexor muscles (overactive) | Lengthen flexor carpi radialis, flexor carpi ulnaris, palmaris longus, flexor digitorum superficialis, flexor digitorum profundus, and pronator radii teres |
| Extensor muscles (normal strength) | Extensors (extensor carpi radialis longus to flexor pollicis longus or flexor digitorum profundus); or flexor carpi radialis or flexor carpi ulnaris |

\* Information obtained by clinical examination including observing the patient's functional capabilities, testing and recording individual muscles as accurately as possible, determining the sensibility of the palmar surface of the hand, grading the degree of spasticity, athetosis, or overall type of cerebral palsy, and determining a method of management and the general principles that control the final treatment.

Note that the flexor muscles are all overactive in varying degrees, and the extensor muscles vary from weak wrist, fingers, and thumb in class 2, in which the flexors are overactive and the extensors have 50% of their normal strength, and class 3, in which the flexors are overactive and the extensors have normal strength.

**Fig. 14–2**  Postoperative position of the thumb and wrist (A) and wrist and fingers (B) after simultaneous multiple procedures.

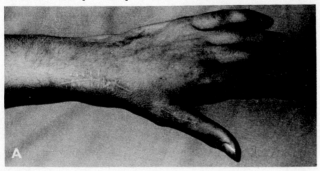
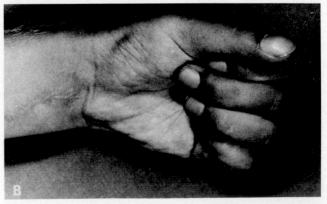

wrist and fingers; arthrodesis of the metacarpophalangeal joint of the thumb; release of excessive forearm pronation.

Figure 14–2, A and B shows the postoperative position of the wrist, thumb, and fingers after simultaneous multiple procedures: arthrodesis of the metacarpophalangeal joint of the thumb; lengthening of the flexor pollicis longus and reinforcement with the brachioradialis; plication of the abductor pollicis longus and extensor pollicis brevis (1 cm); rerouting of the extensor pollicis longus and formation of a new pulley for that tendon; transfer of the pronator radii teres to the extensor carpi radialis brevis; transfer of the extensor carpi ulnaris to the base of the fourth metacarpal. Persistent wrist motion, in flexion and extension, allows thumb and finger extensor reinforcement by both the tenodesis effect and by voluntary motion.

Figure 14–3 illustrates that postoperatively grasp was performed without the thumb in palm. The flexor pollicis longus had been lengthened and reinforced with the brachioradialis; the adductor pollicis was released from the proximal phalanx and transferred to the annular ligament of the thumb. The first dorsal interosseous muscle belly was released from the first and second metacarpals proximally and allowed to recede distally. The abductor pollicis longus tendons were plicated. After this procedure, the fingers flexed voluntarily, and in the position of flexion assisted in elevation of the wrist. The digits also extended slowly as wrist flexion was performed.

Figure 14–4 shows the hand of a 12-year-old patient who demonstrated true grasp and release postoperatively, but the action was slow, deliberate, and affected by overflow. When he performed alone or with family members, his grasp and release were

**Table 14–2**
**Classification and treatment of thumb-in-palm deformity in cerebral palsy**

| Anatomic Part | Treatment Alternatives |
|---|---|
| Extrinsic muscle/tendon | Reinforce extensors and lengthen or lengthen and reinforce flexors |
|   Extensor pollicis longus | Reroute radially; reinforce with flexor digitorum superficialis or brachioradialis; new annular ligament |
|   Extensor pollicis brevis | Shorten and reinforce |
|   Abductor pollicis longus | Shorten or shorten and reinforce |
|   Flexor pollicis longus | Lengthen or lengthen and reinforce; tenodesis to radius |
| Intrinsic muscle | |
|   Adductor pollicis (static or dynamic) | Recess or lengthen; local transfer to sesamoid or metacarpal neck, dorsal web incision |
|   First dorsal interosseous, two heads | Recess from first and second metacarpals; maintain nerve and blood supply |
|   Abductor pollicis brevis | Recess from origin if spastic; reinforce with palmaris longus or flexor digitorum superficialis |
|   Flexor pollicis brevis (two heads deep; differentiate from flexor pollicis longus) | Release insertion through web incision; preoperative muscle block to differentiate one intrinsic from another if spasticity is severe |
| Joints (stability) | |
|   Metacarpophalangeal (thumb) | Arthrodesis if flexion beyond 45 degrees or if hyperextension is severe; capsulodesis if hyperextension is pathologic; arthrodesis if capsulodesis fails or if spasticity is moderate to severe; arthrodesis needed if flexion deformity is the major problem; lengthen and/or reinforce flexor pollicis; extensor plication for flexion deformity if other problems are not severe |
|   Interphalangeal joints | |
|     Flexed | Lengthen flexor digitorum superficialis or flexor digitorum longus; extensor tenodesis for hyperflexed position |
|     Hyperextended | Tongue-in-groove lengthening of combined extensor-intrinsic tendons (intrinsics and common extensor) of middle phalanx (least complex way to treat hyperextension of proximal interphalangeal joint) |
|   Severe hyperextension of proximal interphalangeal joint | Flexor tenodesis for severe deformity; capsulodesis, retinaculum and one-half flexor digitorum superficialis tenodesis; tongue-in-groove; arthrodesis if severe and cartilage damage has occurred or if contracture does not correct with soft-tissue release |
| Class 4* (combined procedures) | |
|   Extrinsic muscles | Reroute and reinforce; lengthen if contracted |
|   Intrinsic muscles | Recess (release and reattach); supplement by muscle strengthening; capsulodesis; arthrodesis |

* Flexor and extensor procedures may be performed during the same operation. Balance is achieved by lengthening contracted muscles and reinforcing weakened elongated muscles. The metacarpophalangeal and the interphalangeal joints are stabilized by tenodesis, capsulodesis, or arthrodesis if necessary.

**Table 14–3**
**Classification of thumb deformities in cerebral palsy***

| Anatomic Part | Comments |
|---|---|
| Metacarpophalangeal joint | Hyperflexed, extended, or neutral |
| Flexor pollicis longus | Active strength with static contracture; weakness with contracture; neutral |
| Interossei | Spastic or contracted, causing a tight thumb web; mild or severe flexion deformity of metacarpophalangeal joint, hyperextension of the interphalangeal joint caused by intrinsic spasticity or contracture |
| Adductor pollicis | If spastic or contracted, may cause narrowing of the thumb web, hyperflexion of the metacarpophalangeal joint, ulnar rotation of the thumb, and limited thumb extension when wrist is flexed; deformity can be mild, moderate, or severe, with varying degrees of spasticity and contracture |
| Extensor pollicis longus | Elongated and weak or spastic, causing contracture of the first metacarpal toward the second metacarpal; the web space is consequently narrow; the muscle belly may be strong, weak, or 50% of normal |
| Abductor pollicus longus-extensor pollicis brevis | This muscle-tendon unit is usually elongated with fair strength; strength must be determined by clinical testing and by defining the effect of the action on the first metacarpal |
| Palmar intrinsic muscles of thumb | Abductor pollicis brevis and flexor pollicis brevis may show fair or good strength but may be spastic, maintaining first metacarpal and proximal phalanx of the thumb in the palm |
| Skin contracture | Occurs in very old deformities, but in the author's experience, only about 10% of the thumbs treated have required z-plasty and/or skin grafting |

* This classification is based on anatomic alterations and degree of severity. Each anatomic element is tested, described, documented while function is attempted, and graded for severity. This requires an assessment of the anatomic-pathologic condition of the involved areas of the thumb complex.

both helpful and satisfactory. However, when he was in the doctor's office or working with a new therapist, the overflow affected his reaction time and diminished the speed of grasp and release.

The surgical procedures completed were as follows: (1) lengthening of the flexor carpi radialis and flexor carpi ulnaris; (2) transfer of the flexor digitorum superficialis ring finger to the extensor pollicis longus, for which a new pulley was formed from the retinaculum. The flexor superficialis was passed under the abductor prior to suturing the flexor to the extensor; (3) arthrodesis of the metacarpophalangeal joint of the thumb; (4) transfer of the flexor digitorum superficialis of the long finger through the interosseous space to extensor carpi radialis brevis. Grasp and pinch were improved both in speed and strength.

Figure 14–5 shows the hand of a 10-year-old child with spastic hemiparesis. Prior operative procedures were fusion of the metacarpophalangeal joint of the thumb, plication of the abductor pollicis longus, release of the adductor insertion, and origin and reattachment of the adductor insertion to the annular ligament. However, because of persistent overaction of the flexor pollicis longus, continued weakness of the abductor pollicis longus and extensor pollicis longus, the metacarpal rolled palmarward, and the thumb could not be controlled during flexion.

The plan of treatment was to weaken the thumb flexors and reinforce the extensors and abductor pollicis longus in order to control position of the thumb as the wrist was flexed and extended.

Note the incision in the thumb web through which the following procedures were accomplished: (1) recession of the insertion of adductor to the annular ligament of the thumb; (2) release of the origin of the adductor pollicis from the third metacarpal; (3) recession of the first dorsal interosseous from the first and second metacarpals; (4) plication of the abductor pollicis longus; (5) arthrodesis of the metacarpophalangeal joint of the thumb.

Figure 14–6 shows this same patient postoperatively. After the thumb has been reinforced and the flexor pollicis longus lengthened, the thumb abducts and extends when the wrist is flexed. Sufficient strength remains to allow use of the thumb in both grasp and pinch activities.

As shown in Figure 14–7, when full flexion was performed postoperatively, the thumb and fingers moved away from the palm and provided a wide surface for the patient to grasp large objects. Smaller objects were managed by less wrist flexion and by control of thumb and finger motion so that excessive abduction and extension were avoided.

Figure 14–8 illustrates that the patient's control of grasp and release was voluntary and strong. The

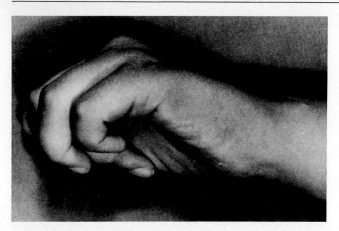

**Fig. 14–3**   Postoperative grasp without the thumb in palm.

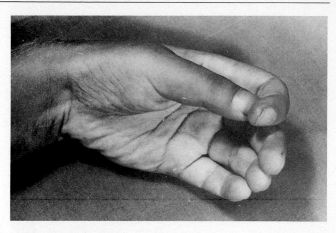

**Fig. 14–4**   True grasp and release performed postoperatively by a 12-year-old patient.

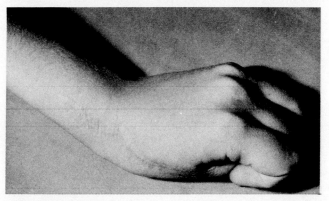

**Fig. 14–5**   The hand of a 10-year-old child with spastic hemiparesis, preoperative position.

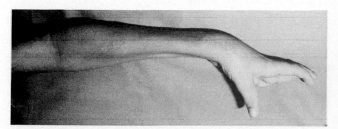

**Fig. 14–6**   The same patient postoperatively after thumb reinforcement and lengthening of flexor pollicis longus.

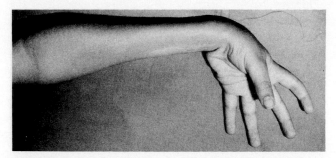

**Fig. 14–7**   This same patient postoperatively with full flexion being performed.

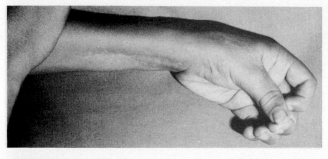

**Fig. 14–8**   The same patient with voluntary, strong grasp and release.

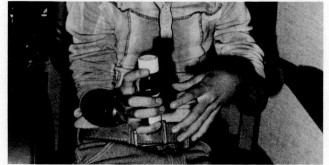

**Fig. 14–9**   Active flexion and ulnar deviation of the wrist in this patient.

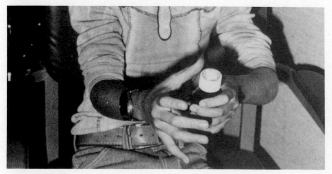

**Fig. 14–10**   The object in Fig. 14–9 has been passed from the right hand to the left hand.

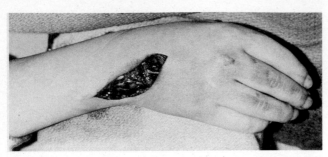

**Fig. 14–11**  Surgical exposure for secondary transfer of the extensor carpi ulnaris to the extensor carpi radialis brevis.

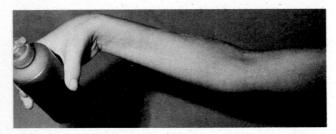

**Fig. 14–12**  Postoperative position of the hand, demonstrating how the patient receives or grasps a large object.

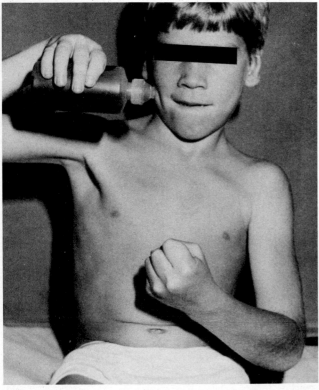

**Fig. 14–13**  Postoperative function of the right extremity after multiple tendon transfers and lengthenings.

thumb was out of the palm when grasp was performed slowly. As the fingers were voluntarily flexed, the wrist extensors were contracting actively and grip was strong. The thumb remained out of the palm if the fingers assumed a position of flexion before the thumb flexed. Occasionally, however, the thumb moved into the palm before the fingers were flexed.

Analysis of the deformity resulted in a plan of treatment that would lengthen the flexor pollicis longus and reinforce it with the brachioradialis; lengthen the flexor digitorum superficialis of the long and ring fingers; transfer the pronator radii teres to the extensor carpi radialis brevis through the interosseous space to improve both supination of the forearm and dorsiflexion of the hand; transfer one half of the extensor carpi ulnaris to the extensor carpi radialis brevis.

Figure 14–9 shows the patient able to flex the wrist actively and to deviate it to the ulnar side; perform a release of the thumb and fingers; and prepare the left hand for receiving an object from the uninvolved right hand. In Figure 14–10, the object has been passed from the right hand to the left hand. The thumb and fingers are flexed, grasp is performed, and the object is held firmly while the wrist is dorsiflexed. This position provided maximum strength. Release is possible by flexing the wrist and contracting the abductor-extensor tendon complex of the thumb and extensor digitorum communis of the fingers. At the same time, the wrist extensors are relaxed and wrist flexors are contracted.

Figure 14–11 illustrates the surgical exposure for secondary transfer of the extensor carpi ulnaris to the extensor carpi radialis brevis. One half of the extensor carpi ulnaris tendon remains attached to the fifth metacarpal. This segment is sutured proximally to the annular ligament to prevent excessive radial deviation. The proximal muscle-tendon unit is routed subcutaneously and woven into the extensor carpi radialis brevis. With the hand in neutral position, the tendon is sutured at 60% of its measured excursion.

Figure 14–12 shows the postoperative position of the hand, demonstrating how the patient receives or grasps a large object. The voluntary wrist flexion method of acquiring an object is relatively easy. Voluntary finger and thumb flexion results in wrist elevation and improved strength and endurance. When release is necessary, the patient flexes the wrist rather than initiating finger extension.

The several incisions used for lengthening and transferring the wrist flexors, arthrodesis of the thumb, release of the thumb web contracture, reinforcement and realignment of the wrist and finger extensors, and release of the elbow contracture are hardly visible and have faded. Subcuticular sutures or skin tapes or both would eliminate the objectionable cross-hatching that occurs when multiple incisions are closed with wide horizontal sutures.

Figure 14–13 illustrates function of the right upper extremity after multiple tendon transfers and lengthenings. The child has the ability to hold both large and small objects, and to initiate voluntary grasp and release. Training should include awareness of the eye-hand reflex and reinforcement by simultaneous use of the opposite extremity in order to achieve maximum function and endurance of the involved extremity.

Figure 14–14 illustrates the postoperative condition of the hand and digits in a 16-year-old male after multiple simultaneous procedures. The thumb is away from the palm, in an abducted position. The fingers are extended with less flexion deformity than existed preoperatively. The wrist flexors have been lengthened, and the flexor digitorum superficialis of the long finger was transferred to the extensor pollicis longus through the pronator quadratus and interosseous space. The flexor digitorum superficialis of the ring finger was transferred to the extensor digitorum communis tendon. Grasp and release are voluntary and reasonably rapid.

Figure 14–15 is a radiograph of the hand of a 14-year-old patient showing arthrodesis of the metacarpophalangeal joint with two 0.045-inch fixation pins. The pins have been in place for two years and

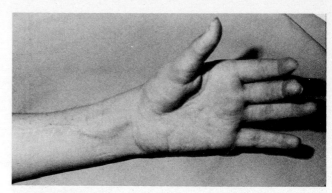

**Fig. 14–14**  Postoperative condition of the hand and digits in a 16-year-old patient after multiple simultaneous procedures.

will be removed. The thumb is in neutral position and rotated so that the tip is opposite the radial aspect of the index finger. This arthrodesis lessens the thumb-in-palm position and augments control of the entire thumb after the abductor pollicis longus and extensor pollicis brevis are shortened.

Figure 14–16 is a preoperative demonstration of contracture of the flexor pollicis longus and static and dynamic deformity of the index, long, and ring fingers as dorsiflexion is performed. The flexor carpi radialis shows moderate contracture.

As shown in Figure 14–17, after the thumb is

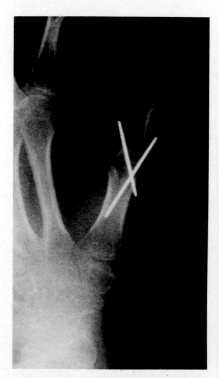
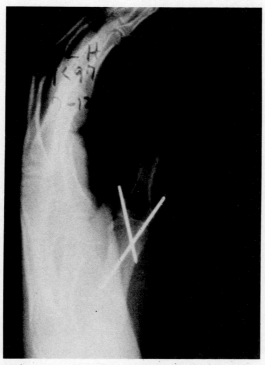
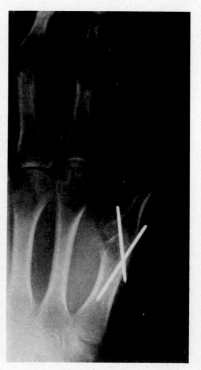

**Fig. 14–15**  Radiograph of the hand of a 14-year-old patient showing arthrodesis of the metacarpophalangeal joint with two 0.045-in fixation pins.

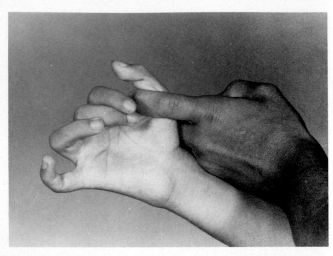

**Fig. 14–16**   Preoperative demonstration of contracture of the flexor pollicis longus and static and dynamic deformity of the index, long, and ring fingers, as dorsiflexion is performed.

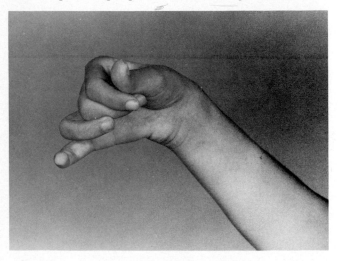

**Fig. 14–17**   Hyperextension of the distal joint of the thumb after thumb release and slight wrist flexion.

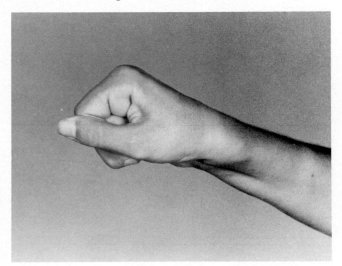

**Fig. 14–18**   Postoperative grasp performed voluntarily; as the fingers were flexed, the wrist was elevated.

released and the wrist is flexed slightly, the overactivity of the spastic abductor pollicis brevis and the tenodesis effect of the extensor pollicis longus cause hyperextension of the distal joint of the thumb. The flexor pollicis longus pulls the first metacarpal toward the palm and the spastic intrinsics also cause the thumb-in-palm deformity. The thumb in this position interferes with grasp of the index and long fingers. Overactivity of the extensor carpi ulnaris and flexor carpi ulnaris is evident as flexion occurs. The plan of treatment will depend on individual analysis of the thumb deformity and the concept that weakened muscles should be reinforced and overactive muscle-tendon units should be lengthened and, if necessary, reinforced.

Postoperatively, as shown in Figure 14–18, grasp was performed voluntarily, and as the fingers were flexed the wrist was elevated. The finger flexors were lengthened and the tendon transfers have been performed both to the thumb and the wrist extensors. The hand is useful for dressing, playing, and other activities of daily living. However, the child is predominantly right-handed and uses the left hand only as a helping hand.

The patient whose hand is shown in Figure 14–19 had deformities of hyperextension of the proximal interphalangeal joints of the fingers, elevated thumb-in-palm position, and thumb web space contracture. The hyperextension of the interphalangeal joint is being corrected by capsular plication, proximal placement of the retinacular flap, and tenodesis of the segment of the flexor digitorum superficialis to the fibro-osseous canal. A probe is under the flexor superficialis and the joint capsule is in the clamp. This method of correcting hyperextension will not cause a fixed contracture and will prevent hyperextension and locking of the interphalangeal joints. Maximum flexion persists and maximum extension is possible. The surgical procedure is usually performed through lateral incisions on both the radial and ulnar aspects of each digit.

After reinforcement and plication of the abductor pollicis longus, the thumb remains out of the palm, the wrist is extended, and the fingers are flexed. Arthrodesis of the metacarpophalangeal joint of the thumb and improved muscle-tendon control of the first metatarsal will prevent the thumb from crossing into the palm during voluntary extension.

Figure 14–20 shows release of an elbow contracture performed through an "S" incision that started just medial to the origin of the brachioradialis, extended obliquely across the anterior aspect of the elbow almost parallel with the skin creases, and passed distally over the flexor carpi ulnaris. Through this incision, the radial nerve was isolated with a rubber tape around the nerve after the nerve had been identified with an electrical stimulator. A second

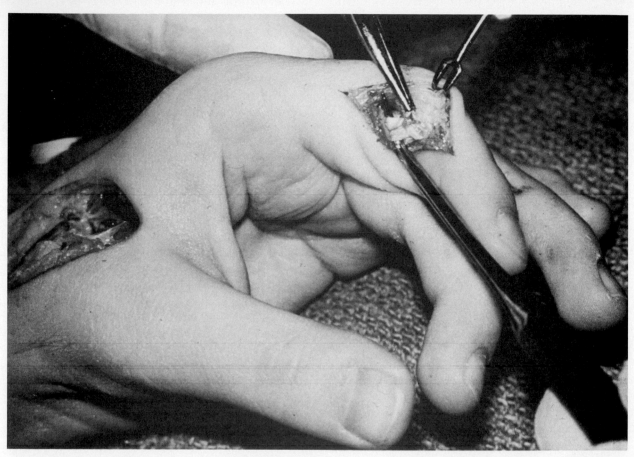

**Fig. 14–19**   Hyperextension of the interphalangeal joint being corrected by capsular plication, proximal placement of the retinacular flap, and tenodesis of the segment of the flexor digitorum superficialis to the fibro-osseous canal.

**Fig. 14–20**   Release of elbow contracture performed through an "S" incision.

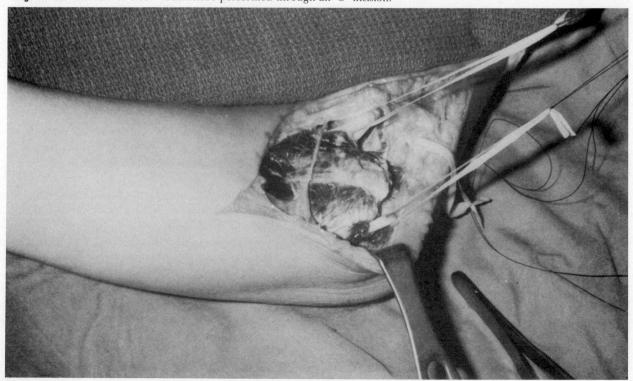

tape was passed around the ulnar nerve and a third tape around the median nerve. The flexor muscle mass was released from the humerus. This included the palmaris longus, flexor carpi radialis, pronator radii teres, and the superficial half of the flexor carpi ulnaris.

The biceps tendon was lengthened and the brachialis was released from the ulna. Controlled recession of the muscle origins was performed and measuring lengthening was completed so that proper tension persisted and recovery of flexion was assured.

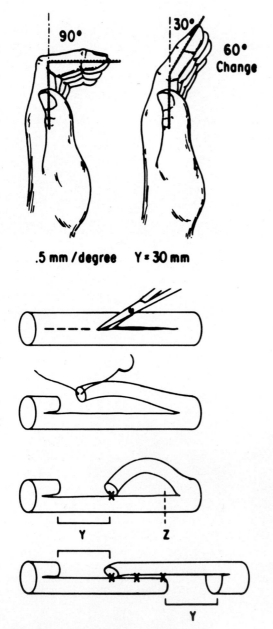

**Fig. 14–21** Schematic representation of the method designed for controlled lengthening of the flexor digitorum superficialis tendons, and for all other tendons that require lengthening.

The method illustrated in Figure 14–21 was designed for controlled lengthening of the flexor digitorum superficialis tendons, and for all other tendons that require lengthening. The static contracture is measured at 90 degrees, and the desired correction is to 60 degrees. The concepts established in the Magnus-Blix curve have resulted in an observation that 0.5 mm of lengthening per degree of correction will maintain appropriate tension on the muscle bellies for drawn contracture. This method of controlled lengthening prevents the muscle belly from retracting and thereby maintains sufficient tension on the muscle belly unit to maintain satisfactory strength and function after lengthening has been performed.

To elucidate further the concepts presented in the first part of this discussion, several case histories will be presented that delineate the individual deformity and examination; the original diagnosis; functional impairment; the surgical procedures that were performed; the postoperative management; and the results.[9,10]

### Case 1

**Examination** The right upper extremity of a 12-year-old boy with an original diagnosis of spastic hemiplegia showed dynamic wrist flexion, thumb-in-palm deformity, and flexed digits when he attempted to elevate the wrist. When more effort was expended and an attempt was made to elevate the fingers, hyperextension of the interphalangeal joints of the index, long, ring, and little fingers occurred.

**Functional Impairment** The patient had difficulty in grasping and receiving an object because of the thumb-in-palm. Also, the hyperextended fingers locked in hyperextension as digit straightening was attempted. Voluntary flexion was limited because of digit hyperextension. Once the hyperextended position was released by manipulation with the opposite hand, strong finger flexion was possible.

**Analysis of Deformity** Hyperextension of the proximal interphalangeal joints was caused by overactivity of the intrinsic muscles; overpull of the extensor digitorum communis associated with a wrist flexion deformity and hyperextension of the metacarpophalangeal joints; and a stretched volar capsule of the interphalangeal joints (Fig. 14–19).

The thumb-in-palm was associated with overactive flexor pollicis longus and weak extensor pollicis longus (Fig. 14–5).

Pronation and supination of the forearm were balanced, elbow flexion and extension were performed voluntarily and well controlled, and stereognosis of the hand was good.

Voluntary extension of the hand was possible with the extensor carpi radialis longus, extensor carpi radialis brevis, and extensor carpi ulnaris. This action was possible when the fingers were flexed, because the principal cause of wrist flexion deformity was overactivity and contracture of the flexor digitorum superficialis muscles of the four fingers and of the flexor pollicis longus. When the flexor muscles were contracting, the voluntary action of the extensor muscles became apparent.

**Plan of Treatment** Release the contractures of the thumb and fingers. Reinforce the extensor-abductor action of the thumb, and stabilize the metacarpophalangeal joint to maintain the thumb out of the palm. Correct the abnormal hyperextension of the interphalangeal joints of the fingers.

**Surgical Procedures** The flexor pollicis longus tendon was lengthened 2 cm at the wrist. The technique for all tendon lengthenings is shown in Fig. 14–21. The ratio of 2:1 describes the joint angle of correction and the amount of lengthening of the tendon. For example, a 45-degree joint angle requires a 22-mm lengthening of the flexor tendon. The tendon is usually split at least a one-third distance longer than the lengthening, i.e., a 30-mm split for a 20-mm lengthening. A nonabsorbable suture is used.

A 2-cm lengthening of the flexor digitorum superficialis of the long finger at the wrist-forearm level is performed.

A transfer of the flexor digitorum superficialis to the rerouted extensor pollicis longus was performed. The technique was as follows: perform a tenotomy of the flexor digitorum superficialis of the ring finger at the wrist level with the tendon under tension, in order to obtain a long segment of the tendon. This was equivalent to doing a tenotomy of the tendon in the midpalm or at the base of the finger.

This proximal tendon was transferred to the extensor policis longus that has been released from its fibro-osseous canal and redirected to the radial side of the first metacarpal. The muscle belly and the tendon remain connected.

The flexor digitorum superficialis tendon was directed deep to the abductor pollicis longus, which formed a readymade pulley that prevented the redirected extensor pollicis longus from functioning as an opponens pollicis. This condition does occur if the extensor pollicis longus is allowed to migrate excessively toward the palmar surface of the thumb.

Arthrodesis of the metacarpophalangeal joint of the thumb was performed by removing the articular cartilage, maintaining the convex surface of the metacarpal head, and deepening the concave surface of the proximal phalanx. The bone segments were realigned with the phalanx in 10 degrees of flexion and sufficient rotation to direct the pulp of the hand to the radial aspect of the index fingertip. Fixation was provided with two 0.062-inch fixation pins, either parallel or crossed. These were cut off subcutaneous-

ly. Thumb adduction and flexion were further decreased by transferring the adductor pollicis to the neck of the first metacarpal, and by segmental shortening of the abductor pollicis longus-extensor pollicis brevis tendons just distal to the musculocutaneous junction. The annular ligament is opened by a Z incision and repaired in an elongated fashion to avoid bowstringing and subluxation of these tendons (Fig. 14–19).

Hyperextension of the interphalangeal joints of the fingers is treated by tongue-in-groove lengthening of the radial and ulnar intrinsic tendons and the central tendon of the extensor digitorum communis over the proximal phalanx. The tongue is 2 cm long and the lengthening is 1 cm long. This procedure is performed on the index, long, ring, and little fingers. Dynamic correction occurred and palmar tenodesis or capsulorrhaphy at the proximal interphalangeal joint was unnecessary. If static tenodesis is desired, then the capsulorrhaphy and tenodesis are necessary.

**Postoperative Care** A compression dressing was applied with the wrist in neutral position and the thumb abducted 5 cm from the index finger. The entire palm of the hand is visible and the thumb is not hyperextended or flattened. The interphalangeal joints of the digits were flexed 45 degrees and maintained in that position by a dorsal plaster splint that extended from the fingertips to the elbow. A second sugar-tong splint was applied around the elbow to prevent slippage of the hand and forearm splint, to maintain the elbow at right angles to avoid dependent swelling, and to relax the flexor and extensor muscles of the hand and digits. Drains were removed from the palmar incision in 24 hours, without removing the plaster splint. The plaster splint remained in place for four weeks, after which a removable dorsal splint was constructed for the fingers and an abduction web splint for the thumb. These splints were removed for one hour three times a day and the patient initiated wrist elevation, finger flexion, and wrist flexion-finger extension maneuvers. The entire effort is aimed at improving grasp and release, and maintaining the thumb out of the palm. After the second month, the splints were removed for two hours three times a day and during the third month they were used only at night. The flexed position of the interphalangeal joints and the abducted position of the thumb were protected for three months, after which acrylic or other kinds of night splints were used to maintain the interphalangeal joints in flexion and the thumb in abduction. Protective splinting continued for six months from the time of the operation.

**Results** Functional improvement is based on alteration of the original anatomic deformity, on the rapidity of grasp and release, and on the patient's ability to handle objects with greater ease and improved endurance. The results in this particular patient were as follows: The wrist and fingers could be extended through a greater range of motion more easily, and the flexed position of the wrist and fingers was eliminated. The thumb remained out of the palm during wrist extension and flexion and even under stress the thumb did not migrate into the palm. The patient had active flexion and extension of the first ray without interfering with placement or reception of objects in the palm. Hyperextension of the fingers was eliminated during active wrist and finger extension. When the digits were under stress while holding objects, the interphalangeal joints did not lock in hyperextension, although they did assume a mild hyperextended position. Manipulation of the locked interphalangeal joints of the involved hand with the opposite normal hand was unnecessary because hyperextension did not occur when forceful extension of the involved fingers was attempted. Objects could be handled more rapidly, and different-sized objects were manipulated with relative ease. Finally, the appearance of the hand was greatly improved and the patient's attitude toward appearing in public and toward performing activities at school was dramatically altered.

## Case 2

A 9-year-old girl was diagnosed as having spastic hemiplegia caused by a cerebral problem at birth.

**Functional Impairment** Moderate flexed position of the hand, thumb-in-palm, and limited supination were the usual positions of the involved extremity. The thumb was in the way when objects were shifted from the uninvolved left hand to the affected hand. Digit release was performed slowly because of limited abduction and extension of the thumb. Extension of the wrist was also performed slowly. Elbow extension and flexion were performed without difficulty. Supination of the forearm was possible through only 30 degrees and pronation through 40 degrees.

**Analysis of Deformity** The metacarpophalangeal joint of the thumb was hypermobile, with 80 degrees of excessive flexion. Extension of the first metacarpal and of the proximal phalanx of the thumb was incomplete. The extensor pollicis longus was weak. Both the wrist and the finger extensor muscles were strong. However, a contracture of the flexor carpi radialis prevented rapid extension of the hand and caused a persistent moderate dynamic flexion deformity.

**Plan of Treatment** Maintain the thumb out of the palm and improve active and passive extension of the first ray. Improve the speed of wrist extension by decreasing the flexion contracture caused by the flexor carpi radialis longus.

**Surgical Procedures** Arthrodesis of the metacarpophalangeal joint of the thumb in 10 degrees of flexion was performed with the thumb pad rotated to meet the radial aspect of the index finger. Fixation was with two 0.045-inch fixation pins.

The abductor pollicis longus and extensor pollicis brevis were shortened approximately 1 cm in order to abduct and extend the first metacarpal at the carpometacarpal joint.

The flexor digitorum superficialis of the ring finger was transferred through the pronator quadratus and the interosseous space to the realigned extensor pollicis longus. The tendon of the extensor pollicis longus was not separated from its muscle belly. In its new radial location, a stabilizing pulley for the extensor pollicis longus was prepared from a segment of the dorsal retinaculum.

The flexor carpi radialis was lengthened 20 mm to correct a 40-degree palmar angulation of the wrist.

**Special Comments Concerning Case 2** The flexor carpi radialis is the most frequently contracted muscle-tendon unit of the palmar aspect of the forearm. Arthrodesis of the metacarpophalangeal joint rather than capsulodesis was selected because the joint was hypermobile in both flexion and extension. Preoperative muscle testing indicated that the abductor pollicis longus had good strength, but the extensor pollicis longus showed poor strength. The strength of the wrist extensors was readily determined by having the patient close the fingers and elevate the hand. Once the hand was extended, the examiner could palpate the extensor tendons of the wrist and could detect both resistance and strength of the extensor carpi radialis longus and brevis by this maneuver. In such a case, if the flexor carpi ulnaris is transferred to the extensor carpi radialis brevis, or even to the extensor digitorum communis, the result will always be over-correction and may lead to a fixed dorsiflexion contracture, which interferes with finger extension. Only those muscles that are definitely weakened should be reinforced by tendon transfer.

**Postoperative Care** The tourniquet was released and bleeding points coagulated. A compression dressing was applied with the wrist at neutral position, the thumb abducted and extended, and the fingers protected by a bulky, soft, compression dressing. A dorsal plaster splint was used extending from the fingertips to the wrist to protect the lengthened flexor carpi radialis, and a second splint on the dorsum of the thumb and wrist was used to hold the thumb in abduction extension. A sugar-tong splint was placed around the elbow to maintain elevation and to stabilize the dressings.

Twenty-four hours after the operation the soft dressings were split, the plaster splint was left in place, and the Penrose drains removed. Compression dressing was reapplied and the cast splint was left in place for four weeks. At that time a new removable dorsal splint was made for both the thumb and the wrist, and active exercise one hour at a time was initiated with the splint off three times a day. The protective splint was used for an additional four weeks, after which it was used only at night for an additional four months. The plaster is replaced as necessary; or a half shell Lite cast is used; or an Orthoplast splint is constructed. The functional and active exercise program is primarily related to activities of daily living and improving speed and strength of both grasp and release.

**Results** The patient showed significant improvement in voluntary use of the hand. Objects could be released quickly, they could be received rapidly from the other hand, and the involved hand was used more frequently in activities of daily living, such as dressing, eating, and school activities. The thumb was out of the palm and did not bypass the index finger while grasp was performed.

Active wrist extension was rapid, and the wrist could be elevated to 30 degrees of dorsiflexion without difficulty. The patient was followed for ten years without evidence of recurrent deformity or alteration after the growth plate had closed spontaneously.

### Case 3

An 18-year-old male was diagnosed as having severe spastic hemiplegia involving the left upper extremity due to cerebral palsy.

**Examination** The extremity showed flexion deformity of the wrist, thumb-in-palm, flexion of the metacarpophalangeal joint, and excessive pronation of the forearm. Proprioception and stereognosis of the hand were diminished, compared with the opposite normal hand.

**Functional Impairment** The thumb was in the palm and could not be extended and abducted voluntarily. The wrist was flexed and, as extension of the hand was attempted, the fingers were flexed, the thumb became tighter in a position of palmar flexion, and objects could not be grasped or retrieved. The excessive pronation prevented access to the palm when the patient had objects in the other hand or even when the involved hand was manipulated as a helping hand. Both grasp and release of the affected hand required manipulation by the normal hand, and voluntary use of the involved hand and forearm was minimal.

**Analysis of Deformity** The wrist flexor muscles were contracted and overactive and were the major cause of the flexed position of the hand. The wrist extensors, however, were rated at 80% of normal strength when tested while the fingers were flexed and the wrist and hand were extended. The extensor carpi radialis longus, brevis, and extensor carpi ulnaris could be palpated and their strength demonstrated. Excessive ulnar deviation had resulted in displacement of the extensor carpi radialis longus and extensor carpi radialis brevis tendons to the ulnar side of the wrist; the extensor carpi ulnaris was acting as a wrist flexor because the extensor annular ligament was stretched and had allowed the extensor carpi ulnaris to shift to the ulnar palmar aspect of the wrist.

**Plan of Treatment** Weaken the wrist flexors by lengthening the tendons. Indirectly strengthen the wrist extensors without transferring a flexor to an extensor muscle. Stabilize extensor muscles of the thumb and redirect the thumb out of the palm. Maintain abduction and extension of the thumb, in addition to stabilizing the metacarpophalangeal joint. Mobilize the distal radial ulnar joint by resection of a short segment of the distal ulna and by resection of the pronator quadratus. Also, transfer the pronator radii teres through the interosseous space to a new insertion on the extensor surface of the radius.

**Surgical Procedures: Dorsal Wrist Surgery** Three quarters of the extensor carpi ulnaris was transferred to the insertion of the extensor carpi radialis brevis. The extensor carpi ulnaris was split into one-quarter and three-quarter segments. One quarter of the tendon was used to stabilize the proximal ulna by placing it through a drill hole in the proximal ulna and the three-quarter segment was transferred to the extensor carpi radialis brevis after it passed under the extensor digitorum communis tendon.

The distal 2 cm of the ulna was resected. The periosteal sleeve was maintained, the triangular fibrocartilage was intact, and the annular ligament and local soft tissue were repaired to stabilize the proximal ulna and to prevent radial deviation of the hand at the wrist joint.

The extensor carpi radialis longus and brevis were centralized in line with the third metacarpal and an annual ligament was constructed from the dorsal retinaculum to prevent shifting of the extensor tendons toward the ulnar side.

The extensor indicis proprius of the index finger was transferred to the extensor digitorum communis of the long finger, which showed incomplete extension, where the index finger had excessive extension.

**Palmar Wrist Surgery** The flexor carpi radialis was lengthened 1 cm. The contracture and overactivity were about 25 degrees, which required lengthening of the flexor carpi radialis approximately 12 mm.

The flexor carpi ulnaris was lengthened 15 mm, since this muscle-tendon unit was pulling the hand in ulnar deviation and was slightly tighter than the flexor carpi radialis.

The pronator radii teres was released through the proximal end of the forearm incision and transferred to the flexor pollicis longus, which was lengthened 1 cm.

The pronator quadratus was released from the ulna to diminish the excessive pronation deformity.

**Correction of Thumb Deformity** The flexor pollicis longus was lengthened 1 cm and reinforced with the brachioradialis in neutral position.

Arthrodesis of the metacarpophalangeal joint of the thumb in 10 degrees of flexion and sufficient rotation was performed to allow the thumb pulp to match with the radial side of the index finger.

Plication of the abductor pollicis longus-extensor pollicis brevis 1.5 cm proximal to the pulley was performed.

The extensor pollicis longus was released from the annular ligament and the tendon was rerouted toward the first metacarpal. The extensor pollicis longus was then reinforced with the brachioradialis, and the flexor pollicis longus was lengthened 2.0 cm.

The pronator radii teres was released from the radius, transferred through the interosseous membrane, and resutured to the radius in a new location after the forearm was supinated.

Accessory excisions were made as follows: The pronator quadratus muscle belly was excised about 60%; the distal ulna was mobilized by releasing the pronator quadratus and the other wrist muscles.

**Postoperative Care** The tourniquet was released; all bleeding points were coagulated. A compression dressing and a ten-thickness dorsal plaster splint were applied, holding the wrist at 10 degrees of dorsiflexion, the thumb in abduction, the forearm supinated about 60 degrees, and the elbow flexed at right angles.

The splint remained in place for four weeks, but drains were removed 24 hours after surgery. At four weeks, the splint was removed for one hour three times a day for a month. During the third month, it was removed for two hours, three times a day.

The hand and wrist are protected for approximately six months by night splints of Lite cast or Velcro. The wrist is at neutral, the thumb is abducted and extended, and the fingers are relatively free.

**Results** Eight years after this group of procedures was completed, the patient had active supination of 25 degrees and active pronation of 40 degrees. The hand could be elevated voluntarily, the fingers extended without assistance from the opposite hand, and the thumb was out of the palm. Grasp and release were possible with relative ease. The patient could receive and retrieve primarily both small and large objects.

The speed of grasp and release was increased,

voluntary control of the thumb and finger extensors was improved and the wrist extensor muscles maintained the hand in either a neutral or elevated position after the flexor tendons had been lengthened and thereby weakened.

Extension of the thumb and fingers was improved by the patient's ability to flex and extend the wrist voluntarily. The tenodesis effect augmented thumb and finger movement.

The elbow did involuntarily flex through 30 degrees when the patient was walking and affected by anxiety and stress but, otherwise, the patient could relax and control elbow motion in both flexion and extension.

The patient has been observed for eight years following the original surgical procedures, and no additional surgical treatment has been necessary.

### Case 4

An 18-year-old woman had hemiparesis caused by a cerebral vascular lesion that occurred during childhood: the left upper extremity showed thumb-in-palm, a flexed wrist, pronation of the forearm, and moderate static and dynamic alterations of the elbow joint. Dynamic involuntary flexion occurred with certain stressful activities.

**Examination** The upper extremity showed persistent wrist flexion to 70 degrees, thumb-in-palm when the wrist was extended and flexed, finger flexion with the wrist in neutral and the flexed position, forearm pronation constantly, and a static elbow flexion position at 45 degrees, which was aggravated by activity. Grasp and release were active, but active extension of the hand and fingers was limited by myoclonus and spasticity of the flexor pollicis longus and flexor digitorum superficialis muscles.

**Analysis of Deformity** The thumb-in-palm position occurred because of overactivity of the flexor pollicis longus and weakness of the extensor pollicis longus. The abductor pollicis longus-extensor pollicis brevis was overstretched and unable to control the first metacarpal because of the greater strength of the flexors when compared to the abductor-extensor muscle group. The metacarpophalangeal joint was hyperflexed.

The wrist flexor muscles and the pronator radii teres and pronator quadratus were overactive and caused hand flexion and excessive pronation of the forearm. The supinator muscles were unable to neutralize the flexion pronation muscle strength and the force of gravity, which augmented both flexion and pronation of the hand and forearm.

**Surgical Procedures** The flexor digitorum superficialis of the index finger was lengthened 20 mm to correct a 45-degree flexion deformity of the interphalangeal joint.

The flexor superficialis of the long finger was detached from its distal segment at the wrist and passed through the interosseous space in the region of the pronator quadratus and sutured to the extensor digitorum communis and the extensor index proprius. A split segment of this superficialis was also transferred to the extensor digiti quinti.

The flexor superficialis of the ring finger was detached from its distal segment at the wrist level and transferred to the extensor pollicis longus through a subcutaneous route. The wrist was at neutral position, the thumb abducted 5 cm from the index finger, and the tip of the thumb was rotated opposite the radial aspect of the index finger. The metacarpophalangeal joint was fused in 10 degrees of flexion and held with two 0.062-inch fixation pins.

The flexor digitorum superficialis was mobilized on the palmar surface about 6 cm proximally so that its course was deep to the abductor pollicis longus in its course to the extensor pollicis longus, which acted as a pulley and stabilized the transfer of the flexor superficialis to the extensor pollicis longus.

### Arthrodesis of the Metacarpophalangeal Joint of the Thumb

The convex surface of the metacarpal head and the concave surface of the proximal phalanx were denuded of cartilage, held together by manual compression and fixed with two 0.062-inch fixation pins. The position was 10 degrees of flexion and 30 degrees of radial rotation so that the pulp of the thumb made contact with the radial aspect of the index fingertip. Sufficient tension was placed on the sagittal bands of the thumb and the extensor tendon so that the distal joint is in 10 degrees of flexion when the wrist is neutral or dorsiflexed and in 10 degrees of extension when the wrist is flexed.

The abductor pollicis was recessed by releasing the insertion from the proximal phalanx and transferring the tendon to the annular ligament or sesamoid tendon. The web space was loosened by incising the superficial fascia and releasing the first dorsal interosseous muscle bellies from the first and second metacarpals and the adductor pollicis origin from the third metacarpal.

The abductor pollicis longus-extensor pollicis brevis complex was shortened 1 cm by a Z incision, which removes tendons so that the staggered ends of the tendons are reapproximated with a 3-0 nonabsorbable suture. The incision was made distal to the annular ligament and, after the tendons were repaired, a segment of the annular ligament was removed to avoid impingement of the tendons on the annular ligament.

The extensor pollicis longus was released from its annular ligament opposite Lister's tubercle and routed toward the radial side of the wrist and thumb. The flexor digitorum superficialis of the ring finger was then buttonholed into this redirected tendon in order to improve both abduction and extension of the first ray.

The flexor pollicis longus was lengthened 2 cm at the wrist in order to correct for a 45-degree static contracture of the distal phalanx. The lengthened tendon was then reinforced with the brachioradialis, which had been released from its origin and mobilized proximally.

**Wrist Procedures** One half of the extensor carpi ulnaris was separated from its attachment into the base of the fifth metacarpal, mobilized to the musculotendinous junction proximally, transferred deep to the extensor digitorum communis, and sutured to the extensor carpi radialis brevis under the same tension as that of the segment that remains attached to the fifth metacarpal. This transfer reinforces wrist extension, lessens ulnar deviation, and obviates the need for a transfer of a strong wrist flexor to a wrist extensor that has fair strength.

The preoperative assessment of muscle strength of the extensor carpi radialis brevis showed it to be 60% of normal. An additional transfer of the extensor carpi ulnaris would bring the strength of wrist extension to 80% to 85% of normal and prevent a flexed wrist deformity.

**Postoperative Care** The tourniquet was released, bleeding points were coagulated, compression dressings applied, Penrose or suction drains were placed in both the dorsal and volar wounds, and dorsal plaster splints were applied.

The drains were removed in 24 hours, after which a new dorsal splint was used to stabilize the wrist in 20 degrees dorsiflexion, the fingers in 30 degrees flexion at the interphalangeal joints and 0 degrees at the metacarpophalangeal joints, the thumb web was spread, and the thumb was abducted and extended. This splint remained in place for one month, after which a removable splint was made for use during the second month. During this time, the supervised home exercise program was arranged so that the splint was removed for one hour three times a day, during which time arm and hand voluntary motions were initiated.

A night splint was used for four months after the original procedure had been completed. This splint provided stabilization of the thumb in abduction-extension, the wrist in 20 degrees extension and the interphalangeal joints in flexion. The pins remained in the thumb at the site of the fused metacarpophalangeal joint for at least one year.

### Case 5

A 14-year-old girl with hemiparesis showed deformity of the right hand and upper extremity. The right hand and fingers were flexed, the thumb was in the palm, the extensor carpi radialis longus and brevis were rated 40% of normal strength, the thumb extensors were 25% of normal strength, and the flexor pollicis longus was contracted.

The elbow showed a static flexion contracture of 45 degrees, and dynamic flexion of 70 degrees was observed while the patient was either walking or under moderate emotion stress.

**Functional Impairment** The flexion deformity of the elbow resulted in diminished hand function. The flexed position of the wrist and the thumb-in-palm interfered with grasp. When grasp was attempted, the dorsiflexed position of the wrist and the flexed fingers interfered with the patient's ability to receive objects or to assist the left hand with the uninvolved right hand.

**Analysis of Deformity** Elbow flexion was caused by overaction of the biceps, brachialis, and muscle bellies of the wrist flexors and the brachioradialis. The triceps strength was good, and the wrist flexor muscles could be voluntarily activated.

The thumb deformity was caused by a hypermobile metacarpophalangeal joint, an overactive flexor pollicis longus, and weakness of the extensor pollicis longus, extensor pollicis brevis, and abductor pollicis longus.

The extensor muscles were elongated and weak, and these deficiencies affected hand elevation, thumb extension, and active supination.

**Plan of Treatment** Improve extension of the elbow by lengthening the biceps humerus, recession or myotomy of the brachialis, release of the forearm flexors from the humerus, incision of the lacertus fibrosis and the fascia in the upper arm in order to avoid compartment compression, and, if necessary, release the origin of the brachioradialis. Correct thumb-in-palm deformity, stabilize the metacarpophalangeal joint. Reinforce the weak extensors of the fingers, the thumb, and the wrist.

**Surgical Procedures: Left Palmar Forearm and Hand** The long finger flexor digitorum superficialis was passed through the interosseous space to the base of the fourth metacarpal under proper tension to improve wrist dorsiflexion.

The ring finger flexor digitorum superficialis was transferred to the rerouted extensor pollicis longus. The course of the transferred flexor tendon was on the palmar surface of the flexor carpi radialis and under the pulley formed by the abductor pollicis longus tendon.

The flexor pollicis longus was lengthened 20 mm to correct a 45-degree statis contracture.

**Thumb Reconstruction** The metacarpophalangeal joint of the thumb was fused in 10 degrees of flexion and

sufficient rotation to allow the thumb to make direct contact with the radial aspect of the pulp of the index finger. The bone segments were held together by two crossed 0.062-inch fixation pins.

The abductor pollicis longus and the extensor pollicis brevis tendons were shortened 1 cm either proximal or distal to the annular ligament depending on the severity of the deformity, and the annular ligament was partially excised to prevent the site of the tendon suture from impinging on it.

The flexor pollicis longus was lengthened but not reinforced because its strength was adequate for voluntary flexion.

**Extensor Region Muscle Reinforcement** The extensor digitorum communis tendons of the index, long, ring and little fingers were reinforced by the brachioradialis muscle. This muscle was mobilized and redirected to the extensor surface.

Ninety percent of the extensor carpi ulnaris tendon was detached from the fifth metacarpal, mobilized proximally, and transferred to the extensor carpi radialis brevis insertion. The 10% of the tendon that remained attached to the fifth metacarpal was sutured proximally to the annular ligament of the extensor carpi ulnaris while the wrist was held in neutral position. This tenodesis prevented excessive radial deviation after the extensor carpi ulnaris muscle was relocated.

**Elbow Contracture Correction** The multiple operations about the elbow were performed through an S-contoured incision beginning on the lateral border of the arm and extending to the medial aspect of the elbow joint. The biceps tendon was lengthened 2 cm to correct a 45-degree static contracture.

A brachialis muscle was released from the coronoid process and sutured to the undersurface of the lengthened biceps tendon.

The pronator radii teres muscle origin, the origin of flexor carpi radialis, and one half of the muscle belly of the flexor carpi ulnaris were released from the medial humeral condyle, recessed distally 1.5 cm, and sutured to the surrounding periosteum.

**Postoperative Management** The tourniquet was released, Penrose drains or small suction drains were inserted at the wrist and elbow wounds, and a compression was applied, over which dorsal plaster splints were added to prevent motion. The drains were removed in 24 hours and the splints were continued for four weeks. At that time an active assistive exercise program was initiated. All tendon transfers and tendon lengthenings at the elbow, wrist, thumb, and hand were protected by removable splints. The splints were taken off for one hour three times a day for two weeks and then two hours three times a day for the next two weeks. During the third month, the splints were taken off during the day, the home exercise program was continued, and the splints were reapplied only at night.

**Results** Grasp and release were improved. Objects could be placed into the palm without being obstructed by the thumb. Grip strength was improved, and release could be performed with the wrist in neutral position rather than in flexion; this indicated better action of the digit extensor muscles. Elbow activities were improved as noted by more rapid extension of the forearm, active flexion was performed with greater ease than preoperatively, and there as no obvious weakness during this motion. When the patient walked, the extremity was held in a natural position since the acutely flexed position was eliminated.

### Surgical Procedures Performed in Special Situations

Lengthening of the flexor digitorum profundus muscles at the wrist is performed after the flexor digitorum superficialis tendons have been lengthened. Both groups of flexors are lengthened if the initial elongation of the flexor digitorum superficialis tendons does not diminish both the existing contracture and spasticity. Maximum voluntary control of extension is necessary and occasionally both groups of flexors require lengthening. After the flexor superficialis tendons are lengthened, the tension on the proximal interphalangeal and distal interphalangeal joints is tested while the wrist is at 10 degrees of dorsiflexion. If the finger tips show a flexed position of 90 degrees when the wrist joint is at neutral and the proximal interhalangeal joints are extended to zero degrees, a severe contracture of the flexor produndus tendons is present, and lengthening of the tendons of the long, ring, and little fingers is necessary. The index finger is usually not contracted and does not require lengthening.

Tenodesis of the extensor digitorum communis to the extensor carpi radialis brevis is necessary if digit extension is weak or slow and if an available active motor is insufficient to elevate the finger extensors.

The transfer of the flexor carpi ulnaris by way of either the ulnar aspect of the wrist or through the interosseous space to the extensor carpi radialis brevis will reinforce the strength of wrist and hand extension. This procedure is performed if other transfers, such as the extensor carpi ulnaris or the flexor digitorum superficialis muscles, are either not available or are too weak to restore wrist extension. This transfer is appropriate if the extensor carpi radialis longus and brevis are not functioning. If the wrist extensors show only partial weakness, the transfer of the flexor carpi ulnaris to the extensor carpi radialis brevis will usually cause overcorrection and result in a fixed dorsiflexion deformity.

Partial carpalectomy consists of excision of the carpal scaphoid, the lunate, and the triangularis. This procedure is performed when the flexion contracture is static and ancient and when forceful elevation of the hand may cause stretch of the median and ulnar nerve and the radial and ulnar arteries. Carpalectomy is augmented by multiple tendon lengthenings on the palmar aspect of the wrist, tendon transfers to the thumb and fingers, and release of the volar capsule at the wrist if necessary. The proximal carpalectomy shortens the forearm 10 mm and results in an improvement of approximately 25 degrees of dorsiflexion without increased tension on the flexors.

The release of antebrachial fascia of the forearm from elbow to wrist is performed in conjunction with multiple tendon transfers and tendon lengthenings. The antebrachial fascia functions as a compartment encasement and may cause excessive compression of muscle bellies and a primary muscle ischemia after multiple transfers are performed. A fascial release is performed as a prophylactic for the prevention of compartment syndrome.

Reinforcement of the flexor digitorum profundus muscles after the flexor digitorum superficialis muscles have been lengthened is occasionally necessary to maintain strong flexion strength. If the flexor digitorum profundus muscles require lengthening, then the resulting weakened muscles will be reinforced by the flexor digitorum superficialis tendons. Furthermore, if the flexor digitorum profundus muscles do not require lengthening but are inherently weak, then the lengthened flexor superficialis tendons are buttonholed into the flexor profundus muscles and sutured side to side.

The formula for determining the tension on a transferred muscle tendon unit is obtained as follows: (1) The range of passive excursion of the muscle-tendon to be transferred is determined by direct measurement during the operation. (2) Sixty percent of this excursion is the proper tension for the muscle-tendon unit after it has been transferred and sutured in place. (3) The recipient muscle-tendon unit is adjusted so that the segment it controls is in neutral position when the wrist is at zero degrees and the metacarpophalangeal joints are flexed 45 degrees. This tension has demonstrated that Blix's curve is accurately portrayed when the tension of the donor and the recipient matches these figures.

The extensor carpi ulnaris is transferred to the base of the fourth metacarpal and sutured into drill holes into bone; or, the extensor carpi ulnaris is transferred to the insertion of the extensor carpi radialis brevis at the base of the third metacarpal. A strip of tendon from the extensor carpi ulnaris remains attached to the base of the fifth metacarpal and is detached from the muscle belly and then sutured to the annular ligament to prevent radial deviation. This procedure is designated as a tenodesis.

The pronator radii teres is released from the radius, the tendon-muscle unit is mobilized, and the tendon is transferred through the interosseous space to the shaft of the radius with the forearm in supination. This muscle may also be used to reinforce the extensor carpi radialis longus and brevis or the flexor pollicis longus.

Plication of the retinacular ligament of the proximal interphalangeal joint is performed by advancing the volar segment proximally and the dorsal segment distally. Another option is advancement of the capsule proximally and plication of a capsule to the proximal capsular flap and the periosteum; also, tenodesis of one fourth of the flexor superficialis to the fibro-osseous canal on the radial and ulnar aspects of the proximal interphalangeal joint can be performed. This procedure is used as an alternate technique to the tongue-in-groove lengthening of the lateral bands and central extensor tendon.

The following variations of tendon lengthenings, muscle belly releases, and tendon transfers can also be performed:

(1) The origin of the brachioradialis is released when an elbow flexion contracture is severe. The radial nerve and the motor branches of that nerve to the brachioradialis are identified by electrical stimulation just prior to initiating the muscle belly release.

(2) The mobilized distal end of the brachioradialis is transferred to the flexor pollicis longus to reinforce a lengthened flexor tendon; or the brachioradialis is transferred to the extensor pollicis longus to reinforce a weakened extensor muscle of the thumb.

(3) The brachioradialis is mobilized and transferred to the extensor digitorum communis when this muscle group is weak and requires strengthening. The brachioradialis should be mobilized for approximately 8 cm proximal to its insertion. Although the excursion is limited, the muscle is effective provided that a long excursion is unnecessary for movement of the unit that is being reinforced.

(4) The flexor carpi radialis is lengthened in either the young child or the adult. This tendon is usually lengthened rather than transferred, as it is essential as an active wrist flexor and also to prevent dorsiflexion deformity.

(5) Resection of the distal ulna is performed if the pronation deformity is severe, if a flexion contracture of the wrist is static, and if subluxation of the ulna has occurred because of prolonged displacement associated with the pronated forearm. The remaining proximal ulna is stabilized with one half of the extensor carpi ulnaris. It is placed through a drill hole in the distal end of the proximal ulna to aid in stabilizing the ulna and provide a collagen base for reconstruction of the periosteal and fascial sleeve, which extends to the carpal bones.

(6) The radial head is resected in the adolescent or adult if chronic dislocation of the proximal radius has occurred from excessive pronation deformity of the forearm and unrecognized dislocation of the radial head. Resection is performed proximal to the attachment of the biceps tendon to the radial tubercle.

(7) Osteotomy of the radius and ulna is performed to correct fixed supination or pronation contracture in the adolescent or adult in an attempt to realign the severe contracture that has been present since childhood. Four-hole intermediate compression plates are used to obtain firm fixation and to avoid displacement.

Arthrodesis of the radial carpal and second and third metacarpal joints is performed in the following special situations:

(1) A severe flexion deformity of the wrist is present and there are no active flexor or extensor muscles functioning. Also, a severe flexion contracture of the fingers is present and tenotomy or lengthening of the finger flexors is necessary for repositioning the digits. Even in certain instances when the digits are not moving, positioning of the hand in a neutral position in order to elongate the forearm is desirable. The arthrodesis is performed between the radius, the carpals, and the second and third metacarpals. If excessive tension is present on the median and ulnar nerves, a proximal-row carpalectomy diminishes the tension on the forearm and hand by shortening the bony structures 1 cm. Also, the distal ulna is resected to allow a forearm and hand to be placed in a neutral position.

(2) Arthrodesis of the wrist is selected after other efforts have been attempted to balance the flexor-extensor motions of the hand, wrist, and forearm. If extension movement continues to be weak after tendon transfers have been attempted; if overactive extensors are present, or if, when the hand is held in neutral position, the patient has voluntary flexion and extension of the fingers, then arthrodesis of the wrist is helpful. The stiff wrist will not detract from efficient grasp and release provided that wrist movement is not essential in assisting extension or flexion of the digits. However, if arthrodesis of the wrist is performed as the initial procedure before tendon lengthenings or tendon transfers or a combination of these, then the benefit of wrist motion in providing the flexor-extensor action will be lost. Furthermore, extension or flexion tenodesis of the thumb is eliminated by wrist fusion. An independent mobile thumb is essential before arthrodesis of the wrist is considered.

The flexor carpi ulnaris is transferred through a large opening in the interosseous membrane to the extensor carpi radialis brevis to diminish a long-standing flexion deformity and to reinforce hand and wrist extension. The flexor carpi ulnaris is mobilized on the palmar aspect of the wrist and passed through a large opening in the interosseous membrane. The extensor carpi radialis brevis is shortened by transferring the flexor carpi ulnaris to the extensor brevis tendon as far distally as possible. The flexor carpi ulnaris may require elongation of its tendon by a 6- to 8-cm free graft in order to insert the tendon into the distal segment of the wrist extensor.

The flexor carpi radialis that functions actively is lengthened but not transferred, as its continued action as a wrist flexor is essential to balance the hand and forearm.

The extensor digitorum communis muscle should either be active or reinforced by tendon transfer to avoid a flexed position of the fingers, as dorsiflexion of the hand occurs by the transfer of the flexor carpi ulnaris.

Release and recession of the abductor pollicis brevis and flexor pollicis brevis is occasionally necessary to decrease the thumb-in-palm deformity. This deformity is detected by having the examiner test the intrinsic thumb muscles while the patient is attempting to grasp. Also, a flexion deformity of the metacarpophalangeal joint and hyperextension of the distal joint of the thumb occur because of spastic thumb intrinsic muscles. After these muscles are released, opposition may be weakened and a tendon transfer is occasionally but rarely necessary to restore abduction-opposition.

## References

1. Goldner JL: Reconstructive surgery of the hand in cerebral palsy and spastic paralysis from injury to spinal cord. *J Bone Joint Surg* 1955;37A:1141–1154.
2. Goldner JL, Ferlic DC: Sensory status of the hand as related to reconstructive surgery of the upper extremity in cerebral palsy. *Clin Orthop* 1966;46:87–92.
3. Goldner JL: Reconstructive surgery of the upper extremity affected by cerebral palsy or brain or spinal cord trauma. *Curr Pract in Orthop Surg* 1966;3:125–138.
4. Green WT, Banks HH: Flexor carpi ulnaris tendon transplant and its use in cerebral palsy. *J Bone Joint Surg* 1962;44A:1343–1352.
5. Inglis AE, Cooper W: Release of the flexor pronator origin for flexion deformities of the hand and wrist in spastic paralysis. *J Bone Joint Surg* 1966;48A:857–867.
6. Swanson AB: Surgery of the hand in cerebral palsy, in Flynn JE (ed): *Hand Surgery*, ed 3. Baltimore, Williams & Wilkins Co, 1982, pp 476–488.
7. Zancolli EA: Surgical management of the hemiplegic spastic hand in cerebral palsy. *Surg Clin North Am* 1981; 61:395–406.
8. Goldner JL: Upper extremity tendon transfers in cerebral palsy. *Orthop Clin North Am* 1974;5:389–414.
9. Goldner JL: Upper extremity surgical procedures for patients with cerebral palsy. American Academy of Orthopaedic Surgeons *Instructional Course Lectures, XXVIII*. St. Louis, CV Mosby, 1979, pp 37–66.
10. Goldner JL: Surgical treatment for cerebral palsy, in Evarts-Burton (ed): *Surgery of the Musculoskeletal System*. New York, Churchill-Livingstone Inc, 1983, vol. 1, p 439.

## Acknowledgment

Figures 14–2A, 5, 6, 8, and Figures 11 through 14 were reproduced with permission from Goldner JL: Upper extremity surgical procedures for patients with cerebral palsy, in American Academy of Orthopaedic Surgeons *Instructional Course Lectures, XXVIII*. St. Louis, CV Mosby Co, 1979, pp 37–66.

# Treatment of Hip Problems in Cerebral Palsy

Leon Root, MD

## Introduction

Although treatment of cerebral palsy must concentrate upon the entire patient, a special area of concern is the hip. Not only can deformities of the hip prevent ambulation and even interfere with sitting ability, they can also cause disabling pain. Therefore, the etiology of hip deformity must be understood so that a logical method of prevention and correction can be employed.

Hip problems can be divided into two areas: (1) gait abnormalities and (2) hip instability. Often these are interwoven; i.e., instability leads to poor gait patterns, and, in nonambulatory patients, an unstable hip can hinder sitting.

## Gait Patterns

Specific patterns of standing and walking are frequently associated with specific types of involvement. The spastic diplegic child walks with thighs adducted and internally rotated, hips and knees flexed, and feet in equinus (Fig. 15-1). An analysis of muscle function reveals that hip flexors and adductors overpower hip extensors and abductors, that excessive femoral anteversion is present, that spastic hamstrings prevent full knee extension, and that the triceps surae muscles cause persistent heel elevation.

A patient who is spastic hemiplegic walks with the involved hip slightly abducted, the knee in extension, and the foot and ankle in equinovarus (Fig. 15-2). Analysis reveals satisfactory muscle balance about the hips, mild tightness of hamstrings, but overpowering triceps surae and posterior tibial muscles. Hip deformity is rare in the hemiplegic, but common in diplegic and quadriplegic patients. The difference is caused by muscle imbalance, which is always present in the diplegic but hardly ever in the hemiplegic. Obviously, there are exceptions to these broad statements: All diplegics are subject to hip deformity. "Beware of the hip in the diplegic."

The person with mild quadriplegic or total body involvement resembles a diplegic patient and can have similar hip problems. The moderate to severe quadriplegic will almost invariably be confined to a wheelchair so that the treatment goal is good sitting, which requires a straight spine, stable hips and a flexion-extension arc of approximately 90 degrees.

The same muscle involvement and femoral anteversion that can deform the diplegic hip, can wreak havoc on the quadriplegic hip.

Although the problems of hip dislocation will be discussed later, at this point it should be stressed that the muscle imbalance described above can and does cause hip dislocation in a significant number of cases. Therefore, not only should walking ability be improved and sitting preserved, but hip stability should be ensured.

Gait or motion analysis studies have been a great help in evaluating muscles while walking. However, these sophisticated procedures are not universally available. Careful observation of gait, measurement of range of motion, and radiographs remain the basic tools by which the cerebral palsy patient is evaluated in order to determine a treatment program. These evaluation tools are the basis for this discussion.

## Gait Abnormalities

The child whose thighs rotate internally while walking can have tight adductor muscles, tight medial hamstrings, femoral anteversion, or all three. If examination reveals normal anteversion, then the muscles alone must be responsible.

### Adductor Tightness or Contracture

Testing abduction in both flexion and extension is important. With slow stretching, a maximum range can be established. With rapid stretching, the reflex is stimulated and a functional range can be determined (Fig. 15-3). In either case, if abduction is less than 30 degrees the child will scissor when walking.[1] Surgery is necessary in order to correct this condition. Passive stretching and braces have not been helpful in the author's experience. Two techniques exist for adductor surgery: the classic tenotomy and obturator nerve neurectomy[2,3] or the adductor transfer.[4-6] In the ambulating child or the child who has the potential for ambulation, the author recommends transferring the adductors (longus, brevis, gracilis) to the ischial tuberosity, leaving the obturator nerve intact (Fig. 15-4). The transferred muscle not only provides an increased range of abduction, but also maintains hip stability and aids in hip extension. The technique is simple, relatively bloodless, takes approximately 45 minutes and requires only three weeks in a spica cast.

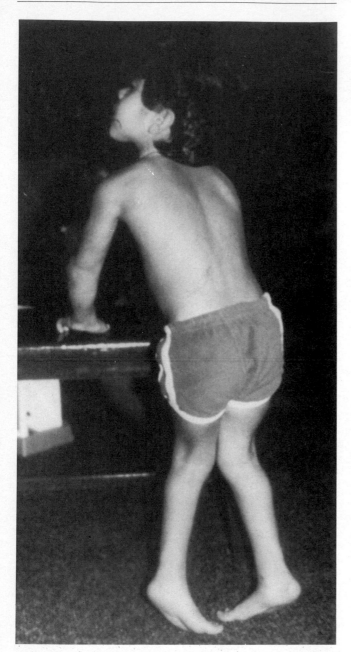

**Fig. 15–1**   Spastic diplegic child with typical adducted, internally rotated thighs, knee flexion and equinus.

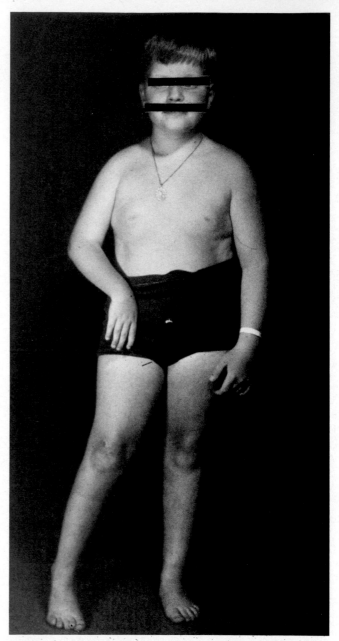

**Fig. 15–2**   Hemiplegic child with hip abducted, knee in extension and foot in equinovarus.

The author uses adductor tenotomy and obturator neurectomy in nonambulatory patients who are confined to a wheelchair, and in some of these patients, especially those under the age of 6, even a transfer is advisable because of its effectiveness in preventing hip flexion contracture.

### Medial Hamstring Tightness (Contracture)

In 1959, Phelps[7] described the internal rotation function of the gracilis muscle. He also believed it had a strong influence upon hip stability. However, the semitendinous and semimembranous muscles also can internally rotate the thigh.[8] If straight leg raising is less than 70 degrees and the leg internally rotates as it is being elevated, then the medial hamstrings are tight or contracted (Fig. 15–5). If so, they should be treated surgically. Proximal release of the hamstring muscles is not advised in the ambulatory patient because of frequent increase in lumbar lordosis following this procedure.[9] The author approaches them through a small longitudinal incision placed over the semitendinous tendon proximal to the flexion crease of the knee. The semitendinous tendon is transected, leaving a few filaments of tenosynovium intact. The gracilis is treated similarly, but only the aponeurosis of the semimembranous muscle is incised. Since the procedure is done with the patient supine, straight leg raising after the releases will stretch apart the aponeurosis of the semimembranous muscle, obtaining the desired length. It is not necessary to achieve more than 70 to 80 degrees of straight leg raising.

Postoperative immobilization should last two weeks, after which night extension splints are used for 6 to 12 weeks depending on the severity of the underlying spasticity.

### Hip Flexion Contracture

The crouched gait is often associated with tightness of the hip flexors, i.e., tensor fascia lata, rectus femoris, and iliopsoas muscles. If the patient has greater than 25 degrees of hip flexion contracture, exaggerated lordosis while walking, and a strongly positive Ely (or Duncan) test, then the hip flexors should be released or lengthened. In general, unless there is radiographic evidence of hip instability, the author does not lengthen the iliopsoas tendon.[10] Through a short, oblique incision distal to the anterior superioiliac spine, the tensor fascia lata muscle is identified and the aponeurosis and tight muscle fibers are transected.[11] Deeper in the wound, the straight and reflected heads of the rectus femoris are detached from their origins (Fig. 15–6). If hip instability is present, the psoas tendon can be easily isolated over the pubic ramis beneath the muscle mass of the iliacus and recessed by transecting the tendon. Postoperative cast immobilization is not necessary, and resumption of therapy and ambulation can begin as soon as the patient is comfortable.

### Femoral Anteversion

The cardinal sign of excessive femoral anteversion is an internal rotation walking pattern with inward deflection of the patella in the stance phase of gait. The second most telling clinical feature is an increased range of internal rotation in the prone position. These children characteristically sit in the "W" or "TV" position. Hip rotation is tested with the patient prone and the knees flexed (Figs. 15–7 and 15–8). Normal hips have a greater range of external rotation and usually the sum of both approximates 90 to 100 degrees. Thus, 60 degrees of external rotation and 30 degrees of internal rotation would be considered normal. In the diplegic or quadriplegic child, increased femoral anteversion is universal. Internal

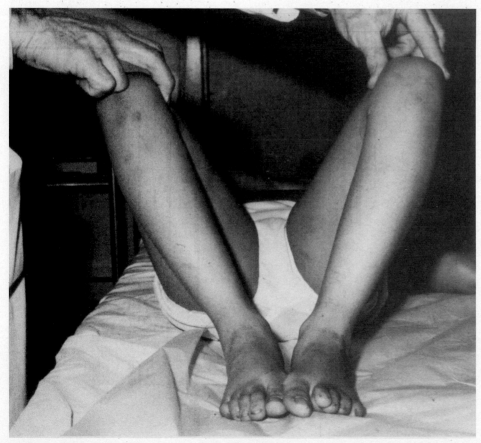

**Fig. 15–3** Maximum passive abduction of 20 degrees on right and 30 degrees on left.

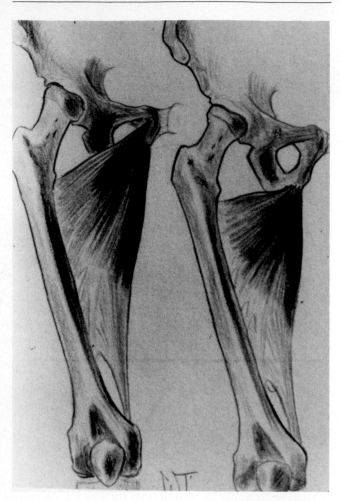

**Fig. 15–4**  Schematic drawing of position of transferred adductor muscles.

rotation can be from 50 to 90 degrees with external rotation being 40 to 0 degrees respectively. The excessive femoral anteversion is thought to be caused by delayed weightbearing and persistent muscle imbalance about the hips. Radiographs are helpful in measuring the degree of anteversion.[12-14] More recently the use of computed tomography has improved the accuracy of measurement of femoral anteversion. However, the author does not rely upon the "numbers." The important consideration is the axis of the femur in walking. The neutral knee that is slightly externally rotated provides for a smoother gait, not only for the hips but also for the knees and feet. In the author's experience, persistence of internal rotation of the thigh can lead to compensatory external tibial torsion and to severe pes valgus. Braces and therapy have been ineffectual in correcting femoral anteversion. If the child is over 6 years of age, the author recommends a derotation intertrochanteric osteotomy and usually adds a slight varus component. The goal is to provide adequate external rotation of the hip while leaving approximately 20 degrees of internal rotation to allow for normal hip internal rotation during gait.[15] The posterior approach to the hip is preferred, which allows excellent visualization of the osteotomy site and functional determination of the degree of rotation.[16]

### Hip Instability (Hip Subluxation and Dislocation)

Hip instability, which can lead to subluxation and dislocation (S/D), will not only interfere with walking abilities, but will create difficulties for the wheelchair

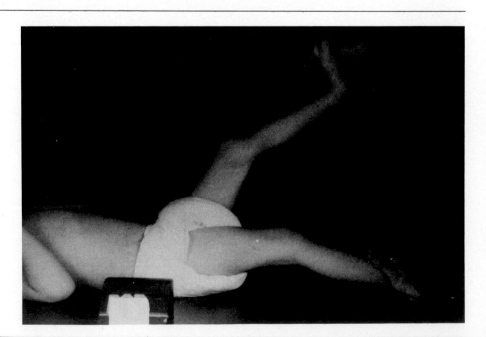

**Fig. 15–5**  Note tendency for internal rotation of thigh with passive straight leg raising caused by tight medial hamstring muscles.

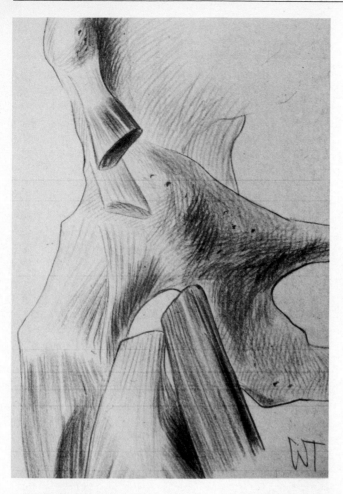

**Fig. 15–6**   Diagrammatic view of release of rectus femoris and sartorius (the latter is rarely necessary).

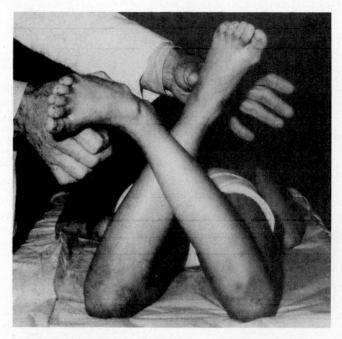

**Fig. 15–7**   Testing rotation of the hip prone. External rotation 20 degrees bilaterally.

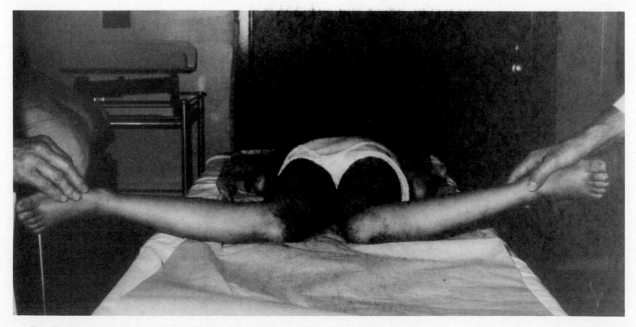

**Fig. 15–8**   Internal rotation 90 degrees bilaterally.

**Table 15–1**
**Incidence of hip dislocation in cerebral palsy**

| Study | Year | Percent |
|---|---|---|
| Gherlinzoni and Pais[24] | 1950 | 4.6 |
| Mathews et al[22] | 1953 | 2.6 |
| Tachdjian and Minear[25] | 1956 | 4.2 |
| Pollock and Sherrard[21] | 1958 | 23.0* |
| Phelps[7] | 1959 | 17.0 |
| Baker et al[26] | 1962 | 28.0 |
| Samilson et al[23] | 1972 | 28.0* |

*Represents subluxation and dislocation.

patient and eventually may lead to pain in both groups. Hip deformities in cerebral palsy rank second in frequency only to talipes equinus.[17-21] The incidence has been reported to be from as low as 2.6%[22] to as high as 28%.[23] See Table 15–1.[7,21-26] Baker and associates,[26] Samilson and associates,[23] and Hoffer and associates[27] have reported higher incidences of hip subluxation and dislocation in the patient with severe or total body involvement. Phelps[7] reported 17% and Pollock and Sharrard[21] reported 23% hip S/D in a general population. Although the incidence of hip S/D in the totally involved patient is greater, hip instability occurs with significant frequency in the paraplegic and diplegic patient.

### Etiology

Hip instability in the cerebral palsy patient is an acquired condition and the conditions that lead to this

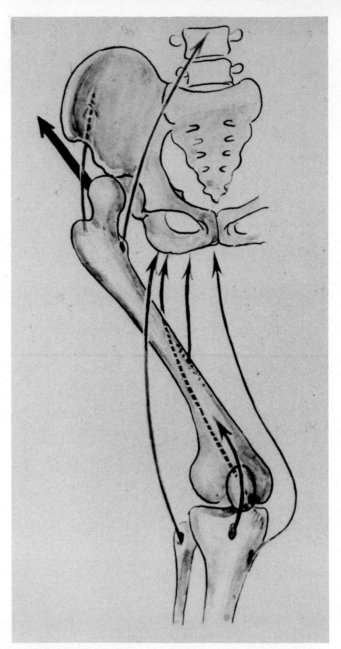

**Fig. 15–10** Muscle forces of the adductor pulling medially, iliopsoas in flexion and external rotation, and proximal pull of the quadriceps and hamstrings.

abnormality are present early. Initially there is exaggerated fetal femoral neck valgus and increased femoral anteversion that persists, especially when weight-bearing is delayed. Most important is the muscle imbalance caused by strong hip flexors, and adductors overpowering weaker hip abductors and extensors. Pelvic obliquity and scoliosis are often associated with hip dislocation. Samilson and associates[23] incriminated retained neonatal reflexes as another cause of abnormal posturing that leads to pelvic obliquity and hip instability.

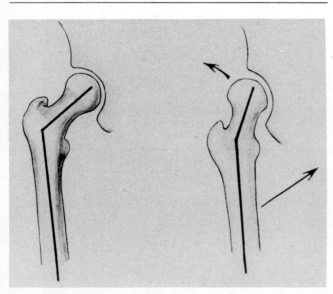

**Fig. 15–9** Schematic drawing of abnormal femoral anteversion and apparent coxa valga, positioning femoral head superiorly in the acetabulum with the hip in extension.

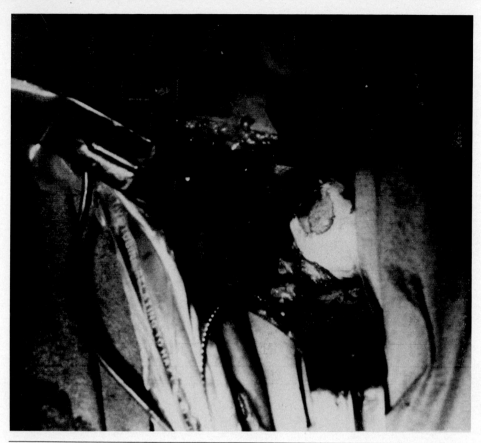

**Fig. 15-11** Superior lateral notching of the femoral head caused by pressure from overlying capsule and spastic abductor muscles.

## Natural History

If the muscle imbalance is not corrected and the thighs are adducted and flexed, the femoral head rotates to the superior margin of the acetabulum, and the anteverted position of the femoral head allows gradual subluxation of the hip (Figs. 15–9 and 15–10). In addition to the iliopsoas and the adductors exerting a dislocating force, the hamstrings, quadriceps and abductors pull the femoral head proximally. Once the femoral head escapes from the protection of the acetabulum, it is subjected to tremendous pressures by the overlying capsule and spastic abductor muscles. The growing femoral capital epiphysis develops classic notching of the superiolateral portion of the femoral head, which is pathognomonic of spastic dislocation (Fig. 15–11). In addition, the ligamentum teres is stretched and becomes hypertrophied, causing medial notching of the femoral head (Fig. 15–12) as described by Samilson and associates.[23] The deformed head often becomes painful in early adolescence or in young adulthood. If the hip dislocation is unilateral, pelvic obliquity occurs and pre-existing scoliosis can be accentuated.

## Treatment

Great emphasis has been placed upon physical therapy and abduction braces as a method of preventing hip deformities in patients with cerebral palsy. With mild spasticity these methods may indeed be helpful, but in the severely involved child bracing or positioning has not been found effective by the author. Children with severe involvement may benefit by a good physical therapy program, but if the muscle imbalance is severe, the hip will subluxate or dislocate despite these measures.

The only reliable prevention is surgery designed to balance the muscle power about the hips before subluxation occurs. If the adductors are tight, i.e., less than 40 degrees of abduction, these muscles should either be released or transferred. In the presence of a broken Shenton's line or mild subluxation, the iliopsoas muscle should either be recessed, transferred to the hip capsule, or released, depending upon the particular situation. Finally, if a fixed hip flexion contracture is present, the rectus femoris and tensor fascia lata muscles should be released. The iliopsoas tendon can be detached from the lesser trochanter through the same approach as the adductor muscle release or transfer (Fig. 15–13) or it can be reached through an anterior incision over the hip joint, isolated over the brim of the pelvis beneath the iliac muscle, and then transected.

Once subluxation occurs, particularly if the child is over 4 years of age, muscle releases alone will not

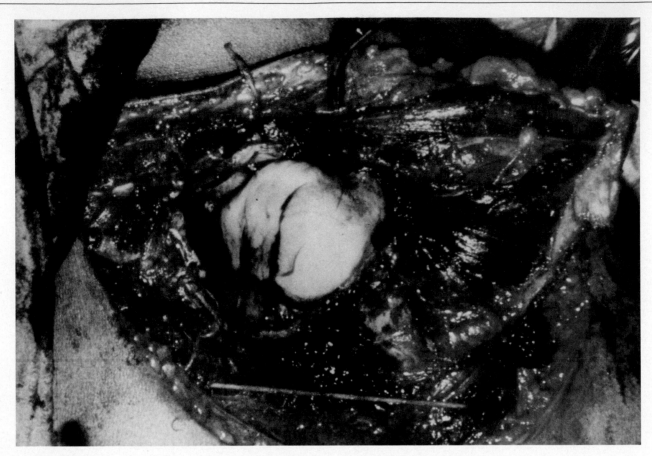

**Fig. 15–12** Hypertrophied ligamentum teres with underlying medial femoral head defect.

suffice to reduce the hip. Subluxation of the hip is a bony deformity. The axiom that a bone deformity cannot be corrected with a muscle transfer holds true. Naturally, appropriate muscle releases or transfers should be done, i.e., adductor release or transfer, hip flexor release including the iliopsoas tendon. At the same time the patient should have a varus rotation osteotomy (VRO) to direct the femoral head into the acetabulum (Fig. 15–14).

A VRO is a complex procedure. It is essentially a three-plane operation in which the surgeon must decrease the neck shaft valgus to approximately 115 degrees; must correct for anteversion, yet allow 20 degrees of internal rotation; and finally must avoid placing the hip in either an exaggerated flexed or extended position. In performing a VRO, it is essential that the osteotomy be at the level of the lesser trochanter and that firm internal fixation be used so that correction is not lost. This author prefers the posterior approach for this procedure, which allows the osteotomy site to be easily visualized. A postoperative hip spica cast is necessary for only three weeks. Its main purposes are to protect the hip, control muscle spasm, and make the patient more comfort-

able. After the cast is removed, the patient is started on active range of motion exercises and may be allowed to sit. At six weeks, a radiograph is taken and, if the osteotomy is well healed, ambulation can begin.

Three specific problems can occur in the postoperative period: (1) if the VRO is unilateral, it may cause shortening of the involved extremity (Fig. 15–15); (2) if the procedure is bilateral, it may take one year to regain preoperative levels of ambulation; (3) compensatory external tibial torsion often develops, and after the external femoral rotation, the tibia may have to be rotated internally in order to correct the external attitude of the foot (Fig. 15–16). The author performs this correction at the same time the hip plates are removed, approximately one year following VRO.

In late S/D, increased acetabular obliquity may prevent adequate reduction and stability even after a VRO. In these instances a pelvic osteotomy is required. Radiographs taken with the patient standing (if able), and an anteroposterior view of the pelvis with the hips in neutral and abduction are helpful in determining whether or not the acetabulum is sufficient. When the femoral head does not reduce well in the abducted position, a VRO will not suffice. In this case, a combined procedure consisting of an open reduction of the hip, a VRO with femoral shortening, and a pelvic osteotomy are necessary (Figs. 15–17 and 15–18). Numerous pelvic osteotomies have been described, but the author's experience has been with the Salter innominate osteotomy,[28,29] the Chiari osteotomy,[30,31] and the Sutherland double osteotomy.[32] In the younger child in whom there is a pliable pelvis, the Salter innominate osteotomy is preferable because the acetabular cartilage remains intact. In general, the acetabulum is larger than the femoral head so this option is acceptable. In unilateral cases with pelvic obliquity, the Salter innominate osteotomy is helpful in restoring leg length.

The Chiari osteotomy is preferable in children over 8 years of age. It provides good coverage but not

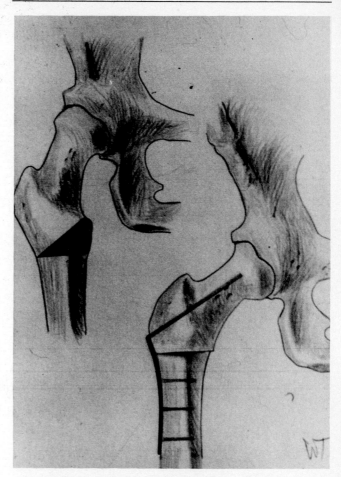

**Fig. 15–14** Schematic view of varus rotation osteotomy redirecting the femoral head centrally into the acetabulum.

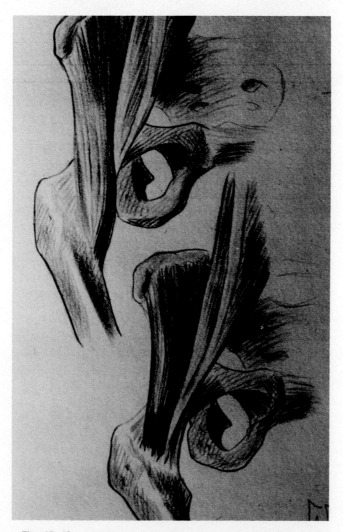

**Fig. 15–13** Recession of the iliopsoas tendon through medial approach with reattachment to the anterior portion of the hip capsule.

normal articular cartilage. The Sutherland double osteotomy attempts to rotate the entire hemipelvis over the femoral head, which is a technically difficult operation, but if done well, will provide good coverage.

Whatever pelvic osteotomy is performed, it is essential to shorten the femur in order to prevent excessive pressure on the femoral head. Although some believe these procedures should be done separately, the author's experience demonstrates that it is best done combined.[33] In 27 combined procedures in 23 patients, reduction was achieved in 75%. In the other 25%, some subluxation persisted but did not progress. Most importantly, after one year the hips of all patients were painless, although many patients experienced pain during the first year. Of 23 patients, 21 had generalized moderate to severe body involvement, whereas the other two were diplegic. The subluxated or dislocated hip should be reduced as long as there is any growth potential.

For the patient over 18 years of age with a painful

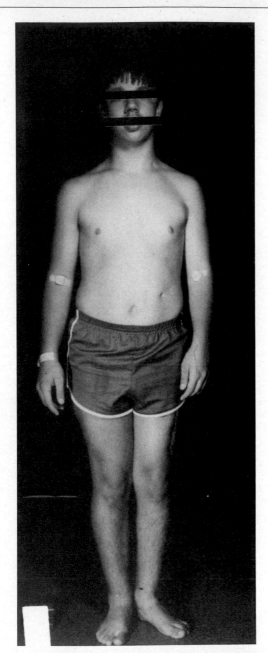

**Fig. 15–15**  Shortening of the left lower limb following varus rotation osteotomy.

excess muscle is sutured around the proximal end so that it does not articulate with the acetabulum. The author has performed this procedure only once, and follow-up is too short for comment. Causes for concern are the excessive difference in leg length if done unilaterally and whether or not the procedure will decrease the patient's ability to sit.

Valgus osteotomies have been advocated by both Samilson and associates[23] and Evans.[37] The femur is

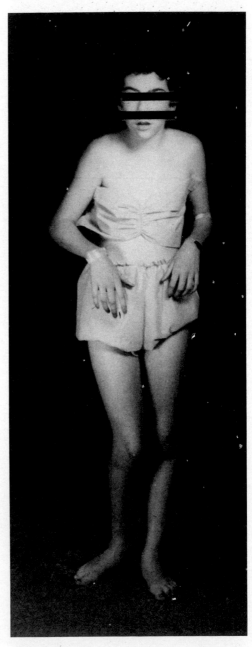

**Fig. 15–16**  The right thigh is in marked internal rotation caused by femoral anteversion, and the leg is externally rotated in an attempt to compensate for the proximal deformity.

S/D hip, the options are limited. The combined osteotomies will not be successful. The author's experience with head-neck resections (Girdlestone operations) has been poor, with patients continuing to have pain. Hoffer and associates,[27] Bleck,[34] and Samilson[35] also have reported poor results with the Girdlestone operation. A modified procedure consisting of proximal femoral resection with interposition of soft tissue has been described by Castle and Schneider.[36] Essentially, the upper third of the femur is excised and the

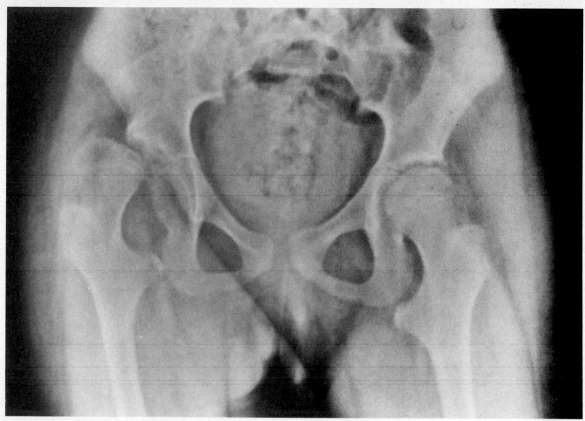

**Fig. 15–17**   An 8-year-old spastic quadriplegic girl with right hip subluxation and a very shallow acetabulum.

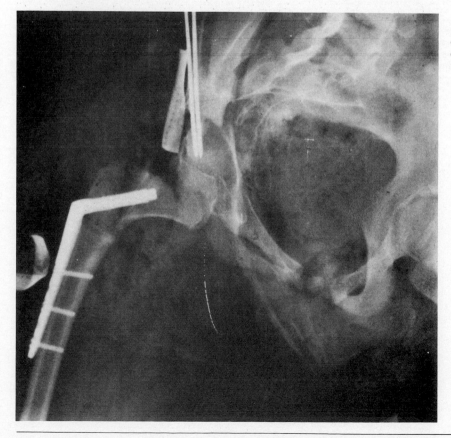

**Fig. 15–18** An interoperative radiograph demonstrating the combined pelvic osteotomy and femoral varus rotation osteotomy with shortening. The femoral head is well covered.

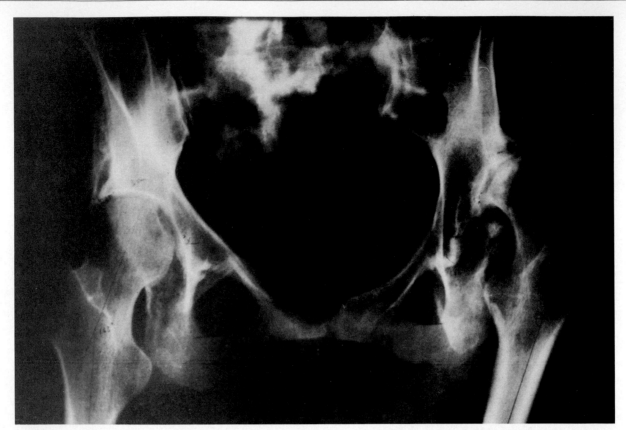

**Fig. 15–19**  A 28-year-old spastic quadriplegic woman with painful left hip subluxation.

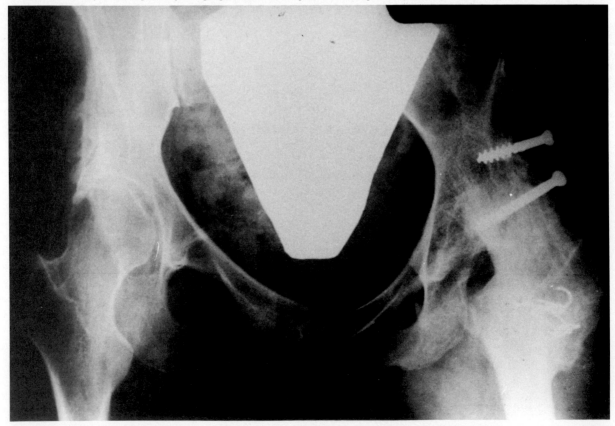

**Fig. 15–20**  The same patient four years following fusion. There is no pain and sitting is comfortable.

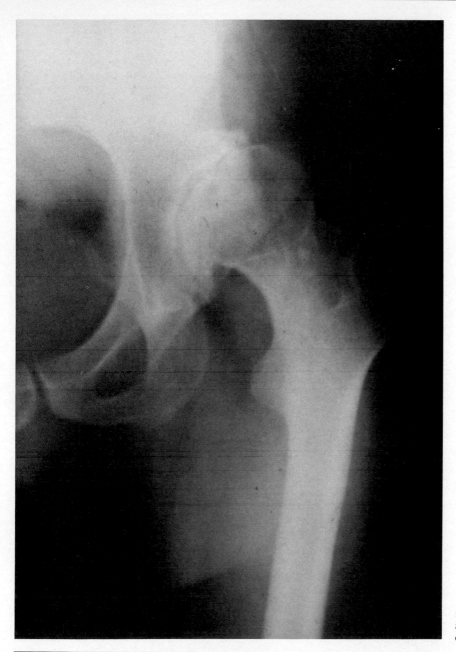

**Fig. 15–21** A 42-year-old spastic diplegic man with painful subluxation of the left hip and evidence of degenerative osteoarthritic changes.

abducted after an osteotomy is performed in the intertrochanteric region. The proximal femoral component is then allowed to rest against the pelvic brim. The author has had no experience with this method, but Samilson and associates did state[23] that with the hips in abduction, it is often difficult to have the patient sit comfortably in a wheelchair.

As salvage procedures for the painful S/D hip, the author has performed and recommends either hip arthrodesis or total hip replacements.[38] Both of these are major procedures but nevertheless have proved successful. With a solid hip arthrodesis, a patient can obtain a painless stable hip and have minimal restriction of activities (Figs. 15–19 and 15–20). An ideal candidate for a hip fusion is one who has unilateral hip instability and has no lower spine abnormality and generally would be a younger patient, either ambulatory or confined to a wheelchair. In the eight cases reported by the author, only two patients required repeat surgery for pseudoarthrosis.[38]

Total hip replacement is also reliable in relieving pain and improving mobility. Initially, it was feared that the patient with cerebral palsy would not tolerate a total hip replacement, and it would loosen quickly

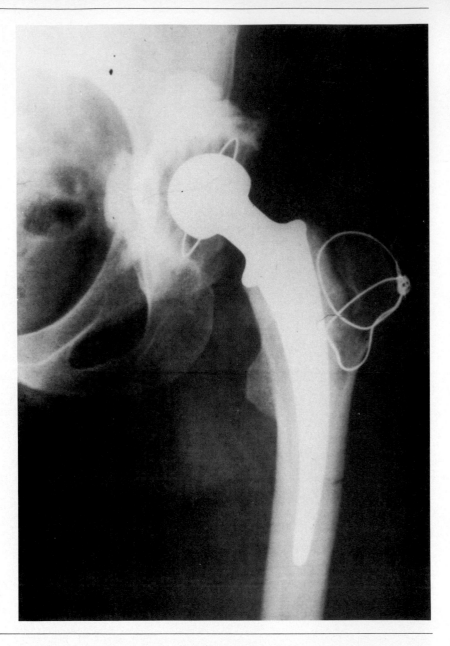

**Fig. 15–22**   The same patient one year following left total hip replacement. Patient is asymptomatic and has resumed walking with crutches.

and fail. However, in 15 cases with a minimum of a 2.6-year follow-up, only one case showed evidence of loosening, and that was seven years following surgery (Figs. 15–21 to 15–23).

## Summary

The two major problems of the hip in cerebral palsy relate to gait abnormalities and hip instability. Gait abnormalities are a result of muscle imbalance and should be corrected with appropriate muscle transfers and releases. Frequently, femoral anteversion may be associated with internal rotation of the limb, and if severe, should be corrected.

Hip instability leading to S/D is a very serious problem in cerebral palsy and is usually worse in the more severely involved patients. Early muscle releases should be done before the hips subluxate. Once subluxation occurs, muscle releases must be combined with a varus rotation osteotomy. If acetabular insufficiency is present, pelvic osteotomy is necessary to obtain stability. In the older patient who has a painful S/D hip, the author recommends either a hip arthrodesis or a total hip replacement.

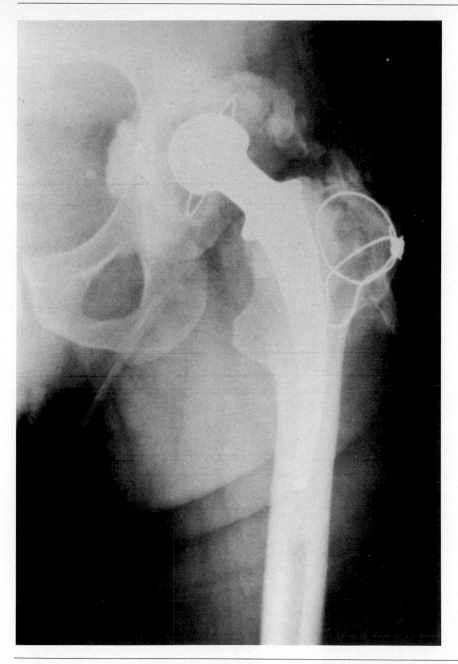

**Fig. 15–23** The same patient ten years following left total hip replacement. Prosthesis remains in good alignment without evidence of loosening. The formation of heterotopic bone has not caused pain or decreased function.

## References

1. Sharrard WJW, Allen JMH, Heaney SH: Surgical prophylaxis of subluxation and dislocation of the hip in cerebral palsy. *J Bone Joint Surg* 1975;57B:160–166.
2. Banks HH, Green WT: Adductor myotomy and obturator neurectomy for correction of the hip in cerebral palsy. *J Bone Joint Surg* 1960;42A:111–126.
3. Keats S: Combined adductor-gracilis tenotomy and selective obturator-nerve resection for correction of adduction deformity of the hip in children with cerebral palsy. *J Bone Joint Surg* 1951;33A:698.
4. Couch WH, DeRosa GP, Throop FB: Thigh adductor transfer for spastic cerebral palsy. *Dev Med Child Neurol* 1977;19:343–349.
5. Griffin PP, Wheelhouse WW, Shievi R: The adductor transfer for adductor spasticity: A clinical and electromyographical gait analysis. *Orthop Trans* 1977;1:76.
6. Root L, Spero CR: Results of the adductor transfer as compared to adductor tenotomy neurectomy in cerebral palsy. *J Bone Joint Surg* 1981;63A:767.
7. Phelps WM: Prevention of acquired dislocation of the hip in cerebral palsy. *J Bone Joint Surg* 1959;41A:440.
8. Sutherland DH, Schottstaedt ER, Larsen LJ, et al: Clinical and electromyographic study of seven spastic children with internal rotation gait. *J Bone Joint Surg* 1969;51A:1070.
9. Drummond DS, Rogala E, Templeton J, et al: Proximal hamstring release for knee flexion and crouched gait in cerebral palsy. *J Bone Joint Surg* 1974;56A:1598.
10. Bleck EE: Surgical management of spastic flexion deformities

of the hip with special reference to iliopsoas recession. *J Bone Joint Surg* 1971;53A:1468–1488.

11. Roosth HP: Flexion deformity of the hip and knee in spastic cerebral palsy: Treatment by early release of spastic hip-flexor muscles. Technique and results in thirty-seven cases. *J Bone Joint Surg* 1971;53A:1489–1510.

12. Dunlap K, Shand AR, et al: A new method for determination of torsion of the femur. *J Bone Joint Surg* 1953;35A:289.

13. Magilligan DJ: Calculation of the angle of anteversion by means of horizontal lateral roentgenography. *J Bone Joint Surg* 1956;38A:1231.

14. Muller ME: Ischiometric and radiologique. *Rev Chir Orthop* 1956;42:124–133.

15. Murray MP, Drought AB, Kory RC: Walking patterns of normal men. *J Bone Joint Surg* 1964;46A:335.

16. Root L, Siegal T: Osteotomy of the hip in children: Posterior approach. *J Bone Joint Surg* 1980;62A:571–575.

17. Bleck EE, Holstein A: Iliopsoas tenotomy for spastic hip flexion deformities in cerebral palsy. Presented at the Annual Meeting of the American Academy of Orthopaedic Surgeons, Chicago, 1963.

18. Bleck EE: Orthopaedic management of cerebral palsy. *Saunders Monograph in Clinical Orthopaedics.* Philadelphia, WB Saunders, 1979.

19. Nelson KB, Ellenberg JH: Epidemiology of cerebral palsy, in Schoenberg BS(ed): *Advances in Neurology.* New York, Raven Press, 1978, vol 19, p 421.

20. Pollack GA: Surgical treatment of cerebral palsy. *J Bone Joint Surg* 1962;44B:68.

21. Pollock GA, Sharrard WJW: Orthopaedic surgery in the treatment of cerebral palsy, in Illingworth RS (ed): *Recent Advances in Cerebral Palsy.* London, J & A Churchill, 1958, p 286.

22. Mathews SS, Jones MH, Sperling SC: Hip derangements seen in cerebral palsied children. *Am J Phys Med* 1953;32:213–221.

23. Samilson RL, Tsou P, Aamoth G, et al: Dislocation and subluxation of the hip in cerebral palsy. *J Bone Joint Surg* 1972;54A:863–873.

24. Gherlinzoni G, Pais C: Trattamento della lussazione patologica dell'ance: Indicazioni, tecnica e resultati lontani. *Chir Organi Mov* 1950;34:335–437.

25. Tachdjian MO, Minear WL: Hip dislocation in cerebral palsy. *J Bone Joint Surg* 1956;38A:1358–1364.

26. Baker LD, Dodelin ND, Bassett FH: Pathological changes in the hip in cerebral palsy; incidence, pathogenesis, and treatment. *J Bone Joint Surg* 1962;44A:1331.

27. Hoffer MM, Abraham E, Nickel VL: Salvage surgery at the hip to improve sitting posture of mentally retarded, severely disabled children with cerebral palsy. *Dev Med Child Neurol* 1972;14:51.

28. Salter RB: Innominate osteotomy in the treatment of congenital dislocation and subluxation of the hip. *J Bone Joint Surg* 1961;43B:518.

29. Salter RB, Dubos JP: The first fifteen years' personal experience with innominate osteotomy in the treatment of congenital dislocation and subluxation of the hip. *Clin Orthop* 1974;98:72–103.

30. Chiari K: Medial displacement osteotomy of the pelvis. *Clin Orthop* 1974;98:55–71.

31. Salvati EA, Wilson PD: Treatment of irreducible hip subluxation by Chiari's iliac osteotomy: A report of results in 19 cases. *Clin Orthop* 1974;98:151–161.

32. Sutherland DH, Greenfield R: Double innominate osteotomy. *J Bone Joint Surg* 1977;59A:1082–1091.

33. Root L, Brourman SN: Combined pelvic osteotomy with open reduction and femoral shortening for dislocated hip. Presented at the Annual Meeting of the Pediatric Orthopaedic Society, San Antonio, Texas, 1985.

34. Bleck EE: Hip deformities in cerebral palsy, in American Academy of Orthopaedic Surgeons *Instructional Course Lectures, XX.* St Louis, CV Mosby Co, 1971, pp 54–82.

35. Samilson R: Dislocation of the hip in cerebral palsy. Presented at the Annual Meeting of the American Academy for Cerebral Palsy and Developmental Medicine, Houston, Texas, October 1970.

36. Castle ME, Schneider C: Proximal femoral resection-interposition arthroplasty. *J Bone Joint Surg* 1978;60A:1051.

37. Evans EB: Personal communication, 1986.

38. Root L, Goss JR, Mendes J: The treatment of the painful hip in cerebral palsy by total hip replacement or hip arthrodesis. *J Bone Joint Surg* 1986;68A:590–598.

# The Orthopaedic Management of the Ankle, Foot, and Knee in Patients With Cerebral Palsy

Neil E. Green, MD

## Introduction

Cerebral palsy results from a nonprogressive cerebral lesion acquired in the perinatal period. Clinical manifestations depend upon the area or areas of the brain that have been damaged. This discussion will be devoted primarily to spasticity, the most common of the physical manifestations resulting from the cerebral insult.

If only one cerebral hemisphere has been injured, the patient will manifest a spastic hemiplegia involving the upper and lower extremities on the side opposite the cerebral lesion. In patients with a spastic diplegia, the lower extremities are involved, with generally very minor upper extremity involvement, which may only be detectable with fine motor testing. A child with spastic quadriplegia will manifest involvement of all four extremities.

## The Ankle

### Equinus Deformity

An equinus deformity of the ankle is the result of muscular imbalance between the triceps surae and the anterior tibialis. Although the anterior tibial muscle is frequently functional, it may be overpowered by a very spastic triceps surae. A child with spastic cerebral palsy will begin ambulation as a toe walker because of an imbalance between the plantar flexors and the dorsiflexors of the ankle. The age at which the child begins walking will depend upon the type of cerebral palsy and the severity of the neurologic damage. Children with a spastic hemiplegia will usually begin walking between the ages of 18 and 21 months, unless the lesion is severe. Children with spastic diplegia will usually begin walking by the age of 48 months, and those with spastic quadriplegia will generally walk later, if at all.[1]

In children with cerebral palsy, the equinus deformity is the most common deformity requiring care. Early attempts at bracing this deformity will be futile. A short-leg brace with a high-top shoe will effectively hide it. A plastic solid ankle-foot orthosis may provide more control of the ankle, but it will not usually prevent the child from toe walking. None of these devices will prevent the development of an equinus deformity requiring surgical release. Some authors have tried short-leg (inhibitive) casting with short-

term success; however, Achilles tendon lengthening will usually be required to correct the equinus deformity and is, therefore, the definitive treatment.[2]

The timing of this procedure depends upon other problems in the lower extremities and the overall physical abilities of the child. The equinus deformity may worsen the child's balance. A heel cord lengthening is indicated to reduce the stretch reflex and to reduce a fixed contracture in an ambulatory child, but it should be noted that any muscle lengthening will weaken that muscle. Heel cord lengthening may also be performed in a child who is cruising (walking holding onto an object) and who might be able to walk independently if not for the equinus deformity. It is also frequently performed in conjunction with other procedures of the lower extremities. In fact, it is preferable to perform all procedures on the legs of a spastic child at one time, as this approach allows the child to continue ambulating and also avoids the repeated hospitalization of the child.[1,3] At one time, it was common practice to stage surgical procedures on children with cerebral palsy, performing one operation each year—a practice which served only to increase the hospital census.

The triceps surae may be lengthened in three ways: (1) lengthening the gastrocnemius fascia only, (2) anterior translocation of the heel cord, and (3) lengthening of the heel cord itself.

Each type of selective gastrocnemius lengthening (e.g., Vulpius, Strayer, and Baker) lengthens the gastrocnemius while leaving the soleus intact.[1,4,5] Until recently, the decision to perform a selective gastrocnemius lengthening has been based on results of the Silfverskiöld test. Because the gastrocnemius muscle originates on the distal femur and can thus be relaxed if the knee is flexed, Silfverskiöld hypothesized that if a heel cord was tight with the knee both extended and flexed, the soleus and the gastrocnemius were both responsible for the heel cord contracture; if the heel cord was tight when the knee was extended but not flexed, only the gastrocnemius was responsible for the Achilles tightness. Unfortunately, Perry and associates[6] have shown this hypothesis to be unreliable. In addition, the recurrence rate of heel cord contracture is 30% with gastrocnemius lengthening only versus 10% with complete heel cord lengthening.[1]

Anterior translocation of the heel cord requires complete detachment of the insertion of the heel cord from its insertion on the os calcis, with reinsertion of the tendon into the os calcis anterior to the original insertion.[7] This procedure has yielded good results, although it involves much more dissection than does a simple Achilles tendon lengthening.

The Achilles tendon may be lengthened by performing either a Z lengthening or a sliding lengthening. The Z lengthening is frequently used for the correction of club feet, and the sliding lengthening is generally preferred for the correction of heel cord tightness resulting from spastic conditions. The sliding lengthening provides better control of the tendon than does the Z lengthening, since the tendon retains continuity, making suturing of the tendon unnecessary. Overlengthening is, therefore, much less likely with a sliding lengthening than with a Z lengthening.

Several types of heel cord lengthenings have been employed. The triple lengthening described by Hoke is easily performed and yields good reproducible results (Fig. 16–1). In this procedure, the Achilles tendon is exposed through a posterior medial incision made halfway between the medial malleolus and the most posterior aspect of the heel cord. The position of the incision will keep the scar away from the heel of the shoe and should prevent the development of a painful scar. The sheath of the Achilles tendon is split longitudinally and preserved. Three transverse half-cuts are made in the tendon; the most proximal and most distal cuts are made medially, and

the middle cut is made laterally. A 15-gauge knife blade is inserted longitudinally into the Achilles tendon in the exact midportion of the tendon. The first proximal cut is placed just distal to the musculotendinous junction. The knife is turned medially and the medial half of the tendon is completely severed. This same procedure is repeated as far distally in the tendon as possible. The final cut is made midway between these two medial cuts. This middle cut is directed laterally. Once these cuts have been made, the foot is dorsiflexed just to neutral, allowing the tendon ends to slide on themselves. The tendon retains its continuity and no suturing is necessary. Postoperatively, a long-leg plaster cast is applied with the foot dorsiflexed to neutral and the knee straight but not hyperextended. Full weightbearing is allowed as soon as the plaster is dry. This cast may be changed to a short-leg cast in two or three weeks. The short-leg cast is worn for three to four weeks.

Postoperative bracing may be required to prevent recurrence of the equinus deformity if the patient does not have a functioning anterior tibial muscle. If the anterior tibial muscle functions voluntarily and has good strength, the postoperative gait will most likely be good and the equinus contracture should not recur. If the anterior tibial muscle functions only with the withdrawal reflex (flexion of the hip, knee, and ankle simultaneously), the gait will be improved,

**Fig. 16–1** Hoke triple cut Achilles tendon lengthening. Two half cuts are made on the medial side of the tendon, and one is made between these two cuts on the lateral side, also cutting one half of the diameter of the tendon. When the foot is dorsiflexed, the tendon ends slide on themselves, thereby lengthening the Achilles tendon but maintaining continuity in the tendon itself so that suturing is not necessary. (Reproduced with permission from Bleck EE: *Orthopaedic Management of Cerebral Palsy.* Philadelphia, WB Saunders, 1979, p 121.)

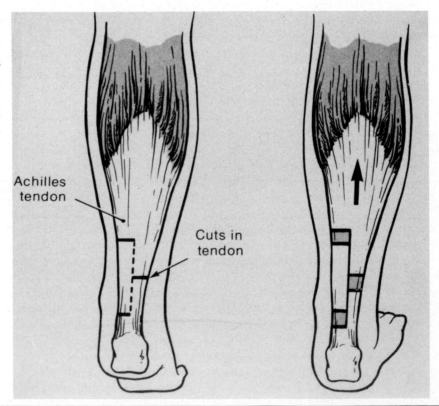

Achilles tendon

Cuts in tendon

but a steppage gait will continue. In this instance, since dorsiflexion can be accomplished only with a withdrawal, the hip and knee are flexed more than normal during swing to enable the foot to be dorsiflexed. These patients without volitional control of the anterior tibial muscle may require postoperative bracing to prevent recurrence. However, the child with no function in the anterior tibial muscle will require prolonged bracing to prevent recurrence of the equinus contracture. Bracing is usually accomplished with a solid plastic ankle-foot orthosis.

Complications of heel cord lengthening are rare, but a calcaneus deformity may occur. It may result from an overlengthened heel cord but is more commonly seen after an inappropriate Achilles tendon lengthening, in which a hamstring lengthening is not performed, or when a spastic posterior tibial tendon is transferred to the dorsum of the foot at the same time a heel cord lengthening is performed, or in patients with athetosis.

Because of their continuous movements, patients with athetosis will rarely develop a fixed joint deformity. A patient with tension athetosis may not, however, exhibit these gross movements and therefore may not be recognized as having athetosis. Lengthening of the heel cord in such a patient may result in a calcaneus deformity because the balance of the plantar flexors and the dorsiflexors of the foot has been changed. The weakened triceps surae is unable to balance the athetoid foot dorsiflexors, and a calcaneus deformity results.

A varus deformity of the foot is commonly seen along with an equinus deformity in patients with hemiplegia. The posterior tibial muscle is frequently the cause of the varus deformity, and transfer of this muscle to the dorsum of the foot in combination with a heel cord lengthening may result in a calcaneus deformity. This deformity will be discussed further in the section dealing with pes equinovarus.

In patients with hamstring tightening, failure to lengthen the hamstring muscles at the time of heel cord lengthening is the second most common cause of calcaneus deformity after heel cord lengthening. It should be remembered that the entire leg is involved in the spasticity. For example, the crouched gait may be caused by multiple joint contractures. A crouched gait may develop in a child who walks with bilateral equinus contractures and who undergoes only a heel cord lengthening. Preoperatively, this child will have kept the knees extended despite significant hamstring tightness and spasticity, because equinus position of the feet forces the knees into extension during the stance phase of gait. Once the heel cords have been lengthened, the knees are no longer forced to extend during stance, but instead remain flexed because of significant tightness of the hamstrings, causing the child to crouch. The crouched position forces the

tibia forward at the ankle, producing a calcaneus posture, which can be prevented by performing a hamstring lengthening at the same time the heel cord is lengthened.

## The Foot

### Pes Equinovarus

A varus hindfoot will usually occur in conjunction with an equinus deformity, although varus is occasionally seen without a concomitant equinus deformity, especially if only a heel cord lengthening is performed in a patient with a spastic equinovarus deformity. The varus hindfoot usually occurs in patients with a hemiplegia, although it is occasionally seen in a patient with a quadriplegia, especially if the spasticity is very asymmetrical. This level of involvement is frequently referred to as a bilateral hemiplegia because of the asymmetry.

The cause of the varus deformity is muscle imbalance. The peroneal muscles are usually weak in patients with a hemiplegia, and either the posterior tibial muscle or the anterior tibial muscle is spastic. A gait study is sometimes required to determine which of these two muscles is the cause of the varus deformity. In children with a hemiplegia secondary to perinatal causes, the spasticity of the posterior tibial muscle usually produces the varus deformity. In these patients, the anterior muscle is frequently weak or nonfunctional. A hemiplegia that occurs later in life may result in overactivity of the anterior tibial muscle with resultant pes varus.

If the varus deformity is the result of overactivity of the anterior tibial muscle with the resultant midfoot varus, a split anterior tibial tendon transfer (SPLATT) will correct the deformity.[8] The split anterior tibial tendon transfer is performed by first exposing the insertion of the anterior tibial tendon and splitting it longitudinally, leaving the medial half of the tendon attached to the foot (Fig. 16–2A). A second longitudinal incision is made over the musculotendinous junction of the anterior tibial muscle, and the split in the tendon is continued all the way to the musculotendinous junction. A third incision is made over the cuboid, exposing the entire bone. Two drill holes spaced as far apart as possible are made in the cuboid. These holes are connected within the substance of the cuboid so that the tendon may be passed through the holes to be sutured onto itself. The split lateral portion of the anterior tibial tendon is passed subcutaneously distally to exit into the incision that was previously made over the cuboid. The tendon is then passed through the holes in the cuboid and sutured onto itself under moderate tension (Fig. 16–2B). The foot should lie in neutral position (Fig. 16–2C). The foot is immobilized in a long-leg cast if

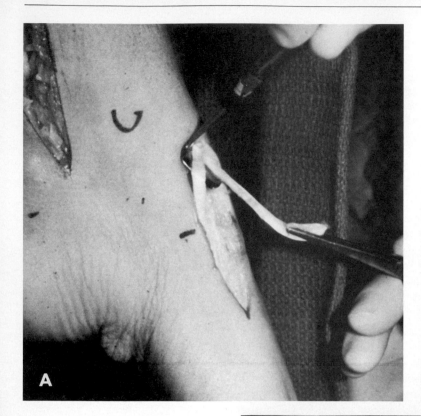

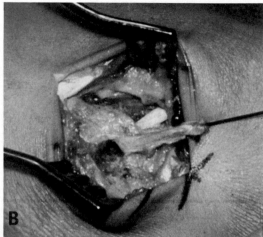

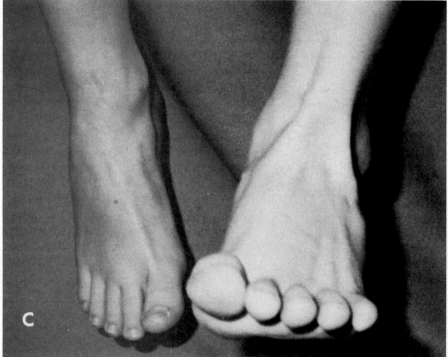

**Fig. 16–2**   Split anterior tibial tendon transfer (SPLATT). **A:** The first incision exposes the insertion of the anterior tibial tendon, and the tendon is split longitudinally as far proximally as possible. The medial half of the tendon is left attached to the first metatarsal and first cuneiform, but the lateral half is detached from its insertion. The forceps holds the detached lateral half of the anterior tibial tendon. The retractor is underneath the medial half of the tendon. The medial malleolus is outlined. **B:** The anterior tibial tendon is split as far proximally as the musculotendinous junction. The split lateral half of the tendon is then passed subcutaneously into the incision made over the cuboid. It is then passed into the holes made in the cuboid, and sutured to itself under moderate tension. The split lateral portion of the anterior tibial tendon is seen passing through the drill holes in the cuboid. The ankle is to the right of the photograph and the toes are to the left. **C:** The split anterior tibial tendon transfer serves as a sling to maintain the midfoot and forefoot in neutral, because the pull of the muscle is equally split between the medial and lateral halves of the tendon. Notice the equalization of pull on both ends of the tendon so that the forefoot is dorsiflexed into a neutral position.

the heel cord has been lengthened, or a short-leg cast if not. Immobilization is continued for six weeks.

The most frequent cause of hindfoot varus in the child with spastic cerebral palsy is the spastic posterior tibial muscle. Many solutions have been proposed to treat the varus deformity secondary to the spasticity of this muscle. A simple tenotomy of the posterior tibial tendon is easily performed, but as this procedure usually results in a valgus deformity with breakdown of the longitudinal arch, it should not be performed. Anterior transposition of the posterior tibial tendon as described by Baker and Hill[9] involves rerouting the tendon anterior to the medial malleolus, decreasing its plantar flexor force. Although the posterior tibial muscle is effectively lengthened by this technique, the deformity may not be corrected because the muscle retains its varus pull. In addition, if the muscle is continuously spastic, a calcaneus deformity may result because the posterior tibial muscle has been converted into an ankle dorsiflexor as a result of the transposition.[10]

Anterior transfer of the posterior tibial muscle through the interosseous membrane is a very attractive procedure, because it removes the actual deforming force and balances the absent or weak anterior tibial and peroneal muscles. This procedure is effective in patients with nonspastic paralytic equinovarus deformities of the foot. Some surgeons have reported successful treatment of the spastic foot by performing an anterior transfer of the posterior tibial muscle, but others have reported that it produces a calcaneovalgus deformity.[11,12] To understand this discrepancy, it must be realized that in some spastic feet the posterior tibial muscle is continuously spastic, whereas in others it is a phasic muscle. In those feet in which the posterior tibial muscle is phasic, the muscle fires appropriately and will not likely cause a calcaneus deformity if transferred. A continuously spastic posterior tibial muscle, on the other hand, will maintain its constant spasticity when transferred, and if a heel cord lengthening accompanies the anterior transfer of the posterior tibial muscle, a calcaneus deformity will likely result. A gait study can reveal whether the posterior tibial muscle is continuously firing or phasic. Because the results of this transfer are so variable, it is difficult to recommend it for the treatment of the varus hindfoot in the spastic patient.

Lengthening of the posterior tibial tendon has produced good results according to those who have reported this procedure.[1,13] The only problems reported have been the occasional recurrence in the very spastic foot, and the production of a calcaneovalgus foot if the tendon is lengthened excessively at the same time a heel cord lengthening is performed. The tendon is best lengthened by performing a sliding or fractional lengthening, which is accomplished by making two transverse or oblique cuts completely through the tendon. These cuts must be made well proximal to the musculotendinous junction. By performing the oblique cuts within the musculotendinous portion of the tendon, the muscle fibers that insert into the tendon distal to the level of the cuts prevent complete transection of the musculotendinous unit. The lengthening is therefore well controlled.

Split posterior tibial tendon transfer (SPOTT) may be performed to balance the flexible spastic varus foot[14,15] and is an attractive alternative to lengthening, because with it the plantar flexion power of the posterior tibial muscle is retained, thereby decreasing the chance of a calcaneus deformity. In addition, because half of the tendon is transferred to the lateral side of the foot, the weak peroneal muscles are balanced; and because half of the tendon is left in its original insertion, a valgus deformity should not occur.

Three or four incisions are required for performing the split posterior tibial tendon transfer—two medial and either one or two laterally. The first medial incision is made over the insertion of the posterior tibial tendon on the tarsal navicular, extending proximally for about 3 cm. The posterior tibial tendon is split longitudinally and the plantar half of the tendon is detached from its insertion on the navicular, leaving the dorsal half of the tendon intact. The longitudinal split is continued as far proximally as the wound permits. A second incision is made posterior to the medial malleolus (Fig. 16–3A). In most instances, a heel cord lengthening is performed simultaneously, and this second incision is the one used for that purpose. The longitudinally split tendon is brought into this wound, and the longitudinal split is continued to the level of the musculotendinous junction (Fig. 16–3B). The split portion of the tendon is then passed posterior to the tibia and fibula but anterior to the neurovascular structures, and anterior to the toe-flexor muscles and the heel cord. A third incision is made on the lateral side of the foot just posterior to the lateral malleolus. This incision may curve distally following the peroneal muscles, or it may be interrupted and two separate incisions used. The slit tendon is passed into the lateral wound and then passed distally with the peroneus brevis muscle. The split posterior tibial tendon is passed in and out of two or three small splits made in the peroneus brevis tendon and sutured to this tendon under maximal tension (Fig. 16–3C). At the end of the procedure, the foot should lie in neutral to slightly valgus position, because the split tendon itself serves as a dynamic sling to balance the spasticity of the posterior tibial muscle (Fig. 16–3D).

The split posterior tibial tendon transfer should correct a hindfoot varus if the deformity is flexible. If the hindfoot has a fixed deformity, a lateral closing

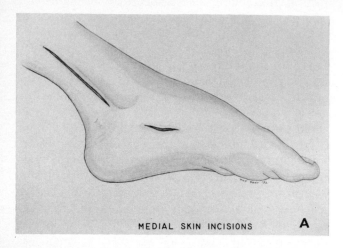

MEDIAL SKIN INCISIONS    **A**

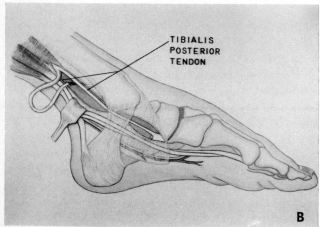

TIBIALIS
POSTERIOR
TENDON

**B**

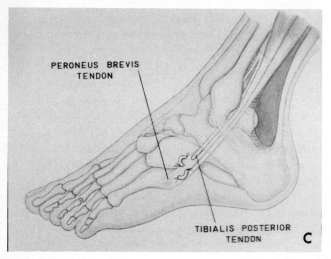

PERONEUS BREVIS
TENDON

TIBIALIS POSTERIOR
TENDON    **C**

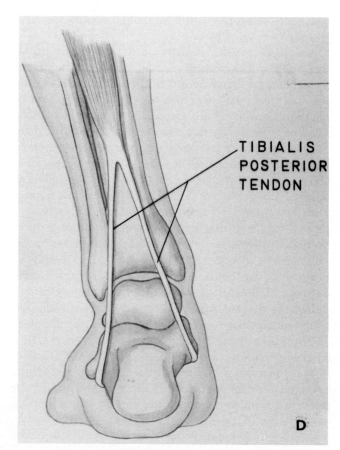

TIBIALIS
POSTERIOR
TENDON

**D**

**Fig. 16–3**    The split posterior tibial tendon transfer (SPOTT). **A:** Two medial incisions are used to expose the posterior tibial tendon. The first is made distally over the insertion of the tendon on the navicular. The second is a longitudinal incision made posterior to the medial malleolus. It is situated halfway between the medial malleolus and the posterior aspect of the heel cord. This is the incision used for a heel cord lengthening, which is usually performed in conjunction with a split posterior tibial tendon transfer. **B:** The posterior tibial tendon is split longitudinally as far proximally as the musculotendinous junction. One half of the tendon is left attached to the navicular, but the other half is detached and brought into the proximal wound. **C:** The split portion of the posterior tibial tendon has been passed posterior to the tibia and fibula but anterior to the neurovascular bundle and tendons to exit just posterior to the lateral malleolus. The tendon is passed usually distally with the peroneus brevis tendon, and then sutured to it by weaving the posterior tibial tendon through the peroneus brevis tendon under maximal tension. **D:** The two ends of the posterior tibial tendon balance each other so that when the posterior tibial muscle contracts, the tendons pull equally on the medial and lateral side of the foot, thereby preventing the development of a varus or valgus deformity. (Reproduced with permission from Green NE, Griffin PP, Shiavi R: Split posterior tibial tendon transfer in spastic cerebral palsy. *J Bone Joint Surg* 1983;65A:748–754.)

edge osteotomy of the os calcis must be performed at the same time as the split posterior tibial tendon transfer to correct the bony deformity.

### Pes Valgus

The etiology of pes valgus is complex in the child with spastic cerebral palsy. Whereas the varus hindfoot occurs more commonly in the patient with a hemiparesis, a valgus deformity of the foot is usually the result of a spastic diplegia or quadriplegia. Children with a pes valgus will usually have an associated equinus deformity that may be either dynamic or fixed. In addition, in order for a valgus deformity to develop, the child must have inherent ligament laxity. If laxity is not present, the foot with an equinus deformity would remain in equinus. If ligament laxity is present, then although the hindfoot remains in equinus, the midfoot and the hindfoot deviate into valgus and the midfoot dorsiflexes, allowing the foot to be plantargrade. This situation occurs at the expense of breakdown of the midfoot. It is not, however, the only cause of the valgus foot. Spasticity of the peroneal muscles tends to pull the foot into valgus. In 1982, Bonnett and associates[16] reported the results of gait analyses of the feet and legs of patients with spastic diplegia and found that the posterior tibial muscle was either very weak or nonfunctional in patients who also had a pes valgus.

The evaluation of the equinovalgus foot requires a thorough physical examination. The amount of equinus and whether it is flexible or rigid must be determined. In addition, the degree of valgus deformity must be determined. This deformity may also be either flexible or rigid. Radiographs are helpful in assessing the degree of the valgus deformity; however, they should be taken with the patient in the standing position to simulate weightbearing. In addition, a standing anteroposterior radiograph of the ankle must be obtained to determine if the valgus deformity is in the foot or in the ankle joint (Fig. 16–4).

The physical consequences of a valgus deformity are usually less severe than those of a comparable varus deformity, since the valgus position of the foot is not unstable for the child. If the deformity is severe, a painful callus may develop over the head of the talus, which is prominent in the middle of the depressed longitudinal arch. In addition, since the midfoot is in valgus, the patient bears weight on the medial border of the great toe, which tends to force the proximal phalanx into a valgus position, producing a hallux valgus. Pain may develop on the medial side of the head of the first metatarsal or on the medial side of the interphalangeal joint of the great toe.

The treatment of pes valgus depends on the severity of the deformity and the symptoms it has pro-

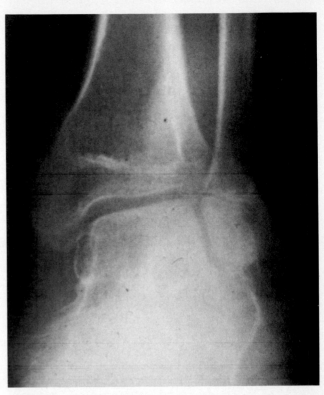

**Fig. 16–4**  Standing anterior-posterior radiograph demonstrating valgus in the ankle joint. Before performing any procedure at the level of the subtalar joint to correct an angular deformity, one must obtain a standing radiograph of the ankle to be certain that it is not deformed.

duced. Although an associated equinus deformity is usually present, heel cord lengthening alone will not generally correct a pes valgus. To correct an equinovalgus deformity of the foot, other procedures must be performed in addition to a heel cord lengthening.

Peroneus brevis tendon lengthening has been reported to provide correction of a valgus deformity of the foot.[17] In the author's experience, good results have been obtained with lengthening only the peroneus brevis, if done before the adaptive changes in the bones of the hindfoot have become severe. Lengthening of the peroneus brevis should be performed as an intramuscular fractional lengthening to prevent overlengthening. Lengthening of both peroneal muscles, which has yielded poor results, should not be performed. Anterior transfer of the peroneal tendons also has not yielded good results and therefore cannot be recommended.

Bonnett and associates[16] reported on the results of transfer of the peroneus brevis to the posterior tibial muscle in patients with a spastic pes valgus. Noting that these patients exhibited inactivity of the posterior tibial muscle, they therefore believed that the valgus deformity was caused at least in part by the posterior tibial absence. Bonnett and associates' results have not been adequately evaluated through long-term follow-up, nor have they been confirmed by others.

A Grice subtalar extra-articular arthrodesis is the procedure that has yielded the most consistently good results for the correction of the valgus foot in the spastic child.[18-21] This procedure has produced some unsuccessful results, however. Proper patient selection and careful performance of the technique are of utmost importance. In order to perform a Grice procedure, the valgus deformity must be flexible. If the foot is rigid, a triple arthrodesis is the only means of correction.

The technique as first described by Grice involved the use of a bone graft from the anterior cortex of the proximal tibia, although others have used fibula or bank bone. This bone graft must be inserted into the sinus tarsi so that the graft is perfectly parallel with the longitudinal axis of the tibia. Since the graft serves as both a graft and a means of internal fixation, if the graft is not parallel it may dislodge, resulting in loss of correction. Another complication of this procedure is the development of a varus hindfoot, which tends to be less satisfactory than the original valgus deformity. It is important to insert a graft of proper length so that the hindfoot remains in neutral to slight valgus. It is better to err on the side

of too much valgus than to attempt to obtain a perfectly neutral heel and risk the development of a varus hindfoot. Another method of performing a subtalar arthrodesis was reported by Dennyson and Fulford.[22] Their technique combines the use of a screw across the subtalar joint for internal fixation with an iliac crest bone graft placed in the sinus tarsi (Fig. 16–5). Other authors have reported good results with this procedure.[23] The sinus tarsi is approached in the same manner as in a standard Grice procedure. With the foot held in the corrected position, a screw is inserted into the dorsum of the neck of the talus and drilled across the subtalar joint and into the os calcis. This provides excellent internal fixation and allows the amount of correction of the subtalar joint to be measured more accurately. The iliac crest is regarded as superior to the tibia for grafting purposes.

If the valgus deformity of the foot is rigid, correction is possible only with a triple arthrodesis. The object of this operation is to obtain a solid arthrodesis in a corrected position. A triple arthrodesis is usually performed only in the mature or nearly mature foot, since considerable growth retardation results if the procedure is performed in the young foot. In addition, since much of the surface area of the skeletally immature tarsal bone is made up of cartilage, less

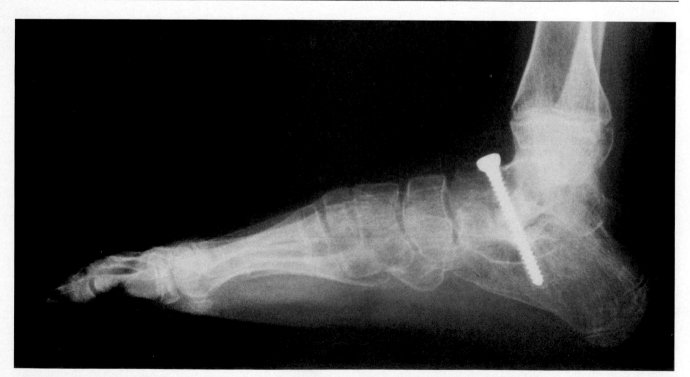

**Fig. 16–5** Dennyson and Fulford described a subtalar arthrodesis in which the subtalar joint is stabilized with a screw that is inserted into the neck of the talus. The screw crosses the subtalar joint into the os calcis. The foot is held in the desired amount of correction while the screw is inserted. The foot should be in a few degrees of valgus.

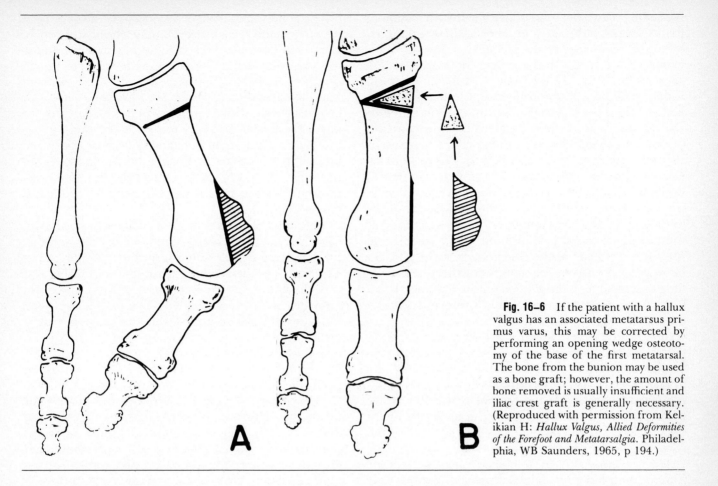

**Fig. 16–6**  If the patient with a hallux valgus has an associated metatarsus primus varus, this may be corrected by performing an opening wedge osteotomy of the base of the first metatarsal. The bone from the bunion may be used as a bone graft; however, the amount of bone removed is usually insufficient and iliac crest graft is generally necessary. (Reproduced with permission from Kelikian H: *Hallux Valgus, Allied Deformities of the Forefoot and Metatarsalgia.* Philadelphia, WB Saunders, 1965, p 194.)

bone surface is available for fusion, resulting in a higher rate of nonunion than is found in the older child's foot.

The operation is performed through an incision in the sinus tarsi, exposing all three joints. The sinus tarsi is first exposed by carefully reflecting distally the short toe-extensor muscles. Underneath will be found fat that occupies the sinus tarsi. This fat should be completely debrided so that all three joints are fully exposed. The valgus position may be corrected by removing appropriate wedges, which allows the foot to be placed in the desired position, which is, however, usually quite difficult in the rigid valgus foot. Hoke recommended removing the entire head of the talus, then denuding the subtalar joints and calcaneocuboid joints of cartilage down to bleeding bone, and replacing the talar head after also denuding it down to raw bone. Although these techniques have worked for some, in the author's experience better results are obtained by first restoring, as far as possible, the normal architecture of the hindfoot before fusing it. This restoration is done by completely releasing the three joints with very wide capsulotomies. The capsular releases are continued systematically until the hindfoot is mobilized. At this point, the triple arthrodesis may be performed without the use

of wedges by denuding the joint surfaces down to bleeding bone, so that as much contact as possible is made between all the joint surfaces to increase the likelihood of obtaining a solid arthrodesis. The use of internal fixation is preferred in the spastic foot. Either staples or Steinmann pins may be used.

### Hallux Valgus

The etiology of hallux valgus in the spastic foot is varied. As in the nonspastic foot, a metatarsus primus varus may exist as the primary deformity. However, even in the absence of this deformity, the child with a spastic diplegia or spastic quadriplegia is at risk for the development of a hallux valgus. Two mechanisms account for this fact. The first is the equinovalgus posture of the foot, which causes the medial border of the great toe to be forced against the floor, producing a lateral thrust on the proximal phalanx of the great toe. In time, the proximal phalanx of the great toe is deviated laterally, producing the valgus deformity of the metatarsophalangeal joint. A third cause of the hallux valgus is the spasticity of the adductor hallucis muscle, which pulls the proximal phalanx into valgus.

The need for treatment of a hallux valgus will depend upon the symptoms present. Many different procedures have been described for the correction of hallux valgus, although a number of these are directed to the correction of the metatarsus primus varus, which may not exist in the spastic foot with a hallux varus. The Mitchell osteotomy is probably the most widely performed procedure for the correction of hallux valgus and has been used in the correction of the spastic foot. If a metatarsus primus varus is present, an opening wedge osteotomy of the base of the first metatarsal may also be used. Care must be taken to protect the physis of the first metatarsal, which is located at the proximal end of the metatarsal. The osteotomy should therefore be placed just distal to the physis. If a large amount of bone is removed at the bunion site and it is of good quality, it may be used for the graft in the osteotomy site (Fig. 16–6). However, because in the adolescent there is usually little excess bone at the bunion on the first metatarsal head, iliac crest graft is usually preferred for the opening wedge osteotomy.

Recurrence of the deformity is a definite possibility. The most common cause for recurrence is the presence of an uncorrected equinovalgus deformity of the foot. If this deformity is present, it must be corrected before or at the time of correction of the hallux valgus. In addition, the spastic adductor hallucis muscle must be lengthened to help prevent recurrence of the deformity.

The development of a hallux varus is another complication of hallux valgus surgery. It may occur if the abductor hallucis is spastic and is tightened too much or if the adductor hallucis is transferred to the neck of the metatarsal. In the latter case, a spastic abductor hallucis is unopposed and will provide a hallux varus.

Because of the risk of recurrence of the hallux valgus or of the development of a hallux varus, Renshaw and associates[24] investigated the use of the McKeever arthrodesis for the correction of spastic hallux valgus. They reported good results with this procedure and noted that in their experience, it yielded consistently better results than did other procedures. In performing this procedure, the metatarsal phalangeal joint must be fused in 5 degrees of dorsiflexion to aid in push-off.

## The Knee

### Crouched Gait

In the spastic child the crouched gait may be the result of a hip flexion deformity, a knee flexion deformity with hamstring spasticity, a calcaneus deformity of the foot, or a combination of any of these problems. Therefore, before attempting to correct the crouched gait surgically, the possible mechanisms of the deformity itself must be fully understood.

The child with an uncorrected hip flexion contracture may stand erect by developing a lumbar lordosis. If the hip flexion contracture becomes severe and is too great for the lumbar lordosis to allow complete compensation, the child will have to walk with the hips flexed. If the hips alone are flexed, the child will be unbalanced, with a tendency to fall forward. If the knees are flexed to compensate for the hip flexion, the child will be better balanced because the force line will fall closer to the ankle joint. In this scenario, the child does not have hamstring tightness, but rather is flexing the knees to compensate for the hip flexion deformity.

The most obvious and most common cause of a crouched gait in the spastic child is hamstring spasticity. Hamstring tightness may be evaluated in two ways. The first is by performing a straight leg raising test with the knees extended. The end point of the exam is the degree at which the pelvis begins to move as the hip is flexed. In order to tell when the pelvis begins to move with continued straight leg raising, the examiner must place one hand on both anterior superior iliac spines of the pelvis. The other hand is used to perform the straight leg raising maneuver.

The second method of assessing the amount of hamstring tightness is by holding the hip flexed to 90 degrees and fully flexing the knee. One hand keeps the hip flexed at 90 degrees, and the other hand extends the knee. The point at which the hamstring tightness limits further knee extension marks the amount of hamstring tightness.

A calcaneus deformity is another cause of the crouched gait in the spastic child. The only way a child with a calcaneus deformity will be able to place the forefoot on the ground is by flexing the knees. It is important to remember, however, that the most common cause of a calcaneus deformity is iatrogenic, occurring in the patient with both hamstring and heel cord tightness who undergoes only a heel cord lengthening. As a result of the persistent hamstring spasticity, the child crouches, which pushes the tibia forward, thereby producing the calcaneus deformity. The treatment of the spastic crouched gait, therefore, requires knowledge of the possible causes and a thorough evaluation of the patient. Although a hip flexion deformity by itself is seldom the sole cause of a crouched gait, it may contribute to its development. The iliopsoas muscle is frequently spastic in the child with a spastic diplegia, and it should be carefully evaluated. If the patient has a fixed hip flexion deformity of 30 degrees, consideration should be given to a fractional lengthening of the iliopsoas. A tenotomy of the psoas should probably not be performed, because the spastic muscle may retract proximally, greatly weakening hip flexion.

Hamstring lengthening must be performed in any child undergoing heel cord lengthening who also has significant hamstring tightness. The hamstrings should be lengthened if there is a fixed flexion contracture of the knees. A hamstring lengthening should also be performed if the child walks with the knees flexed more than 15 or 20 degrees at their straightest, and in addition has significant hamstring tightness on static testing. Hamstring tightness will also limit the stride length of the gait, which is best assessed in a gait laboratory.

The goal of treatment for hamstring tightness is to weaken the muscles and to decrease their stretch reflex, which can be accomplished with hamstring tenotomy, transfers of the hamstrings, and lengthening of the hamstrings both proximally and distally.

Tenotomy should probably not be performed because of the possibility of producing a genu recurvatum deformity. Tenotomy of the semitendinosus, however, is occasionally performed along with lengthening of the other hamstrings. The other muscles are left in continuity, and this procedure seems to yield satisfactory results. Transfer of the hamstrings to the femur to aid in hip extension or to change the rotational pull of these muscles has not proved successful in the long term and is usually not performed.

Lengthening of the hamstrings has been the most successful means of weakening the hamstrings and decreasing their stretch reflex. This procedure will also produce a correction of the flexion contracture of the knee, a more erect posture by eliminating the crouched gait, and a lengthening of the stride. The hamstrings may be lengthened either proximally or distally; however, the proximal release as proposed by Seymour and Sharrard[25] should probably be performed only for patients with severe extension contracture of the hips secondary to hamstring tightness. These patients find it difficult to sit because of the posterior inclination of the pelvis, which produces a lumbar kyphosis. Releasing the hamstring muscles proximally from the ischium seems to improve these patients' ability to sit.[26]

Lengthening of the hamstrings distally has been the most widely accepted procedure and the one that yields the best results. In patients with mild hamstring tightness, the medial hamstrings alone may be lengthened. In the patient with severe tightness, both the medial and the lateral hamstrings should be lengthened, which is most easily accomplished with the patient prone, although if the adductor muscles or the iliopsoas muscles or both are being lengthened at the same time, the hamstrings may be lengthened with the patient supine. If the medial hamstrings alone are to be lengthened, the incision is placed posteromedially. If both medial and lateral hamstrings are to be lengthened, the incision is placed directly posteriorly. The incision is a straight longitudinal one that begins about 5 cm proximal to the popliteal crease and continues proximally for about 7.5 to 10 cm. The semimembranosus, semitendinosus, and gracilis tendons are identified at their musculotendinous junction. A fractional lengthening of each is performed by making two transverse or oblique cuts in the tendon well proximal to the musculotendinous junction. As the knee is extended, the tendon will slide on itself, lengthening the muscle. If there is a knee flexion contracture or if the hamstrings are very tight, the biceps femoris muscle is lengthened also. This is accomplished in the same manner, by cutting the tendon transversely, well proximal to the musculotendinous junction, producing a fractional lengthening.

Postoperatively, the patient is placed in a cylinder cast if no other surgery has been performed. If the heel cord has been lengthened, a long-leg cast is applied. The knee is immobilized for approximately three weeks; however, the patient is allowed to walk in the cast immediately postoperatively. Once the cast is removed, the patient is begun on quadriceps strengthening and active range of motion exercises.

One of the complications of hamstring lengthening is the development of a genu recurvatum deformity. This deformity may result from tenotomy of all the hamstring tendons, but most commonly it results from lengthening only the hamstrings in the face of an equinus deformity. In this instance, the hamstring spasticity that prevented recurvatum preoperatively is removed, and the knees are forced backwards by the hyperextension moment of the plantarflexed foot. It is therefore important to assess carefully the entire patient when performing any surgery on a child with spasticity, because each joint is intimately related to the adjacent joint. In this instance, lengthening of the heel cord contracture would prevent the development of genu recurvatum.

Another major component of the spastic gait is the stiff-kneed gait. Children with a spastic diplegia or a spastic quadriplegia frequently walk without flexing their knees sufficiently to allow their feet to clear the floor. The toes of their shoes therefore scrape the floor during the swing phase of gait. This is well demonstrated on slow-motion video analysis of the gait cycle. The stiff-kneed gait is caused by to a lack of knee flexion during swing and not by a lack of foot dorsiflexion, although this may also contribute to the dragging of the foot. Spasticity of the quadriceps femoris muscle limits knee flexion and also results in a high-riding patella. The Ely test will be positive in a patient with quadriceps spasticity, although this may test may not be specific for the quadriceps, since the psoas may fire with knee flexion. The Ely test, which is performed with the patient prone, was designed to measure the amount of rectus femoris contracture. The knee is flexed slowly, and if the quadriceps is tight, the ipsilateral pelvis will rise because of the quadriceps tightness.

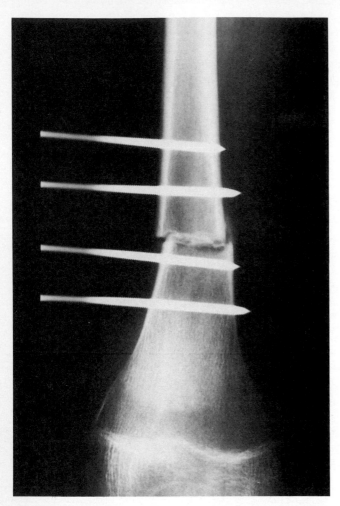

**Fig. 16–7** A femoral derotation osteotomy may be performed in the distal femur. The osteotomy is held with either one or two pins proximal and distal to the osteotomy. The pins are incorporated into a cylinder cast.

Proximal release of the rectus femoris has not been successful in increasing knee flexion during gait; however, Gage[27] has recently reported a new procedure that has significantly improved knee flexion. In this procedure, the rectus femoris is dissected free from the quadriceps tendon distally and then cut, leaving the vastus lateralis, the vastus medialis, and the vastus intermedius intact and still inserted into the quadriceps tendon. The rectus femoris tendon is exposed by making a transverse incision on the anterior aspect of the thigh approximately 4 to 5 cm proximal to the proximal pole of the patella. The incision is shaded to the medial side of the rectus tendon if the rectus is to be transferred to the sartorius, which will be performed if the patient toes in. On the other hand, the incision is shaded to the lateral side if the rectus tendon is to be transferred to the fascia lata, which is the procedure to be performed in the case of the toed-out gait. Postopera-

tively, patients are immobilized for comfort with the knee extended. They are begun on active range of motion exercises and on ambulation without splints within two weeks. The early results of this treatment have been very promising.

Toeing-in is a major problem for the child with spastic diplegia or spastic quadriplegia. Many muscle transfer procedures have been tried with little long-term success. Adductor tenotomy and iliopsoas lengthening will not affect the amount of in-toeing. Two procedures have been specifically designed for the correction of the toed-in gait. The first was described by Baker and Hill.[9] It consists of transfer of the semitendinosus tendon to the lateral side of the femur during hamstring lengthening. The results have unfortunately been unpredictable. The second procedure is the anterior transfer of the gluteus medius proposed by Steel.[28] The gluteus medius is the main internal rotator of the lower extremity but is even more important as a stabilizer of the pelvis. By transferring the gluteus medius anteriorly, a Trendelenburg gait may be produced.

The major cause of in-toeing in the spastic child is femoral anteversion. In the neurologically unimpaired child, the amount of femoral anteversion is greatest in infancy and slowly decreases during growth until the child is approximately 9 years of age. In the spastic child, this decrease in the amount of femoral anteversion does not occur, and the child is therefore left with persistence of the infantile posture of the configuration of the upper end of the femur.

Because the spastic child has difficulty clearing the floor with the feet, in-toeing in this child will be a problem because the toe of one shoe will catch on the heel of the opposite shoe. Since the internally rotated gait is caused by femoral anteversion, it is best corrected by performing a derotation osteotomy of the femur. This procedure is indicated in the child over the age of 9 years who toes in significantly during gait and in whom the in-toeing is hindering ambulation. On static testing, this child will usually exhibit at least 80 degrees of internal rotation of the hips with the hips extended and 20 degrees or less of external rotation of the hips.

The femoral osteotomy may be performed either proximally in the intertrochanteric region of the femur or distally in the area just above the supracondylar region of the femur. The proximal derotation intertrochanteric osteotomy is performed when the amount of valgus angulation of the femoral neck is being altered. If, on the other hand, only a derotation osteotomy of the femur is being performed, it is technically easier to perform it distally in the supracondylar region of the femur. In addition, morbidity is much less with this procedure, and the recovery time is shorter.[29] The distal femoral osteotomy is performed by making a longitudinal incision that begins 2 cm proximal to the flare of the femoral condyle and continues proximally for 4 to 5 cm. The femur is exposed subperiosteally, and the level of the osteotomy is determined radiographically. The femur is cut three quarters of the way across at this level. Next, one or two large Steinmann pins are inserted into the fragment just proximal to the osteotomy site. They are inserted into the femur parallel to the floor with the patient supine and the patient's leg extended and in neutral rotation. Two distal pins are then inserted just distal to the osteotomy (Fig. 16–7). These pins are inserted at an angle to the proximal pins that is equal to the amount of correction desired. If, for example, 35 degrees of increased external rotation of the leg is desired, the distal pins will be inserted at an angle of 35 degrees to the proximal pins. The femoral osteotomy is then completed, and the proximal femur is stabilized while the distal fragment is externally rotated until the proximal and distal pins are parallel. The osteotomy may be stabilized by incorporating the pins in an external fixator or a cylinder cast.

Postoperatively, weightbearing is not allowed until early union is achieved, which usually occurs in approximately four weeks. At this time, the pins are removed and the leg is placed in a cylinder cast. The child is allowed to walk in the cast until union is complete, which usually takes another four to six weeks.

## Summary

The surgical treatment of children with spastic cerebral palsy should be directed at all the problems of the child rather than focusing on one problem area at a time.[3] Although the difficulties encountered by these children can be divided into separate areas for discussion, treating one problem without consideration of the others will result in unnecessary additional hospitalization for subsequent operations. In addition, since each joint is intimately linked to another, surgical treatment of one joint problem may lead to worsening of an adjacent joint deformity unless it too is addressed. Thus, the surgical care of the lower extremities in spastic cerebral palsy requires that the entire patient be evaluated and all necessary surgical procedures be coordinated.

## References

1. Bleck EE: *Orthopaedic Management of Cerebral Palsy.* Philadelphia, WB Saunders, 1979.
2. Duncan WR, Mott DH: Foot reflexes and the use of the inhibitive cast. *Foot Ankle* 1984;4:145–148.
3. Norlin R, Tkaczuk H: One stage surgery for correction of lower extremity deformities in children with cerebral palsy. *J Pediatr Orthop* 1985;5:208–211.
4. Strayer LM: Recession of the gastrocnemius. *J Bone Joint Surg* 1950;32A:671–676.
5. Baker LD: A rational approach to the surgical needs of the cerebral palsy patient. *J Bone Joint Surg* 1956;38A:313–323.
6. Perry J, Hoffer M, Giovan P, et al: Gait analysis of the triceps surae in cerebral palsy. *J Bone Joint Surg* 1974;56A:511–520.
7. Throop FB, DeRosa G, Reech C, et al: Correction of equinus in cerebral palsy by the Murphy procedure of tendo-calcaneus advancement: A preliminary communication. *Dev Med Child Neurol* 1975;17:182–185.
8. Hoffer MM, Reswig J, Garrett A, et al: The split anterior tibial tendon transfer in the treatment of the hindfoot in childhood. *Orthop Clin North Am* 1974;5:31–38.
9. Baker LD, Hill LM: Foot alignment in the cerebral palsy patient. *J Bone Joint Surg* 1964;46A:1–15.
10. Bassett FH, Baker LD: Equinus deformity in cerebral palsy. *Curr Pract Orthop Surg* 1966;3:59–74.
11. Root L, Kirz P: The result of posterior tibial tendon surgery in 83 patients with cerebral palsy. *Dev Med Child Neurol* 1982;24:241–242.
12. Bisla RS, Louis HJ, Albano P: Transfer of tibialis posterior tendon in cerebral palsy. *J Bone Joint Surg* 1976;58A:497–500.
13. Banks HH, Panagakos P: The role of the orthopaedic surgeon in cerebral palsy. *Pediatr Clin North Am* 1967;14:495–515.
14. Green NE, Griffin PP, Shiavi R: Split posterior tibial tendon transfer in spastic cerebral palsy. *J Bone Joint Surg* 1983;65A:748–754.
15. Kling TF, Kaufer H, Hensinger RN: Split posterior tibial tendon transfers in children with cerebral spastic paralysis and equinovarus deformity. *J Bone Joint Surg* 1985;67A:186–194.
16. Bonnett G, et al: Varus and valgus deformities of the foot in cerebral palsy. *Dev Med Child Neurol* 1982;24:499–503.
17. Nather A, Fulford G, Stewart K: Treatment of valgus hindfoot in cerebral palsy by peroneus brevis lengthening. *Dev Med Child Neurol* 1984;26:335–340.
18. Grice DS: An extra-articular arthrodesis of the subastragalar joint for correction of paralytic feet in children. *J Bone Joint Surg* 1952;34A:927–940.
19. Keats S, Kouten J: Early surgical correction of the planovalgus foot in cerebral palsy. *Clin Orthop* 1968;61:223–233.
20. Ross PM, Lyne ED: The Grice procedure: Indications and evaluations of long-term results. *Clin Orthop* 1980;153:194–200.
21. Root L: Varus and valgus foot in cerebral palsy and its management. *Foot Ankle* 1984;4:174–179.
22. Dennyson WG, Fulford R: Subtalar arthrodesis by cancellous grafts and metallic fixation. *J Bone Joint Surg* 1976;58B:507–510.
23. Barrasso JA, Wile PB, Gage JR: Extraarticular subtalar arthrodesis with internal fixation. *J Pediatr Orthop* 1984;4:555–559.
24. Renshaw T, Sirkin R, Drennan J: The management of hallux valgus in cerebral palsy. *Dev Med Child Neurol* 1979;21:202–208.
25. Seymour N, Sharrard WJW: Bilateral proximal release of the hamstrings in cerebral palsy. *J Bone Joint Surg* 1968;50B:274–277.
26. Drummond DS, Rogala E, Templeton J, et al: Proximal hamstring release for knee flexion and crouched posture in cerebral palsy. *J Bone Joint Surg* 1974;56A:1598–1602.
27. Gage J: Presented at the meeting of the Pediatric Orthopaedic Society of North America, Boston, May 1986.
28. Steel H: Gluteus medius and minimus insertion advancement for correction of internal rotation gait in cerebral palsy. *J Bone Joint Surg* 1980;62A:919–927.
29. Hoffer M: Supracondylar derotation osteotomy of the femur for internal rotation of the thigh in the cerebral palsied child. *J Bone Joint Surg* 1981;63A:389–393.

# The Orthopaedic Care of Children With Muscular Dystrophy

Neil E. Green, MD

## Introduction

The muscular dystrophies are a group of hereditary disorders of skeletal muscle. They are noninflammatory, but produce progressive degeneration of skeletal muscle with associated weakness.

## Classification

The true muscular dystrophies are classified according to their genetic patterns of inheritance. The X-linked dystrophies are the most common, and are the ones discussed in this chapter. They are Duchenne's muscular dystrophy and Becker's muscular dystrophy. The two differ primarily in severity. Duchenne's muscular dystrophy is a much more severe form of the disease than Becker's muscular dystrophy, which has a better prognosis. The two main autosomal recessive muscular dystrophies are limb-girdle muscular dystrophy and congenital muscular dystrophy. Finally, fascioscapulohumeral muscular dystrophy is inherited as an autosomal dominant trait.

## Duchenne's Muscular Dystrophy

### History

Duchenne's muscular dystrophy was first described by Meryon in 1852. In 1868 Duchenne de Boulogne noted that calf pseudohypertrophy was associated with this disease, which now carries his name. Because of its X-linked recessive inheritance, this disease occurs in males, and in females with Turner's syndrome. It is reported to occur in one in 3,000 live births. There is a family history in 60% of patients, and the disease is thought to occur as a result of a spontaneous mutation in 30% of patients.

### Clinical Features

Infants with Duchenne's muscular dystrophy may initially be thought to be "floppy," but they reach their early motor milestones at appropriate times. They may, however, be late in achieving independent ambulation and initially they may be toe walkers. They are also physically slower and weaker than their peers. Parents usually know something is` wrong before the children reach the age of 4 or 5 years. Calf pseudohypertrophy gives the appearance of above-average strength, whereas these children are really much weaker than their peers. They find climbing difficult or impossible, and they are not able to run or jump. The diagnosis is usually obvious by the age of 5 or 6 years when severe weakness is manifest.

The proximal musculature is affected first. In the early stages of the disease, there is weakness of the hip extensors and the quadriceps. Because of the quadriceps weakness, these children find it difficult to rise to a standing position from the floor. To do this, they place their hands on their anterior thighs to help extend their thighs, thereby overcoming the quadriceps weakness. This action keeps the knees from buckling, and has been referred to as Gower's sign. The gait is subtly altered. There is an increase in hip flexion during the swing phase of gait, with a concomitant decrease in ankle dorsiflexion. The cadence of the gait is also decreased. As the disease progresses, gait worsens. There is progressive equinus positioning of the feet during gait. This is actually beneficial to children with Duchenne's muscular dystrophy, because the equinus posture helps force the knees into hyperextension, thereby locking them. If the equinus deformity is removed by performing a heel cord lengthening, the tendency to force the knees into hyperextension is lost, and the knees will buckle because of the weakness of the quadriceps.

These children maintain ambulation with extreme difficulty as the disease progresses. Maintaining the upright position requires an alteration in the position of the trunk. The quadriceps muscles are weak and become progressively weaker. The hip extensors are also extremely weak. As a result, the patients develop flexion contracture of the hips. As the flexion contracture worsens, the hips are kept flexed when the children are supine. Because they cannot keep their legs upright, the hips drop into abduction and flexion. This "frog" position becomes the normal supine position in children with advancing weakness, which in turn contributes to the development of severe flexion and abduction contracture of the hips. To compensate for the flexion contracture, marked lumbar lordosis develops. The lumbar lordosis progresses to frank hyperextension of the back, which is also biomechanically necessary to enable these children to lock their hips in extension and prevent collapse, since they lack strength in the hip extensor musculature. At this point, almost anything that disturbs this delicate balance means an end to ambulation. The hyperextension of the back also represents an attempt to keep the vertical force line behind the center of the hip joint; at the same time, however, the force line must be kept in front of the knee to lock the knee joint in extension.[1] As muscle strength continues to decrease, the force line moves closer to the hip and

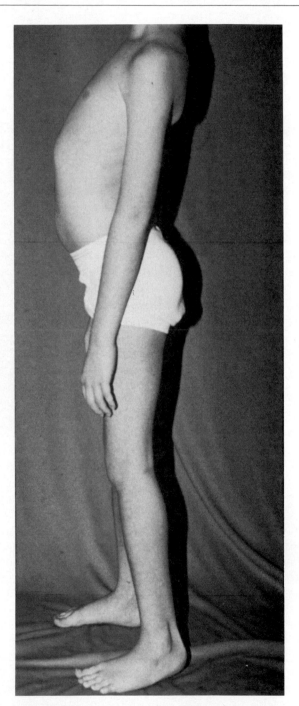

**Fig. 17-1** This 7-year-old child with Duchenne's muscular dystrophy shows a very characteristic posture. Note the lumbar lordosis and the hyperextension of the upper spine. In addition, the neck is extended and the chin is tucked in to help keep as much weight as possible posterior to the hip.

knee joints. The chin is tucked in and the neck extended in an attempt to maintain balance (Fig. 17-1). The arms are held away from the body, and the gait is wide-based to improve balance. The iliotibial tract tightens, contributing to the progressive hip abduction contracture. This contracture of the iliotibial band helps to stabilize the pelvis and the knee. Once no further compensatory mechanisms are available, the children stop walking. This may be a dramatic event, since just before ambulation stops, compensation is maximal.

### Diagnosis

The diagnosis of Duchenne's muscular dystrophy depends on good history-taking and the physical examination. Muscular weakness and calf pseudohypertrophy should suggest the diagnosis. A positive family history increases the probability of the diagnosis, as it is present in 60% of patients.

Patients with Duchenne's muscular dystrophy initially have markedly increased creatine phosphokinase levels (at least ten times normal in young patients and frequently more than 10,000 U/L). These very high levels of creatine phosphokinase decrease as the disease progresses and muscle mass is lost.

Muscular biopsy, which is usually performed in these patients to confirm the diagnosis, demonstrates a nonspecific myopathy. Early in the course of the disease, significant fibrosis develops and degenerating muscle fibers show marked variations in fiber size. As the disease progresses, these fibers are replaced by connective tissue and fat.

### Physical Findings

The degree of muscular weakness depends on the age of the patient. Orthopaedic surgeons may be called upon to make the initial diagnosis of muscular dystrophy since children with muscular dystrophy may be referred because they exhibit a clumsy gait or experience difficulty in walking. Orthopaedic consultation may also be sought because of toe walking. At this stage, muscular weakness is certainly evident, although it is not as severe as it will be in two or three years.

Because proximal muscles become weak before distal muscles, examination of the lower extremities demonstrates an essential absence of gluteal muscle strength. In addition, the quadriceps is very weak, and Gower's sign is present because of the patient's need to stabilize the knee to prevent buckling when standing.

Calf pseudohypertrophy is present (Fig. 17-2). The calves are enlarged because of infiltration of the musculature by fat and fibrosis, and they have the consistency of hard rubber. Distally the extrinsic musculature of the foot and ankle retains strength for a longer period than does the proximal musculature of the upper leg. The anterior tibial muscle, however, becomes weak early, followed by the peroneal muscles. The posterior tibial muscle retains its strength the longest. As a result of this pattern of weakness, the foot develops an equinovarus deformity.

Weakness is not limited to the lower extremities. The shoulder girdle musculature also becomes extremely weak, leading to the so-called Meryon sign, which is elicited by lifting the child with one arm encircling the child's chest. A child with good muscle strength in the shoulder girdle contracts the muscles about the shoulder to increase shoulder stability, thus facilitating the lifting. The child with muscular dystrophy, however, is unable to do this because of severe muscle weakness. As the patient is lifted, his arms abduct until they eventually slide through the examiner's arms, unless the chest is tightly encircled. As the weakness of the upper extremities increases, the child eventually becomes unable to move his arms. Although the patient's hands retain some strength longer than do the arms, the use of the hands is limited because the weakness of the arms makes it difficult to change the position of the hands.

Duchenne's muscular dystrophy is purely a muscle disease with no neurologic involvement, and sensation is therefore normal. Patients usually have IQs approximately 20 points below the mean. In addition, the weakness of the facial musculature limits facial expression, contributing to the impression of intellectual dullness. These children also develop cardiomyopathy that may become severe. Cardiologic evaluation, including an echocardiogram, should be considered before any surgical procedure is performed.

As muscular weakness progresses, significant contractures develop about the lower extremities. Severe hip flexion and abduction contracture are present but difficult to elicit unless the pelvis is manually stabilized by the examiner; the child is unable to do so because of muscle weakness. The Thomas test for hip flexion contracture is performed with the patient supine. One hand is placed on the anterior pelvis to stabilize it. An assistant is needed to flex the opposite leg maximally to flatten the lumbar spine and reduce the lumbar lordosis. The examiner then maximally flexes the hip to be examined, at which point it is adducted before being extended. Although adduction of the hip is a most important part of the examination, it is frequently neglected because the contribution of the tensor fascia femoris muscle to the development of the flexion contracture is not widely recognized. The tensor fascia femoris muscle is very contracted and contributes greatly to the hip flexion and abduction contracture. If the hip is not adducted as it is extended, the amount of hip flexion contracture will be underestimated because of increasing

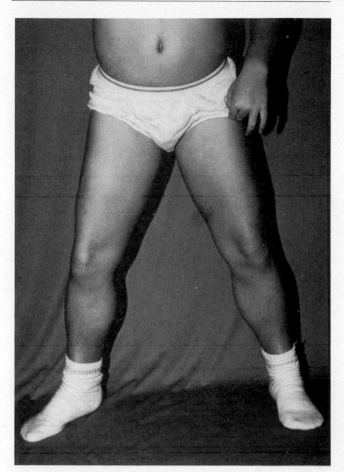

**Fig. 17–2** This 6-year-old boy with Duchenne's muscular dystrophy demonstrates the characteristic calf pseudohypertrophy.

abduction. If the hip is held in adduction while it is extended, there is usually a flexion-adduction contracture of more than 60 degrees. It is very important, however, that the opposite hip be maintained in maximum flexion and the pelvis stabilized to prevent the pelvis on the opposite side from rising and thereby negating the adducted posture of the examined hip (Fig. 17–3).

The Ober test, which is an assessment of the amount of abduction contracture of the hip, is performed with the patient in the lateral position. During this examination, it is imperative to flex the opposite hip fully and to stabilize the pelvis to prevent it from tilting as the leg being examined is brought into adduction. The abduction contracture is usually greater than 30 degrees. The tensor fascia femoris muscle and the fascia lata itself are the main contributors to the abduction contracture.

As long as the child is still walking or at least standing, flexion contracture of the knee does not develop; however, flexion contracture begins to develop in the knee as soon as the child ceases ambulation. The ankle is in equinus, which is necessary for

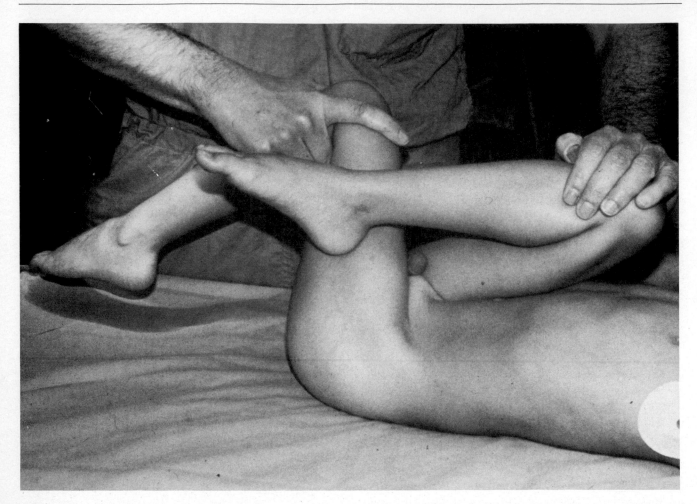

**Fig. 17–3** Examining the hip flexion and abduction contracture requires that the opposite hip be fully flexed onto the patient's abdomen. The hip being examined is first flexed and then adducted to assess the tensor fascia femoris muscle, the tightness of which is a major cause of the flexion and abduction contracture. The hip is then extended while the adduction thrust is maintained. The end point is felt when the hip tends to abduct as it is extended. The amount of hip flexion remaining at this point represents the true amount of contracture.

ambulation because the equinus position of the foot helps to hyperextend the knee, thereby lessening the tendency of the knee to collapse because of the extreme weakness of the quadriceps muscles. The posterior tibial muscle retains its strength longer than the other extrinsic muscles of the foot, and will, therefore, eventually produce a varus deformity of the foot if neglected.

**Prognosis**

Duchenne's muscular dystrophy is a progressive disease that usually confines the patient to a wheelchair by the age of 12 or 13 years and much earlier if contractures are not relieved. Death ensues by or before the early third decade as a result of pulmonary or cardiac failure. Nevertheless, the quality of the patient's life can be improved by maintaining the ability to stand and walk for as long as possible. Once

walking is no longer possible, the patient can use a chair as long as significant scoliosis does not develop. Once scoliosis develops, it usually becomes relentlessly progressive and soon makes sitting impossible.

Although the prognosis is guarded, it is important for the child with muscular dystrophy to continue walking for as long as possible. A patient who receives no treatment at all usually stops walking before the age of 10 years and frequently before the age of 9 years. Appropriate therapy can allow the patient to walk until the age of 12 or 13 years.

**Treatment**

The major goal of early treatment is to maintain functional ambulation as long as possible. This entails the prevention or retardation of the development of contractures of the lower extremity. Once children with Duchenne's muscular dystrophy cease ambulation, they are susceptible to the development of scoliosis. For this reason, the spine must be carefully monitored. In addition, patients and their families require psychological support, which should be provided by the members of the muscular dystrophy clinic team.

Early in the course of the disease, while the child can still ambulate without difficulty, contractures of the lower extremities develop; eventually these will prevent ambulation. The equinus contracture of the feet should not be corrected early in the course of the disease, since the equinus position of the foot helps to force the knee into extension which, in turn, helps to prevent buckling of the knee secondary to the severe weakness of the quadriceps. To prevent the equinus deformity from becoming severe, stretching exercises and night-time bracing should be employed. The flexion and abduction contracture of the hips, however, impedes effective ambulation and should be minimized. The patient's family, therefore, should be taught exercises designed to stretch out the patient's hips. In addition, the child should sleep with lower extremity braces that prevent him from assuming the "frog" position during sleep. This position is a major factor in the development of the flexion and abduction contracture of the hips.

As the child with muscular dystrophy becomes older, ambulation becomes increasingly difficult because of muscular weakness and hip contracture. The force line of the body, which the child attempts to keep behind the center of rotation of the hip, gradually moves closer to both the center of the hip and the front of the knee, causing the hip and knee to give way during ambulation. If this anterior shift of the force line is allowed to continue unchecked, the child will probably stop walking before the age of 9 or 10 years. Continued ambulation is important for both physical and psychological reasons. The earlier the child becomes permanently wheelchair-bound, the greater the risk that scoliosis and severe contractures of the lower extremities will develop. In addition, pulmonary function, which deteriorates fairly rapidly in these children because of muscular weakness, deteriorates at an even faster rate if the child is not ambulatory and scoliosis develops as a result.

When the child finds ambulation increasingly difficult because of muscle weakness and contractures, surgical intervention becomes necessary. The timing of surgery is critical. It should not be performed too early, since the child should not be put in braces until absolutely necessary. Conversely, if one waits too long, the patient will stop walking. It is easier to keep patients walking than to induce them to resume walking once they have stopped. Surgery is best performed when the child finds unassisted ambulation very difficult and falls increasingly often. At this point, the patient requires bracing anyway, to replace the essentially absent quadriceps muscles. However, severe hip flexion and abduction contractures and equinus deformities make bracing difficult. All of these deformities should be corrected simultaneously. Since the child will be braced postoperatively, the knee extension moment provided by the equinus deformity will no longer be required, and the Achilles tendon should be lengthened.

Surgical treatment consists of releasing the contractures of the hip and ankle.[2] In most thin children, percutaneous incisions can be used. Percutaneous incisions greatly reduce postoperative discomfort, thereby hastening postoperative mobilization.[3] The child must be mobilized immediately after surgery to prevent or limit the rapidly progressive weakness caused by prolonged periods in bed.

The hip flexion and abduction contracture is released percutaneously. The sartorius, tensor fascia femoris, and rectus femoris muscles should be released along with the fascia lata about the hip lateral to the anterior superior iliac spine. This is done with the opposite hip held in maximum flexion to flatten the lumbar spine. The hip to be released is first flexed and then extended, with the hip held in adduction to place tension on the muscles to be released. A No. 15 knife blade is inserted percutaneously just medial and just distal to the anterior superior iliac spine (Fig. 17–4). The sartorius is released first; then, while the knife is still inserted, the tensor fascia femoris muscle is released. The knife is pushed laterally and subcutaneously, without cutting the skin, to release the fascia completely. The knife is brought to the original point of insertion and pushed deeper to release the rectus femoris completely. Obviously, great care must be taken to avoid the neurovascular structures of the anterior thigh. A thorough knowledge of the anatomy of the region is imperative. The second portion of the "Ober-Yount" fasciotomy is then performed. Approximately 3 to 4 cm proximal to the upper pole of the patella, the fascia lata is released percutaneously through a stab wound made in the mid portion of the fascia lata. In addition, the knife is pushed almost to the bone to release the lateral intermuscular septum completely.

The next part of the procedure is the Achilles tendon release, which is also performed percutaneously. The tendon may be cut without repair since the patient will be continuously braced postoperatively. Although the posterior tibial tendon is not tight at this stage of the disease, it will become so because it retains its strength longer than any other tendon in the lower extremity. The tendon may be sectioned through a very small incision just proximal to the insertion of the posterior tibial tendon. Some surgeons prefer to transfer the posterior tibial tendon through the interosseous membrane to the dorsum of the foot.[4] This helps to prevent the recurrence of the equinovarus deformity; however, this procedure requires considerable dissection and increases postoperative pain.

After surgery, the legs are placed in long-leg casts. The heels of the casts must be well padded to prevent the development of pressure ulcers. The feet must not be put into a calcaneous posture that would make the development of heel ulcers more likely. The child is transferred from the operating table to a Circo-electric bed, which allows the patient to begin standing the afternoon of the operation. If the patient can tolerate more, he is allowed to take a few steps. The patient quickly progresses to walker-assisted ambulation. Once transfer is achieved, the patient is placed in a regular bed and physical therapy is continued.

The casts are bivalved and bilateral long-leg orthoses are fitted. The casts may be worn at night in place of the orthoses. The orthoses are usually custom-molded plastic models that are lighter than the metal braces previously used. The patient is discharged from the hospital as soon as he can ambulate independently with the aid of a walker.

The release of contractures usually enables these children to walk for at least another two to three years. By the age of 12 or 13 years, however, muscle weakness is so great that they can no longer walk. It is at this point that spinal deformity becomes a threat.

Scoliosis affects approximately 90% of children with Duchenne's muscular dystrophy. In most, although not all, cases the curve is progressive. The scoliosis produces a pelvic obliquity that makes sitting increasingly difficult until the ability to sit is lost

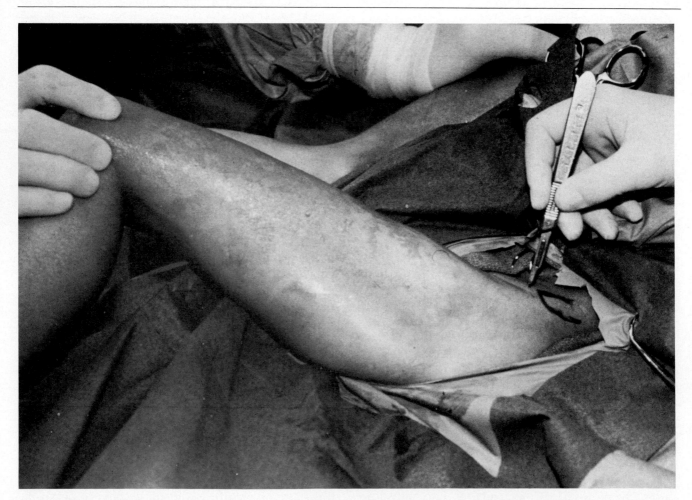

**Fig. 17–4** This intraoperative photograph demonstrates the technique of percutaneous release of the hip flexors, the tensor fascia femoris, and the fascia. The opposite hip is fully flexed while the hip being released is extended but maintained in an adducted position to tighten both the hip flexors and the tensor fascia femoris muscle. The anterior superior iliac spine is outlined. The knife is inserted just distal and just medial to the anterior superior iliac spine. One must be careful to remain lateral to the neurovascular structures on top of the iliacus muscle. The sartorius muscle, the tensor fascia femoris muscle, and the fascia lata are released first. The rectus femoris muscle is then released.

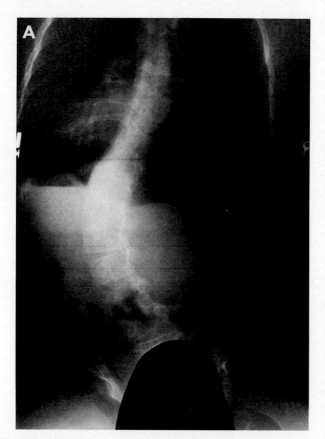
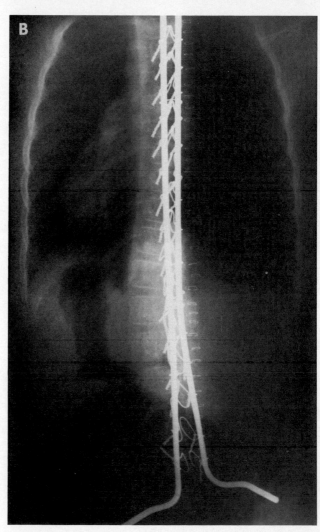

**Fig. 17–5**   Anteroposterior radiographs of the spine of a 13-year-old boy with Duchenne's muscular dystrophy who underwent posterior spinal fusion. Stabilization was accomplished with Luque rods segmentally wired to the spine from T2 through to the sacrum. Fixation to the pelvis was done by the Galveston technique. **A:** Progressive scoliosis with an associated pelvic obliquity. **B:** The same patient after the posterior spinal fusion. The curvature and the pelvic obliquity have been eliminated.

completely. The progressive muscular weakness itself causes a steady decrease in pulmonary function, and scoliosis causes even more rapid deterioration because of restrictive lung disease. Because of the potential loss of sitting balance and the deterioration of pulmonary function, most surgeons recommend spinal fusion for progressive scoliosis. Bracing is usually not recommended, since at best it only slows the progression of the curve. Unfortunately, there is a very narrow time frame in which spinal surgery can be performed safely. The forced vital capacity (FVC) of the lungs should be 50% or more to reduce pulmonary complications to an acceptable level. Once a spinal curvature is detected, pulmonary function is already below normal. If a brace is used, the curve

progression is only slowed, not arrested. Once the progression of the scoliosis makes the need for surgical stabilization clear, the FVC is too low for safe surgical correction of the spinal curvature.[5,6]

Most investigators, therefore, recommend posterior spinal fusion once the curve reaches 35 degrees if the FVC is adequate. The recommended procedure is fusion of the entire thoracolumbar spine. The fusion must extend to the top of the thoracic spine to prevent postoperative kyphosis above the fusion. In addition, most surgeons recommend extension of the fusion to the sacrum. The best current technique involves using Luque rods which are segmentally wired to the spine and fixed to the pelvis by the Galveston technique.[7] The sublaminar passage of the wires is accomplished at each level through a small laminotomy in the midline. The wires are passed under each lamina from T2 or T3 through L5. The Luque rods are bent to conform to the sagittal architecture of the spine and are passed into the pelvis through predrilled holes made in the posterior superior iliac spines. The wires are then tightened around the rods. This provides extremely secure fixation, obviating the need for postoperative immobilization. Autogenous iliac graft is usually scarce and its use is compromised by the iliac insertion of the Luque rods; an allograft is therefore usually employed (Fig. 17–5). The patient is mobilized as soon as he is comfortable, usually within four or five days. Sitting balance is immediately improved.The child can now sit in a chair without slumping into an almost leaning position. In addition, transfers from bed to chair are much easier because of greater spinal stability.

## References

1. Sutherland DH: *Gait Disorders in Childhood and Adolescence*. Baltimore, Williams and Wilkins, 1984, pp 152–157.
2. Johnson EW, Eyring EJ, Burnett C: Surgery in muscular dystrophy. *JAMA* 1972;222:1056–1057.
3. Siegel IM, Miller JE, Ray RD: Subcutaneous lower limb tenotomy in treatment of pseudohypertrophic muscular dystrophy. *J Bone Joint Surg* 1968;50A:1437–1443.
4. Drennan JC: *Orthopaedic Management of Neuromuscular Disorders*. Philadelphia, JB Lippincott, 1983, pp 10–41.
5. Kurz LT, Mubarek SJ, Schultz P, et al: Correlation of scoliosis and pulmonary function in Duchenne muscular dystrophy. *J Pediatr Orthop* 1983;3:347–353.
6. Sussman MD: Advantage of early spinal stabilization and fusion in patients with Duchenne muscular dystrophy. *J Pediatr Orthop* 1984;4:532–537.
7. Allen BL Jr, Ferguson RL: The Galveston technique of pelvic fixation with L-rod instrumentation of the spine. *Spine* 1984;9:388–394.

# Orthopaedic Management of the Lower Extremities in Spina Bifida

Elizabeth A. Szalay, MD

## Introduction

Spina bifida is one of the most common birth defects today; its incidence is approximately 1 in 2,000 live births.[1] Improved management has led to survival of most affected infants, with a marked increase in adolescents and adults who have myelodysplasia.

Realistic goal-setting is the key to overall management. The maximum potential of each child must be realized, without placing undue emphasis on achieving unrealistic goals. Surgery should be avoided, if possible, but when surgery is necessary, hospitalization time and the amount of school missed should be minimized.

## Ambulation

Normal childhood development involves progression through a series of motor milestones: a child sits at approximately 6 months of age, pulls to stand at 10 months, and begins to walk at 12 to 14 months. If possible, myelodysplastic children should pass these milestones at approximately the same ages.

The goal for management of lower extremity function is ambulation for most children, and mobility for the teen and adult. Ideal mobility is defined as the ability to get from one place to another with minimum energy expenditure. As the myelodysplastic child wearing braces and using crutches gets older, increasing body weight increases the energy expended in walking. Depending upon the degree of paralysis,[2] many children cannot meet the long-term energy requirement for independent ambulation; for these children, ideal mobility is achieved by using a wheelchair. A child or adolescent in a wheelchair may perform many normal activities, including participation in sports, which cannot be done with braces and crutches.

Nevertheless, ambulation is a goal for most children because in the very young child, intellectual and motor development is assisted if the child can be taught to stand and walk independently, even though such activity may be limited to the years of early childhood. The upright position diminishes postural contractures such as talipes equinus and knee flexion. The upright, weightbearing position enhances normal bone density and growth.[3] Perhaps most impor-

tantly, parents more readily accept the ambulatory limitation of their child if they believe that a reasonable effort at ambulation has been made.

### Nonorthopaedic Determinants of Ambulation

Intelligence, sense of balance, weight, and motivation all affect the degree of ambulation. Intelligence and balance are most influenced by neurosurgical care. A child who has appropriate shunting of hydrocephalus and careful monitoring of the central nervous system will be given the greatest opportunity for ambulation. In the older child, weight is perhaps the most limiting factor in achieving ambulation. Children who have myelodysplasia are often severely overweight; dietary consultation and early family intervention are important in preventing this complication. Finally, the motivation of the child and the family is also a crucial factor in achieving ambulation.

### The Primary Orthopaedic Determinant of Ambulation

The level of neurologic involvement determines the degree of ambulation achieved. For long-term ambulation, strong quadriceps and medial hamstring function are required (involvement no higher than the level of the fourth lumbar vertebra). Ambulation is facilitated by deformity-free limbs that may be easily brought to a braceable position and so maintained with orthotics. To enable efficient bracing, fixed joint contractures must be corrected either by stretching or by surgical manipulation.

## Spasticity: Causes and Concerns

Spina bifida is a multisystem disease. The degree to which the central neurologic axis is involved is reflected in the level of peripheral neurologic functioning.

In an Australian study of 109 patients, 54% were found to have flaccid paralysis, while 46% exhibited either upper extremity, lower extremity, or combined spasticity.[4] A non-spastic child with involvement at a lower lumbar neurologic level has a 100% chance of ambulation, while a spastic child with involvement at the same neurologic level has only a 78% chance of ambulation. Thus, spasticity must be considered an important determinant of ambulation.

Almost all children who have myelodysplasia exhibit an Arnold-Chiari malformation; progressive spasticity, upper extremity involvement, or bulbar

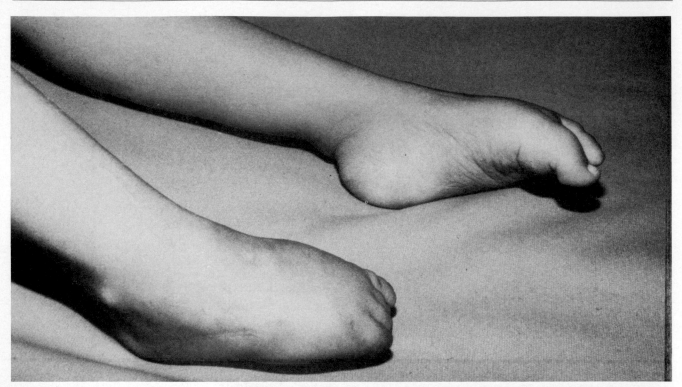

**Fig. 18–1** Patient with L5 level spina bifida. Following tibialis anterior transfer to the heel cord, she developed progressive spasticity and equinus contracture, which recurred even after heel cord tenotomy.

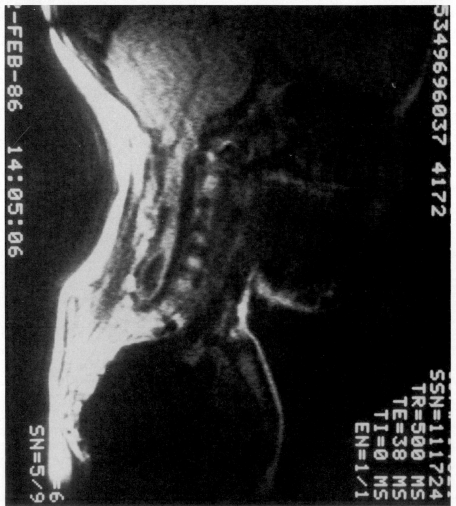

**Fig. 18–2** Magnetic resonance image of the cervical spine in patient illustrating a large syringomyelia, which may be causing spasticity.

involvement should suggest tonsilar compression and may be benefited by foramen magnum decompression.

Eighty-five percent of children with spina bifida have some degree of hydrocephalus. Decompensated hydrocephalus, complications of shunt surgery, infection, hydromyelia, or syringomyelia may produce spasticity.

Twenty-one percent of children with myelodysplasia will have additional congenital anomalies of the spine[5]; up to 5% of children who have congenital scoliosis have diastematomyelia.[6]

In all children who exhibit loss of neurologic function, increased spasticity, or rapid progression of scoliosis, diastematomyelia, or other causes of spinal cord tethering, such as lipomatous infiltration of the spinal cord or a low-lying cord from a tight filum terminali, must be sought.

Thus, serial neurologic examinations must be performed on every myelodysplastic child; a change in neurologic function, however subtle, may indicate a correctable lesion (Figs. 18–1 and 18–2).

## Orthopaedic Management

In managing a child who has spina bifida, the orthopaedic surgeon must (1) establish and record the level of neurologic involvement in the newborn period; (2) educate the parents regarding prognosis, ambulatory potential, and expected problems; (3) maintain the limbs and spine as deformity-free as possible; (4) prescribe and supervise the use of orthotics or wheelchair for optimal mobility; and (5) monitor neurologic function over time.

In the newborn or perinatal period, a careful motor examination must be performed to determine the exact neurologic level of function. This examination provides important baseline information and can be used to educate parents as to the ultimate prognosis for their child's functioning. Determination of

neurologic level also identifies deformities that can be expected to develop and dictates the stretching exercises and positioning necessary to prevent such deformities (Table 18–1).

## Orthotics

Orthotics are expensive and cumbersome, and their effective and economical use requires an understanding of what they can and cannot do. Bracing can stabilize weak joints, help prevent contractures by maintaining the body in a weightbearing position, and provide lower extremity and trunk stability that promotes independent upper extremity activity, which will build confidence and increase environmental interaction. These goals are achieved, however, at considerable financial expense. Furthermore, braces can be hot and encumbering, and improper brace fit may cause pressure sores in insensate skin.

Bracing cannot correct fixed joint deformities. A joint must be flail or able to be placed in a suitable position prior to bracing. Bracing also cannot increase the energy available for ambulation. Braces function by decreasing the number of joints that must be controlled for ambulation, but available energy is not increased.

### Types of Orthotics

With advances in plastic technology, the art of bracing has taken on new dimensions. Polypropylene braces can be fashioned to conform exactly to a deformed limb and are useful in providing a total contact orthosis. They are more cosmetic than the older metal braces, primarily because shoe wear can be varied to include tennis shoes and other "normal"-appearing shoes. However, plastic braces are hotter than metal braces to wear, especially in southern climates. Importantly, they are not as sturdy as metal braces and may not be suitable for a very heavy child. Disadvantages of metal braces include increased

**Table 18–1**
**Level of paralysis predicts ambulatory potential and deformities**

| Level of Paralysis | Affected | Prognosis | Problems |
|---|---|---|---|
| Thoracic | Flail hips, knees, feet | With or without childhood ambulation; wheelchair by adolescence | "Frog" contracture; poor trunk control/positional feedback; scoliosis/kyphosis |
| High lumbar (L1–L3) | Hip flexors/adductors | Ambulation in childhood; wheelchair by adolescence | Hip flexion/adduction contracture; hip dislocation; knee extension contracture; lordosis/scoliosis |
| Low lumbar (L4–L5) | Quadriceps; medial hamstrings with or without tibialis anterior | May be long-term ambulators | Hip subluxation/dislocation; torsional problems; calcaneous deformity |
| Sacral | Lacks only foot intrinsics | Independent ambulation | Cavus deformity; claw toes |

weight and the need for attachment to unsightly "orthopaedic" shoes.

## Principles of Bracing in Spina Bifida

In some neuromuscular diseases such as cerebral palsy, the long-term goal is joint stabilization or muscle balancing to achieve brace independence; in myelodysplasia, however, brace independence is often an unrealistic goal. It is difficult to balance muscles across a joint when antagonistic muscles are absent. To this end, it is most practical to render the joint flail to allow optimal positioning for bracing and then to stabilize the flail joint with a brace.

With a very young child, approximately 10 to 18 months of age, the first developmental milestone to

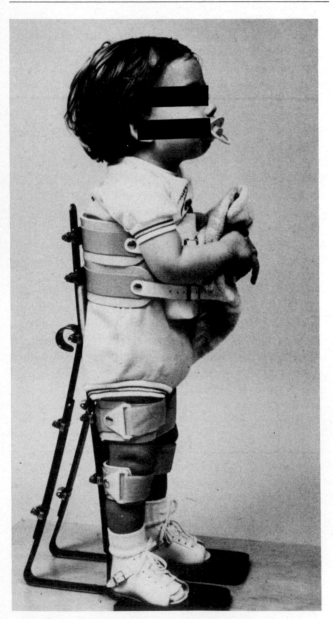

**Fig. 18–3** The standing frame, or parapodium.

be achieved is that of independent standing. The parapodium, or standing frame, provides stable support to enable upright positioning.[3] Standing serves to encourage head control, allows independent bimanual activity, and helps the child develop confidence in achieving a stable, upright position (Fig. 18–3). As the child gains confidence in the standing position, some parapodia can be modified for swivel gait, or the child may be switched to ambulatory braces.

In all but the child with involvement at a very low neurologic level, children most often benefit by a process of progressive brace weaning. They begin ambulation with a swivel or a swing-to gait with the hips locked using a hip-knee-ankle-foot orthosis, i.e., long leg braces with a pelvic band, locked hips, and locked knees (Fig. 18–4). This allows the child to learn progressive control of joints. As the child gains confidence in the upright position and learns the use of a toddler's walker, the hips may then be unlocked for ambulation. The use of the pelvic band at this stage can help control torsional problems such as a tendency to in-toe or out-toe. As the child gains experience in hip control, the pelvic band may be discarded. When quadriceps strength is sufficient, the child may then be taught to walk with knee hinges unlocked; following mastery of this stage, the thigh pieces may then be removed. This weaning process allows progressive learning in ambulation, and control of each joint can be independently achieved. The ultimate level of bracing is determined by the level of paralysis, with a child paralyzed by upper lumbar involvement usually requiring long leg braces, while a child with a lower lumbar level involvement requiring only a short leg brace or ankle-foot orthosis (AFO).

### Specific Problems by Anatomic Region

#### Hip

In children with myelodysplasia, hip problems have several causes. Children with very high level paralysis develop positional contractures. Involvement at levels below the first lumbar vertebra usually causes hip problems that stem from muscle imbalance, as hip flexors and adductors are usually innervated while extensors and abductors remain flaccid. Spasticity, caused by a central nervous system injury or anomaly, is yet another source of hip problems. Children who have spastic hips can have any of the problems that a child with cerebral palsy might exhibit.

A "frogleg" deformity is often seen in children with paralysis at the thoracic level because of the tendency of the flail hip to fall into postural abduction. When involvement is at levels of the first to the fourth lumbar vertebrae, the most common contracture

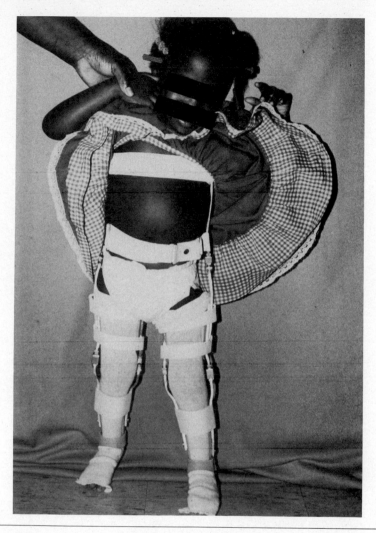

**Fig. 18–4**  Full-control braces (HKAFO) are used to begin ambulation.

about the hip is a flexion/adduction contracture, caused by unopposed hip flexors and adductors. This contracture may progress to produce a posterosuperior subluxation or dislocation (Fig. 18–5). A much rarer contracture can be seen, either as a spontaneous occurrence or following adductor/flexor release, in the face of spasticity: a hyperextension/abduction contracture may produce an anterior subluxation or dislocation of the hip.

Whether or not to treat the posterior myelodysplastic hip dislocation remains controversial. Unlike children who have cerebral palsy, a myelodysplastic child with a dislocated hip is usually not in pain.[7] A hip dislocation does not prevent bracing or ambulation.[7] Surgical procedures for treatment of hip dislocations are often extensive, and dislocations have been seen to recur postoperatively in as many as 45% of cases.[8] For these reasons, a dislocated hip should not be treated if a child has paralysis at a very high level, or if the child is not considered to be a good candidate for long-term ambulation because of obesity, poor

sense of balance, poor motivation, or other factors.

Surgical treatment of the dislocated hip may be considered in the child with excellent long-term ambulatory potential, i.e., involvement at the level of the fourth lumbar vertebra or below with no spasticity. It should be considered especially if the dislocation is unilateral, as a limb length discrepancy and pelvic obliquity may result.

The role of unilateral hip dislocation in the production of pelvic obliquity and scoliosis has not been clearly defined. According to one study, children who have a pelvic obliquity of greater than 25 degrees tend to be nonambulators, but these children also tend to have a higher neurologic level of involvement.[9] However, another study indicated that more ambulatory patients had dislocated or subluxated hips than did nonambulatory patients, reflecting a high incidence of dislocations in children with lumbar level paralysis.[10] It has not been shown that treatment of a subluxating or dislocating hip will affect the development of scoliosis.

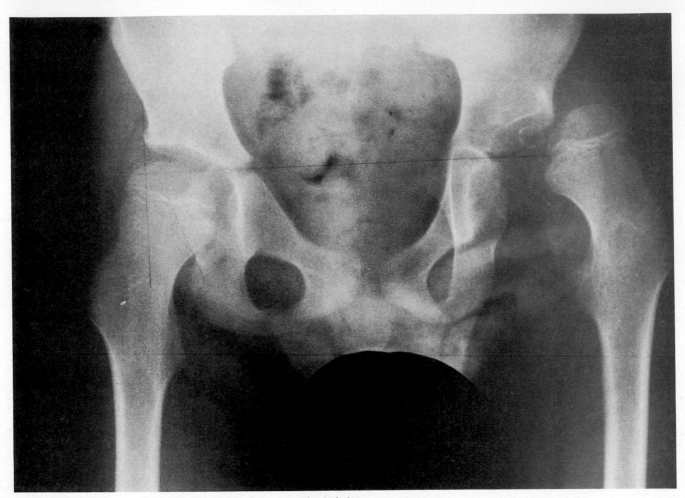

**Fig. 18–5** Progressive subluxation of left hip from muscular imbalance.

In a very young child or a child with minimal subluxation, soft-tissue releases of hip flexors and adductors may be combined with prolonged postoperative night bracing in a position of extension and abduction. The Sharrard iliopsoas transfer has been used to remove the deforming force of hip flexion and to restore hip extensor power; some authors believe it has a place in the treatment of paralysis at the level of the fourth lumbar vertebra. The Sharrard procedure is a difficult surgical endeavor, cannot be performed in a young infant, often functions as a tenodesis rather than active tendon transfer, and alters pelvic anatomy to make pelvic osteotomy difficult should it become necessary. For these reasons, many believe that iliopsoas tenotomy achieves much the same end with significantly lower surgical morbidity.[11]

Bony procedures may be considered in the older child or in the child with more significant subluxation or frank dislocation. Since these dislocations usually occur after considerable acetabular development has taken place, a varus femoral osteotomy may be sufficient to maintain reduction (Fig. 18–6). In children with a deficient or dysplastic acetabulum, an acetabuloplasty may be required. The Chiari innominate osteotomy provides coverage posteriorly as well as superiorly, and may be the most efficient in providing a buttress effect to prevent redislocation.

The very rare extension contracture, which may produce anterior hip dislocation, should always be treated to prevent loss of sitting ability. Treatment requires soft-tissue release of extensor and abductor muscles; femoral shortening may also be needed.[12]

### Knee Deformity

As in the hip, knee deformities in those who have myelodysplasia can be caused by positional contractures, muscle imbalance, or spasticity. The knee flexion contracture is generally positional, caused by prolonged sitting or crawling. In children with spasticity, it may result from a hamstring spasticity. In the ambulatory child, a knee flexion contracture decreas-

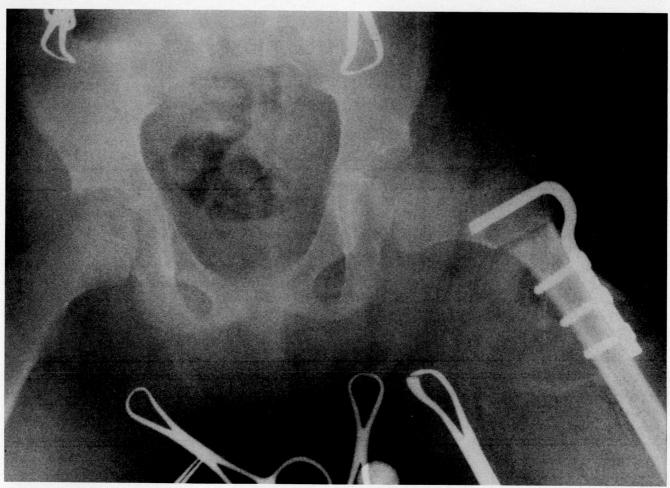

**Fig. 18–6**  With muscle releases and varus osteotomy, reduction of hip is achieved.

es quadriceps efficiency and makes bracing difficult.

Treatment of the knee flexion contracture may consist of stretching or soft-tissue release early or both. In a longer-established deformity, radical soft-tissue release is necessary[13]; if internal or external tibial torsion is concomitant, an extension/derotation osteotomy of the proximal tibia may significantly facilitate bracing and ambulation.

When the defect is at the level of the third lumbar vertebra, the child has strong quadriceps and flail hamstring muscles, which may produce a rigid extension contracture of the knee. In the neonatal period, gentle manipulation and splinting can lead to improvement. The extended position of the knee is a braceable position; flexion must not be gained at the expense of extension.

In the wheelchair-dependent child, a position of rigid knee extension makes sitting difficult and may predispose the child to fractures of the lower extremities. Surgical release of a rigid extension contracture may be indicated in a wheelchair-dependent child to achieve a proper sitting position. In the ambulatory child, V-Y quadricepsplasty,[13] or quadriceps release and even patellectomy may be necessary to achieve sufficient flexion for sitting.

### Rotational Deformities of the Leg

In myelodysplasia, in-toeing may be caused by femoral anteversion; spasticity; hamstring imbalance produced when medial hamstrings are functional and lateral hamstrings are flail; internal tibial torsion; or foot deformities.[14] The first step in treating in-toeing deformities is to identify the cause. Surgical correction, if appropriate, may consist of adductor or hamstring release or both, femoral osteotomy, or tibial osteotomy. Twister cables applied to braces have been used in the past and are seen to have improved the gait in some children, but they necessitate increased energy consumption. As energy limitation is one of the foremost causes of ambulatory failure, twister cables are not advocated.

Normal gait requires a dorsiflexion of the foot

during swing phase to allow clearance of the ground. Out-toeing occurs in the individual who has limited dorsiflexion, such as when the ankle is fixed in a short leg cast; the leg is often externally rotated to facilitate clearance of the foot in swing phase. Many children who have myelodysplasia exhibit external tibial torsion or a plano valgus foot, which often results from heel cord contracture.

External tibial torsion may be associated with a valgus deformity of the ankle joint[15] (Fig. 18–7). Orthotic fitting becomes difficult because pressure sores develop on the medial aspect of the ankle. External tibial torsion may also be associated with increased femoral anteversion.

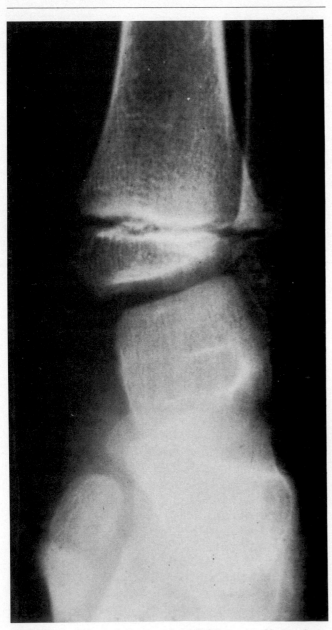

**Fig. 18–7** Valgus deformity of ankle joint, with fibular shortening.

External tibial torsion may be treated by supermalleolar derotational osteotomy, with correction of ankle valgus as needed. Ankle valgus may also be corrected by physeal stapling or hemiepiphysiodesis of the medial aspect of the ankle, providing sufficient growth is remaining to correct the deformity.

**Foot Deformity**

Sixty-three percent of myelodysplastic children exhibit a deformity of the foot.[16] These deformities must be classified as to cause in order to facilitate treatment. The first group includes congenital anomalies, such as clubfoot and vertical talus. The second group is caused by muscle imbalance, such as a calcaneus deformity from unopposed tibialis anterior function, and pes cavus or claw toes from paralysis of the intrinsic foot muscles. The third group of deformities is caused by spasticity and may include any of the above-mentioned deformities, as well as talipes equinus or valgus caused by peroneal spasm.

Treatment of a congenital deformity such as clubfoot consists of surgical release very similar to that employed to treat the nonparalytic foot. A standard posteromedial release is used and, in contrast to treatment of the neurologically normal foot, unopposed tendons are not repaired. If peroneal function is absent, the tibialis posterior and long flexors may be cut rather than lengthened.

Serial casting is employed by some in an attempt to decrease the deformity and minimize skin problems at surgery. The author, however, does not employ serial casting because the skin is insensate and the deformity is often quite rigid, ultimately requiring surgery regardless of nonoperative treatment. However, a percutaneous heel cord lengthening may often be done in early infancy without anesthesia, and may significantly reduce the apparent deformity while not precluding the need for surgery. In the severely deformed foot or in the older child, talectomy may be required to allow proper shoe fitting (Fig. 18–8). Anomalous vascularity or dysvascularity of the foot or both may exist. Skin closure may be difficult after correction of a rigid deformity; therefore, one must be prepared for skin grafting.

In deformities caused by muscle imbalance, treatment may be aimed at rendering the affected joint flail or at balancing musculature about the foot. The calcaneus deformity produced by an unopposed tibialis anterior can produce severe gait problems as well as ulcerations from weightbearing on the point of the heel. In patients with involvement at the level of the fourth lumbar vertebra who have grade 3 strength of tibialis anterior, treatment consists of tibialis anterior tenotomy with subsequent bracing. Transfer of the tibialis anterior through the interosseous membrane to the calcaneus, followed by bracing, is useful in children with involvement at the level of the fifth

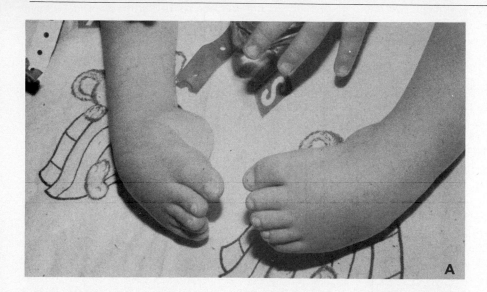

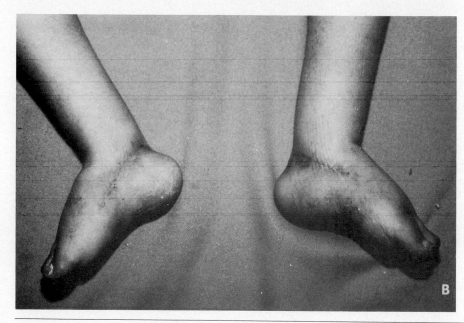

**Fig. 18–8   A:** Rigid clubfoot deformity. **B:** After treatment with talectomy to enable shoe wear.

lumbar vertebra with strong dorsiflexors and no spasticity.[17]

Deformities caused by spasticity must be individually considered. Increasing spasticity or a changing neurologic picture may indicate a correctable central nervous system lesion; if the spasticity cannot be treated, the deformity produced by spasticity must be corrected. Muscle balancing may be cautiously attempted by such means as split anterior tibial transfer, which may be combined with split posterior tibial transfer. As is true for patients with cerebral palsy, tendon transfers in patients with myelodysplasia must be carefully considered to preclude development of an opposite deformity.

### Fracture

Children with myelodysplasia are prone to frac-

tures caused by disuse and osteopenia. Fractures often occur in the postoperative period, after cast immobilization has been discontinued. For this reason, postoperative casting should be minimized, with rapid transition to brace protection of operative sites. In addition, the positioning of casts to allow standing and weightbearing is to be encouraged.

Fractures occurring in insensate limbs are difficult to diagnose. The child will often appear slightly ill, mildly febrile, with a swollen, hot extremity. Significant sequelae of fractures may include fat embolism, pulmonary embolism, or hypovolemia from bleeding about the fracture site.[18] Younger children may develop physeal changes from repeated microtrauma to the physis. This so-called Charcot physis must be distinguished from a neoplasm or other growth disturbance. Once the problem has been identified, the physis must be protected to allow healing.[19] In the management of myelodysplasia, a high index of suspicion for a fracture must be maintained.

## Obesity

Obesity is a major problem in children with myelodysplasia. It decreases ambulatory capacity, impairs self-image, endangers overall health, and increases surgical risks. Orthopaedists should play as active a role as any primary care physician in educating parents early and encouraging compliance with dietary regimen.

## Skin Ulceration

The insensate skin in spina bifida is particularly prone to breakdown in areas of weightbearing, especially where there is an underlying bony prominence. Prevention or correction of deformity, especially that producing an imbalance of weightbearing on insensate skin, can help to prevent the devastating effects of skin ulceration and osteomyelitis. Education of parents and children is important and must begin when the child is young. Children should be taught to inspect their skin daily, to maintain proper hygiene, and to take other measures that will decrease the likelihood of ulceration.

## Summary

Myelodysplasia is a multisystem disease that requires a multidisciplinary approach. The orthopaedist is often the first to identify a changing neurologic picture or deformity and must work closely with neurosurgical colleagues to identify correctable neurologic lesions.

The role of the orthopaedist begins at the birth of the child with spina bifida. At this time, the level of neurologic involvement can be determined. Education of the parents can then begin by outlining the expected ambulatory potential of the child, and predicting deformities or complications that might be anticipated depending on the level of neurologic involvement. The orthopaedist must also emphasize the extreme importance of neurosurgical care in preventing deterioration of neurologic function, so that goals for ambulation and musculoskeletal function can be achieved.

As the child gets older, motor milestones paralleling those of a normal child should be sought with use of a corner chair or sitting device, followed by the use of a standing frame if needed. If appropriate, the child will then progress to full-control braces, with weaning as determined by neurologic level of involvement. Long-term mobility may be achieved by bracing or by the use of a wheelchair. A realistic approach must be taken in goal-setting, so that a child is not pressured to achieve unrealistic goals yet is enabled to achieve full functional capacity.

## References

1. McLaughlin J, et al: Management of the fetus and newborn with neural tube defects. *J Perinatol* 1984;4:3–11.
2. Waters RL, Lunsford BR: Energy cost of paraplegic locomotion. *J Bone Joint Surg* 1985;67A:1245–1250.
3. Menelaus MB: *The Orthopaedic Management of Spina Bifida Cystica*, ed 2. Edinburgh, Churchill-Livingstone Inc, 1980.
4. Mazur JA, et al: The significance of spasticity in the upper and lower extremities in myelomeningocele. *J Bone Joint Surg* 1986;68B:213–217.
5. Brown HP: Management of spinal deformity in myelomeningocele. *Orthop Clin North Am* 1978;9:391–402.
6. Winter RB, Haven JJ, Moe JH: Diastematomyelia and congenital spine deformities. *J Bone Joint Surg* 1974;56A:27–39.
7. Barden GA, Meyer LC, Stelling FH: Myelodysplastics: Fate of those followed for twenty years or more. *J Bone Joint Surg* 1975;57A:643–647.
8. Bazih J, Gross RH: Hip surgery in the lumbar level myelomeningocele patient. *J Pediatr Orthop* 1981;1:405–411.
9. Kahanovitz N, Duncan JW: The role of scoliosis and pelvic obliquity in functional disability in myelomeningocele. *Spine* 1981;6:494–497.
10. Stillwell A, Menelaus MB: Walking ability in mature patients with spina bifida. *J Pediatr Orthop* 1983;3:184–190.
11. Breed AL, Healy PM: The midlumbar myelomeningocele hip: Mechanism of dislocation and treatment. *J Pediatr Orthop* 1982;2:15–24.
12. Szalay EA, et al: Extension-abduction contracture of the spastic hip. *J Pediatr Orthop* 1986;6:1–6.
13. Dias LS: Surgical management of knee contractures in myelomeningocele. *J Pediatr Orthop* 1982;2:127–131.
14. Dias LS, Murali JJ, Collins P: Rotational deformities of the lower limb in myelomeningocele. *J Bone Joint Surg* 1984;66A:215–223.
15. Dias LS: Valgus deformity of the ankle joint: Pathogenesis of fibular shortening. *J Pediatr Orthop* 1985;5:176–180.
16. Duckworth T: Management of the feet in spinal dysraphism and myelodysplasia, in Jahss MD (ed): *Disorders of the Foot*. Philadelphia, WB Saunders, 1982.
17. Banta JV, et al: Anterior tibial transfer to the os calcis with Achilles tenodesis for calcaneal deformity in myelomeningocele. *J Pediatr Orthop* 1981;1:125–131.
18. Anschuetz RH, Freehafer AA, Shaffer JW, et al: Severe fracture complications in myelodysplasia. *J Pediatr Orthop* 1984;4:22–24.
19. Wenger DR, Jeffcoat BT, Herring JA: The guarded prognosis of physeal injury in paraplegic children. *J Bone Joint Surg* 1980;62A:241–246.

# Neuromuscular Spine Deformities

John E. Lonstein, MD

Thomas S. Renshaw, MD

## Introduction

Successful orthopaedic management of neuromuscular spinal deformities includes assessment and treatment of the total patient, with particular attention to individual priorities. This approach usually is best accomplished by using a multidisciplinary health care team. Scoliosis or kyphosis is often difficult to control by orthotic means, although an orthosis may slow curve progression and allow further growth to occur prior to definitive correction and fusion of the spine.

Recent technical advances in spinal instrumentation, particularly those incorporating segmental fixation devices, have rapidly improved and expanded the scope of surgical spinal correction. Nevertheless, all of the neuromuscular disease processes are unique. Each requires a thoroughly skilled and individualized approach to management.

Priorities of patients with severe neuromuscular diseases are as follows: the ability to communicate with other people; the ability to perform many activities of daily living; mobility and ambulation.[1] The orthopaedic surgeon's role in the achievement of these priorities includes (1) prescribing orthoses for lower extremity control to facilitate transferring to and from wheelchairs; (2) preventing or correcting joint contractures; and (3) maintaining appropriate standing or sitting postures. Spinal deformity control is particularly important because of the high prevalence of scoliosis and kyphosis associated with the various neuromuscular diseases (Table 19–1). This chapter will discuss neuromuscular spinal deformities

in general, as well as some of the specific variations of the more common disease processes.

## The Cause of Scoliosis in Neuromuscular Diseases

The specific biomechanical explanation of the genesis and progression of scoliosis in patients with neuromuscular diseases does not exist. One hypothesis is that spinal stability (or freedom from deformity) is directly proportional to the condition of the end support of the spine and inversely proportional to both spinal flexibility and to the approximate square of spinal column length. The amount of tolerable load on a flexible helical column before it buckles can be increased by firm support of the lower and upper ends of the column and decreased by increasing the column's flexibility or its length. It follows that loss of muscle strength or voluntary muscle control, or loss of sensory abilities such as proprioception, when occurring in the relatively flexible and elongating spinal column of a juvenile or adolescent with neuromuscular disease, may be a factor in the development of scoliosis (Fig. 19–1).

## Characteristics of Neuromuscular Scoliosis

In addition to neuromuscular involvement, which is not seen in persons with idiopathic scoliosis, there are other differences between these two types of scoliosis. Neuromuscular scoliosis usually develops at a younger age than does the idiopathic type. Even small curves may progress beyond skeletal maturity and throughout life. In patients with neuromuscular disease, a larger percentage of curves are progressive as compared with the idiopathic type. In addition, many patients with neuromuscular disease have pelvic obliquity, hip joint contractures, and lower extremity asymmetry, which can affect the lumbar spine. Progressing neurologic or muscular disease may also interfere with normal trunk stability. These patients are also usually not as tolerant of orthotic treatment because of discomfort or skin problems. Spinal surgery in this group may be more difficult because of increased bleeding, less satisfactory bone stock, and the frequent necessity to fuse from the upper thoracic region to the pelvis.

**Table 19–1**
**Prevalence of spinal deformities in various neuromuscular disorders**

| Neuromuscular Disorder | Percent With Spinal Deformity |
| --- | --- |
| Cerebral palsy | 25 |
| Myelomeningocele | 60 |
| Infantile quadriplegia | 100 |
| Preadolescent quadriplegia | 90 |
| Duchenne's muscular dystrophy | 95 |
| Spinal muscular atrophy types I, II, and III | 100 |
| Friedreich's ataxia | 95 |

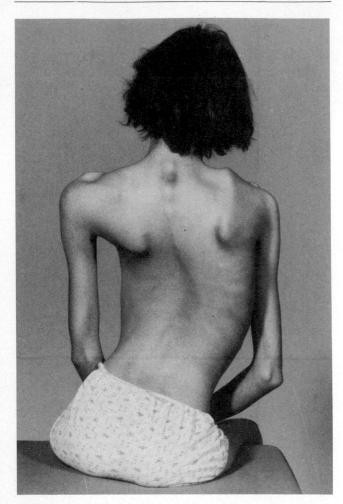

**Fig. 19–1** This 13-year-old girl with neuromuscular scoliosis demonstrates pelvic obliquity (poor lower end support), neck and shoulder muscle atrophy (poor upper end support), rapid growth (increased column length), and reasonable flexibility. They may all be factors in the genesis of her spinal deformity.

## Observation

Not all neuromuscular spine deformities require immediate treatment. Two groups of deformities can be observed for progression before active treatment is started: small curves under 30 degrees must be carefully followed for progression before treatment is instituted; large curves in markedly retarded patients in which the spine deformity has caused no loss of functional status may also be followed. These patients are observed for both progression of their spine deformity and loss of functional status. If the curve progresses, treatment is started. If functional ability is lost or changes, treatment is started. These changes in functional status include a decrease in or loss of walking ability, or a change in sitting ability, e.g., more support may be required to maintain an upright sitting position, or sitting ability may be completely lost. In progressive neuromuscular diseases, loss of function may be caused by progression of the disease or increase in the neuromuscular spine deformity or both.

## Orthotic Treatment

Progressive scoliosis in a very young patient with neuromuscular disease is best approached by an attempt at orthotic control. Even though the scoliosis often continues to progress despite orthotic treatment, usually the rate of progression is slowed by the orthosis, and this temporizing measure can allow further spinal growth to occur before definitive arthrodesis is done. In patients in whom orthotic control appears to halt curve progression permanently, it is difficult, if not impossible, to determine whether or not this phenomenon stems from the natural history of the deformity in those patients.

Infants with neuromuscular diseases may develop significant scoliosis, necessitating orthotic treatment during the first year of life. If the child is large enough, a custom-molded, total contact, thoracolumbosacral orthosis (TLSO) may be used; however, it is often helpful to begin treatment with a Kalibis splint, which applies the principle of three-point fixation to treat the curve.[2] This type of splint is extremely helpful when the infant's trunk contour will not accommodate a more standard TLSO (Fig. 19–2). Older children with scoliosis who have poor voluntary trunk-muscle control are best treated with passive, total contact TLSOs (Fig. 19–2), whereas those who have adequate trunk control may tolerate a "dynamic" form of TLSO, such as a Boston or Milwaukee orthosis. Patients with severe involvement who have no sitting balance and poor head control are often best managed by custom fabricated seating devices such as chair inserts. Another device, the thoracic suspension orthosis, has been helpful in the rare situation in which severe respiratory compromise or problems with skin breakdown can be alleviated by suspending the patient from his thoracic cage using this wheelchair-type of orthosis[3] (Fig. 19–3).

In severe cases in which external orthotic control has failed, but the patient is too young for definitive spinal fusion, use of an internal orthosis, the so-called "rod without fusion," is a valuable alternative.[4,5] This type of surgery involves the insertion of a strong metallic rod, or rods, usually either a Harrington, Moe, or Luque system (Fig. 19–4). Spinal fusion is not performed, and an external orthosis is necessary to support the internal fixation. The hope is that the curve magnitude can be controlled until the patient is old enough for definitive fusion.

## Seating

In clinics at which a large number of cerebral palsy patients are treated, help with seating is an important part of the nonoperative treatment provided. Pa-

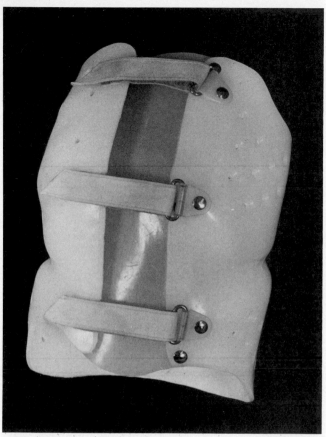

**Fig. 19–2** A polypropylene, anterior opening, total contact thoracolumbosacral orthosis (TLSO) commonly used for the orthotic treatment of neuromuscular scoliosis.

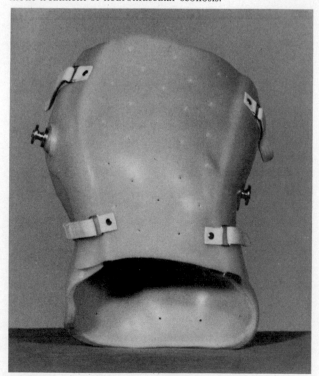

**Fig. 19–3** A bivalve thoracic suspension orthosis. The metal side-spools allow placement on suspension hooks attached to the wheelchair.

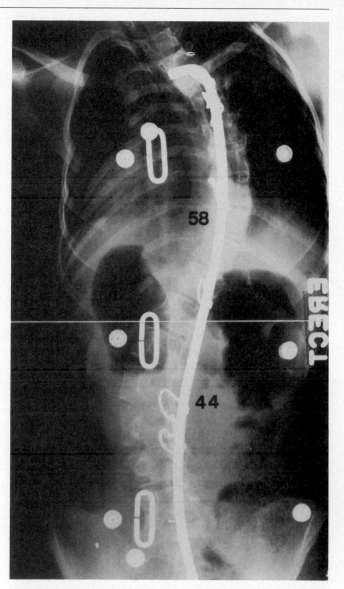

**Fig. 19–4** This 8-year-old girl had double structural neuromuscular curves of 84 degrees and 72 degrees and was deemed too skeletally immature for definitive spinal fusion. A single 0.25-inch L-rod was inserted by exposing only the convex side of each curve and attaching double sublaminar wires at the curve ends and apices. Postoperative orthotic support was essential. After two years of further spinal growth, a fusion was performed.

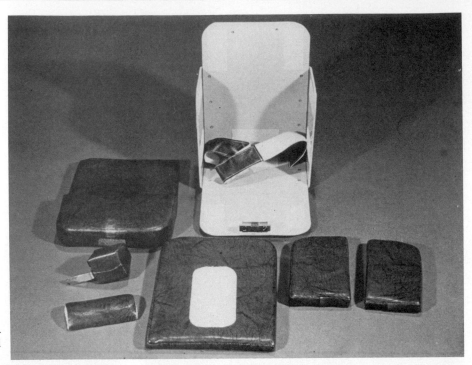

**Fig. 19-5** Upholstered sitting support orthosis with plastic frame and pads to be added.

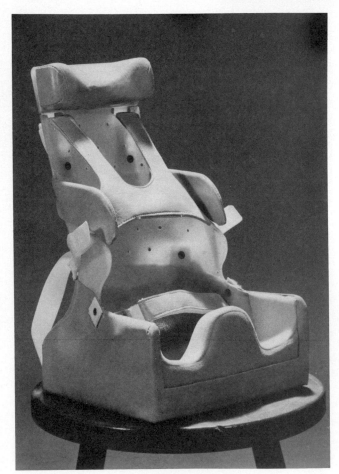

**Fig. 19-6** "Gillette" molded sitting support orthosis.

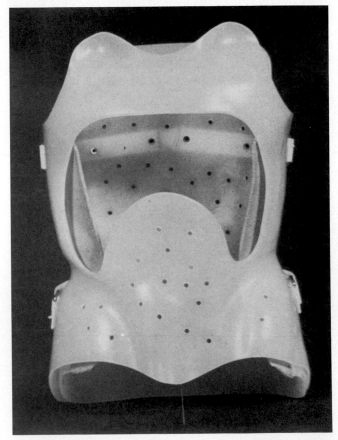

**Fig. 19-7** Two-piece TLSO consisting of interlocking anterior and posterior shells. (Reproduced with permission from Lonstein JE: Deformities of the spine in children with cerebral palsy. *Orthop Rev* 1981;10:33–44.)

tients with absent or reduced sitting balance need help to achieve and maintain a balanced, upright sitting posture. This group includes patients with cerebral palsy or those with paralysis or muscle weakness. The latter group are able to sit with hand support, but in patients with upper extremity weakness this support is not possible. The use of the hands to help with seating turns these paraplegic patients into functional quadriplegics, as the hands are used for sitting support and not for normal upper extremity functional activities.

### Types of Seating Devices

Many devices are available to supply sitting support.[6] The seating devices available are the Tumbleform seat, commercial chairs, the upholstered sitting support orthosis, and the molded sitting support orthosis. These are either commercially made or custom fitted to each individual. The commercial supports have the advantage of easy availability and some adjustment with growth. The disadvantage is that spine control is not optimal and difficult seating situations cannot be treated. The custom-fitted supports give better spine support but take time to fabricate and are not as adjustable for growth.

**Tumbleform Seat** This seat is foam molded and comes in three sizes. It is used for infants and small children and is very effective in supporting these flexible spines; it becomes less effective as the child grows and becomes taller and heavier. A lap belt can be added and the seat can be placed in a stroller or placed on the floor.

**Commercial Chairs** Many chairs are available, specific brands being obtainable in different parts of the country. Examples are the Transporter chair, McClarren buggy, Orthokinetic chair, Responder chair and Mulholland chair. These chairs generally have a pelvic support, abduction pillow, thoracic support, and head support and are useful for flexible, easily controlled spines. They tend to be less effective for larger individuals or where more spine control is necessary. These chairs also are bulky.

**Upholstered Sitting Support Orthosis (SSO)** The upholstered SSO consists of a padded base (seat and back) made of wood or plastic (Fig. 19–5). In all cases, a lap or pelvic strap is added to stabilize the pelvis and a thoracic vest used when thoracic support is necessary. This SSO is placed in a wheelchair to which it is secured. This support is easily adjustable by adding to the base (wood or plastic) and altering the padding. In addition, the pelvis can be controlled with the addition of lateral pelvic supports.

**Molded Sitting Support Orthosis (SSO)** The molded SSO is a plastic custom-fitted support made from a mold taken from the patient.[7] It extends from the distal thighs to the upper back with extensions around the pelvis and thorax (Fig. 19–6). A lap (pelvic) belt is attached to maintain the pelvic position. A thoracic vest is added to hold the trunk back in the support, and a head support is added when necessary. Because of the custom fit and added pelvic and thoracic supports, this SSO supplies maximal sitting support and is used for difficult seating problems. Some adjustment for growth is possible with the addition of plastic to the seat or back portion and widening of the orthosis.

The main principle of any sitting support is progressive trunk and spine control. As with any tall structure, the support of the base is first. This involves lateral pelvic support and a lap belt that holds the pelvis back in any seat. The spine and trunk are controlled by lateral thoracic supports and the thoracic vest. The head is supported with appropriate head supports. The amount of support needed depends on the sitting balance of the patient. If controlling the pelvis allows a good sitting posture, this minimal support is all that is necessary. If, on the other hand, the trunk is still unstable with pelvic support, then thoracic support is necessary. If on fitting the sitting support the head is not controlled, a head support is added. This support is usually accompanied by tilting back of the whole sitting support, which aids in head control.

The tendency of an unstable column, e.g., the spine, to collapse is shown by Euler's law, which gives the critical load able to be supported. In a column with the lower end stabilized and the upper end free the formula is: $\pi EI/4L^2$

Where E = elasticity of the column, I = the area moment of inertia, and L = the length of the column. If the length increases, or the weight increases (smaller area moment of inertia) the critical load able to be supported decreases and the column is more unstable. This law explains why the spine becomes more difficult to support and curves more difficult to control when a child becomes taller and heavier.

What are the results of the use of sitting support? A study of the molded SSO has shown that postural curves are corrected, with no effect on structural curves. Functionally if hand use is present, in the SSO this use is improved. The greatest effect was seen in nursing care. Less care was necessary, as less time was needed for constant repositioning of the patient. In addition, transportation was easier, as an upright position was maintained in the sitting support since the support (with or without its base) could be easily placed in a car or van.

### Thoracolumbosacral Orthosis (TLSO)

The two-piece custom-molded TLSO is important in curve control of neuromuscular spine deformities (Fig. 19–7). It is used to control and correct the scoliosis or kyphosis during the growing years. In this way spine growth is allowed to occur without increasing the deformity. The TLSO is removed for skin care, especially if there is insensate skin. It is usually worn only when the child is upright during the day and is removed at night. Thus, spinal growth is maximized, the curve is controlled, and fusion is needed only at the onset of puberty.

### Surgical Principles

The goal of spinal surgery in patients with neuromuscular scoliosis is to produce a solid arthrodesis of a balanced spine, in the frontal and sagittal planes, over a level pelvis. To accomplish this goal requires a long fusion, usually from the upper thoracic region to either the lower lumbar region or the pelvis, with strong and rigid internal fixation and massive bone grafting. Autogenous bone almost always requires augmentation by bone bank allograft. The development of the L-rod technique (Fig. 19–8) and other forms of segmental spinal fixation has been responsible for a significant advance in the treatment of these difficult deformities.

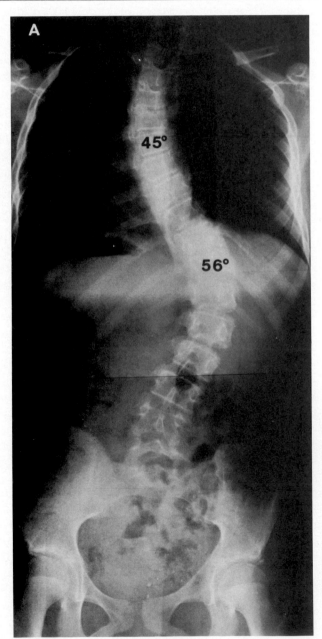
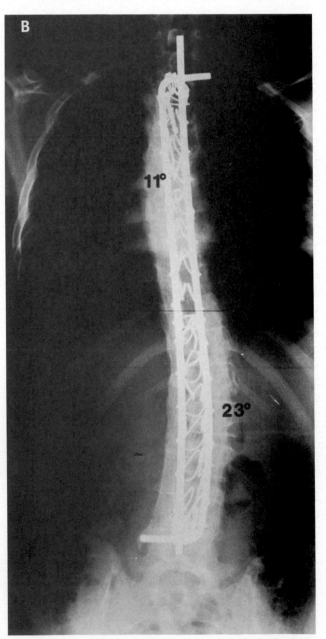

**Fig. 19–8** Preoperative and postoperative views of neuromuscular scoliosis operated on using the L-rod techniques and spinal fusion.

## Preoperative Considerations

Preoperative considerations must include a thorough general medical workup, focusing not only on the musculoskeletal and neurologic systems, but also on the patient's cardiac and pulmonary status and general nutrition. Preoperative hyperalimentation can be a valuable adjunct to the successful surgical management of scoliosis. Gastrointestinal problems such as hiatal hernia or esophageal reflux are common in patients with neuromuscular disease and should be corrected preoperatively if thought to be significant. Many conditions such as Duchenne's muscular dystrophy and Friedreich's ataxia have associated cardiac involvement, which must be carefully evaluated. Most patients with neuromuscular disorders have diminished pulmonary functions. Assessment of the pulmonary status, particularly forced vital capacity and one-second forced expiratory volume, are important. Measurement of arterial blood gases may also be useful in preoperative respiratory evaluation of patients with severe involvement.

Assessment of the patient's ambulatory status is important, since a marginal walker with a progressive disease will probably not walk again following spinal surgery. In such cases, if the surgery should not be deferred, the patient and the parents must understand this fact. Assessment of pelvic obliquity and hip contractures is important, not only for balancing the spine at surgery but also to plan for intraoperative positioning of the patient. Rigid spinal decompensation in the sagittal plane is usually corrected by anterior release and posterior contouring of segmentally attached rods. Decompensation in the frontal plane may require such procedures as vertebrectomy, anterior spinal releases with or without instrumentation, and pelvic osteotomies.[8]

Whether or not an anterior fusion will be necessary is an important preoperative consideration. Anterior fusion should be performed (1) when anterior release is necessary for further correction of severe kyphosis, lordosis, or pelvic obliquity; (2) when scoliosis is severe and rigid and cannot be corrected by traction or bending to an acceptable magnitude (usually less than 60 degrees); or (3) when posterior elements are deficient, such as in patients with myelomeningocele or patients who have had extensive laminectomies performed.

It is important to assess the biplanar extent of the fusion. Most patients with neuromuscular disease require fusion at least as cephalad as the second thoracic vertebra to prevent or minimize the later development of kyphosis above the level of the fusion. The caudal extent of the spinal fusion is usually the pelvis if there is fixed obliquity (greater than 10 to 15 degrees of L4 or L5 tilt relative to the interiliac crest line) and in cases of complete paralysis, such as occurs in patients with myelomeningocele or spinal cord injury.

The type of instrumentation must be determined preoperatively. In neuromuscular scoliosis, segmental instruments are preferable to single distraction rods for posterior fixation. Whether or not anterior instrumentation is necessary depends upon the deformity and the type of posterior fixation planned. Internal fixation of the anterior part of the spine is employed most often in cases of severe lordosis and in scoliosis with deficient posterior bony elements.

The source of bone graft is another important consideration. Many patients with neuromuscular disease have insufficient autogenous bone, either iliac or rib, available for the development of an adequate fusion mass; therefore, augmentation with allografts such as freeze-dried bone or bone from frozen femoral heads is usually necessary.

Techniques to minimize blood loss are important. These may include the judicious use of electrocautery, hypotensive anesthesia, and hemodilution techniques. Use of a cell-saver can reduce the requirement for homologous blood transfusion. Because chronic anemia and poor nutrition are common in patients with scoliosis caused by neuromuscular disease, most are not suitable candidates for preoperative auto-donation of blood.

Finally, it is extremely important to remember that a thorough, detailed, in-depth discussion with the patient's family of the alternative forms of treatment, the planned surgical procedure, its benefits, its risks, and its problems, is essential prior to surgery. Such a discussion must be documented in the patient's medical record.

## Operative Considerations

Neuromuscular spinal surgery should be performed by an experienced, skilled operating team using modern monitoring techniques such as arterial blood gases, central venous pressure, patient core temperature, urine output, and careful measurement of blood loss from suction and weighed sponges. Spinal cord monitoring by means of somatosensory evoked potentials appears to be a valuable technique for patients in whom it is appropriate, e.g., patients with sufficient lower extremity neurologic function. Relative hypothermia often occurs in a lengthy spinal operation in which a large area of tissue is exposed. Heating and humidifying anesthetic gases are the most effective means of preventing this problem.[9]

The surgical technique includes meticulous cleaning of the posterior elements of the spine, with removal of all soft tissue that might interfere with consolidation of the fusion mass. Most surgeons believe that facet joint ablation is important, although those who advocate simply the application of a massive bone graft appear to have good results.[10] A massive bone graft is important to any spinal fusion; in fact it has been stated that as long as the fascia can be closed, then too much bone has not been added. The surgical instrumentation must include balancing the spine to the best extent possible in both the frontal and sagittal planes.

### Postoperative Considerations

In the postoperative period, monitoring of arterial blood gases, central venous pressure, fluid intake and output, body temperature, and hemoglobin and hematocrit should continue. Pulmonary problems are likely complications in the immediate postoperative period and should be prevented or minimized by providing expert pulmonary care, including ventilatory support if needed. Such techniques as periodic suctioning, the use of Spiro-care or blow-bottles and intermittent positive pressure breathing may be appropriate.

Careful attention should be given to the patient's fluid balance. Following spinal surgery, particularly in patients with neuromuscular scoliosis, the antidiuretic hormone levels usually increase profoundly.[11] This increase accounts, in part, for the third space shifts, fluid retention, and oliguria commonly seen in the first 12 to 48 hours. Fluid overload, particularly in patients with impaired renal function or pulmonary compromise, should be avoided.

Once the patient's pulmonary status and fluid balance have been stabilized, mobilization should begin as rapidly as possible by simply elevating the head of the patient's bed, getting the patient to sit up in a chair as soon as tolerable, and resuming ambulation if this was the patient's preoperative status. Rehabilitation, in fact, should begin preoperatively with exercises to maintain upper and lower extremity strength and mobility.

### Complications

Death may result from neuromuscular spinal surgery either because of anesthetic problems or, more commonly, postoperative pulmonary deterioration. Major complications include paralysis, which may occur from an intraoperative traumatic event or from ischemia secondary to thrombosis or edema; pulmonary complications such as atelectasis, pneumonia, or embolic phenomena; infection; and pseudarthroses with instrument failure.

Neurologic injury, other than that which results from inadvertent technical error, occurs most commonly when correcting scoliotic curves of initial magnitudes greater than 90 to 100 degrees. Such large curves are frequently best managed by anterior release followed by careful halo traction to obtain safe, monitored correction and then definitive posterior stabilization after the correction has been obtained. If

one-stage correction of severe scoliosis is carried out in patients with intact spinal cords, spinal cord monitoring, either by somatosensory evoked potentials or the "wake-up" test, is important.[12,13] Although these tests may detect neurologic injury "after-the-fact," the more rapid the detection and treatment of the problem the better the chance for neurologic recovery.

Infection is always a potential problem in the metabolically compromised host, particularly when a temporally and anatomically lengthy spinal fusion operation has been necessary. Patients with myelomeningocele and cerebral palsy appear to have the highest infection rates.

Deep infections can be treated by opening the entire length of the wound down to the instruments and thoroughly debriding and irrigating the wound and washing the bone graft. The graft is replaced and the instruments are left in place. If on debridement the wound is clean, primary closure over irrigation and suction tubes is carried out, leaving the tubes in for five to seven days and prescribing appropriate antibiotic coverage. If after debridement the wound is not healthy or the infection is severe, the patient is treated with repeat debridement and dressing changes with antibiotic coverage until the infection is controlled. Careful delayed primary closure may be carried out, or if appropriate, granulation tissue is allowed to form over the instruments, with healing by secondary intention. The occurrence of a deep infection does not appear to compromise the ultimate healing of the arthrodesis.

Pseudarthrosis formation, with subsequent instrument failure, can be a late postoperative problem. If a pseudarthrosis is suspected because of pain or instrument failure, such techniques as oblique radiographs, recumbent bending radiographs, or tomograms may be helpful. Technetium 99m bone scans are also occasionally valuable in detection of a pseudarthrosis. If the patient with a pseudarthrosis has pain or loss of correction has occurred, repair will probably be necessary. On the other hand, an asymptomatic pseudarthrosis without curve progression can be appropriately managed by observation.

## Spinal Deformity in Specific Neuromuscular Conditions

### Cerebral Palsy

The general principles delineated above will be applied to the spine deformities of cerebral palsy, which are used as an example of neuromuscular deformities. Thereafter, other causes will be described and their treatment plan given, showing how they differ from cerebral palsy. Whereas deformities secondary to poliomyelitis used to be the most common neuromuscular spine deformities, the advent of vaccines has all but eliminated this disease. Today, spine deformities associated with cerebral palsy are the most common neuromuscular deformities in the Western world.[14-16]

The incidence of spine deformities in cerebral palsy varies depending on the degree of neuromuscular involvement.[17] In an ambulatory population of spastic hemiplegics the incidence is under 10%,[14] whereas in a population of total-care spastic quadriplegics, the incidence is nearly 70%.[18] These deformities can be treated by observation, seating, orthoses, or surgery depending on their severity and the age of the child.

**Observation** Certain curves are observed in the child with cerebral palsy. These are small curves under 30 degrees in the growing child or larger curves up to 45 or 50 degrees in the skeletally mature patient. Larger curves are treated, depending on the patient's mental status. If the growing child has normal or near-

normal intelligence, curves over 30 degrees are immediately treated. In the skeletally mature child, on the other hand, larger curves are handled in the same manner as in idiopathic scoliosis, with fusion of curves greater than 45 to 50 degrees.

In the child with moderate to marked mental retardation, curves over 30 degrees are observed. The child is followed at four- to 12-month intervals depending on the skeletal maturity. The magnitude of the curve and its effect on the functional status of the child are followed. If curve increase has been documented or if the curve changes the functional status of the child, treatment is instituted. It can be either nonoperative or operative depending on the magnitude of the curve and the maturity of the child.

In cerebral palsy, there are two broad categories of spinal deformities. Firstly, kyphosis or scoliosis may be present because the child has not developed normal sitting balance. If placed in a sitting position,

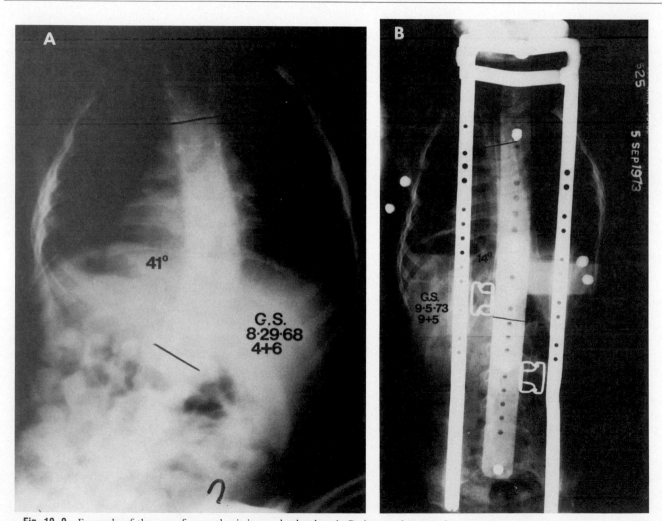

**Fig. 19–9**   Example of the use of an orthosis in cerebral palsy. **A:** Patient at the age of 4 years, 6 months with a 41-degree right thoracic scoliosis. She was ambulatory. **B:** A Milwaukee brace was fitted, which controlled the curve during her growth; a 14-degree curve at the age of 9 is shown. (Reproduced with permission from Lonstein JE: Deformities of the spine in children with cerebral palsy. *Orthop Rev* 1981;10:33–44.)

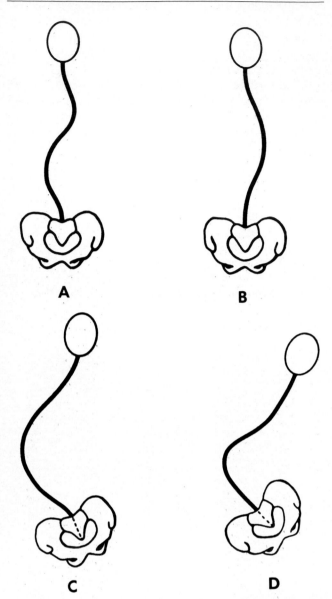

**Fig. 19-10** Curve patterns in cerebral palsy. **A and B** show a group I curve with a level pelvis, **A** being a double curve and **B** a single thoracic curve. **C and D** are examples of group II curves with pelvic obliquity, the sacrum being part of the curve. (Reproduced with permission from Lonstein JE and Akbarnia BA: Operative treatment of spinal deformity in patients with cerebral palsy or mental retardation—an analysis of 107 cases. *J Bone Joint Surg* 1983;65A:43–45.)

the child will fall forward into a total spinal kyphosis or sideways with scoliosis. Secondly, a structural curve, usually scoliosis, may be present. The collapsing spine seen in neuromuscular deformities is not seen in cerebral palsy.

As cerebral palsy is a result of a traumatic, infectious, anoxic, or hemorrhagic insult to the brain, all aspects of cerebral function must be evaluated: mental status, hand function, developmental stage, muscle tone, vision, hearing and communication ability. With reference to the spinal deformity, evaluation of the type and magnitude of deformity, as well as of the functional, ambulatory or sitting status of the child is important.

**Seating** In a cerebral palsy clinic, seating is the most common form of nonoperative treatment used.[6,7] Because of the delay in physical and mental development, sitting ability is retarded or absent. The exact choice of seating device depends on the individual's age and sitting ability, and follows the principles above. Many children require sitting support into adulthood, the molded SSO being ideal for this purpose because of its durability, its close fit, which minimizes skin pressure problems, and its ability to control the pelvis and spine of a larger patient.

**Orthoses** Orthoses[19] are used for curve control during growth usually in a child who is ambulatory with or without assistance or who has independent sitting ability (Fig. 19–9). Children who are dependent sitters occasionally need an orthosis for curve control during growth. The orthosis of choice is a TLSO, either one with a one-piece back opening or more commonly one with a two-piece bivalved design. A Milwaukee brace is generally poorly tolerated by children with cerebral palsy, but may be used occasionally.

As functional curves are more common than structural curves in cerebral palsy, the use of seating devices is more common than the use of orthoses for curve treatment and control. It is rare for a child whose curve is controlled by a seating device to require an orthosis. If the curve, functional or structural, increases in the seating device, it occurs at the time of the pubertal growth spurt. At this stage, surgery is usually the treatment of choice rather than a TLSO.

In some cases the TLSO controls the curve initially, but subsequent curve increase occurs despite a well-fitting orthosis that is worn as prescribed. In these cases, instrumentation without fusion can be used to control the curve during growth, allowing spinal growth and postponing spinal arthrodesis until puberty. This program is used in cerebral palsy, but it seems to be less effective than in other neuromuscular deformities, which may be because of the structural nature of the scoliosis as well as the retarded growth rate in these children.

**Surgery** The indications for surgical correction[20–22] and stabilization of spinal deformities depend on the mental state of the individual with cerebral palsy. In children with normal or near-normal intelligence, the indications are similar to those for idiopathic scoliosis, i.e., curves of 40 to 45 degrees or greater during puberty, curves over 50 to 60 degrees in the young adult, progressive curves or those that do not respond to nonoperative treatment. In children with moderate to marked mental retardation, the indica-

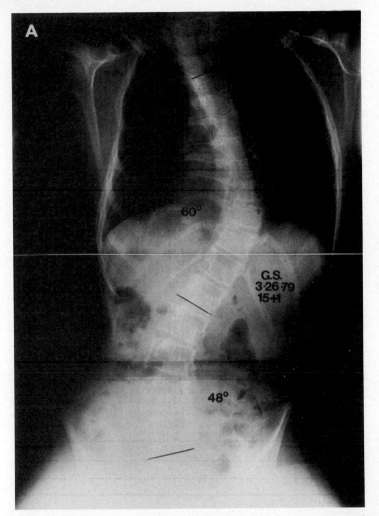
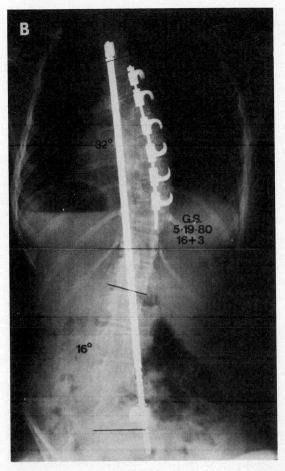

**Fig. 19–11**  (Continuation of Fig. 19–9) **A:** Patient at the onset of puberty showed curve increase to 60 degrees. **B:** A posterior fusion with Harrington instrumentation of both curves was performed and the fusion is solid a year postoperative. (Reproduced with permission from Lonstein JE: Deformities of the spine in children with cerebral palsy. *Orthop Rev* 1981;10:33–44.)

tions tend to be more conservative. In these children, the indications are failed nonoperative therapy, such as in children whose curves progress despite a seating program or an orthosis. Larger curves are treated if they cause a change in functional status, with alteration in sitting or walking ability. An 80-degree curve in a child who is a supported sitter is thus operated on if it progresses or changes the child's sitting ability, i.e., if more support is needed for sitting, sitting tolerance is reduced, or the ability to sit supported is lost.

Two questions must be answered in planning surgery once it is indicated: (1) should the arthrodesis include fusion to the sacrum; and (2) what is the best surgical approach—posterior alone, or a combined anterior and posterior approach? As with all cases of neuromuscular spinal deformities treated surgically, rod contouring in the sagittal plane to preserve thoracic kyphosis and lumbar lordosis is essential. In

addition, since the iliac crest is small with a poor supply of autogenous bone graft, the use of banked allograft bone is fairly routine in these cases.

In considering the extent of surgery and the surgical approach, it should be noted that the scoliosis in cerebral palsy falls into two groups[22] (Fig. 19–10). A group I curve is characterized by a level pelvis, with the curve patterns similar to the curves of idiopathic scoliosis. The patient is commonly ambulatory, being taken care of at home, with pure mental retardation, without spasticity predominating. The more common group II curve is a long lumbar or thoracolumbar curve that extends into the sacrum, which is a part of the curve. Pelvic obliquity is thus common in this group. In addition, the individual is less commonly ambulatory, is usually not cared for at home, and is more likely to have classic cerebral palsy with spasticity rather than pure mental retardation.

Group I curves (Fig. 19–11) require a posterior

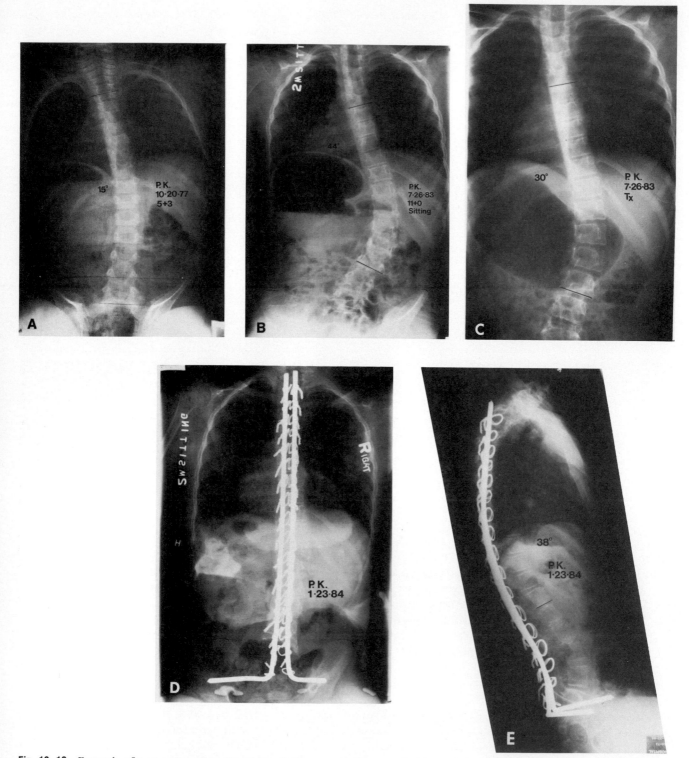

**Fig. 19–12** Example of a one-stage posterior approach for a group II curve. **A:** The patient, a totally involved dependent sitter with cerebral palsy presented at the age of 5 years, 3 months. She was placed in a molded SSO which supported her spine. **B:** At the age of 11, curve increase was noted and when she sat without support the scoliosis was 44 degrees. **C:** A traction radiograph showed correction to 30 degrees with a level pelvis and balanced spine. **D:** A one-stage posterior fusion was performed with Luque instrumentation with excellent curve correction. **E:** The lateral view shows the rod contouring to maintain the thoracic kyphosis and lumbar lordosis.

fusion alone. As the pelvis is level and not a part of the curve, fusion to the sacrum is not necessary. In rare cases in which a large lumbar curve is present, an anterior release and fusion of the lumbar curve aids correction and reduces the rate of pseudarthrosis.

In general, group II curves require long fusion to the sacrum because the sacrum is a part of the curve, with pelvic obliquity present. In the rare case of a level pelvis in a group II long thoracolumbar curve, fusion to the sacrum is still necessary. These patients have no sitting balance, and thus the spine must be stabilized to the pelvis to treat the scoliosis adequately. Luque instrumentation with Galveston pelvic fixation is ideal in these cases, as it supplies a corrective force for these long curves as well as providing excellent internal stabilization by means of the segmental sublaminar wiring.

In these group II curves, the surgical approach can be either a posterior fusion alone or a combined two-stage anterior and posterior fusion. The choice between these two approaches is made using a traction radiograph. This radiograph is best taken on the Risser/Cotrel frame using a head halter, pelvic straps, and lateral convex Cotrel strap. A traction radiograph taken on the X-ray table has proved less useful because of the spasticity present, which prevents an adequate appreciation of the flexibility of the deformity. The radiograph must show the pelvic level, and balance of the spine and torso over the pelvis (Fig. 19–12). On this traction radiograph, if the pelvis is leveled and the torso is in balance over the pelvis, a one-stage posterior approach is indicated. If, however, the traction radiograph shows residual pelvic obliquity, or the torso is not balanced over the pelvis, a two-stage approach is best.

The one-stage posterior approach is used in group II curves when the traction radiograph demonstrates a level pelvis with the torso in balance over the pelvis. Fusion extends from the second or third thoracic vertebra to the sacrum, even if only a thoracolumbar curve is present. Fusion to the mid or lower thoracic spine will result in kyphosis, as the spine bends over the top of the fusion. Extension to the upper thoracic area prevents this late complication without any loss of motion or increase in the rate of pseudarthrosis. The authors prefer to use large 0.25-inch Luque rods whenever possible, with double 16-gauge wire used at every level.[23] The Galveston pelvic fixation technique has proved the best technique of inferior fixation in these cases.[10] Careful posterolateral fusion technique is necessary in the lumbar and especially lumbosacral area to ensure an adequate arthrodesis.

The two-stage approach is used if on the traction radiograph the pelvis does not become level or the torso is not balanced over the pelvis (Fig. 19–13). The anterior approach is via a thoracoabdominal exposure of the convexity of the thoracolumbar (or lumbar) curve. The intervertebral disks are completely removed throughout the extent of the curve, extending to the lumbosacral joint whenever possible. To aid in correction, a wedge of vertebral endplate is removed when the intervertebral space is narrow. The disk space is packed with morseled rib bone, supplemented by banked allograft bone where necessary. Instruments are rarely used anteriorly, as sufficient loosening is achieved by complete disk excision. In addition, segmental instrumentation anteriorly (Dwyer or Zielke) has been found to block additional posterior correction at the second stage.

After a week of bed rest, the patient undergoes the posterior stage of the operation. Traction is not used between the stages. The anterior stage is a releasing procedure that increases the curve's flexibility, with the correction and stabilization occurring during the posterior approach. No additional correction is obtained with traction. Similarly, traction prior to an anterior release and fusion does not increase the curve's flexibility. The curve's flexibility can be seen on the traction radiograph, and preoperative traction does not result in any additional correction.

The second-stage posterior approach and technique is the same as described above under the single-stage posterior approach, i.e., long fusion from the second thoracic vertebra to the sacrum using a Luque rod and Galveston pelvic fixation technique. Rod contouring to maintain the normal sagittal spinal contours and the use of banked bone are essential.

Pulmonary care is essential in these patients postoperatively, since they cannot cooperate with deep breathing and coughing exercises. To prevent atelectasis and pneumonia, regular change in position combined with suctioning of the nasopharynx and trachea are essential. These procedures help with the control of secretions and also induce a cough reflex. A nursing staff experienced in care of these patients is essential in postoperative care and in preventing postoperative complications.

The use of postoperative immobilization after spinal fusion depends on the activity level of the child and the security of the internal fixation. If the child is a total care patient and the internal fixation is secure, external immobilization in a postoperative TLSO has not been found to be necessary to ensure adequate arthrodesis. If the child is active or the internal fixation is not secure, a postoperative TLSO is used until the fusion is solid. This process may take up to a year as the incorporation and maturity rate in these spinal fusions is slow.

### Duchenne's Muscular Dystrophy

Boys afflicted with this progressive muscle wasting disease usually stop walking between the ages of 9 and 12 and then become progressively weaker, with

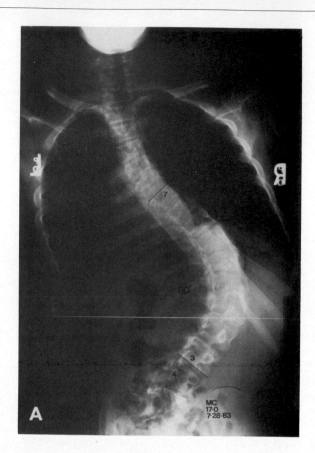

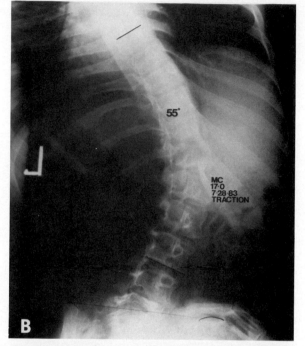

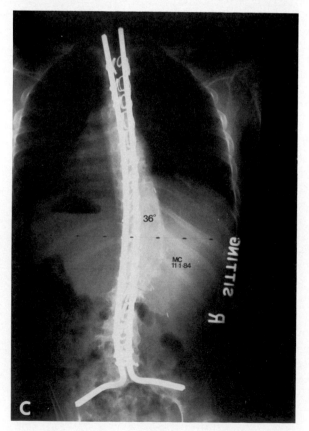

**Fig. 19–13 A:** A patient at the age of 17 with an 80–degree right thoracolumbar curve and loss of sitting balance. **B:** A traction radiograph shows correction to 55 degrees, the pelvis is nearly level but the thorax is not balanced over the pelvis. **C:** A two-stage anterior and posterior fusion was performed. A year later the fusion is solid and a balanced spine over a level pelvis is seen.

death most often occurring in the late teens to early 20s. Therefore, a major goal in the overall management of Duchenne's muscular dystrophy is to prolong walking and standing in knee-ankle-foot orthoses. Soft-tissue surgery may be required to correct hip or knee contractures or, more commonly, equinovarus foot deformities. Then, if standing activities can be maintained, the orthotic prevention of flexion contractures of the knees and hips and control of pelvic obliquity are easier (Fig. 19–14).

More than 90% of the patients with Duchenne's muscular dystrophy will develop scoliosis.[24,25] This spinal deformity usually does not develop until walking has ceased. Then the curve progresses at the rate of approximately 2 to 3 degrees per month in most cases. Some patients with rigid lordosis as a component of their deformity seem to have curve progression at a slower rate or sometimes not at all.

In the past, orthotic treatment of this scoliosis has been attempted, but with minimal success. In the Newington Children's Hospital experience of 31 patients treated with thoracolumbosacral orthoses, 24 (77%) showed continued curve progression. Over the follow-up period, the average progression was 15 degrees per year in the orthosis-treated group as compared with 31 degrees per year for patients not treated with orthotics.[24] It appears from this study and that of Moseley and associates[25] that orthotic treatment of scoliosis in Duchenne's muscular dystrophy can slow progression of the curve, but this delay in progression may be, in fact, buying "false time," since it only defers surgery until a point at which the patient is at greater operative and postoperative risk. Because of this fact, the authors' present indications for spinal fusion in this disease are curves greater than 30 degrees, a forced vital capacity greater than 30% of normal; and a prognosis of at least two years or more of life remaining. The patient should have a functional cough, little or no cardiomyopathy, and should have stopped ambulating independently, since a long spinal fusion in an independent ambulator with severe neuromuscular disease will often remove the compensatory balance mechanisms necessary to walk. In fact, the majority of patients with Duchenne's muscular dystrophy have already stopped walking before they develop significant scoliosis.

In Duchenne's muscular dystrophy, it appears that the results of pulmonary function tests deteriorate at approximately 4% per year after 12 years of age.[26] Also, 10 degrees of curve progression in thoracic scoliosis also appears to decrease pulmonary functions by about 4%. Thoracolumbar and lumbar curves, on the other hand, have little or no effect on pulmonary functions. The percent of forced vital capacity and percent of peak flow rate are the best

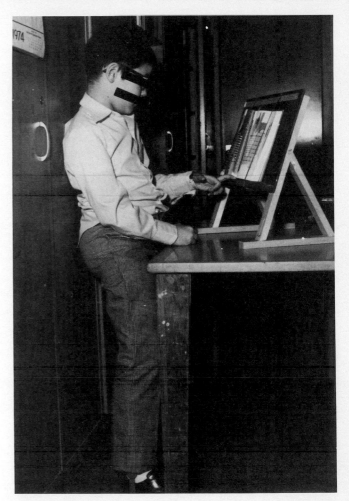

**Fig. 19–14** A boy with Duchenne's muscular dystrophy standing at school with the aid of ischial weightbearing knee-ankle-foot orthoses.

measures of effective pulmonary functions in this condition.

A technique successful in stabilizing these scoliotic spines is L-rod insertion with sublaminar wire fixation from the upper thoracic spine (T2 or T3) to the level of the fifth lumbar vertebra or to the pelvis. It frequently may be unnecessary to fuse to the pelvis. Many surgeons will routinely fuse to the fifth lumbar vertebra if there is no fixed pelvic obliquity. If there is greater than 10 to 15 degrees of fixed pelvic obliquity, then fusion to the pelvis is recommended. It is also important to preserve the patient's lumbar lordosis for good sitting balance. Blood loss can be substantial in these patients. Massive amounts of bone graft are needed. Because rapid postoperative mobilization is important, the Circoelectric bed is very useful in the rapid resumption of upright standing to prevent contractures and excessive loss of strength in the postoperative period.

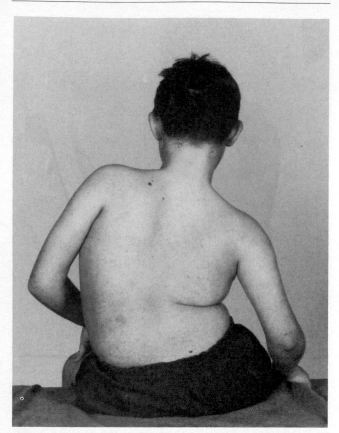

**Fig. 19–15** This boy with Duchenne's muscular dystrophy and severe scoliosis needs to use his right arm and hand for trunk support to maintain sitting balance. He was treated with L-rod spinal fusion.

The use of spinal fusion to treat scoliosis in Duchenne's muscular dystrophy has the following benefits: (1) preservation of or improvement in sitting balance; (2) avoidance of back pain; (3) improvement of spinal decompensation; (4) freeing the arms of the necessity for trunk support; (5) improvement of body image; and (6) possibly slowing the deterioration of pulmonary functions (Fig. 19–15). Some patients have also reported that they sleep better and more comfortably after the scoliosis is corrected.

## Paraplegia and Quadriplegia

The risk of developing spinal deformity after spinal cord injury depends to a significant extent upon the age of the patient. In the preadolescent period the risk of deformity is about 90%, with scoliosis being more common than kyphosis. A cephalad injury and the presence of spasticity caudal to the spinal cord lesion also increase the risk of developing an abnormal curve.

Deformity occurs less often if the patient is injured as an adult. Kyphosis is more common than scoliosis in this group, the most likely causes being progressive kyphotic collapse at the fracture site, particularly if more than half of the vertebral body is compressed, and kyphosis develops secondary to extensive laminectomies above the thoracolumbar junction. If the patient has pre-existing idiopathic scoliosis, progression may occur following spinal cord injury regardless of the patient's age.[27]

Etiologic factors in this type of paralytic scoliosis may include loss of spinal support secondary to motor paralysis, loss of sensory function, hip and suprapelvic contractures, chronic instability of the vertebral column, malunion of vertebral fractures, osteopenia, and the effects of growth. All children with spinal cord injury should be presumed to be developing a paralytic spinal deformity until proven otherwise.

Early preventive treatment of spinal deformity includes perfect reduction and stable healing of the vertebral lesion, prevention of contractures, control of spasticity, and follow-up evaluations throughout the growth period. Once a mild deformity is detected, it should be carefully monitored. While orthotic treatment is rarely definitive, it may help to delay progression and allow for further spinal growth before fusion is necessary. Most insensate patients can tolerate a total-contact TLSO; however, it is important to watch for skin breakdown and problems with thermoregulation. A bivalved orthosis is convenient for ease of donning and doffing. Once a scoliotic curve exceeds 40 degrees or a kyphosis exceeds 60 degrees, surgery should be strongly considered. In either instance, if preoperative radiographs do not show improvement to less than 50 to 60 degrees, then both anterior and posterior spinal fusion may be necessary to obtain adequate correction and to balance the spine.

The fusion technique for this type of deformity includes the strongest possible internal fixation. Stainless steel L-rods 0.25 inch in diameter with sublaminar wiring have proved quite effective. In addition, massive bone graft should be used to pack in as much bone as possible throughout the fusion length while still being able to close the fascia. Both the sagittal and the coronal plane balance of the spine must be maintained with the technique. Fusions should extend from the first or second thoracic vertebra to the pelvis in paralytic scoliosis of this type (Fig. 19–16). Postoperatively, a bivalved TLSO is an excellent way to augment the internal fixation in a paralyzed patient. The authors' practice has been to wean the patient from the orthosis one year postoperatively if the fusion mass appears solid on radiograph.

The paralyzed patient with scoliosis has many potential postoperative problems. These include pulmonary complications such as infection, aspiration pneumonia, and atelectasis; problems with soft-tissue healing secondary to denervated, atropic tissue or poor nutrition; deep wound infection; and pseudarthrosis formation. The fusion mass in this type of scoliosis is often slow to develop and consolidate and many times appears atrophic. Other problems include hypercalcemia, which occurs in approximately 25% of these patients; osteopenia and fractures; autonomic dysreflexia; orthostatic hypotension; spasticity and contractures; pressure ulcerations of the skin; heterotopic bone formation; problems with thermoregulatory mechanisms; gastrointestinal problems, such as prolonged ileus and stress ulcers; genitourinary problems, including urinary tract infections and stone formation; thromboemboli; and finally,

psychosocial problems related not only to the paralysis, but also to the stress of surgery. In-depth discussion of the management of all of these problems is beyond the scope of this chapter.

### Spinal Muscular Atrophy

Although the overall likelihood that scoliosis will develop in spinal muscular atrophy is very high, its incidence varies with the severity of involvement. Virtually all patients with types I, II, and III involvement will develop scoliosis.[28] The onset is usually in childhood around the age of 7 and the majority of

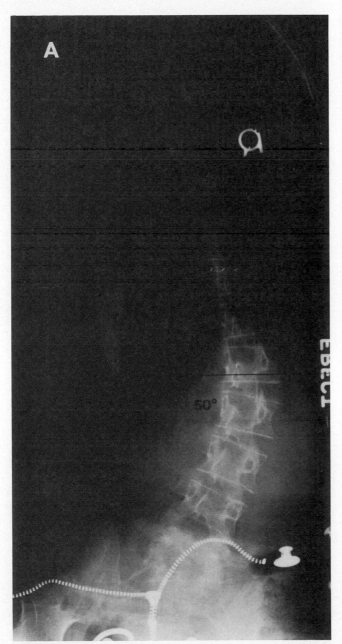
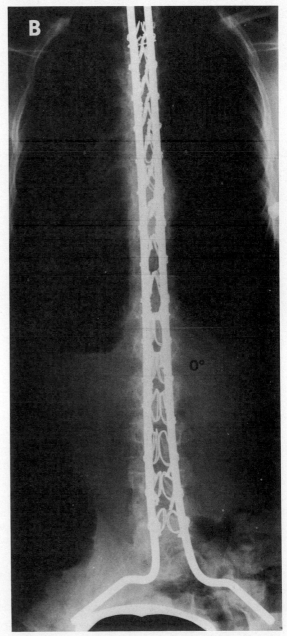

**Fig. 19–16** **A:** A 50-degree right thoracolumbar "paralytic" scoliosis in a 15-year-old girl with C6 quadriplegia. **B:** She was treated by spinal fusion with L-rod segmental instrumentation from T2 to the pelvis and allograft bone grafting.

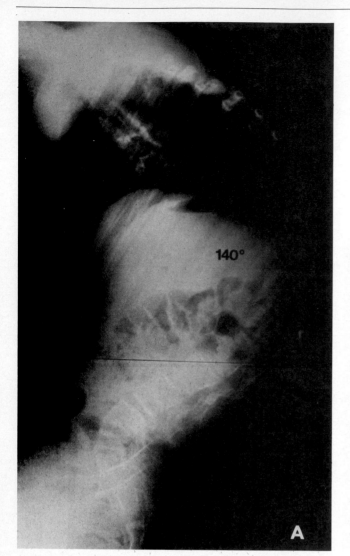
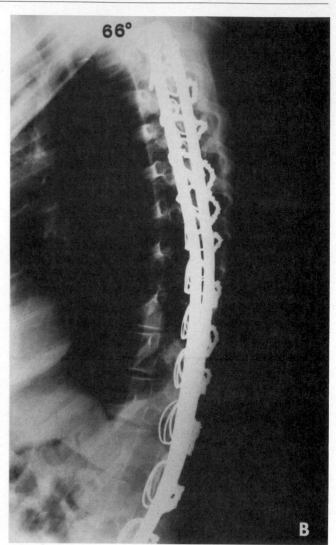

**Fig. 19–17** Preoperative and postoperative lateral radiographs of a 19-year-old man with collapsing kyphosis and Friedreich's ataxia. The internal fixation is a "U-rod" with double sublaminar wires.

curves are progressive.[29] Once a curve reaches 20 degrees in a skeletally immature patient, it may be wise to consider orthotic treatment.[30] A total contact TLSO is well tolerated by patients with spinal muscular atrophy and does not usually impair mobility significantly.

The surgical treatment of scoliosis in spinal muscular atrophy is posterior spinal fusion with internal fixation and adequate bone grafting. When a curve reaches 40 to 45 degrees, surgery is indicated. Patients with type I and type II involvement are nonambulators and should have fusion to the pelvis if any pelvic obliquity is noted.

Patients with spinal muscular atrophy require aggressive postoperative pulmonary care and rapid mobilization. If the pulmonary involvement is such that the forced vital capacity is less than 20% of predicted, the patient is at great risk for postoperative mortality.

### Friedreich's Ataxia

Almost all patients with Friedreich's ataxia will develop scoliosis and more than half will have hyperkyphosis as well[31] (Fig. 19–17). Curve patterns are more likely to resemble those of idiopathic scoliosis than the long "C-shaped" paralytic curves of many neuromuscular disorders.[32] Although more than half the curves develop at or prior to skeletal maturity, many times the scoliosis does not appear until the late teens or early 20s. These latter curves are less likely to be progressive. In addition, curve progression does not appear to be related to the degree of weakness. Successful orthotic treatment of progressive scoliosis in this condition is extremely rare and requires prolonged treatment. Therefore, most physicians elect to follow scoliosis until it reaches about 45 degrees or more and then perform definitive spinal fusion. An effective method is L-rod segmental spinal instrumentation with sublaminar wiring and massive bone graft. It is very important to evaluate cardiomyopathy preoperatively in patients with Friedreich's ataxia. Despite successful spinal fusion and a balanced spine, many of these patients toward the end of their life will require seating orthoses such as custom chair inserts because they have lost effective trunk and head control.

### Myelomeningocele

Overall, 60% of patients with myelomeningocele will develop scoliosis, the incidence being proportional to the neurosegmental level of paralysis. Patients with higher levels are more likely to develop deformity.[33] It is important to remember that 10% to 20% of these patients will also have congenital scoliosis. Scoliosis and kyphosis in myelomeningocele have traditionally been difficult to treat. With advances in internal fixation, however, more successful surgical series are being reported.

In about two thirds of the patients with myelomeningocele and scoliosis, the curves appear before the age of 10 years. These require careful monitoring and may require orthotic treatment for some control initially in order to allow further growth of the spine. Prognostic signs for progressive spinal deformity include early onset, asymmetrical motor paralysis, and the presence of spasticity. The progression of scoliosis may be a sign of tethering of the spinal cord or the development of hydromyelia or a fistula. These problems must be ruled out in any patient with myelomeningocele and progressive spinal deformity.[34]

Treatment of scoliosis in myelomeningocele includes the surgical fusion of any progressive congenital curve, regardless of the patient's age. A total contact TLSO is appropriate for paralytic curves in the range of 20 to 40 degrees. Most curves of 40 degrees should be treated by definitive spinal arthrodesis, which usually requires both anterior and posterior fusion, the latter extending from the upper thoracic region to the pelvis. Care should be taken to obtain biplanar balance of the spine, preserve appropriate lumbar lordosis, and add massive bone graft. It is well to protect the fusion with a postoperative bivalved TLSO for at least one year to allow for strengthening of the fusion mass.

Kyphosis occurring in a patient with myelomeningocele is very difficult to treat. It may be congenital, paralytic, or both. Regardless of cause, it is always progressive and is often accompanied by skin breakdown, restrictive pulmonary impairment, and occasionally by obstructive uropathy. The goals of treatment are to produce a balanced, flat back by means of a large-volume anterior and posterior bony fusion mass and then to maintain the correction. Surgery is technically easier in a patient more than 3 years old, although fusion of progressive severe kyphosis often cannot be delayed. While techniques of vertebral resection and instrumentation differ, common to most successful techniques is some type of vertebrectomy, massive bone graft, and rigid segmental internal fixation followed by postoperative external support.[35,36] Our current preference is for vertebral body resection at or proximal to the apex of the kyphosis and L-rod fixation to the pelvis via the Galveston technique[10] and pedicular wiring. The fusion and instrumentation should extend high into the thoracic region.

### References

1. Bleck EE: *Orthopaedic Management of Cerebral Palsy.* Philadelphia, WB Saunders, 1979, p 87.
2. Moe JH, Bradford DS, Winter RB, et al: *Scoliosis and Other Spinal Deformities.* Philadelphia, WB Saunders, 1978, p 382.
3. Drennan JC, Renshaw TS, Curtis BH: The thoracic suspension orthosis. *Clin Orthop* 1979;139:33–39.
4. Moe JH, Kharrat K, Winter RB, et al: Harrington instrumentation without fusion plus external orthotic support for the treatment of difficult curvature problems in young children. *Clin Orthop* 1984;185:35–45.
5. Rinsky LA, Gamble JG, Bleck EE: Segmental instrumentation without fusion in children with progressive scoliosis. *J Pediatr Orthop* 1985;5:687–690.
6. Letts M, Rang M, Tredwell S: Seating the disabled, in *The Atlas of Orthotics*, ed 2. St Louis, C V Mosby Co, 1985, p 450.
7. Carlson, JM, Winter RB: The "Gillette" sitting support orthosis. *Orthot Prosthet* 1978;32:35.
8. Lindseth RE: Posterior iliac osteotomy for fixed pelvic obliquity. *J Bone Joint Surg* 1978;60A:17–22.
9. Kling TF Jr, Pandit U, Hensinger RN, et al: Efficacy of heated/humidified inspired anesthetic gas in maintaining body temperature during scoliosis surgery. *Orthop Trans* 1986;10:29–30.
10. Allen BL Jr, Ferguson RL: The Galveston technique for L rod instrumentation of the scoliotic spine. *Spine* 1982;7:276–284.
11. Bell GR, Gurd A, Orlowski J, et al: Syndrome of inappropriate antidiuretic hormone (SIADH) secretion in post-operative adolescent spinal fusion patients. *Orthop Trans* 1983;7:17.
12. Engler GL, Spielholz NI, Bernhard WN, et al: Somatosensory evoked potentials during Harrington instrumentation for scoliosis. *J Bone Joint Surg* 1978;60A:528–532.
13. Hall JE, Levine CR, Sudhir KG: Intraoperative awakening to monitor spinal cord function during Harrington instrumentation and spine fusion: Description of procedure and report of three cases. *J Bone Joint Surg* 1978;60A:533–536.
14. Bleck EE: Deformities of the spine and pelvis in cerebral palsy, in Samilson RL (ed): *Orthopedic Aspects of Cerebral Palsy.* Philadelphia, J B Lippincott, 1975, pp 124–144.
15. MacEwen GD: Cerebral palsy and scoliosis in spinal deformities, in Hardy JH (ed): *Neurological and Muscular Diseases.* St Louis, C V Mosby Co, 1975.

16. Drennan JC: *Orthopedic Management of Neuromuscular Diseases.* Philadelphia, J B Lippincott, 1983, pp 253–296.

17. Samilson EP, Bechard R: Scoliosis in cerebral palsy: Incidence, distribution of curve patterns, natural history and thoughts on etiology. *Curr Pract Orthop Surg* 1973;5:183–205.

18. Madigan RR, Wallace SL: Scoliosis in the institutionalized cerebral palsy population. *Spine* 1981;6:583–590.

19. Bunnell WP, MacEwen GD: Non-operative treatment of scoliosis in cerebral palsy: Preliminary report on the use of a plastic jacket. *Devel Med Child Neurol* 1977;19:45–49.

20. Bonnett CA, Brown JC, Grow T: Thoracolumbar scoliosis in cerebral palsy: Results of surgical treatment. *J Bone Joint Surg* 1976;58A:328–336.

21. Stanitski CL, Micheli LJ, Hall JE, et al: Surgical correction of spinal deformity in cerebral palsy. *Spine* 1982;7:563–569.

22. Lonstein JE, Akbarnia BA: Operative treatment of spinal deformity in patients with cerebral palsy or mental retardation–an analysis of 107 cases. *J Bone Joint Surg* 1983;65A:43–55.

23. Luque EA: Segmental spinal instrumentation for correction of scoliosis. *Clin Orthop* 1982;163:192–198.

24. Cambridge WR, Drennan JC: The natural history of scoliosis in Duchenne muscular dystrophy. Read before the 53rd Annual Meeting of the American Academy of Orthopaedic Surgeons, New Orleans, February 24, 1986.

25. Moseley, CF, Koreska J, Miller F: Treatment of spinal deformity in Duchenne muscular dystrophy. Read before the 52nd Annual Meeting of the American Academy of Orthopaedic Surgeons, Las Vegas, January 26, 1985.

26. Kurz LT, Mubarak SJ, Schultz P, et al: Correlation of scoliosis and pulmonary function in Duchenne muscular dystrophy. *J Pediatr Orthop* 1983;3:347–353.

27. Renshaw TS: Paralysis in the child: Orthopaedic management, in Bradford DS, Hensinger RM (eds): *The Pediatric Spine.* New York, Thieme Inc, 1985, pp 118–128.

28. Evans GA, Drennan JC, Russman BS: Functional classification and orthopaedic management of spinal muscular atrophy. *J Bone Joint Surg* 1981;63B:516–522.

29. Hensinger RN, MacEwen GD: Spinal deformity associated with heritable neurological conditions: Spinal muscular atrophy, Friedreich's ataxia, familial dysautonomia, and Charcot-Marie-Tooth disease. *J Bone Joint Surg* 1978;58A:13–24.

30. Shapiro F, Bresnan MJ: Current concepts review: Orthopaedic management of childhood neuromuscular disease: Part I.: Spinal muscular atrophy. *J Bone Joint Surg* 1982;64A:785–789.

31. Cady RB, Bobechko WP: Incidence, natural history, and treatment of scoliosis in Friedreich's ataxia. *J Pediatr Orthop* 1984;4:673–676.

32. Labell H, Tohmé S, Duhaime M, et al: Natural history of scoliosis in Friedreich's ataxia. *J Bone Joint Surg* 1986;68A:564–572.

33. Banta JV, Becker GJ: The natural history of scoliosis in myelomeningocele. *Orthop Trans* 1986;10:18.

34. Bunch WH, Scarff TB, Dvouch V: Progressive neurological loss in myelomeningocele patients. *Orthop Trans* 1976;7:185.

35. Lindseth RE, Stelzer L: Vertebral excision for kyphosis in children with myelomeningocele. *J Bone Joint Surg* 1979;61A:699–704.

36. Lindseth RE: Posterior iliac osteotomy for fixed pelvic obliquity. *J Bone Joint Surg* 1978;60A:17–22.

# Fractures of the Extremities: Diagnosis and Management

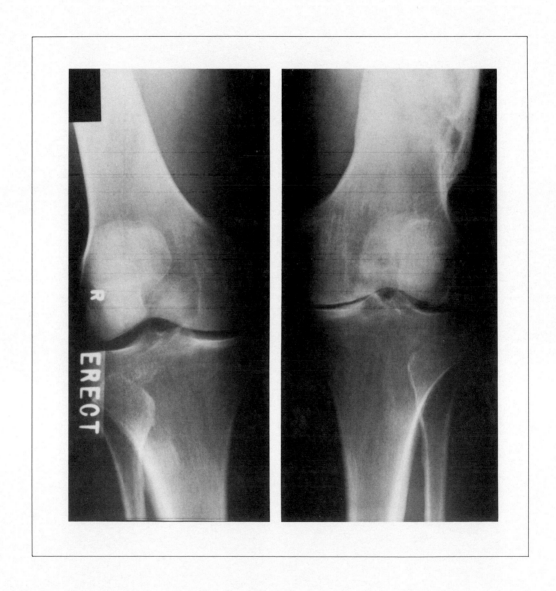

# Flexible Intramedullary Nailing
# of Long Bones

## Introduction

### William R. Dobozi, MD

Flexible intramedullary nails for the treatment of intertrochanteric fractures and proximal one-third fractures of the femur were first introduced by Ender and Simon-Weidner in 1970. In 1977, Pankovich broadened their indications to include fractures of the femoral, tibial, and humeral shafts. Since that time, flexible nails have gained acceptance for treatment of these fractures, offering a nonreamed system as one of their main advantages. Complications have also surfaced with this technique, caused mainly by inexperience on the surgeon's part in performing what was thought to be a "simple" procedure. It is the purpose of this chapter to discuss in detail the proper indications for and surgical technique used in flexible intramedullary nailing of long-bone fractures.

In his discussion of the effects of flexible intramedullary nails on fracture healing, Segal reviews the literature on flexible intramedullary nailing as well as alternative methods of immobilizing long-bone fractures: reamed intramedullary nailing and rigid fixation by compression plates. Segal concludes that flexible nailing is the most efficacious for both biologic and mechanical reasons.

Pankovich gives a general treatment of flexible intramedullary nailing and the clinical misconceptions that have arisen concerning the use of this technique in a variety of clinical settings.

The author discusses the specific use of intramedullary flexible nailing in the treatment of subtrochanteric fractures of the femur. Indications, contraindications, surgical technique, and postoperative management are among the topics covered.

Pankovich then discusses the use of this technique in treating femoral shaft fractures. Acknowledging the technical difficulty of this technique, Pankovich lists fracture types and their suitability for intramedullary nailing. He also discusses special situations such as multiple trauma and noncemented implants, as well as common complications associated with this technique.

Segal details the indications, contraindications, and surgical procedure used in the flexible intramedullary nailing of tibial shaft fractures. Acknowledging

that these fractures are still most often treated by closed reduction and cast immobilization, he discusses the increased use of nailing in situations heretofore reserved for nonsurgical treatment. Citing clinical experience with more than 150 tibial fractures, Segal explains his surgical technique and the clinical results using flexible nailing.

Referring to poor rotational control and the difficulty and occasional hazard associated with flexible intramedullary nailing of humeral shaft fractures, Hall nevertheless argues that surgical treatment is sometimes desirable. Basing his discussion on clinical results from Cook County Hospital in Chicago, Hall discusses indications, surgical technique, and complications.

## Fracture Healing of Long Bones in the Presence of Flexible Intramedullary Nails

### David Segal, MD

Numerous factors affect bone healing, and the orthopaedic surgeon can influence this biologic process by deciding which method of immobilization to use: flexible intramedullary nailing; reamed intramedullary nailing; or rigid fixation by compression plates. The purpose of this brief discussion is to review the effects of immobilization on bone healing and, specifically, the advantages of using flexible intramedullary nailing and its effect on primary long-bone healing.

In 1964 Trueta and Cavadias[1] showed that the periosteal blood vessels in long bones provide blood to only a small portion of the outer cortex; the largest blood supply comes from the nutrient artery. In 1955 the same authors[2] in experiments with nailing of fractures showed that the nail will destroy sufficient branches of the nutrient artery to cause avascularity of the cortex, which can be extensive, persisting even up to eight months. They have also concluded, however, that bone marrow ischemia acts to stimulate periosteal bone proliferation. They concluded that the suppression of the intramedullary blood supply by an undescribed law of compensation causes an increase in the vascularity of the periosteum. This effect of intramedullary nailing was confirmed by MacNab and DeHaas,[3] who have shown that in the adult dog's tibia and probably in the human tibia as well the periosteal blood vessels supply only 10% of the outer cortex. Rhinelander[4,5] has shown that extraosseous blood supply develops immediately after the fracture and persists until the medullary circulation restores normal centrifugal flow of blood through the cortex and the external callus. He concluded that "extensive reaming leads to delay in remodeling of cortical bone" and "it always causes delay in the healing because it greatly limits the formation of medullary bridging callus which produces the early osseous healing."

Thus, reamed intramedullary nails, while causing destruction to the intramedullary blood supply, stimulate a compensatory increase in the extraosseous circulation.[1-6] Another advantage of the reamed nail is its rigid fixation of the fragments. In the normal process of long-bone healing, the bridging callus has zones of fibrocartilage; these zones are fewer and smaller in the presence of rigid fixation. The experimental work of Rhinelander,[4,5] MacNab and DeHaas,[3] and Trueta and Cavadias[1,2] has all pointed to the same conclusion: a fully fitting intramedullary nail, while damaging the intramedullary circulation, also provides a better rigid environment and more rapid healing with smaller areas of fibrocartilage.

In 1949 Danis[7] was the first to propose the use of compression plates for fixing fractures. This idea was further developed by the Arbeitsgemeinschaft für Osteosynthesefragen (AO) group, mostly by Schenck and Willenegger.[8] Compression plating produces "contact healing" or intercortical callus formation. Under compression plates cortex-to-cortex healing takes place without the formation of endosteal or periosteal callus. While this form of healing may produce bony continuity most rapidly, it does not provide the strongest union.

Sarmiento and associates[9] have studied the strength of callus formation in animals. They fixed the fractured long bones with plates and then compared callus strength to that achieved with cast immobilization. Initially the plates provided stability to the fragments, but they noticed that eventually it was the external callus that provided stronger bony union. Similar results[9] have been obtained in experimental work in which long bones were stabilized by intramedullary nails and compared to those stabilized with casts.

In their enthusiasm to use AO principles in fracture treatment, some were led to believe that callus formation is a "bad sign" indicating lack of compression and possible failure of fixation. While this still may be true for compression plating, it is now understood that callus formation is a "good sign" indicative of strong-

er bony healing. This recognition led to a renewed interest in cast bracing and functional bracing, encouraging controlled motion at the fracture site with large callus bridging the fracture.

Cast bracing and functional bracing of the upper and lower extremities have proved valuable in treating long-bone fractures. However, angular and rotational deformities are difficult to control, and it is the latter that limits their use. The author believes that the use of flexible intramedullary nails combines all the advantages associated with long-bone healing: (1) the intramedullary blood supply is only partially damaged, as reaming is avoided and most of the intramedullary circulation remains intact; (2) nonrigid bony stability is obtained, yet compression forces can still act on the fragments; (3) these forces create controlled motion of the fragments resulting in a strong callus and early bony union; (4) the flexible intramedullary nails act as internal splints, reducing the incidence of angular and rotational deformities.

The orthopaedic surgeon has been using intramedullary fixation in the form of Rush pinning since 1934. There was a renewed interest in this fixation method when Dr. Ender described the use of Ender nails in hip fractures. Unfortunately, clinical experience with this method in the United States has not concurred with the positive experience reported from Europe. Nevertheless, the improved alloys and instruments and the variety of flexible intramedullary nails have enabled their successful use in fractures of all the long bones, mostly the femur, tibia, and humerus. Its application in treating fractures of the long bones of the forearm is still in the experimental stage.

### References

1. Trueta J, Cavadias AX: A study of blood supply of the long bone. *Surg Gynecol Obstet* 1964;118–3:485.
2. Trueta J, Cavadias AX: Vascular changes caused by Küntscher type nailing. *J Bone Joint Surg* 1955;37B:492.
3. MacNab I, DeHaas WG: The role of periosteal blood supply in the healing of the fractured tibia. *Clin Orthop* 1974;105:27.
4. Rhinelander FW: The normal microcirculation of diaphyseal cortex and its response to fracture. *J Bone Joint Surg* 1968;50A:784.
5. Rhinelander FW: Tibial blood supply in relation to fracture healing. *Clin Orthop* 1974;105:34–38.
6. Trueta J: Blood supply and the rate of healing of tibial fractures. *Clin Orthop* 1974;105:11.
7. Danis R: *Théorie et pratique de l'ostéosynthèse*. Paris, Masson, 1949.
8. Schenck R, Willenegger H: Morphological findings in primary fracture healing. *Symp Biol Hung* 1967;7:75.
9. Sarmiento A, Latta LL, Tarr R: The rationale of functional bracing of fractures. *Clin Orthop* 1980;146:28.

# Twelve Misconceptions About the Use of Flexible Intramedullary Nails

### Arsen M. Pankovich, MD

## Misconception 1: Intertrochanteric Fracture

Since their introduction by Ender[1] in 1969, flexible nails have been advocated primarily, indeed, almost exclusively, for intertrochanteric and some subtrochanteric fractures. In Europe, intertrochanteric fracture is still the primary indication for flexible intramedullary nailing.

In the author's experience, the intertrochanteric fracture, particularly one that is unstable, is the worst indication for fixation with flexible nails. Final instability, which is not uncommon in unstable fractures, often leads to failure of fixation. This experience is shared with many North American surgeons who have used the technique.

Therefore, it is important to emphasize that nailing of intertrochanteric fractures with flexible nails is a difficult procedure that is likely to fail when done by an inexperienced surgeon.

## Misconception 2: Rotational Instability

Rotational instability must be defined as permanent rotational malposition of fracture fragments after insertion of the nails in proper rotational alignment. When rotational force is applied, motion of fixed fragments does not lead to permanent rotational displacement when the fixation device is capable of springing back to its original position. Kyle[2] showed that flexible nails (Ender type) in femoral shafts have less torsional resistance (1.71) than locked rigid nails (8.3), yet they possess significant springback (92%) and thus maintain the original alignment almost as well as locked rigid nails (100% springback), unlike AO rods (39% springback with a torsional resistance of 1.0). In other words, the rotation of fragments around each other when rotational force is applied does not produce permanent displacement.

The bad reputation of Ender nails in intertrochanteric fractures is the result of the frequency of postoperative external rotation deformity. The author has observed that a patient whose intertrochanteric fracture has been fixed with Ender nails tends to keep the leg in external rotation to relieve the pain experienced when the leg is in the neutral position. This pain is obviously caused by motion at the fracture site. If the leg is kept in external rotation for an extended period, as is often the case in elderly patients, external rotation contracture of the hip develops even though there is no rotational misalignment. Of course, intertrochanteric fractures often occur in elderly patients with osteoporotic bone and comminuted fractures, and rotational misalignment can and does develop, particularly when too few nails are driven into the femoral head.

Rotational misalignment in femoral shaft fractures occurs during reduction of the fracture and before nail insertion. It can be corrected only by removing the nails and repositioning them after the rotation is corrected and never by forceful derotation of the fragments. This can cause additional fractures at the fracture site and at the portals.

## Misconception 3: Bending Instability

Tencer and associates[3] and Kyle[2] showed that the stiffness of Ender nails was significantly lower than that of rigid rods (0.14 for Ender nails and 1.0 for AO rods). The author's experiments showed that springback after bending of a shaft fracture was significant. Bending of a cadaver femur to 40 degrees did not produce permanent deformation of the nails or fracture site. The author has seen only two cases in which bending deformation occurred and required renailing. Therefore, bending stability is quite good and is of no clinical significance in terms of permanent deformation or ambulation.

## Misconception 4: Sliding Fracture Fragments

It is clear that fractures with bicortical comminution cannot be fixed properly by simple rigid nailing without adjunctive measures. Winquist and Hansen[4] showed that Küntscher nails alone can be used only in transverse and short oblique fractures in the midshaft of the femur, in fractures with unicortical comminution (type II), and in simple segmental fractures. More comminuted fractures and those in the proximal and distal parts of the femoral shaft require locked nails or alternative methods. The indications for flexible nails are the same. Therefore, the idea that fracture fragments fixed with flexible nails slide because of poor fixation is a misconception. After fixation with flexible or rigid nails, various degrees of pistoning of fracture fragments occur. In simple, stable fracture configurations, fracture fragments slide toward each other but produce no shortening. In unstable fracture configurations, the primary fracture fragments slide until they meet each other. The shortening thus produced is often equal to the length of the comminuted segment (Fig. 20–1).

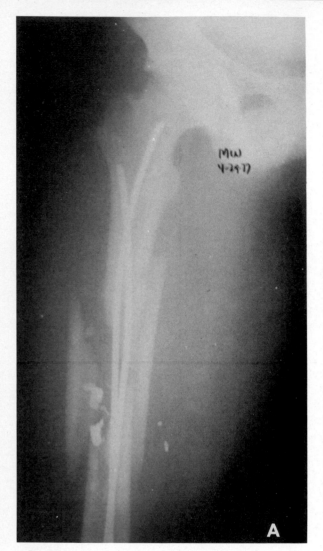
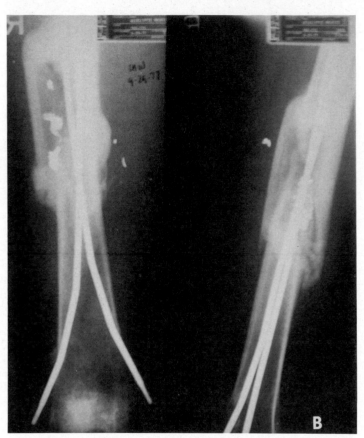

**Fig. 20–1** Simple nailing of a fracture with bicortical comminution inevitably leads to sliding of main fracture fragments and consequent shortening of the femur. **A:** Roentgenograms taken immediately after surgery. **B:** The fracture fragments have slid toward each other and the nails have pulled out because postoperative traction or other adjunctive measures were not used. Shortening of the femur resulted.

### Misconception 5: Antegrade Nailing Through a Portal in the Piriform Fossa

Flexible nails precured for three-point fixation must be straightened before being inserted through the piriform fossa. Thus, they lose their springback and no longer control rotation. Fixation is poor and the nails tend to slide out.[5]

### Misconception 6: Knee Pain

When the nails are properly inserted and positioned flat on the cortex of the distal femur (Fig. 20–2) and locked with a screw (Fig. 20–3), knee pain should not be expected after the wounds have healed.

Obviously, when nails slide or protrude out of the bone, local pain is inevitable (Fig. 20–4).

### Misconception 7: Simplicity

Although this method appears to be simple, it requires experience, surgical skills, and judgment. This is a demanding technique (Fig. 20–5).

### Misconception 8: Locking

Kolmert and associates[6] showed in an experimental model that Ender nails coupled to cancellous screws provided reliable stability in supracondylar femoral fractures. Perry and associates,[7] in a series of commi-

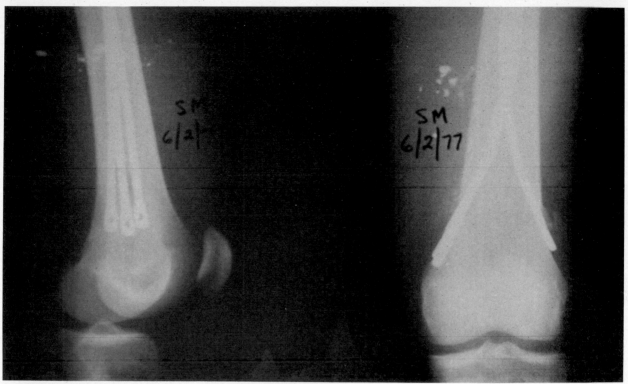

**Fig. 20–2** Whenever possible, nails are inserted through portals at the level of the proximal pole of the patella. The portal holes should be drilled close to the posterior cortex.

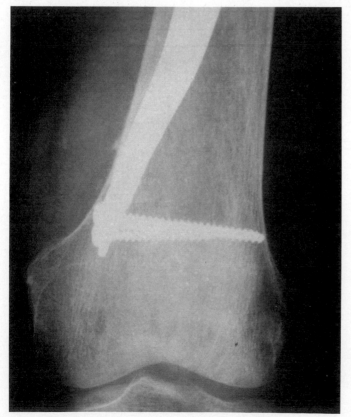

**Fig. 20–3** Locked nails after fixation of an intertrochanteric fracture.

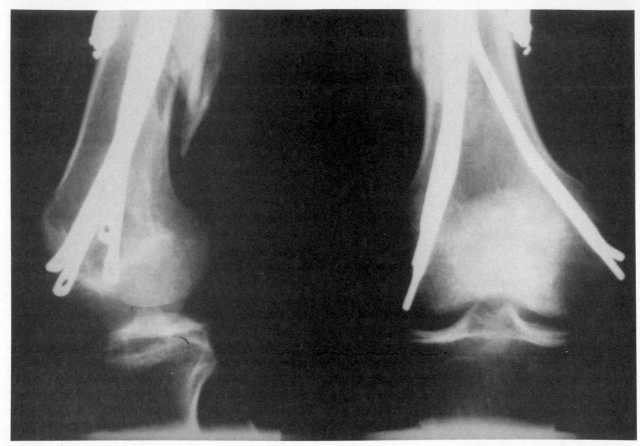

**Fig. 20–4** Protruding nails are a consequence of a faulty technique.

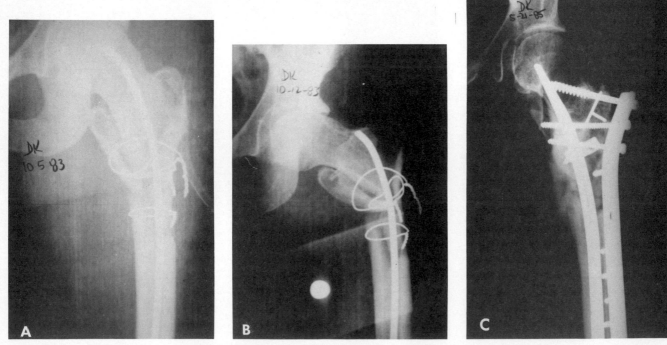

**Fig. 20–5** Judgment, skill, and experience are required when fixing a complex fracture. **A:** Immediately after surgery the roentgenograms show good alignment but little fixation. Postoperative traction was mandatory. **B:** When the patient was allowed to get up, displacement of the fracture was inevitable. **C:** An extensive procedure with bone grafting was required to fix this complex fracture.

nuted femoral fractures, demonstrated that nails tied distally with multiple wires do not need proximal locking if the proximal metaphyseal bone is dense (as it is in individuals less than 40 to 45 years old). The nails are effectively locked by the dense bone and, once inserted, they do not penetrate.[7]

The author has used locked nails in a variety of femoral fractures and has found fixation to be excellent with screws, cables, and multiple wires.

**Locking With Screws** The nails most often used in femoral fractures are 4.5 mm in diameter. Most eyes allow a 3.5-mm AO cancellous screw to be inserted (Figs. 20–6 and 20–7). This should be verified before insertion of any individual nail. Most nails that are 4 mm in diameter accept 3.5-mm AO cancellous screws; smaller nails accept 2.7-mm AO cortical screws. These smaller nails are used primarily in tibial and humeral fractures.

The width of the distal femur sometimes makes it impossible to reach the opposite cortex with a screw. The author usually uses a screw 45 mm in length in both the femur and the tibia. In the distal humerus, the medullary canal is narrow and screw length must be determined for each nail.

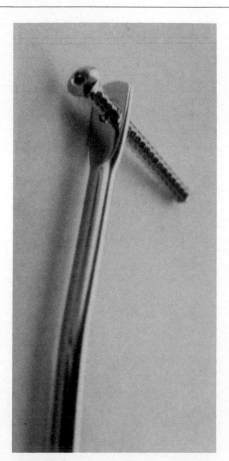

**Fig. 20–6** An AO 3.5-mm cancellous screw inserted through the eye of a nail.

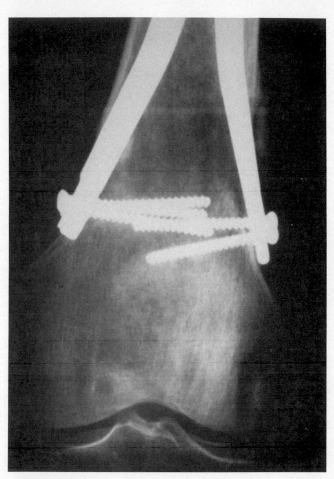

**Fig. 20–7** Each of five nails used in the fixation of a femoral fracture was locked with a screw. Fixation was good.

Although screw locking is suitable for most patients, it should not be used in very overweight individuals. A cable should be used instead.

**Locking With a Cable** Titanium cables can be used if they are removed not later than two months after surgery.

The cable should be inserted through the eye of a nail before it reaches the portal. The cable is then passed through the portal, the bone, and the opposite portal, and through the eye of the nail again before it reaches its final position. The nails are then driven into their final positions and the cable is pulled out as far as possible, cramped, and cut off (Figs. 20–8 and 20–9). Slackness in the cable must be avoided because it would allow the nails to slide.

The surgeon should practice this cable technique to become familiar with insertion problems. Two or three extra cables should be available at the time of surgery.

**Locking With Multiple Wires** If a cable is not available, monofilament wires can be braided together, inserted in the same way as a cable, and tied around the nails' ends (Fig. 20–10).

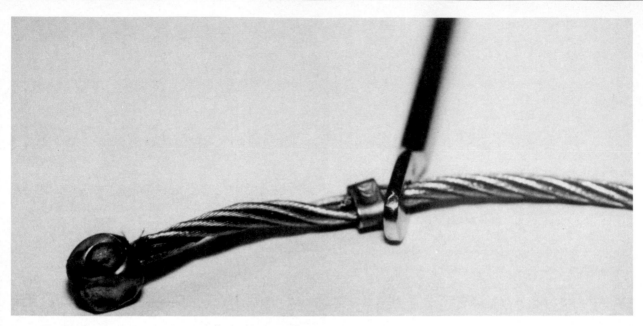

**Fig. 20–8**   The cable was passed through the eye of a nail and cramped with a collar.

**Fig. 20–9**   A femoral fracture was fixed with three nails and a cable passed through the eyes of two nails. The free nail should not migrate since the fracture is stabilized with the locking mechanism.

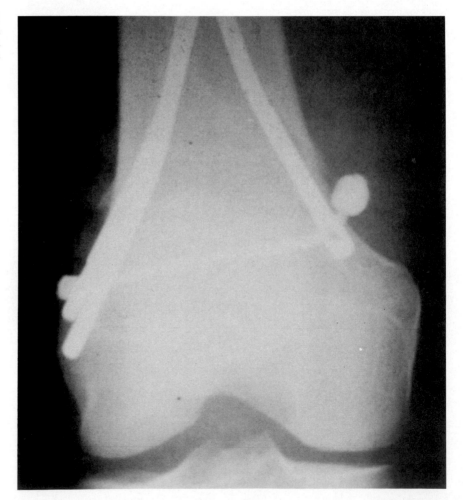

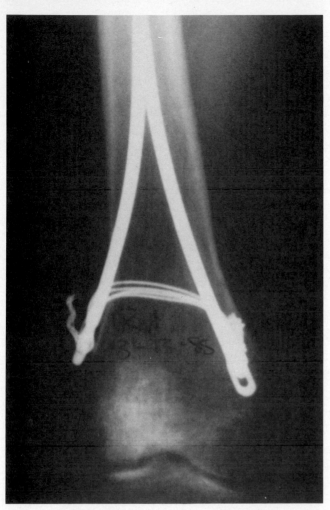

**Fig. 20–10** Multiple wires are used to lock the nails. The wires must be tied securely around the nail ends. (Reproduced with permission of Clayton Perry, MD.)

## Misconception 9: Multiple Trauma

Flexible nails should not be used as a fast, temporary method for fracture fixation. Speed tends to produce inadequate fixation, leading to fixation failure and negating any potential benefits. Furthermore, it may be more difficult to plan permanent procedures after failed fixation and the consequent complications.

If flexible nails are to be used for fracture fixation in patients with multiple injuries, it is imperative that each procedure be executed precisely and in the same way as for single fractures. Although it takes more time to do these procedures properly, the patient will benefit.

## Misconception 10: Open Fracture

Immediate nailing is indicated for some open fractures and is an excellent means of fracture stabilization.

When deciding whether or not to nail an open fracture, it is important to consider the condition of the muscle envelope around the bone. The femur has an excellent muscle envelope; when it is preserved, immediate flexible nailing is indicated even when more complex procedures must be undertaken. In the tibia, there are no muscles on the anteromedial surface. Therefore, the bone must appear viable and the periosteum must be attached before immediate nailing can be undertaken.

## Misconception 11: Pathologic Fracture

Flexible nailing may provide good, temporary fixation of a pathologic fracture or an impending fracture,[8] but the patient's condition and probable life span must be taken into consideration.

## Misconception 12: Nonunion

Rigid fixation of a nonunion is required for healing and flexible nails do not provide such rigid fixation. Rigid nails or plating is preferable for a nonunion.

### References

1. Ender J: Probleme beim frischen per-und subtrochanteren Oberschenkkelbruch. *Hefte Unfallheilkd* 1970;106:2.
2. Kyle RF: Biomechanics of intramedullary fracture fixation. *Orthopedics* 1985;8:1356–1359.
3. Tencer AF, Johnson KD, Johnston DWC, et al: A biomechanical comparison of various methods of stabilization of subtrochanteric fractures of the femur. *J Orthop Res* 1984;2:297–305.
4. Winquist RA, Hansen ST: Closed intramedullary nailing of femoral fractures. *J Bone Joint Surg* 1984;66A:529–539.
5. Browner BD, Burgess AR, Robertson RJ, et al: Immediate closed antegrade nailing of femoral fractures in polytrauma patients. *J Trauma* 1984;24:921–927.
6. Kolmert L, Persson BM, Romanus B: An experimental study of devices for internal fixation of distal femoral fractures. *Clin Orthop* 1982;171:290–299.
7. Perry CR, Pankovich AM, Cohn SL: Locked flexible intramedullary nails in the treatment of unstable femoral fractures. Presented at the 53rd Annual Meeting of American Academy of Orthopaedic Surgeons, New Orleans, Feb 22, 1986.
8. Moehring HD: Closed flexible intramedullary fixation for pathological lesions in long bones. *Orthopedics* 1984;7:829–834.

## P A R T D

# Flexible Intramedullary Nailing of Subtrochanteric Fractures of the Femur

### William R. Dobozi, MD

Subtrochanteric fractures of the femur are often a therapeutic challenge because the bone is osteoporotic or the fracture is severely comminuted, making fixation difficult. Also, muscle forces in this region concentrate high degrees of stress on implants, resulting in a high percentage of failure.

The most commonly used internal fixation device for subtrochanteric fractures is the compression hip screw and side plate. This combination acts as a lateral tension band that resists medial compressive forces in comminuted fractures. Failure rates, on the average, are 20% with this device.[1-3]

In 1966 Zickel introduced intramedullary fixation of subtrochanteric fractures and he and others reported excellent results.[4-7] However, the technique is technically demanding and comminuted fractures may require adjunctive fixation (cerclage wiring). Also, reaming of the proximal fragment may increase comminution and instability.

Flexible intramedullary nailing of proximal femur fractures was introduced in 1970 by Ender and Simon-Weidner.[8] Theirs was a closed method of stabilization that, in most cases, used a nonreamed system. The nails provided favorable mechanical conditions at the fracture site, reducing the stresses applied to them because of their intramedullary position (Fig. 20–11).

## Indications

Almost all subtrochanteric fractures can be treated by flexible intramedullary nailing. Certain fracture configurations, however, may require postoperative traction or adjunctive fixation to prevent shortening or loss of fixation.

Simple transverse and short oblique fractures can be stabilized by closed nailing alone, with no postoperative traction or immobilization needed. Long oblique fractures require adjunctive cerclage wiring before nailing to prevent shortening (Fig. 20–12). Comminuted fractures can be treated by one of two methods. The first involves a closed nailing alone with the nails acting merely as an internal splint to align the fracture. These cases require postoperative traction for three to four weeks before weightbearing

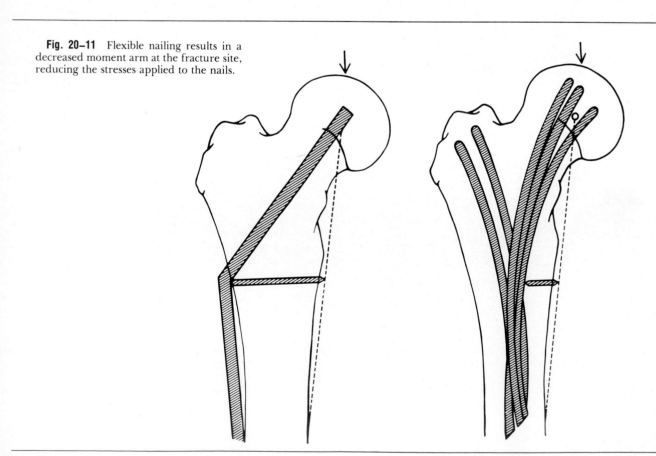

**Fig. 20–11**   Flexible nailing results in a decreased moment arm at the fracture site, reducing the stresses applied to the nails.

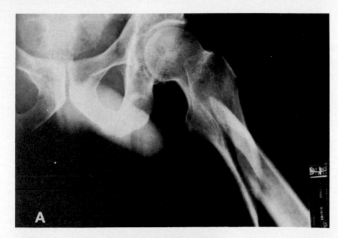

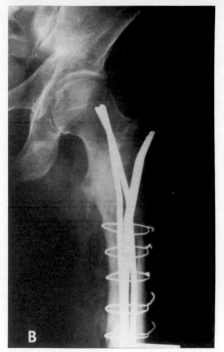

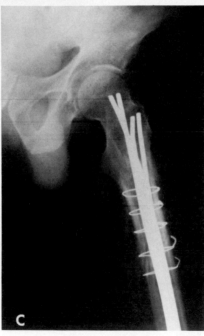

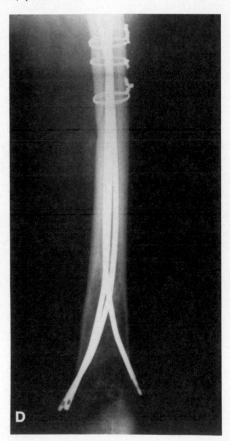

**Fig. 20–12  A:** Long oblique subtrochanteric fracture in a 45-year-old man. **B:** The fracture underwent open reduction with cerclage wires followed by flexible nailing. Anteroposterior radiograph shows good healing at three months. **C:** Lateral radiograph at three months. **D:** Anteroposterior radiograph showing the medial and lateral entry portals used.

is begun. The second approach is adjunctive fixation with cerclage wires to stabilize the fragments before nailing (Fig. 20–13). Bone grafting is not necessary when comminuted fractures are treated with flexible intramedullary nails. Finally, comminuted inter-trochanteric-subtrochanteric fractures are the most difficult to treat in this region. A valgus reduction with unicortical plating and flexible nailing is often necessary (Fig. 20–14). Closed nailing with postoperative traction is an alternative method of treatment for this fracture pattern.

## Preoperative Planning

The fracture pattern is identified on radiographs so that the method of treatment can be planned. The canal diameter is measured at the isthmus on the anteroposterior and lateral views to determine the number of nails to be used. A good rule of thumb is one nail for each 5 mm of canal measured. A minimum of three nails is needed to provide maximum stability.

Surgery is performed as soon after the injury as

possible. If surgery must be delayed, the patient is placed in tibial pin traction. Femoral pin traction is never used because the possibility of pin tract infection in the distal femur would contraindicate flexible nailing. A cephalosporin antibiotic is administered preoperatively and continued for 48 hours postoperatively. Anticoagulation is not routinely used in these patients.

### Surgical Technique

A complete set of 4.5-mm flexible nails and flexible nailing instruments is required. The patient is given either a spinal or a general anesthetic. The patient is then placed on the fracture table in the supine position. The uninjured extremity is widely abducted to allow for free passage of the image intensifier in the lateral projection. The injured extremity is most often positioned in a straight line with the body. The image intensifier is placed superolateral to the injured proximal femur (Fig. 20–15). The fracture is then reduced with traction and internal rotation. Sometimes the injured extremity must be placed in external rotation to achieve a satisfactory reduction and to allow the distal fragment to line up with the externally rotated proximal fragment. The region

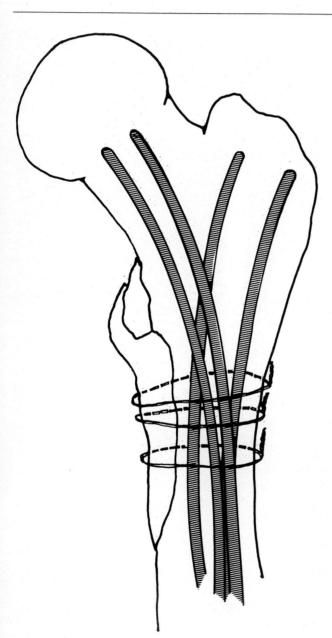

**Fig. 20–13** Comminuted fractures require adjunctive fixation with cerclage wires before nailing to prevent shortening and increase stability.

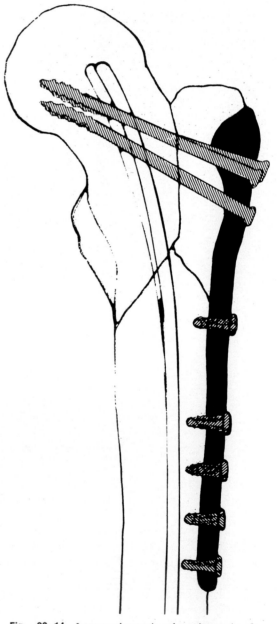

**Fig. 20–14** Intertrochanteric-subtrochanteric fractures may require a unicortical buttress plate plus nailing to increase stability.

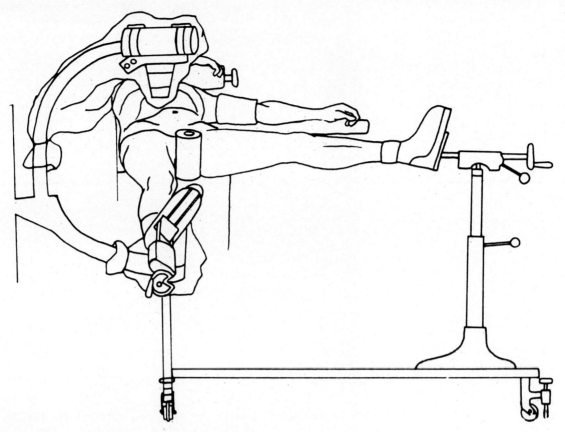

**Fig. 20–15** The image intensifier is placed superolateral to the injured extremity for subtrochanteric and femoral shaft fractures.

from the midtibia to the iliac crest is then prepared in sterile fashion and draped to allow free access to the entire femur.

Medial and lateral entry portals are used for passage of the nails. The medial skin incision begins at the adductor tubercle and is carried proximally for 6 to 8 cm. The fascia is split in line with the skin incision, exposing the vastus medialis muscle. The muscle is gently retracted anteriorly to expose the bone. The medial geniculate vessels running vertically in the periosteum of this region are identified. They serve as landmarks for placement of the entry portal (Fig. 20–16). A 0.25-inch hole is drilled in the bone just proximal and slightly posterior to these vessels. A second hole is drilled 1 cm proximal to the first hole. The hole is enlarged with a Kerrison rongeur to 2 cm long by 1 cm wide (Fig. 20–17). The lateral entry portal is prepared in a similar fashion, with the portal exactly opposite the medial entry portal. An alternative approach is to expose the distal femur simultaneously from both the medial and lateral sides. A through-and-through drill hole is made starting on the lateral side (Fig. 20–18). A second hole is drilled proximal to the first and the entry portals enlarged as described above. A Loman

clamp (optional) is placed proximal to the entry portals and tightened against the bone to prevent longitudinal splitting of the bone when the nails are driven in (Fig. 20–19).

The medial nails are inserted first with their tips directed into the femoral head. C-nails 4.5 mm in diameter are always used. The length of the nails to be used is determined by placing a nail over the anterior thigh with its eyelet opposite the entry portal. The tip of the nail is placed over the femoral head and checked with the image intensifier. A nail of the appropriate length has its tip near the midcervical region (Fig. 20–20). The first nail is driven up to the fracture site and then manipulated across the fracture to drive the tip into the femoral head. The nail is driven to within 1 cm of its final position at this time. The second medial nail is driven up the canal into the femoral head in a similar manner. The tips of the nails should be splayed in the femoral head to provide maximum rotatory stability. The lateral nail or nails are measured with their tips resting over the greater trochanter. At least one nail must be placed from the lateral side. The lateral nail or nails are driven past the fracture into their final positions in the greater trochanter. All the nails are then driven

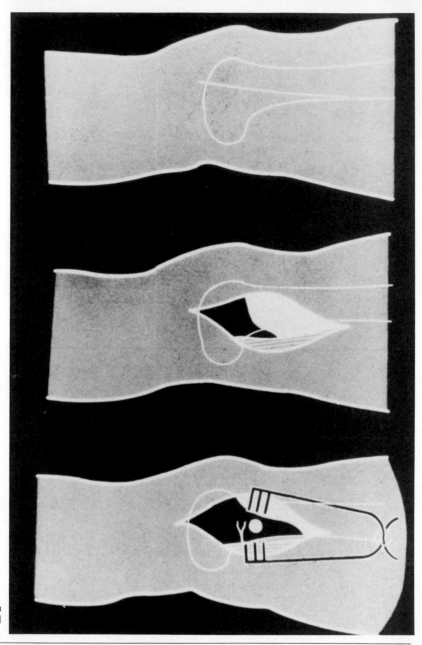

**Fig. 20–16** The geniculate vessels are identified in the periosteum and serve as a landmark for portal placement.

to their final position using the final inserter in the instrument set. The eyelets of the nails should be just visible outside the entry portal; this indicates the correct final placement.

This technique is used for all closed nailings of the subtrochanteric region and for nailings of the femoral shaft. Comminuted fractures require open reduction of the fracture with cerclage wires before this nailing technique can be used. An alternative to cerclage wires is a buttress plate placed laterally with long cancellous screws into the femoral head and short unicortical screws into the shaft below the fracture. The nails are passed from a medial portal

only as far as the screws in the femoral head (Fig. 20–14). If stable fixation has been obtained, the wounds are closed over suction drains and a soft compressive dressing is applied. If traction is to be used postoperatively, a tibial pin is inserted and the patient placed in balanced skeletal traction.

For femoral shaft fractures, C-nails 4.5 mm in diameter are always used. The length of the nails to be used is determined as described above. The nails are inserted from medial and lateral entry portals. The nails are inserted from both sides simultaneously and driven to the fracture site. One surgeon reduces the fracture fragments, while the second surgeon

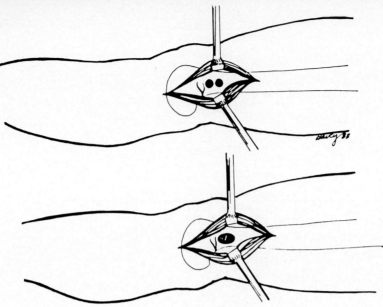

**Fig. 20–17** The holes that are drilled are enlarged with a Kerrison rongeur, completing the entry portal.

## Medial and Lateral Approach

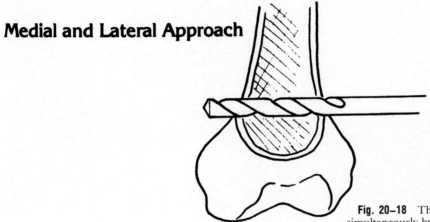

**Fig. 20–18** The medial and lateral entry portals can be made simultaneously by drilling from the lateral side to the medial side.

Skin Protector

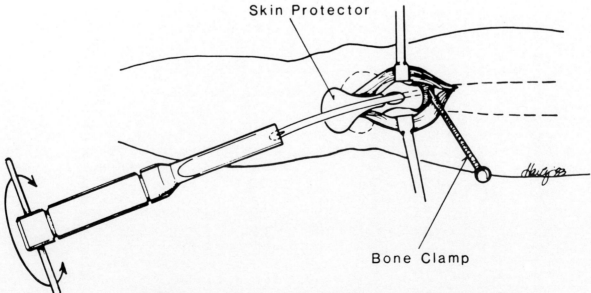

Bone Clamp

**Fig. 20–19** A Loman clamp and skin protector are placed before nail insertion.

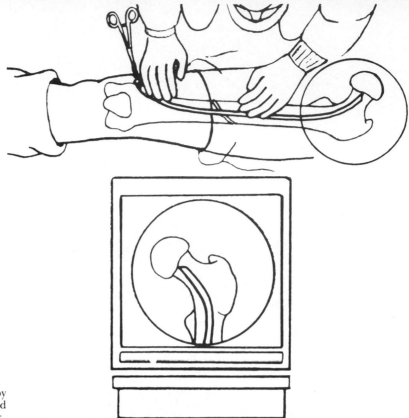

**Fig. 20–20** Nail length is determined by placing a nail over the anterior thigh and checking its length with the image intensifier.

**Fig. 20–21** The fracture can be reduced by manipulation with the tip of the nail if there is minimal displacement.

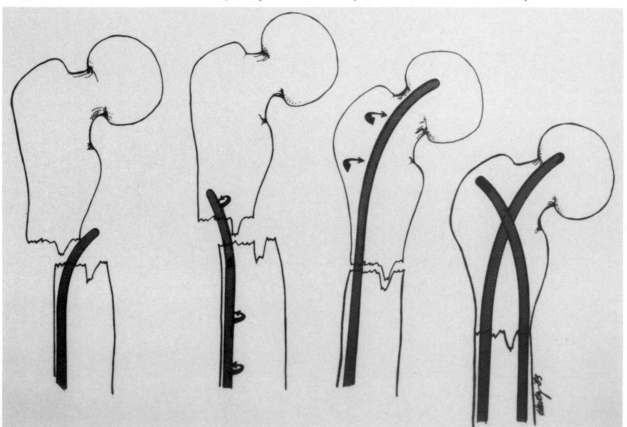

drives the first nail across the fracture site. Rotation of the nail usually reduces the fracture and allows easy passage of the second nail (Fig. 20–21). When the fracture is comminuted, this may be quite difficult to accomplish because curved nails tend to penetrate into the soft tissues. Straightening the nail slightly may help in such cases. The nails are then driven into the proximal fragment until their ends approach the greater trochanter and femoral neck (Fig. 20–22). If more than two nails are to be inserted, care must be taken to prevent the additional nails from pushing previous nails into the medullary canal. This can be controlled by anchoring a towel clip to each nail's eyelet. After all nails are inserted properly, their final positions are checked with the image intensifier. Finally, AO cancellous screws 3.5 mm in diameter and 45 mm in length are inserted through the eye of each nail. The wounds are then closed over suction drains.

After the patient is taken from the fracture table, rotation of both extremities must be inspected and checked. Any significant rotational deformity must be corrected immediately by repositioning the nails surgically. Any attempt at derotation of the extremity is at best dangerous, since a fracture at the entry portals or fracture site may occur and destabilize otherwise stable fixation without correcting the deformity. Furthermore, a stable fracture configuration may be converted into an unstable one. Therefore, the patient should again be placed on the fracture table and the nails should be repositioned after they are withdrawn to just below the fracture site. This is the only way to correct the deformity and should be rather easy to accomplish. The importance of preoperative rotational alignment is evident.

In cases in which fracture fragments are irreducible or nails persistently penetrate outside the bone during insertion, a small incision is made at the fracture site. The fracture fragments are then reduced and the nail's tip is directed into the proximal fragment with a double-gloved finger.

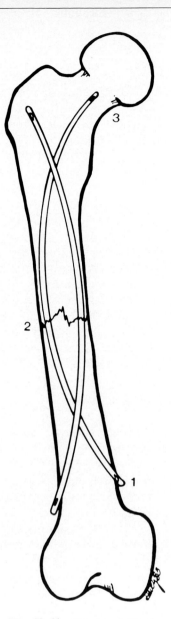

**Fig. 20–22**  Correct nail placement for a femoral shaft fracture. Note the three-point fixation provided by proper placement of the nails.

## Postoperative Management

The major goal of surgery is to obtain fracture stabilization sufficient for early ambulation and weightbearing. Once stable fixation has been achieved, the patient can use a continuous passive motion machine for the knee on the second postoperative day. The machine is used until 110 degrees of motion is obtained, usually in three to four days. The patient is mobilized on crutches or a walker beginning on the third postoperative day. Partial weightbearing gradually progresses to full weightbearing. If fixation is unstable, tibial pin fixation and balanced skeletal traction are used for three to four weeks. During that period, the patient's knee is exercised through daily range of motion by the physical therapy department. When a radiograph shows that the fracture has sufficient callus, the tibial pin is removed. Partial weightbearing is begun and continued for four more weeks. At that time full weightbearing commences. Serial radiographs are obtained at six-week intervals to check the status of healing. The average healing time for subtrochanteric fractures treated by flexible intramedullary nailing is 13 weeks. The nails are removed after complete healing in young patients or in older patients with knee pain secondary to the nails.

## Complications

The major complications encountered with flexible nailing of subtrochanteric fractures are loss of fixation, infection, nonunion, and knee pain.[9-15] Loss of fixation results from inadequate stabilization of comminuted fractures, especially in osteoporotic bone. Motion of the fracture in these cases causes the nails to back out distally, resulting in loss of fixation at the fracture site. This can be prevented by using either postoperative traction or adjunct fixation in these cases. Infections are rare with this technique and respond well to debridement and intravenous antibiotics. Nonunions are also rare with this method of treatment. If one does occur, the nails must be removed and the nonunion stabilized with a compression hip screw and side plate with the addition of an iliac crest bone graft. Knee pain, the most common complication of the flexible nailing technique in the femur, can be prevented by proper placement of the nails well above the flare of the distal femur. Locking the nails with small cortical screws also prevents the nails from backing out distally.

## Conclusions

Flexible intramedullary nailing is a valuable method of treatment for subtrochanteric fractures. The complications of early postoperative mortality, infection, nonunion, and shortening are rarely encountered when this technique is utilized properly. Fatigue failure of the nails is also rare, and, therefore, early ambulation is possible in most patients. Bone grafting of comminuted fractures is unnecessary since biomechanical forces at the fracture site are reduced on the implant when this method of intramedullary fixation is used. Careful preoperative planning and close attention to surgical technique make it is possible to decrease the complications encountered with the flexible nailing technique.

## References

1. Hanson GW, Tullos HS: Subtrochanteric fractures of the femur treated with nail plate devices: A retrospective study. *Clin Orthop* 1978;131:191.
2. Seinsheimer F III: Subtrochanteric fractures of the femur. *J Bone Joint Surg* 1978;60A:300–306.
3. Wile PB, Panjabi MM, Southwick WO: Treatment of subtrochanteric fractures with a high-angle compression hip screw. *Clin Orthop* 1983;175:72.
4. Templeton TS, Saunders EA: A review of fractures in the proximal femur treated with the Zickel nail. *Clin Orthop* 1979;141:213.
5. Zickel RE: An intramedullary fixation device for the proximal part of the femur: Nine years' experience. *J Bone Joint Surg* 1976;58A:866–872.
6. Zickel RE: Subtrochanteric femoral fractures. *Orthop Clin North Am* 1980;11:555.
7. Zickel RE, Mouradian WH: Intramedullary fixation of pathological fractures and lesions of the subtrochanteric region of the femur. *J Bone Joint Surg* 1976;58A:1061–1066.
8. Ender J, Simon-Weidner R: Die Fixierung der trochanterer Brüche mit runden elastischen Condylennägeln. *Acta Chir Austriaca* 1970;1:40–42.
9. Corzatt RD, Bosch AV: Internal fixation by the Ender method. *JAMA* 1978;240:1366.
10. Dobozi WR, Larson BJ, Zindrick MD, et al: Flexible intramedullary nailing of subtrochanteric fractures of the femur. *Clin Orthop*, to be published.
11. Kuderna H, Böhler N, Collon DJ: Treatment of intertrochanteric and subtrochanteric fractures of the hip by the Ender method. *J Bone Joint Surg* 1976;58A:604.
12. Pankovich AM: Adjunctive fixation in flexible intramedullary nailing of femoral fractures: A study of twenty-six cases. *Clin Orthop* 1981;157:301.
13. Pankovich AM, Tarabishy IE: Ender nailing of intertrochanteric and subtrochanteric fractures of the femur: Complications, failures, and errors. *J Bone Joint Surg* 1980;62A:635–645.
14. Raugstad TS, Molster A, Haukeland W, et al: Treatment of pertrochanteric and subtrochanteric fractures of the femur by the Ender method. *Clin Orthop* 1979;138:231.
15. Russin LA, Sonni A: Treatment of intertrochanteric and subtrochanteric fractures with Ender's intramedullary rods. *Clin Orthop* 1980;148:203.

**P A R T E**

# Flexible Intramedullary Nailing of Femoral Shaft Fractures

Arsen M. Pankovich, MD

Although designed by Ender[1] primarily for intertrochanteric and some subtrochanteric fractures, flexible intramedullary nails have been shown to be effective in the fixation of femoral shaft fractures. These new nails differ from the original Rush pins[2] in that they are factory precurved and have a blunt leading end unlike the sharp end of a Rush pin, an important advantage when the nail penetrates into the soft tissues.

Flexible intramedullary nailing is a demanding technique that requires considerable experience, skill, and planning when used in fractures with unstable configurations. It is important for the surgeon to become familiar with the principles of all intramedullary devices, and of flexible nails in particular, before attempting this procedure for the first time. Furthermore, it is important to start with a simpler procedure, such as nailing a transverse midshaft fracture, before undertaking a comminuted or proximally or distally located fracture.

## Fracture Types

It is extremely important to study the fracture carefully. The fracture configuration has to be determined in regard to expected stability after simple nailing.[3]

### Stable Fracture Configurations

These fractures have little tendency to shorten after simple nailing. They include transverse and short oblique fractures, and those with unicortical comminution in which less than 50% of the cortical circumference is involved.

### Unstable Fracture Configurations

Simple nailing of these fractures does not provide longitudinal stability, and shortening is inevitable unless adjunctive measures are taken. Winquist and associates[4] and Chandler[5] discussed the problem of shortening after intramedullary nailing with reamed rigid nails and these principles are applicable to flexible nailing methods as well.

The two basic unstable configurations are long oblique fractures and those with bicortical comminution in which more than 50% of the cortical circumference is involved. Adjunctive measures include postoperative traction, cerclage wiring or unicortical plating of the fracture before nailing, and locking of the nails.

## Management Considerations

### Preoperative Care

After resuscitation and examination of the patient in the emergency room, roentgenograms of the entire femur are obtained and the fracture configuration is determined. The medullary canal is measured at the isthmus to determine the number of nails to be inserted. Generally, for each 5 mm of the medullary space, one 4.5-mm flexible nail can be used. In canals with larger diameters, it is often possible to insert more nails than originally calculated. The surgeon should always plan to use as many nails as possible.

Preoperative skeletal traction is not routine if the procedure is to be done within 24 hours of admission. However, if nailing will be delayed, skeletal traction is advisable to prevent overlapping of fragments and consequent problems with reduction at nailing.

### Timing of Nailing

Optimal timing for nailing is within 12 to 24 hours after the injury. The patient can thus walk within days of surgery and be discharged from the hospital early. Fracture healing is in no way delayed by early surgery, as is true for open rigid nailing of femoral fractures.[6]

### Open Fractures

For purposes of intramedullary fixation and as a guide for planning immediate or delayed fixation of open fractures, the author devised a classification of open fractures that considers the condition of the skin, muscles, bone, and neurovascular system. Each level is given a numeric assignment according to severity of the injury, since each may be differently involved.

Grading of the skin: In grading the skin, it is important to look for quality of the skin and not length of the laceration. 1, puncture wounds and clean lacerations of any length; 2, lacerations that require skin edge excision but consist of viable skin beyond the edge; 3, any laceration with contusion of the surrounding skin that is potentially or actually necrotic or where there is a significant skin loss.

Grading of the muscle: In grading a muscle injury, it is important to recognize that a viable muscle envelope around a bone is an excellent protective layer for the bone. Such muscle envelopes may be damaged, lost, or anatomically nonexistent (as, for example, over the anteromedial surface of the tibia). The grades are as follows: 1, minimal muscle contusion or laceration or both; 2, contusion or laceration of a muscle requiring local muscle debridement, but with enough viable muscle to form a protective envelope over the bone; 3, no muscle envelope (lost or, in some anatomic locations, naturally absent), leaving the bone exposed.

Grading of the bone: In grading a bone, it is important to recognize the condition of the periosteum, its attachment to the bone and bone fragments, and fracture configuration. The grades are as follows: 1, stable fracture configuration, viable bone, and attached periosteum; 2, unstable fracture configuration and no free major fragments devoid of periosteum; 3, stable or unstable fracture configuration in which periosteum is lost from the bone surface or there are free major fragments devoid of periosteum.

Injuries involving major nerves or vessels are assigned grades N (name of the nerve) and V (name of the vessel) or NV if both are involved.

Finally, massive injuries and partial amputations involving skin, muscles bone and, frequently, neurovascular structures are assigned grade A.

An open fracture may be given a numeric assignment of 1,1,1,N for punctured skin, with intact muscle and a transverse fracture, and a nerve injury or 1,3,3,V in cases in which punctured skin covers the medial surface of a very comminuted tibial fracture. At the time of surgery the numeric value may be changed.

### Gunshot Fractures

Low-velocity gunshot fractures are treated by minimal debridement and washing, antibiotic coverage, and immediate nailing as in closed fractures.[3] High-velocity gunshot and shotgun fractures are not suitable for immediate flexible nailing.

### Age of the Patient

Flexible nailing of femoral shaft fractures is indicated in all age groups except children below the age of 10 years. In adolescents, entry portals are made above the distal femoral physis and the trochanteric apophysis is spared.

Fractures in adults aged 20 to 45 years are treated by simple flexible nailing or by nailing with flexible nails locked at portals, unless the bone is osteoporotic or a pathologic fracture is present. Locked nails will not penetrate through the dense metaphyseal bone in the proximal femur in young adults. Otherwise, other adjunctive measures, such as cerclage wiring or unicortical plating, are used.

In patients over 50 years of age, simple nailing of stable fracture configurations is indicated. The fracture canal is stacked and nails locked at the portals to prevent migration out of the bone. Fractures with unstable configurations require adjunctive fixation of the fracture site in addition to locked nails at the entry portals. Locked flexible nails will penetrate proximally in this age group and cannot prevent shortening by themselves.

### Fracture Nailing Methods

#### Nailing of Fractures With Stable Configurations

These fractures are fixed by simple nailing (Fig. 20–23). In most instances nailing is done in retrograde fashion from the supracondylar portals. Although the fracture configuration is stable, it is important to use as many nails as can be inserted easily. It is also advisable to lock nails with screws to prevent their sliding out and causing knee pain. A midshaft transverse or short oblique fracture of the femur is an ideal case. Nailing is usually simple, fixation is excellent, postoperative ambulation and full weightbear-

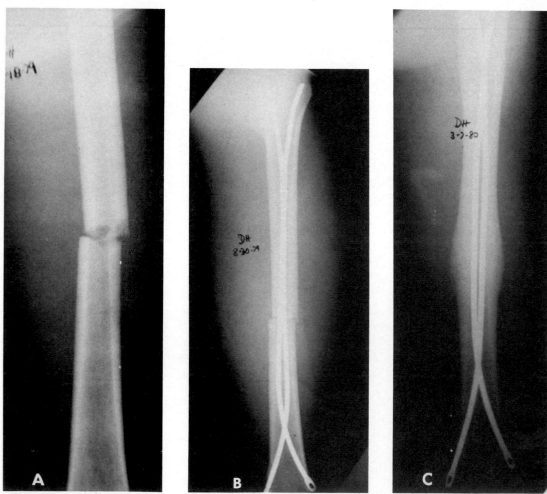

**Fig. 20–23** A 17-year-old youth, known to be hemophiliac, sustained a transverse midshaft fracture of the left femur in a fall from a tree. **A:** Radiograph on admission. **B:** After appropriate preoperative transfusions, the fracture was fixed with two flexible nails. On the second postoperative day, the patient was out of bed and receiving physical therapy for ambulation training and weightbearing as tolerated. **C:** The fracture healed uneventfully.

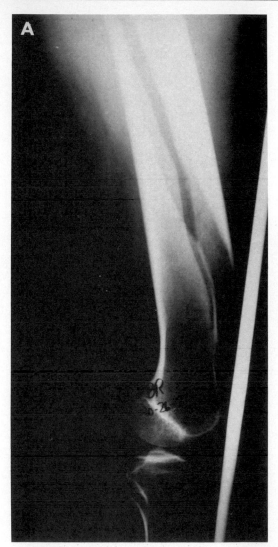
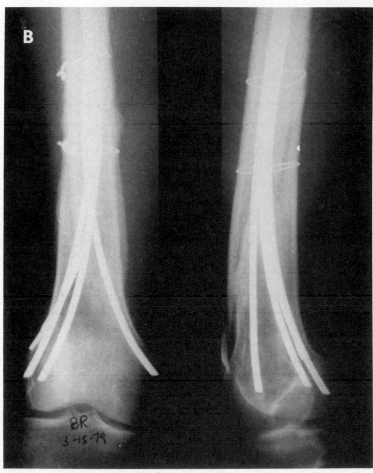

**Fig. 20–24**  A long spiral fracture requires cerclage wiring before nailing. **A:** Initial radiographs. **B:** The fracture was fixed with cerclage wires and antegrade nailing. It had healed at five months.

ing can be started on the day after surgery, and the patient can be discharged within a week.

### Nailing of Fractures With Unstable Configurations

These fractures require adjunctive measures to prevent shortening of the femur.[7]

Long oblique fractures, particularly those located in the upper or lower third of the femoral shaft and in which bone is osteoporotic, should be reduced and fixed with cerclage wires before nailing (Fig. 20–24). A minimum of two or three cerclage wires should be applied; a single wire should never be used. Fixation is effective and early weightbearing is desirable since it actually locks the fragments better. When cerclage wiring is not practical, shortening can be prevented by stacking the canal at the fracture site and locking the nails. This is possible only in young individuals with dense metaphyseal bone that prevents nail penetration.

Fractures with bicortical comminution can and should be stabilized with adjunctive fixation methods in addition to flexible intramedullary nailing. These adjunctive methods are cerclage wiring, unicortical plating, and locking of the nails.

Cerclage wiring is useful in comminuted fractures in the high or low femoral shaft (Fig. 20–25). A delay in weightbearing of several weeks is desirable. The patient should be allowed to ambulate on the unaffected side.

Unicortical plating can be useful in very comminuted bicortical fractures in the upper or lower parts of the femoral shaft. Plating alone does not provide stability, but rather serves as interfragmental fixation and prevents shortening, while flexible nails then enforce this fixation as a neutralization device (Fig. 20–26). Again, early ambulation on the unaffected side, along with delayed weightbearing on the affected side is desirable.

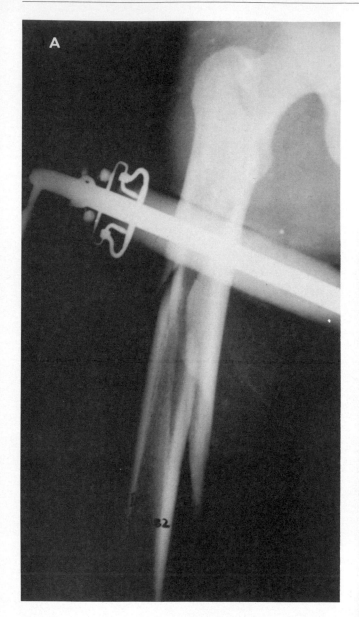

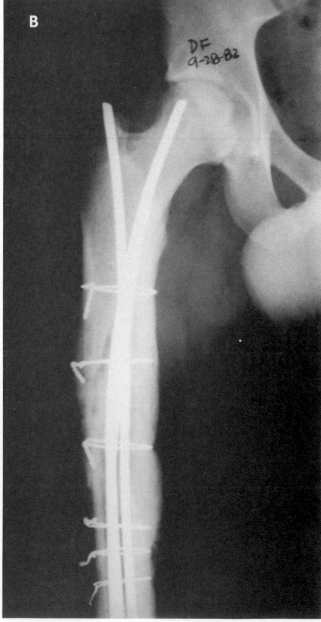

**Fig. 20–25** A fracture with bicortical comminution involving the proximal half of the femoral shaft and intertrochanteric area. **A:** Original radiographs. **B:** Multiple cerclage wires were used before retrograde nailing. The fracture had healed at four months.

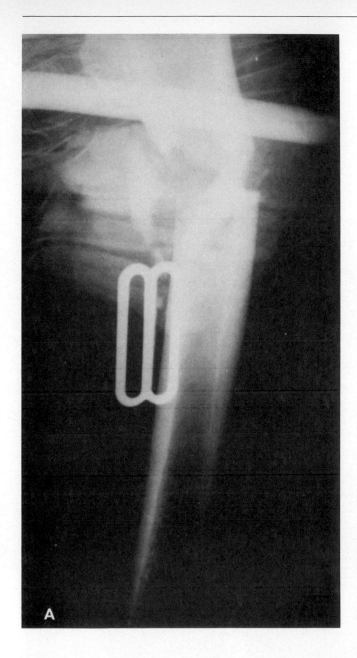

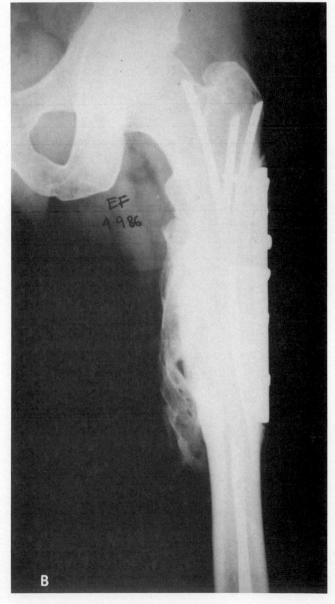

**Fig. 20–26**  An open grade 2,1,2 fracture of the femur was treated immediately with unicortical plating and flexible nailing. **A:** Radiographs on admission. **B:** At five months, the fracture had healed without incident.

Locking the nails prevents shortening in younger adults and provides good rotational and bending stability. Locking can be accomplished with a cable (Fig. 20–27), multiple screws (Fig. 20–28), or multiple wires. Weightbearing on the affected side is not permitted for several weeks postoperatively.

### Femoral Fracture Nailing in Special Situations

**Open Fractures** Some open fractures can be fixed immediately with flexible intramedullary nails because no reaming is necessary. Open fractures with grades 1 and 2 skin, muscle, and bone lesions can be nailed immediately, even if cerclage and unicortical plating are required (Fig. 20–26), although it is clearly preferable to use locked flexible nails whenever possible.

**Gunshot Fractures** Low-velocity gunshot fractures are suitable for immediate nailing (Fig. 20–29). As previously described,[3] only limited irrigation and debridement should be done in the emergency room. Intra-

venous antibiotics, usually a cephalosporin, are administered for three days. The fracture can be fixed on the day of admission or on any subsequent day when the patient's condition permits surgery. Although closed nailing is desirable, as in other fractures, cerclage wiring or unicortical plating can be done immediately in fractures with unstable configurations and when locking of nails is not practical. It must be emphasized that gunshot fractures are usually comminuted and have unstable configurations. Actually, "hidden" fractures (present but invisible on roentgenograms) may be displaced during nailing and contribute to fracture instability.

High-velocity gunshot and shotgun fractures are not suitable for initial nailing because of soft-tissue injury and contamination. Alternative methods of treatment should be used.

**Segmental Fractures** Both fractures may be located on the shaft or may involve the femoral neck or trochanteric or supracondylar parts.[8] It is important to study

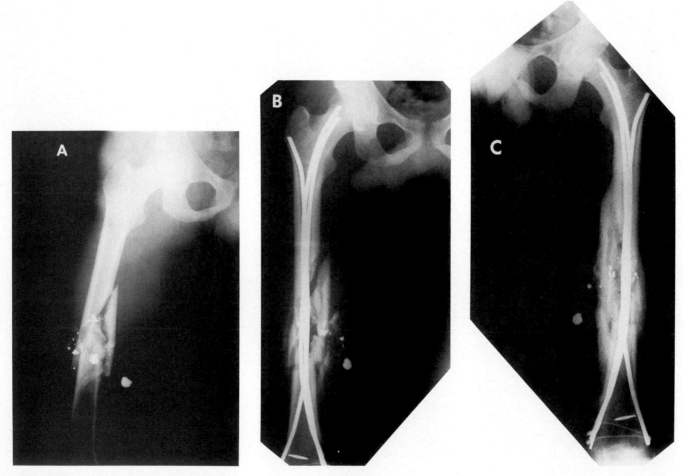

**Fig. 20–27** A gunshot fracture with bicortical comminution was locked with two cables at the portals. (Reproduced with permission from K. Davenport and R. Hall, unpublished.) **A:** Initial radiographs. **B:** Four weeks after nailing, early callus is noted while position of fracture fragments and nails remained unchanged. **C:** Four months after nailing, the fracture healed without shortening of the femur.

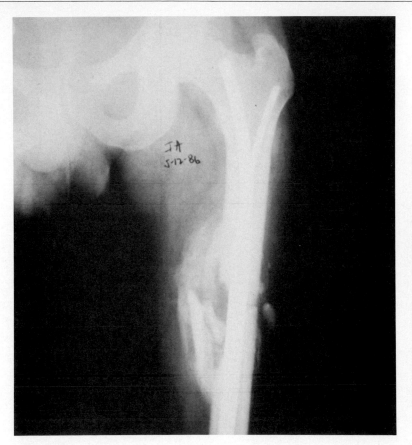
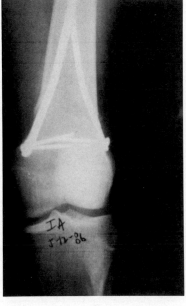

**Fig. 20–28**    A fracture with bicortical comminution was fixed with locked flexible nails in a closed procedure. Nails were locked with multiple screws.

the type of each fracture, paying particular attention to those with unstable configurations.

Simple nailing of a segmental fracture is indicated only when both fractures have stable configurations (Fig. 20–30). Adjunctive measures, particularly locking, must be used when one or both fractures have unstable configurations.

When one fracture involves the femoral neck, the shaft fracture should be fixed first in the same way as any other single fracture. Once the femoral shaft fracture is fixed, the surgeon may fix the femoral neck.

When an intertrochanteric fracture is present, consideration again must be given to methods other than flexible nailing. Whenever possible, the intertrochanteric fracture should be fixed with a hip screw-plate system; if the shaft fracture is in the proximity, a long plate may be used. The stable intertrochanteric fractures often seen in younger individuals are difficult to nail because the medullary canal is narrow and the nails become straight as they are driven up the canal. It is then difficult to negotiate the calcar and penetrate into the femoral head. Conversely, in older individuals, fractures are unstable and difficult to fix with flexible nails. Fixation of the shaft fracture is easy once the intertrochanteric fracture has been fixed.

**Fractures Below Noncemented Implants**    These fractures usually occur through a screw hole at the end of a plate or at the tip of the stem of an endoprosthesis.[9] The fracture can also occur at a distance from the implant. These fractures are ideal for fixation with flexible nails.

When the implant is a plate with screws, three or four nails can often be inserted around the screws (Fig. 20–31). If more nails are to be inserted, one or two screws can be removed through a stab wound under the control of an image intensifier. It is important to insert nails from both the medial and the lateral portals. Often, the first two nails can be inserted to the level of the lesser trochanter while later nails stop penetrating below that level. The nails must be of proper length, and those that are too long must be replaced. These nails should be always locked with screws at the portals.

When the fracture occurs below a noncemented endoprosthesis, it is often possible to insert three or

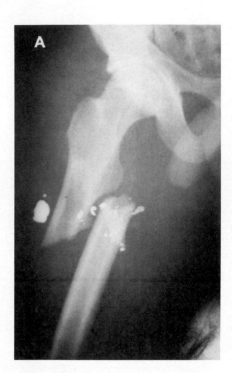 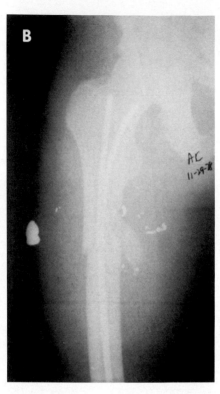 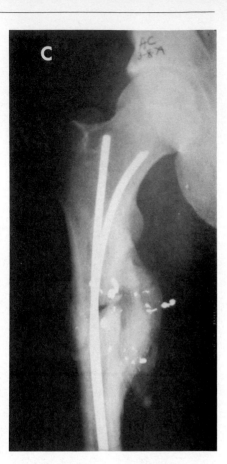

**Fig. 20–29** Gunshot fracture of the femur with minimal comminution was nailed immediately while a patient's gunshot wound of the neck was being explored. **A:** Initial radiographs. **B:** Roentgenograms immediately after surgery. **C:** The fracture was healed at 3½ months.

four nails around the stem (Fig. 20–32). Again, the nails should be inserted from both the medial and the lateral portals and as far proximally as possible. They should be of appropriate length and locked to the femur with screws.

It is also important that fractures with unstable configurations be studied carefully and appropriate adjunctive measures taken during nailing.

**Fractures in Adolescents** These fractures are usually transverse or oblique and less often comminuted. To avoid overgrowth, these procedures should be done in patients more than 10 years old. Two nails can usually be inserted; on rare occasions, three can be used. Nails 4 and 4.5 mm in diameter are inserted from the medial and lateral portals made above the distal femoral physis (Fig. 20–33). The insertion is sometimes quite difficult. Fixation is normally stable, and early weightbearing is possible. The nails are usually not locked. They should be removed six to eight months after insertion.

**Femoral Fractures in Multiple Trauma** Multiple fractures and multisystem injuries are severe injuries, and femoral fractures contribute to the patient's immobil-

ity, leading to the complications of recumbency. Therefore, it is desirable to fix all fractures in the lower extremities, and particularly those in the femur.

There is little place for temporary, fast fixation of the femur with flexible nails in patients with multiple injuries. To mobilize the patient, fixation of femoral fractures must be solid and stable enough to withstand stressing of the extremity. Otherwise, pain from the instability at the fracture site and fixation failure will prevent effective mobility, and contribute to the development of complications. It is the author's view that these fractures should be fixed solidly and permanently if the patient's condition allows for prolonged anesthesia and surgery; this is usually possible. However, when prolonged anesthesia is not advisable, it may be better to postpone bone fixation initially, treat the patient in traction, aggressively treat nonorthopaedic conditions and injuries, and push for as early return to the operating room as possible to fix fractures properly.

**Antegrade Nailing**

This method of flexible nailing is rarely used

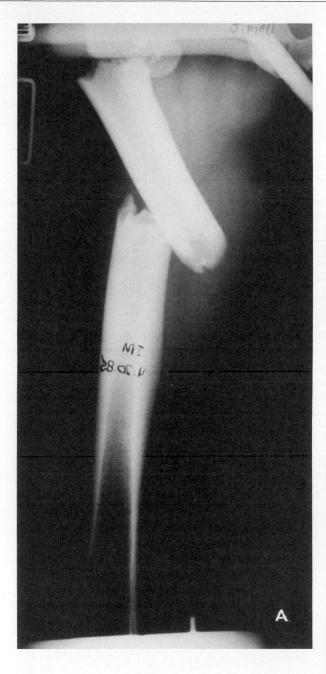

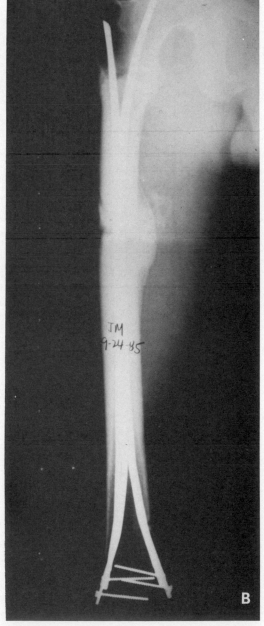

**Fig. 20–30** Stable double transverse segmental fracture was fixed with locked flexible nails. (Reproduced with permission from A. Weber, unpublished.) **A:** Initial radiographs. **B:** At five months, the fracture was healed. Note locked nails.

because of one potential problem—malposition of fracture fragments, particularly in valgus. The technique is demanding.

The prime indication for antegrade nailing is a very low shaft fracture that cannot be fixed by other methods because of local skin and soft-tissue conditions or because of extensive comminution.

The portals must be made at the base or through the greater trochanter. At least one S-nail must be

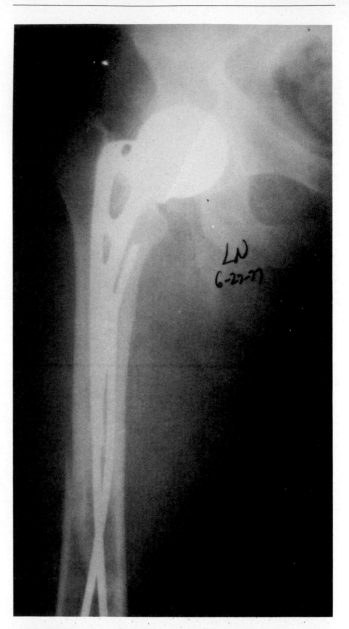

**Fig. 20–32** Long oblique fracture below the level of the stem of an endoprosthesis was fixed with two flexible nails. Fixation was inadequate and sliding of the fragments occurred. Cerclage wires and locked flexible nails would have been more appropriate.

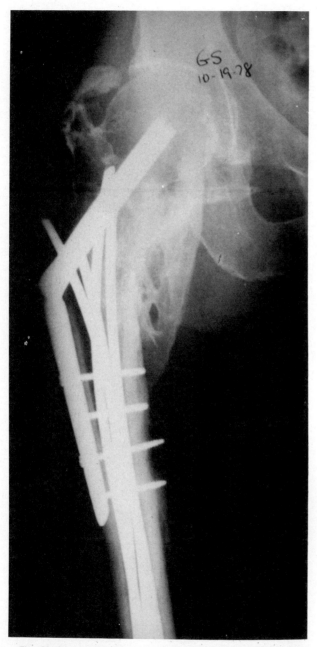

**Fig. 20–31** A fracture in relation to a Jewett nail was fixed with four flexible nails that were easily passed by transverse screws. (Reproduced with permission from Pankovich AM, Tarabishy I, Barmada R: Fractures below noncemented implants: Treatment with Ender nailing. *J Bone Joint Surg* 1981;63A:1024–1025.)

directed into the medial condyle to neutralize the tendency toward valgus malposition.

Browner and associates[10] showed that simple antegrade nailing of comminuted fractures created many complications, as do other intramedullary devices that are not locked or supplemented with adjunctive measures. Furthermore, portals in the piriform fossa often required straightening of the nails, thus losing three-point fixation. Complications included pulling out of nails with consequent loss of fixation and need for reoperations, portal pain, and rotational and angulatory deformities.

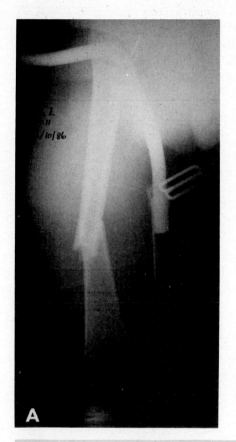

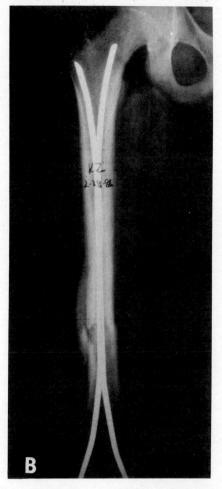

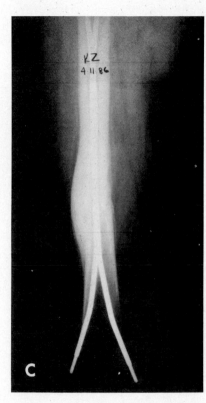

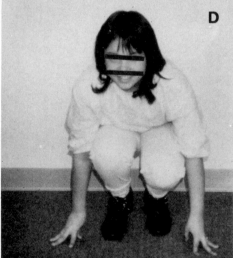

**Fig. 20–33**  Fracture of the femur in a 10-year-old girl. **A:** Original radiographs. **B:** Six weeks after nailing, the fracture is clinically healed. **C:** At three months, the fracture is healed on radiograph. **D:** The patient had full function and walked unsupported five weeks after surgery.

## Complications in Flexible Intramedullary Nailing

### Intraoperative Complications

Malrotation and new intraoperative fractures are the most common complications.

Healing of fractures in internal and external malposition must be prevented. This is best done by preoperative attempts at fracture reduction by matching of bone spikes and obliquity of fragments.

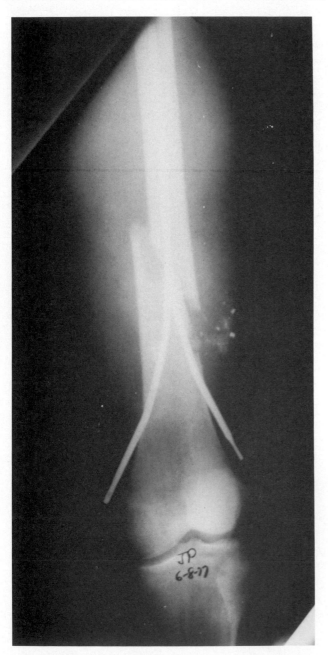

**Fig. 20–34** A long oblique fracture was fixed with two flexible nails. Since no adjunctive measures, such as cerclage wiring or locking, were taken, fracture fragments slid along the nails protruding out of the bone and causing knee pain.

Also, the position of the lesser trochanter should be determined and rotation of the knee adjusted appropriately. After the nails have been inserted, the foot should be rotated to ascertain the appropriate amount of external and internal rotation. Malrotation does not develop after surgery; it occurs before insertion of the nails.

Intraoperative fractures are related to the insertion of nails. If the portal hole is small or the bone thin, longitudinal fractures can and do occur during nail insertion. Although of no consequence to the integrity of the femur, these fractures decrease holding of nails by the bone. If the nails are not locked in these situations, they will pull out easily.

As the nails are driven across the fracture site, they may displace the undisplaced bone fragments which are often not apparent on preoperative radiographs. Displacement of these "hidden" fragments can convert a fracture with a stable configuration into an unstable fracture.

A rare complication is a supracondylar fracture. It occurs through an entry portal, particularly when the portal is too large and when the bone is osteoporotic. The author has encountered this problem only once. Supracondylar fracture should be immediately fixed by wiring the nails' eyes or by fixing fragments with a four-hole plate and leaving the nails in situ.

### Postoperative Complications

Nail migration, nonunion, and infection are the major complications.

Nail migration out of entry portals with accompanying knee pain is most often a complication of retrograde nailing. This complication is the consequence of improper technique. It can occur when too few nails are used, thus allowing slow sliding of the nails out of entry portals, particularly when the portals are large and the bone osteoporotic. This can be prevented by stacking the nails and not making large portal holes. The most effective way to prevent nail migration out of portals is to lock each nail with a screw. Locking the nails is now standard practice in almost all femoral shaft fractures. Another cause of nail migration is settling of fracture fragments if a gap is left between the fragments, even in a fracture with a stable configuration. However, the most common cause of nail migration is failure to use adjunctive fixation measures in simple nailing of a fracture with an unstable configuration (Fig. 20–34). Browner and associates[10] demonstrated this in antegrade nailing. Furthermore, failure of adjunctive fixation, such as breaking of cerclage wires or pulling out of screws from a unicortical plate, will inevitably result in failure of fixation and migration of nails. This is obviously applicable to all intramedullary devices, as clearly described by Winquist and associates[4] for reamed Küntscher nails. Once failure of fixation has

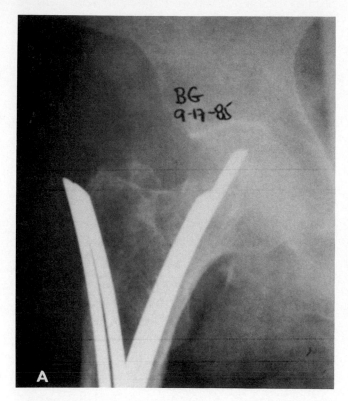
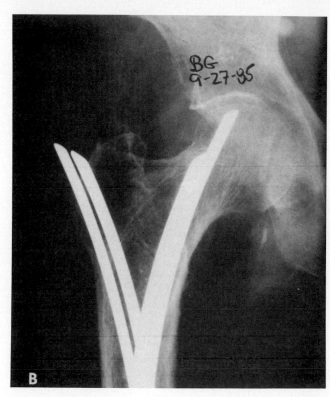

**Fig. 20–35** Proximal migration of locked flexible nails after fixation of a femoral shaft fracture in osteoporotic bone. **A:** Postoperative radiographs. **B:** Ten days later the radiographs showed that all nails had migrated proximally, although in this case they did not penetrate in the joint.

occurred, rotational and even angulatory deformities can develop and renailing may be necessary.

More recently, the extensive use of locked flexible nails has shown, as expected, that locked nails migrate at the leading end when a fracture with an unstable configuration is fixed and when the bone is osteoporotic (Fig. 20–35). This again points to the importance of careful adjunctive fixation of unstable fractures in osteoporotic bone.

The author has seen two nonunions. In the first case, a gunshot fracture of the midshaft was fixed with cerclage wires before nailing. It required removal of a broken nail and plating. The second nonunion, in a fracture below a Jewett nail in osteoporotic bone, was reported previously.[9]

The author is aware of several other nonunions in which nailing was done for fractures in the area of irradiated bone and one nonunion after nailing of a pathologic fracture in a patient with metastatic disease. Finally, nailing of a femoral shaft nonunion with flexible nails failed to achieve bone union.

Nonunion is a rare complication of flexible intramedullary nailing of acute femoral shaft fractures in normal bone.

Osteomyelitis and wound infection are rare complications. The author has seen osteomyelitis in only one patient[3] who underwent immediate plating of the femoral shaft after attempted flexible nailing.

## Summary

Simple flexible intramedullary nailing is a suitable method of fixation of femoral shaft fractures with stable configurations. Complications are rare when nailing is properly executed, and patients are able to ambulate and bear weight within days of surgery.

Problems arise when simple nailing is used to fix femoral shaft fractures with unstable configurations. Sliding of nails out of portals, loss of fixation, malrotation, and knee pain often result. Therefore, adjunctive measures must be used in the fixation of unstable fractures.

The technique of nailing is demanding. The surgeon must be familiar with the principles of intramedullary nailing and should observe several procedures before attempting to do one alone. Furthermore, it is advisable to start with simple nailing of fractures with stable configurations to gain experience and confidence before undertaking a more complex procedure in a fracture with an unstable configuration.

Finally, it must be emphasized that the principles of intramedullary nailing are essentially the same for all intramedullary devices. It must be also emphasized that there is little room for fast, temporary nailings and that there is no substitute for solid, precise fixation. There is no difference between quick insertion of a Küntscher-type rigid nail without reaming and speedy flexible nailing—both are fast and both will result in failure of fixation. The surgeon should resist the temptation to do fast procedures.

### References

1. Ender J: Probleme beim frischen per-und subtrochanteren Oberschenkkelbruch. *Hefte Unfallheilk* 1970;106:2.
2. Rush LV: *Atlas of Rush Pin Techniques*, ed 2. Meridian, Mississippi, The Berivon Co, 1976.
3. Pankovich AM, Goldflies ML, Pearson RL: Closed Ender nailing of femoral-shaft fractures. *J Bone Joint Surg* 1979;61A:222–232.
4. Winquist RA, Hansen ST, Clawson DK: Closed intramedullary nailing of femoral fractures: A report of five hundred and twenty cases. *J Bone Joint Surg* 1984;66A:529–539.
5. Chandler RW: Limitations of conventional nailing. *Orthopaedics* 1985;8:1354–1355.
6. Wilber MC, Evans EB: Fractures of the femoral shaft treated surgically: Comparative results of early and delayed operative stabilization. *J Bone Joint Surg* 1978;60A:489–491.
7. Pankovich AM: Adjunctive fixation in flexible intramedullary nailing of femoral fractures. *Clin Orthop* 1981;157:301–309.
8. Casey MJ, Chapman MW: Ipsilateral concomitant fractures of the hip and femoral shaft. *J Bone Joint Surg* 1979;61A:503–509.
9. Pankovich AM, Tarabishy I, Barmada R: Fractures below non-cemented implants: Treatment with Ender nailing. *J Bone Joint Surg* 1981;63A:1024–1025.
10. Browner BD, Burgess AR, Robertson RJ, et al: Immediate closed antegrade nailing of femoral fractures in polytrauma patients. *J Trauma* 1984;24:921–927.

**P   A   R   T   F**

# Flexible Intramedullary Nailing of Tibial Shaft Fractures

## David Segal, MD

Most tibial fractures are still treated nonsurgically by closed reduction and cast immobilization. Diaphyseal fractures are frequently displaced and unstable and are the result of high-energy trauma associated with damage to the surrounding soft tissues. In many of these fractures, stabilization of the bone is indicated to help soft-tissue healing as well as to prevent angular or rotational deformities. Flexible intramedullary nailing has been used at Boston City Hospital since 1979 with satisfactory results. As experience in treating closed and open tibial fractures increased, indications and contraindications became more defined and flexible intramedullary nailing is now used more often. Presently, the surgical technique used

permits closed nailing with the help of an image intensifier. The indications and contraindications are based on clinical experience with more than 150 tibial fractures, 42 of which were open.

## Surgical Technique

Surgery is performed using general or regional anesthesia after the patient's general condition has been stabilized. The patient is positioned supine on a radiolucent board placed on top of the regular operating table. Its foot portion is lowered so that the image intensifier can be used. A tourniquet is applied to the proximal thigh and the entire leg is prepared and draped free from the knee down to the toes.

A slightly oblique 4- to 5-cm incision is placed along the medial and lateral sides of the proximal tibia. The landmarks on the lateral side are easier to identify, as the incision is placed equally proximal and distal to Gerdy's tuberosity (Fig. 20–36). The incision should be distal to the knee joint; the aponeurosis over the proximal part of the anterior tibial muscles is incised and the muscles are elevated 1 cm off the lateral tibial flare. A 0.25-inch drill hole is placed inferior to Gerdy's tuberosity and is directed medially and posteriorly. The position of the entry portal can be verified by the image intensifier, although this landmark is constant and reliable. The entrance hole is enlarged with an AO awl directed parallel to the long axis of the tibia.

A similar medial incision is done midway between the anterior and posterior borders of the tibia at the medial tibial flare (Fig. 20–37). After the subcutaneous tissues are cut through, the pes anserinus is incised (stab wound) to make room for the drill bit. The medial portal is also enlarged with the awl. A nail of the proper length is then introduced from either side and advanced to the fracture site. The tissues are protected by the skin protector while the nail is advanced. The medial and lateral nails can be advanced simultaneously to the fracture site and then one at a time into the distal fragment or they can be introduced separately. It is important to restore length and rotation as the first nail crosses into the distal fragment and before the fracture is transfixed with the second nail. The flexible nails provide excellent rotational stability. Any malrotation not corrected at the time of surgery will persist.

After the nails reach their final position, the fracture site should be examined once more under the image intensifier to assure that the fragments are not distracted by the nails. The proximal part of the nail (i.e., the eyelet) should be distal to the knee joint. The tourniquet is released and bleeding vessels are coagulated. An anterior compartment fasciotomy through the lateral incision is routinely performed. A suction

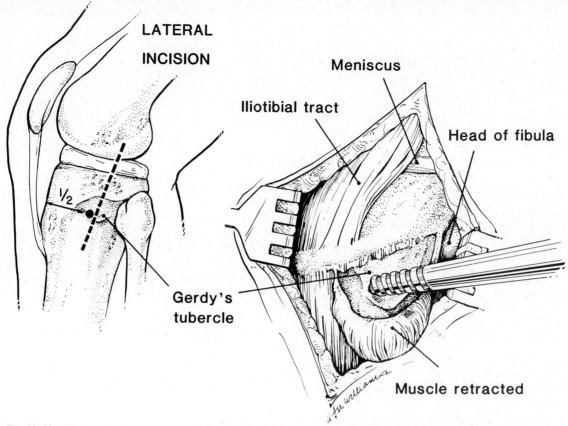

**Fig. 20–36** The surgical approach to the lateral side of the proximal tibia. The knee joint is not explored. Gerdy's tuberosity is a reliable landmark. (Adapted with permission from Wiss DA, Segal D, Gumbs VL, et al: Flexible medullary nailing of tibial shaft fractures. *J Trauma* 1986; 26:1106–1112, Williams & Wilkins.)

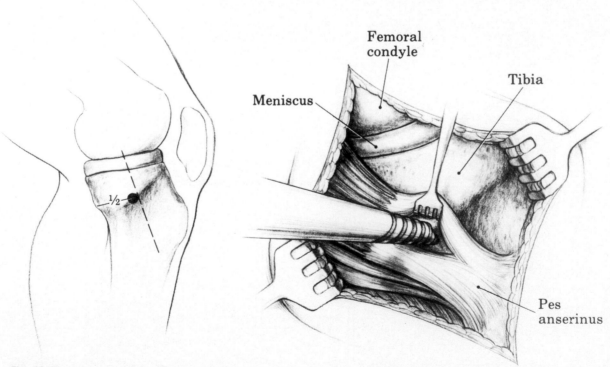

**Fig. 20–37** The surgical approach to the medial side of the proximal tibia. These landmarks are not as well defined. (Reproduced with permission from Wiss DA, Segal D, Gumbs VL, et al: Flexible medullary nailing of tibial shaft fractures. *J Trauma* 1986; 26:1106–1112, Williams & Wilkins.)

drain is left at the lateral incision, the wounds are closed in layers, and the leg is immobilized in a short-leg cast.

## Fracture Reduction

During the reduction of an unstable fracture, the surgeon may find it helpful to tie a non-elastic bandage around the waist so that the distal fragment can be pulled by the surgeon's body weight, leaving both hands free for manipulation (Fig. 20–38). The crossing of the nails into the distal fragment has to be confirmed with the image intensifier on anteroposterior and lateral projections. Whether the medial or the lateral nail should be introduced first can be left to the surgeon except when the fragment is displaced medially or laterally and cannot be manipulated into anatomic alignment. If the distal fragment is displaced medially, it is easier to introduce the medial nail first; the flexible intramedullary nail is C-shaped and will "fall" into the distal fragments when introduced from the medial side into a medially displaced fragment. This, however, only makes reduction impossible by maintaining the displacements. In such a case, the surgeon should introduce the lateral nail first to reduce the distal fragment; the medial nail should be inserted next.

## Nail Size

The length of the nail can be measured on the unaffected tibia or after the fragments are reduced. The nail should bridge the tibia from the entry portal to 1 or 2 cm proximal to the ankle joint. Measuring the unaffected limb from tibial tuberosity down to the ankle joint provides the proper length. The nails come in 4.5-, 4.0-, and 3.5-mm diameters. The author prefers to use the 4.0-mm nails but a combination of 4.0- and 3.5-mm nails can also be used. The 4.5-mm nails are used primarily in femoral fractures and, rarely, in tibial fractures. The diameter of the tibia is measured at its narrowest part. The average adult tibial diameter is 9 to 12 mm and there is room for three to four medium- and small-diameter nails.

## Prebending of the Nails

Intramedullary nails are C-shaped. They can be bent and modified to fit the fracture. Since the nails

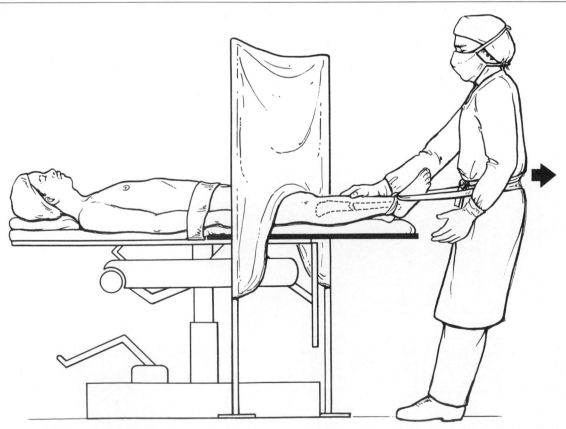

**Fig. 20–38**   The patient is positioned on the translucent board and the lower leg is draped from knee to toes. The surgeon's body weight is used to assist in reducing the fracture.

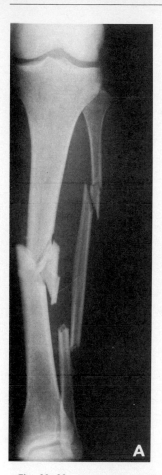
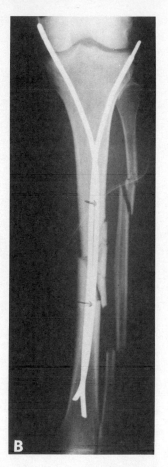
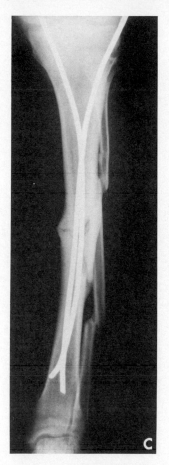
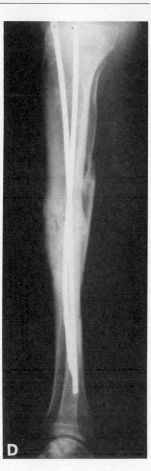

**Fig. 20–39**   Comminuted tibial fracture with a large butterfly fragment. **A and B:** Preoperative and postoperative radiographs. The arrows point to the buttressing effect of the medial nail. **C and D:** Solid healing is apparent at five months. The proximal ends of the nails are too long, causing some discomfort.

provide stability by three-point fixation, their C-shaped configuration should be maintained. As the nail is introduced into the entry portal, it has a tendency to hit the opposite cortex. A slight bend of about 15 to 20 degrees of the most distal centimeter of the nail makes the introduction easier. When the nail has to buttress a large butterfly fragment, it should be prebent so that the convexity of the nail bridges the area of the butterfly fragment or the missing bone (Fig. 20–39).

### Retrograde Nailing

Retrograde nailing, with the flexible nails introduced from the distal fragment into the proximal fragment, is rarely indicated but is occasionally a useful technique. The nails can be introduced from the medial or lateral part of the distal tibia with the eyelet remaining subcutaneous. In the author's experience, this technique has been used primarily to control angular stability in distal-third fractures, es-

pecially in tall individuals with relatively narrow medullary canals. As the flexible nail introduced from the proximal tibia travels through the long tibial shaft, it straightens out. As it reaches the distal third of the tibia, where the canal is wider, the nail loses most of its C-shaped configuration and, thus, its engagement in the distal cortex is not as strong. Adding a retrograde nail restores stability (Fig. 20–40).

Another indication for retrograde nailing is the presence of soft-tissue damage. Figure 20–41 shows a patient with multiple trauma after being struck by a car. The patient had badly bruised tissues around the knee and a displaced but not compounded fracture of the proximal tibia. She also sustained a contralateral grade III open tibial fracture. In this patient retrograde nailing allowed surgery to be performed without cutting through edematous and contused soft tissues. It has been the author's experience that retrograde nailing provides poorer stability than antegrade nailing and that it should be used, therefore, only as a supplementary method in selected patients.

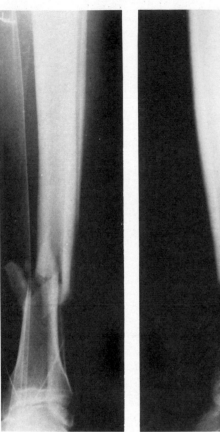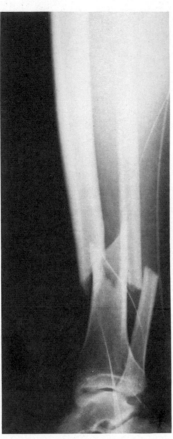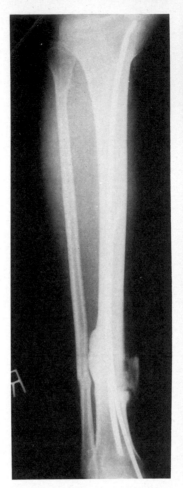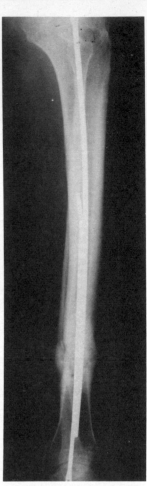

**Fig. 20–40**  Distal-third fracture with comminution. Notice the long and narrow medullary canal. The antegrade nail is supplemented with a retrograde nail to counteract the tendency of the fracture to go into valgus. The retrograde nail is inserted above the medial malleolus. Final radiographs show good healing four months after the injury.

### Nailing of Open Fractures

Intramedullary nailing with flexible nails is now routinely performed on Gustilo's grade I and grade II open tibial fractures. After proper irrigation and debridement, the lower leg is redraped. The surgeons change gowns, gloves, and instruments. The surgical incision used to explore the fracture is closed but the skin laceration is left open. The nail insertion proceeds in routine fashion. The soft-tissue laceration created at time of injury can be used in the reduction and alignment of the fragments provided that further soft-tissue dissection is avoided. Bone grafting, if indicated, is usually postponed for a period of five to ten days. In open tibial fractures, the soft-tissue injuries usually occur through the anterior part of the lower leg where the tibia has little soft-tissue coverage. The author prefers to let the soft tissues recover before applying the local bone graft. Only cancellous bone chips are inserted into the area of the missing bone. This is done either through open

soft-tissue wounds or through a local stab wound. During bone grafting, the adjacent fragments are decorticated; no additional soft tissues are stripped. The bone graft acts as a gap filler. In the author's experience with eight patients in whom this technique was used, the cancellous bone was incorporated without complications. Immediate nailing is done in type I and type II open fractures, but type III tibial fractures should not be treated with immediate intramedullary nailing.

### Indications

The indications for nailing of tibial fractures have gradually been expanded to include tibial fractures previously treated by other methods. Fractures of the tibia 7.5 cm distal to the tibial plateau and 5 cm proximal to the tibial plafond are suitable for flexible intramedullary nailing. Segmental fractures, butterfly fragments, and other fracture configurations associated with instability (e.g., short or long oblique fractures at the distal third of the tibia) are some of the injuries treated with nailing. Patients with failed closed reductions and those who are severely obese are candidates for flexible nailing. A fractured tibia treated with nailing can bear weight earlier than a tibia with a similar fracture treated with a cast without internal fixation.

Tibial nailing can be used in patients who have injuries to other extremities that prevent weightbearing on the contralateral leg or the use of crutches. For example, in a patient with a tibial fracture amenable to treatment in a cast and a contralateral injury to the lower extremity or an injury to the upper extremities making the use of crutches impossible, the surgeon may elect to stabilize the fractured tibia with flexible nails to facilitate earlier ambulation and earlier weightbearing. Patients with multiple trauma, includ-

ing multiple injuries to the long bones, are also candidates for immediate stabilization of the fractures. This facilitates early ambulation. Flexible nails can also be used in patients who have had screws implanted previously. The nails can be inserted as shown in Fig. 20–42.

## Contraindications

Nailing is contraindicated in the presence of infection and in tibial fractures extending to the articular surfaces of either the knee or the ankle. If there is severe comminution or bone loss, flexible nails will not prevent shortening and thus other methods of fixation should be used. Delayed unions and nonunions are also contraindications to flexible nailing since the fragments cannot be rigidly fixed.

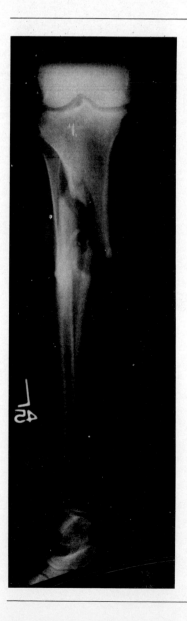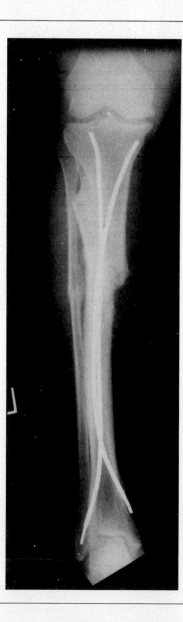

**Fig. 20–41**  Bilateral tibial fractures in a patient with multiple trauma. Notice the preoperative rotational deformity. Retrograde nailing permitted early ambulation and the fracture healed in good alignment.

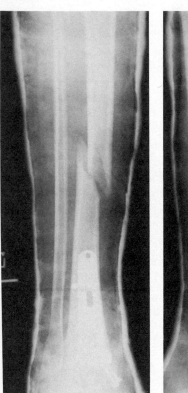
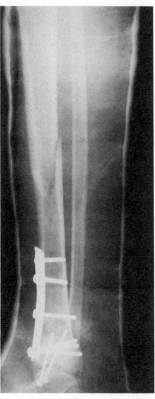
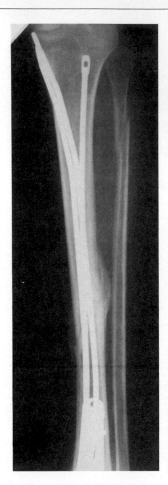
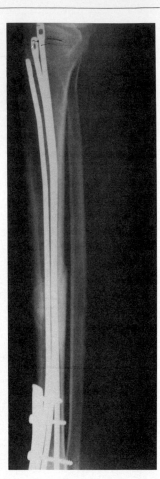

**Fig. 20–42** Midshaft tibial fracture in the presence of an old plafond injury. Three nails were inserted without removing the plate and screws.

Flexible nailing is contraindicated in patients with previous tibial fractures. In the author's experience, previously healed fractures obliterate the medullary canal and prevent advancement of the nail into the distal fragment (Fig. 20–43). In such injuries, careful assessment of the medullary canal is needed before nailing is performed. On two occasions the author failed to advance the nail despite vigorous and repeated attempts.

### Pitfalls and Mistakes

Surgery should be performed when the condition of the soft tissues is ideal. When surgery is postponed for more than seven to ten days, the soft tissues contract and reduction may be difficult. In such late cases the surgeon should use a distraction apparatus to facilitate realignment of the fragments and restoration of the lower leg's proper length. Closed manipulation alone may not enable the surgeon to reduce the fragments to the position desired. Tomograms are occasionally useful to demonstrate that the fracture does not extend to the articular surface. The author found that the worst complications occurred when fractures extending into the proximal metaphysis were first diagnosed at surgery. In these cases, the flexible nails fail to provide the necessary stability.

Proper placement of the entry portals is of the utmost importance. They should be located at the tibial flares, midway between the anterior and posterior border of the tibia. An eyelet placed too anteriorly will irritate the skin when the knee is flexed. The insertion of the nail closely follows the direction of the portal entry. In an opening perpendicular to the long shaft of the tibia, the nail may penetrate or damage the opposite cortex. This can be avoided by placing the drill hole close to the long axis of the tibia.

Advancing the nails inside the medullary canal can be difficult because they occasionally get stuck in the cortex. The surgeon should manipulate the nail by rotating it and advancing it along the path of least resistance. The nails can be rotated 180 degrees, and it is important for the surgeon to know in which direction the distal end points. It is ill-advised to have two nails (medial and lateral) pointing in the same direction. This creates an unbalanced situation and contributes to excessive deformity (varus or valgus) (Fig. 20–44).

In the presence of large butterfly fragments or local comminution, the convexity of the nail should be placed to counteract the weightbearing forces causing the deformity (Fig. 20–39). There is no absolute indication for the nails to extend to the full length of the tibia. As long as the distal part of the nail is properly positioned in the cortex of the distal fragment, a shorter nail is acceptable.

Finally, there are rare situations in which the fragments cannot be reduced or the nail cannot be advanced into the distal fragment. This may happen when a comminuted fragment is stuck inside the canal or if there is soft-tissue interposition. In such rare cases, open reduction of fragments is an alternative provided that soft tissue is stripped only to the extent needed to align and hold the fragments until the nails are in the distal fragment. All incisions are then closed.

## Postoperative Treatment

A suction drain is usually left in the lateral incision for 24 to 48 hours. The patient can begin ambulation and weightbearing as soon as possible. Full weightbearing should be encouraged. Four to six weeks after the injury the cast is removed and a functional brace is applied. This below-knee orthosis permits ankle motion and can be removed for bathing and skin care. The functional orthosis is used until solid healing is obtained (Fig. 20–45).

## Complications

The most common complication is backing out of the nails, although this happens less often than in hip fractures (Fig. 20–46). Irritation caused by the proximal nail is more common when the nails are placed too anteriorly. The nails should never be removed before healing is complete. The nails seldom require early removal. Instructing the patient to limit knee flexion minimizes discomfort. Once fracture healing takes place, the nails can be removed safely. On only one occasion did the author find it necessary to shorten the nail. This can be done with a bolt cutter. It is also possible to interlock the proximal end of the nails by using a 3.5-mm screw inserted directly through the eyelet into the proximal tibia (Fig.

20–47). Interlocking may interfere with the impaction of the fragments. The worst complication occurred when a fracture of a proximal tibia was missed. This made the fixation useless and did not permit immediate weightbearing.

Excessive shortening can occur when comminution is underestimated. The nails do not provide longitudinal stability, and thus allow the fragments to impact, shortening the tibia. Angular stability is also a

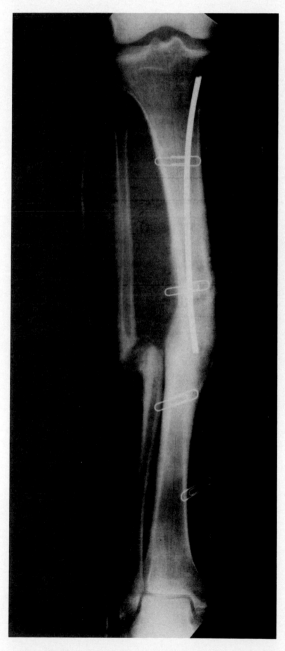

**Fig. 20–43** Patient with multiple trauma who fractured his tibia for the second time. The nail had to be shortened as it failed to advance into the distal fragment because the medullary canal was obliterated by the callus.

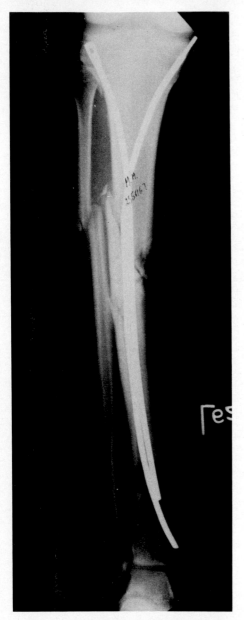

**Fig. 20–44** Segmental tibial fracture stabilized by medial and lateral nails pointing in the same direction. This caused varus deformity in the distal fragment and required wedging of the cast.

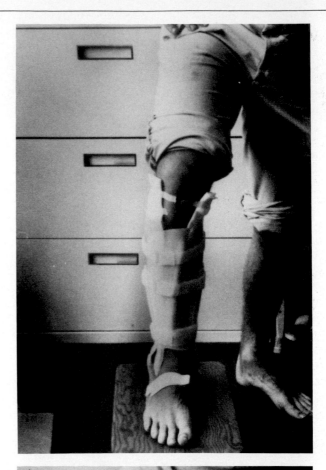

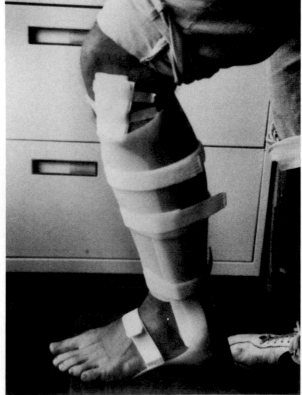

**Fig. 20–45** A below-knee orthosis with a hinged footplate allows ankle motion. It is removed for bathing and skin care and is used until solid union is achieved.

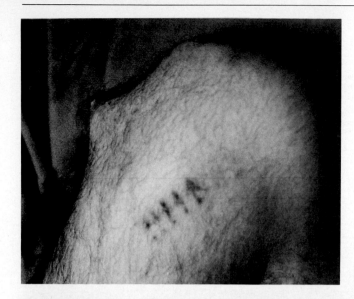

**Fig. 20–46** Nail protruding at the lateral side of the knee. Notice the small surgical incision on the medial side. The nail irritates the skin primarily when the knee is flexed.

**Fig. 20–47** Fractured tibia with flexible nail fixation. The 3.5-mm cortical screws inserted through the eyelet prevent backing up of the nail.

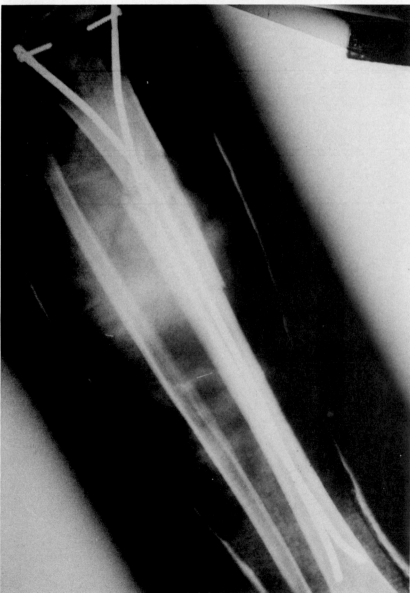

weakness of the system; this is most noticeable in distal-third fractures. The author is using retrograde fixation more frequently to overcome this problem (Figs. 20–40 and 20–41). Malrotation can be a significant problem. The nails provide excellent rotational stability. In malrotation an attempt to derotate the fragments, even with the patient under general anesthesia, will fail. In such a case it is necessary to remove all but one nail, derotate the distal fragment to its anatomic position, and then reintroduce the other nails.

In a series of 120 patients at Boston City Hospital, five patients had nonunions. This occurred early in the series when nailing was not the primary fracture treatment. Some of the patients had either delayed nailing or were immobilized in pins and plaster for as long as four weeks. Delayed unions occur in patients with severe comminution, in which bone is missing or the fibula is not intact, or when weightbearing is delayed. The most gratifying experience is early bony union; this occurs in more than 90% of the patients (Fig. 20–48). The author has found that minimal internal fixation enhances bony union even in complex fractures, with most demonstrating solid union within 16 to 18 weeks (Fig. 20–49).

## Infections

All patients undergoing surgery receive a 48-hour course of antibiotics starting at the time of surgery. Infection is rare and it is usually superficial, occurring at the site of nail insertion and indicating soft-tissue contusion. Local wound care and antibiotics resolve the infection. In the series of 120 patients deep infection developed in two closed fractures. One case was noticed only when the nails were removed after the fracture healed. In both instances the fractures healed solidly and patients responded well to antibiotic treatment. Local infections developed in three patients with open fractures. All three required bony debridement and all eventually healed after local bone grafting. At present, none of the tibial fractures treated with flexible nails at the au-

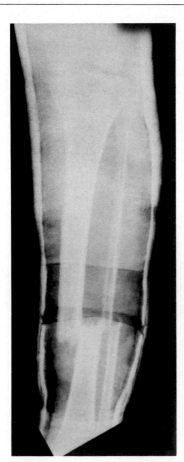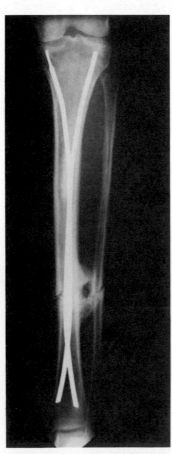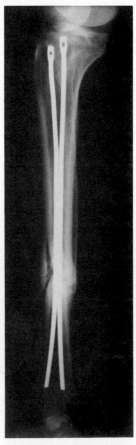

**Fig. 20–48** Comminuted distal-third tibial fracture with good callus and clinical union three months after the injury.

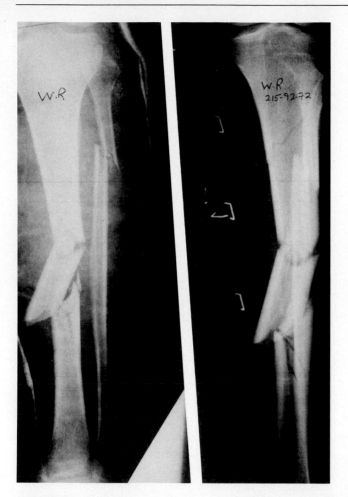
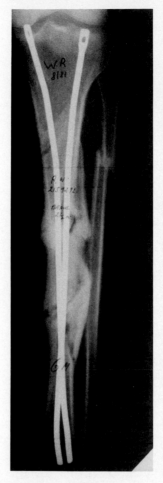
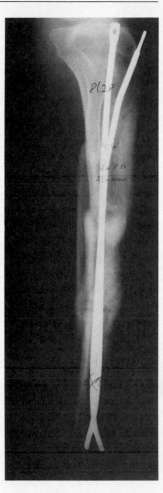

**Fig. 20–49**   Segmental and displaced tibial fracture after failed closed reduction done with the patient under general anesthesia. Solid union was present 17 weeks after the nails were inserted. (Reproduced with permission from Wiss DA, Segal D, Gumbs VL, et al: Flexible medullary nailing of tibial shaft fractures. *J Trauma* 1986; 26:1106–1112, Williams & Wilkins.)

thor's institution has developed a chronic soft-tissue or bony infection.

## Summary

At the author's institution, flexible intramedullary nailing of long bones is most commonly used in tibial fractures. The 4.0-mm nails are most frequently used and are supplemented with the 3.5-mm nails. Over 95% of the nailed tibial fractures are stabilized in the antegrade method directed from the proximal tibia into the distal fragment. Retrograde nailing is done most often to supplement the stability of fractures in the distal third. Surgery can be performed on a standard fracture table with the patient placed on a radiotranslucent board; a biplanar image intensifier is required. Functional bracing is used four to six weeks after surgery. Early solid union is obtained even in comminuted fractures.

**P A R T   G**

# Closed Intramedullary Fixation of Humeral Shaft Fractures

Robert F. Hall, Jr., MD

Intramedullary fixation of long bone fractures was established by Rush,[1] who used flexible pins, and Küntscher,[2,3] who developed rigid rods. More recently, Ender[4] introduced the concept of prebent, multiple, flexible nails for closed fixation of intertrochanteric hip fractures, and Pankovich and associates[5,6] extended their use to femoral and tibial shaft fractures.

Despite amenable bone anatomy, intramedullary fixation of humeral shaft fractures has been investigated only sporadically.[7–16] Poor rotational control[17] has intimidated most surgeons. Further, an entry portal through humeral epicondyles has proven to be impractical, time-consuming, and occasionally hazardous when postoperative supracondylar fracture or ulnar nerve palsy occurs. Proximal entry portal through the greater tuberosity violates the rotator cuff and a prominent nail causes painful shoulder motion.[8,9,14-16]

Although conservative treatment has been effective in the majority of humeral shaft fractures,[18-26] surgical treatment is sometimes desirable. Yet, available methods have proven to be hazardous.[27-30] A closed Ender technique has been effective in the treatment of humeral shaft fractures not responsive to conservative care.

## Material and Methods

Since January 1980, closed, nonreamed nailing of humeral shaft fractures has been performed at Cook County Hospital. During these years, 157 patients with 158 fractures were treated in this manner while 489 fractures were treated with gravity reduction—a surgical percentage of 24%. Of the 157 patients, 52 were women and 105 were men; their ages ranged from 17 to 72 years (mean age, 36 years). The fracture was located in the proximal third of the shaft in 49 cases, in the middle third in 46 cases, and in the distal third in 63 cases. Seven patients were lost to follow-up shortly after surgery. Therefore, this study included 150 patients with 151 humeral fractures. The average follow-up was 11.1 months (range, six to 55 months).

Fractures selected for nailing extended from the surgical neck of the humerus to the distal termination of the intramedullary canal. Other fractures, located more proximally, distally, or within the joint, were excluded. The fracture patterns included 72 transverse, 32 with bicortical comminution, 23 oblique, 20 with a butterfly fragment, and four segmental. The mechanisms of injury included 70 falls, 34 gunshot wounds, 22 cases of blunt trauma, 12 motor vehicle accidents, and six shotgun wounds. Six patients were struck by cars and one by a train.

After the patient's hospital admission, the injured arm was reduced and immobilized with plaster splints. Gunshot wounds were treated with minimal debridement and dressings with povidone-iodine solution. A cephalosporin was administered intravenously for two to three days, followed by an oral antibiotic as described by Elstrom and associates.[31] After the wounds were cultured, open fractures were treated with preoperative antibiotics, immediate surgical debridement, and internal fixation.

The average time from injury to fixation for closed fractures and gunshot wounds was 76 hours (range, eight hours to six days).

Open fractures and shotgun wounds were treated within ten hours of injury. The average time spent in surgery was 76 minutes (range, 25 to 142 minutes). Severely comminuted fractures required longer surgery. Blood loss averaged 75 ml (range, 10 to 460 ml). Blood loss was greater in antegrade roddings, which were not under tourniquet control.

Fifty-nine fractures underwent antegrade nailing and 92 fractures underwent retrograde nailing. One patient underwent antegrade nailing for a proximal-third fracture. A retrograde portal was precluded because of previously implanted plates in an old supracondylar fracture of the humerus.

Of the 34 patients with low-velocity gunshot wounds causing humeral fractures, 31 had grade I wounds and three had grade III wounds. One patient required an iliac bone graft to replace 10 cm of bone loss in a distal-third fracture.

Of the six patients with shotgun wounds, four had been peppered with shot and had grade I injuries. Of the two patients with grade III wounds, one had a lacerated radial nerve with loss of nerve substance. This patient underwent a free flap transfer for soft-tissue coverage and a tendon transfer for radial nerve palsy but the result was a nonunion. The other grade III wound and fracture healed without incident.

Of 111 fractures not associated with missile injuries, 11 were open fractures—ten were grade I wounds and one was a grade III wound. The single grade III fracture underwent adjunctive fixation[32] and an iliac bone graft because of extensive bone loss in the proximal third (Fig. 20–50).

Twenty-eight patients had other injuries in addition to the humeral shaft fractures. These included 13 tibial fractures, nine femoral fractures, six pelvic fractures, six head injuries, four chest injuries, two olecranon fractures, three forearm fractures, two ipsilateral brachial artery lacerations (Fig. 20–51), two wrist injuries, and one hand injury. These patients underwent surgery as soon as possible. The average time from injury to surgery was 14.9 hours (range, eight hours to six days). Those patients who had fractures of both lower and upper extremities were allowed to use platform crutches to aid weight-bearing. The average hospital stay for this entire group with multiple injuries was 24.6 days (range, six to 72 days). No deaths resulted from the initial trauma or pulmonary or fat embolism syndrome.

Radiographs were reviewed for analysis of fracture healing. Specifically, two events were recorded: the earliest appearance of periosteal callus and the appearance of a solid collar of periosteal callus. Union was determined to have occurred when a solid bar of periosteal callus crossed the fracture site and there was no motion or pain on palpation or manipulation of the arm.

Range of motion of the elbow and shoulder was recorded on follow-up visits.

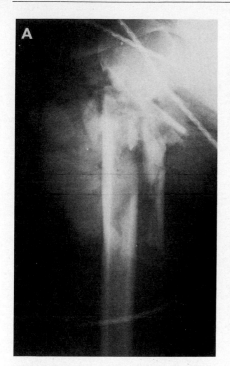
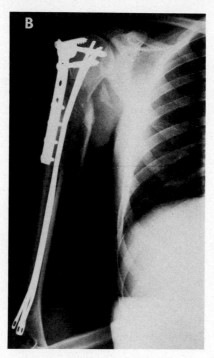
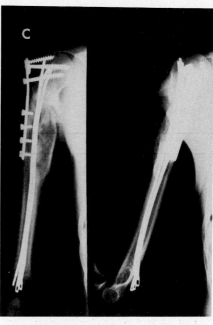

**Fig. 20–50**  **A:** A 22-year-old man suffered a grade III, comminuted fracture of the humerus. **B:** Radiograph taken immediately after surgery shows adjunctive fixation accompanying the intramedullary fixation. An iliac bone graft was added. **C:** One year after injury anteroposterior and lateral radiographs show complete fracture healing and incorporation of the bone graft.

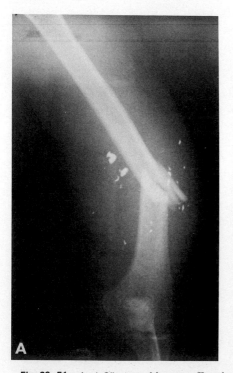
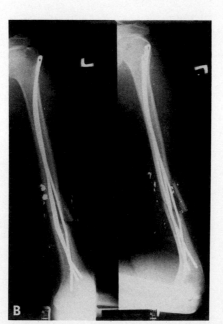
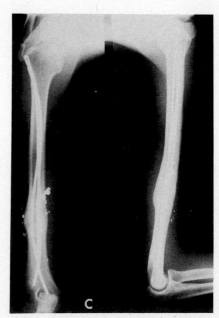

**Fig. 20–51**  **A:** A 35-year-old man suffered a gunshot wound and fracture of the distal third of the humerus along with a laceration of the brachial artery. **B:** Radiographs taken immediately after surgery demonstrate anatomic alignment of the fracture. Note the placement of the proximal nail eyelets below the greater tuberosity and distal distribution in the medial and lateral epicondylar canals. **C:** Fifteen months after surgery, the fracture has healed.

## Indications for Nailing

The indications used in selecting patients with humeral fractures for fixation with flexible intramedullary nails were the following: (1) angulation of 20 degrees remaining in any plane or a transverse fracture in bayonet apposition after closed reduction and plaster immobilization; (2) noncompliance with gravity reduction of fractures (because of senescence, obesity, or behavioral aberration); (3) multiple trauma (associated fractures in the same or another extremity, visceral trauma, and spinal or central nervous system injuries); (4) segmental humeral fractures; (5) bilateral humeral fractures.

## Nail Size Selection

Nails 4.5 mm in diameter were used in the first 17 patients. These were all C-nails. Because these implants were too rigid, more flexible nails 3.2 mm in diameter were used in all the other patients. Both C- and S-nails were used.

## Portal Selection

Proper portal selection is critical to the success of the procedure and depends on the location of the fracture. Fractures of the middle and proximal thirds of the shaft were nailed in a retrograde direction from distal portals, whereas fractures of the distal third underwent antegrade nailing. In general, the portal was placed as far from the fracture as possible. This minimized the risk of fracturing the intervening bone between the portal and the fracture site and later loss of three-point fixation of the intramedullary implants.

## Technique

### Preoperative Preparation

All procedures are done with the patient under general anesthesia. Fractures requiring retrograde nailing are done under tourniquet control. The patient is placed supine on a reversed operating table that provides clearance for an image intensifier. Before draping, fracture alignment is checked under control of an image intensifier and the maneuvers necessary to achieve fracture reduction are rehearsed. The humeral head is visualized in its entirety with the imaging system. A pad is occasionally placed against the chest wall to permit traction on the arm. Finally, the diameter of the intramedullary canal is measured on the radiographs so that the number of nails to be used can be estimated. As a rough guide, a

10-mm canal requires three 3.2-mm nails, a 12-mm canal requires four 3.2-mm nails, and a 14-mm canal requires five 3.2-mm nails.

### Retrograde Technique

A longitudinal incision, about 6 cm in length, is started close to the olecranon fossa and carried proximally. The incision is developed sharply through skin and subcutaneous tissue, the triceps split, and the posterior surface of the humerus exposed. The soft tissue is retracted with Army-Navy retractors. Chandler retractors may produce a radial nerve palsy and should be avoided. A unicortical hole is then placed dorsally with a 6.4-mm drill bit about 2 to 3 cm above the olecranon fossa. Two more holes are placed in tandem and proximal to the first, leaving a 2- to 3-mm bone bridge between holes. A Kerrison rongeur is then used to connect the drill holes and an ellipse fashioned. With the aid of an image intensifier, the length of the nail is estimated by placing it along the surface of the reduced arm. A nail of the correct length should reach the subchondral area of the humeral head. The nail is placed within the osseous canal and driven to the fracture site. The fracture is then reduced with the prearranged maneuvers and a single nail passed across the fracture. Comminuted fractures present some difficulty, and nail manipulation is needed to pass the nail across the fracture. Once it has been captured in the proximal canal, the nail is driven to its final destination. This is the most accurate check of nail length. If the length is satisfactory, the nail is partially withdrawn but kept proximal to the fracture to maintain cylinder alignment. Both C- and S-nails are then added to fill the intramedullary canal snugly. Several centimeters before final impaction, a 1-mm wire is passed through the eyelet of each nail. The nails are then driven within 1 cm of the humeral head so that they protrude no more than 1 cm distal to the edge of the portal. The nails should be distributed in both the humeral head and the greater tuberosity. The cerclage wire through the nail eyelets is then tightened. The soft tissues are closed in layers, and dressings and ace bandages applied about the surgical site.

### Antegrade Technique

Preliminary preparation is the same as in the retrograde technique. Draping should allow access to the shoulder area. An incision is placed over the anterior shoulder, just lateral to the biceps tendon. It starts at the acromion and is carried distally and longitudinally along the proximal humerus for 3.8 cm. The axillary nerve lies just distal to the end of this incision. Sharp dissection exposes the deltoid muscle and blunt dissection exposes bone. Occasionally, the axillary nerve is seen in the distal portion of the wound but it is not routinely exposed. Initially, a

6.4-mm drill hole is placed in the distal portion of the incision. This locates the portal in the metaphyseal flare of the humerus, several centimeters distal to the greater tuberosity. Another drill hole is placed proximal to the first with a 2- to 3-mm bone bridge left between the two holes. Again, a Kerrison rongeur is used to fashion a round portal. The portal should be large enough to accommodate the anticipated number of nails, which are then measured and inserted as in the retrograde technique.

At the end of the procedure, the nail eyelets should be 1 cm distal to the proximal aspect of the greater tuberosity. C- and S-nails should be placed in the lateral and medial epicondylar canals. Fractures between the middle and distal thirds of the humerus should be manipulated with great care because of their susceptibility to postoperative radial nerve injury.

## Postoperative Care

No immobilization is used. Within one day after surgery the patient is allowed to begin active and passive range of motion exercises of the shoulder and elbow without restriction. If the patient cannot be transported to the therapy unit, bedside exercises can be done.

## Results

The behavior of the healing humeral fractures was recorded radiologically. On the average, a periosteal callus appeared in 19.9 days (range, 14 to 28 days). A solid bridge of periosteal callus was apparent at 7.2 weeks (range, six to 11.5 weeks). This correlated well with a decrease in pain at the fracture site and an increase in arm motion. Therefore, callus gradually obliterated the fracture during the next months.

Nine closed fractures had gaps of 1 cm or less of distraction after the surgical procedure but healed at rates similar to those of the others. In two patients with low-velocity gunshot wounds and associated humeral fractures in the middle and distal thirds of the humerus, gaps of 4 and 10 cm of bone loss were present after nailing. The patient with 10 cm of bone loss required an iliac bone graft to restore bone integrity (Figs. 20–52 and 20–53). Both fractures healed without delay.

Range of motion exercises progressed slowly in all patients for 14 days but gradually increased thereafter. A sharp increase was apparent when periosteal bone formation was first noted on the radiograph. After three weeks, motion gradually improved and approached normal by eight weeks. Patients more than 50 years of age consistently progressed more

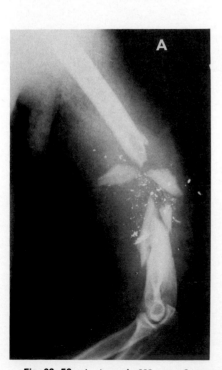
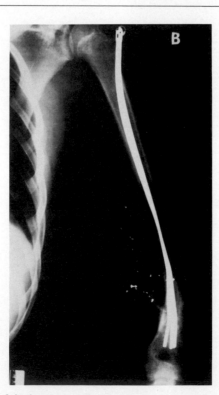
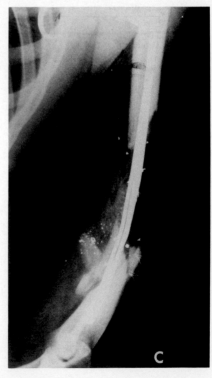

**Fig. 20–52**  **A:** A grade III open fracture of the humerus with loss of bone substance caused by a gunshot wound. The radial nerve was severed but the brachial artery remained intact. **B:** An intraoperative radiograph shows the antegrade placement of three flexible nails and wire cerclage of the proximal nail eyelets. Ten centimeters of distal humeral shaft has been lost while the distal joint was preserved. **C:** Three weeks after iliac bone grafting and wound closure, early calcification of the graft is evident.

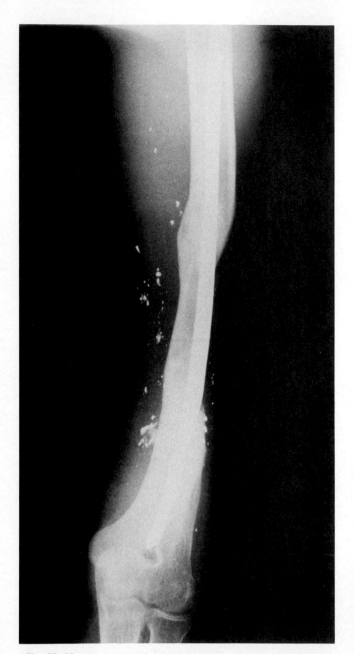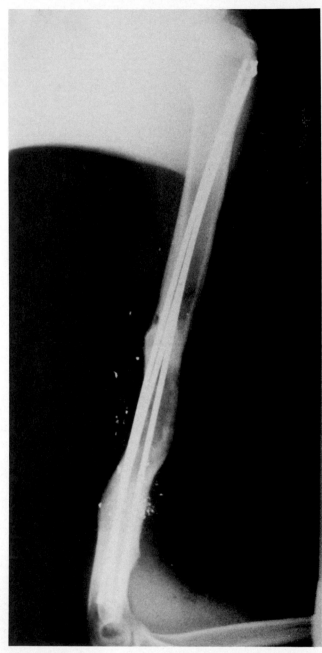

**Fig. 20–53** Two years after injury, the fracture has healed.

slowly. Their preoperative motion was restored, on the average, five months after injury. For the entire series, the average elbow arc of motion was 132 degrees (range, 95 to 150 degrees). All seven patients with extension of 20 degrees or less were more than 50 years of age and had undergone a retrograde nailing. Combined shoulder abduction and external rotation averaged 168 degrees (range, 155 to 178 degrees).

There were 11 preoperative radial nerve palsies related to the initial injuries. Eight were associated with falls, two with low-velocity gunshot wounds, and one with a shotgun wound. All fractures were located between the middle and distal thirds. The patients who suffered falls recovered complete radial nerve function after seven to nine months. Nerve recovery was always heralded by an advancing Tinel's sign. This routinely appeared on the dorsal aspect of the proximal third of the forearm 14 weeks after the injury. In three patients with missile wounds, the radial nerve was severed at the time of injury. One patient's palsy was treated with a sural nerve graft 12 months after injury; the other two had tendon transfers.

## Complications

This series included three nonunions. Two were in grade III open fractures caused by missile injuries and one was in a closed fracture (Fig. 20–54).

No malunions were recorded. Seven patients had residual angulation of 8.5 degrees or less in the anteroposterior plane only.

There were no postoperative wound infections or cases of osteomyelitis.

The largest number of complications were those generated by the nails. Nail retreat proved troublesome and often provoked symptoms. Three patients required revision of the retrograde nailing. The fractures were all located in the middle third and were comminuted. In all three cases an additional nail was added to maintain fracture stability and prevent nail withdrawal.

Combined shoulder abduction and external rotation proved to be intolerant of nail retreat in antegrade nailing. If the eyelet of the nail backed out 4 cm proximal to the greater tuberosity, impingement occurred on the acromion with shoulder abduction.

This occurred in five patients, three of whom required a second surgical procedure. In the other two, the nails were removed at one year.

In cases of nail retreat, at least one nail remained in place. Therefore, starting with the 42nd patient, the eyelets of the nails were captured and grouped together with 1-mm wire. No nail withdrawal occurred thereafter.

Intraoperative problems were limited to three patients who sustained radial nerve palsies. One underwent retrograde nailing of a middle-third transverse fracture with bayonet apposition five days after injury. During surgery, regaining length proved difficult and required strong traction. The postoperative radial nerve palsy disappeared gradually over the next nine months. Since then, all patients with this particular fracture pattern and unsatisfactory reduction have had surgery within 24 hours of admission without incident. The other two patients underwent routine retrograde nailing for oblique fractures in the middle third. Nerve function returned seven months after surgery. None of the nerves were explored when the palsy was discovered postoperatively.

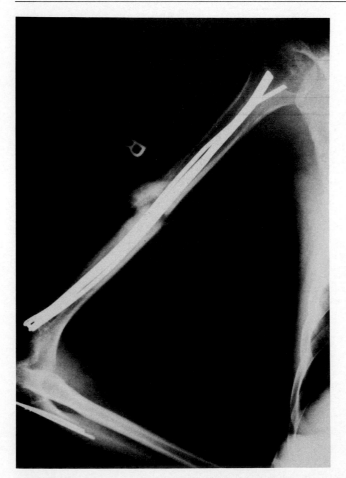
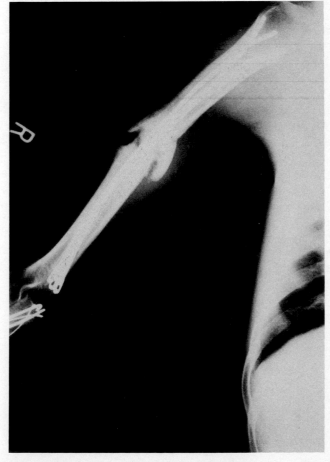

**Fig. 20–54**  One year after intramedullary fixation of a closed midshaft humeral fracture, a nonunion is evident. Subsequent surgery revealed a synovial pseudarthrosis. An ipsilateral olecranon fracture healed without delay.

## Discussion

Caldwell[19] introduced the hanging arm cast treatment of humeral shaft fractures. He created a gravity-dependent, conservative method that has been validated by others.[18-26,33] Although variations have been described, the superiority of a particular method cannot be confirmed. The variations all have a high rate of union, reasonable fracture alignment, and a functional range of motion. One recent innovation, a plaster arm sleeve, effectively immobilizes the fracture while simultaneously allowing range-of-motion exercises.[25] The rate of humeral union is comparable to those in previously reported series in which the arm was immobilized in a traditional manner. Balfour and associates[18] warned that this modality should not be used on a bedridden patient.

Despite this success with nonsurgical methods, surgical intervention is indicated in a fracture unresponsive to closed management or a fracture in a noncompliant patient. Three major problems are traditionally associated with humeral fractures—osteomyelitis, nonunion, and radial nerve palsy. Malunions have not been as well documented because the resilient shoulder joint can functionally correct most malalignment problems. However, Klenerman[34] showed that 30 degrees in the anteroposterior plane and 20 degrees in the lateral plane is unacceptable cosmetically despite adequate function.

Stern and associates[14] reported a series of 70 humeral fractures treated with Rush rod intramedullary fixation. The complication rate was 67%. In general, this type of fixation has been plagued with breakage,[11] restricted range of motion after surgery because of nail impingement,[8,9,14-16] and lack of sufficient nail bulk to support fracture reduction.[15,22] The results of our study using Ender rods show that closed, nonreamed, intramedullary nailing can effectively treat humeral fractures and obtain results similar to those obtained with conservative care.

The recumbent position of the victim with multiple trauma does not allow gravity reduction to align the humeral fracture properly. Cumbersome splints, casts, and traction have led to management problems in the intensive care unit. Loss of reduction and humeral malunion have resulted.[35] Further, these patients have a catabolic physiologic state that places them at risk for nonunions.[14,28] In our series at Cook County Hospital, 28 patients with multiple trauma underwent closed nailing. The average time to union in polytrauma patients was 7.4 weeks, which paralleled healing rates in patients with isolated humeral fractures. In our study it could not be documented that such an adverse physiologic environment actually retarded fracture healing.

Infections are uncommon after closed and open humeral fractures treated conservatively in conjunction with appropriate surgical irrigation and debridement. Plate fixation, previously preferred in open humeral fractures, avoided the potential risk of osteomyelitis along the full length of the intramedullary canal.[36] Further, Stern and associates[14] noted an increased incidence of infection in open humeral fractures treated with open reduction and intramedullary fixation. They concluded that delayed fixation after adequate surgical debridement was more appropriate. In our study, open fractures were not considered a contraindication to immediate closed nailing after irrigation and debridement. Fifty-one open fractures were recorded without a single incidence of wound infection or osteomyelitis.

Although nonunion is an infrequent problem in the conservatively treated humeral fracture, when it does occur an open surgical approach has been advocated. A small number of cases have resulted in residual disability caused by loss of motion, osteomyelitis, radial nerve palsy, and continued nonunion despite surgery.[28,29,37] In particular, transverse fractures in the middle third of the humerus have been documented as vulnerable to nonunion, especially in young adults.[14,21-23,30,34,35] The nutrient artery is located in this area[38] and fracture damage here has poor healing potential.[10,23,34,35,39] Other problems, such as severe comminution, open fractures, surgery, inadequate fixation, and distraction at the fracture site using skeletal traction, have been implicated.[14,23,27-30,33] In the author's series, 24 transverse fractures in the middle third healed promptly. Other vulnerable fracture patterns healed equally as fast. Two patients required bone grafting initially because of extensive loss of bone stock in open wounds. Both healed without delay. In general, flexible intramedullary nails, when inserted under closed conditions and followed by active exercises, do not retard bone healing. Radiographic and clinical union was recorded at 7.2 weeks. This figure was in accord with other studies documenting union between 6.2 and 9.4 weeks after closed, nonsurgical care.[12,18,19,25,30] In the author's study nonunion occurred in two grade III open fractures. In retrospect, an iliac bone graft should have been performed during the initial hospitalization for both patients. The third nonunion occurred in a closed, middle-third fracture of the humerus (Fig. 20–54).

The treatment of humeral fractures associated with radial nerve palsy has been controversial. Some authors recommend nerve exploration and fracture fixation if nerve injury is present.[40-45] However, this may lead to complications.[45] In the author's study, a preoperative radial nerve palsy was not considered an indication for fracture fixation. For other reasons 11 patients with this problem had implants placed and the radial nerves healed spontaneously in eight. The three nerves that did not recover had been severed by missiles. Three patients had radial nerve palsy post-operatively and all three recovered without additional surgery. Pollock and associates[46] documented that 88% of radial nerve palsies associated with humeral shaft fractures are lesions in continuity and therefore should be treated with this in mind. The author's study confirmed Pollock's findings and further demonstrated that intramedullary nailing does not impede nerve recovery. Unfortunately, postoperative radial nerve palsy may not be entirely avoidable with closed nailing because of occasional nerve injury after manipulation of middle- and distal-third fractures.[39,45]

The nails themselves produced the largest group of complications. Rod retreat occurred in eight patients and all proved symptomatic. Revision, with additional nails or nail withdrawal, was required in each instance. Ultimately, the range of motion was not affected by this problem and motion was regained. After the 42nd patient, the nail eyelets were tethered with 1-mm wire to prevent this problem.

Range of motion after humeral fracture treatment has been poorly documented. The range of motion we recorded was comparable to that of the opposite unaffected arm within two months of surgery and coincided with solid periosteal callus at the fracture site. Patients more than 50 years of age progressed more slowly. A similar problem was noted by Spak,[47] who treated humeral shaft fractures in older patients without surgery. In general, the nails maintained bone stability and allowed the patient to regain motion comfortably.

We observed that the humerus heals with some distraction at the fracture when treated with closed nailing. Others have noted the detrimental effect of traction-induced distraction that may lead to nonunion.[23,27,33] However, the preservation of soft tissue and periosteum around the fracture is permitted by closed, nonreamed nailing procedures. Immediate arm exercises allow callus to be deposited generously about the fracture. Therefore, every potential for fracture healing is retained. The literature on humeral fractures reflects this concept by documenting longer healing rates after formal open reduction and internal fixation,[11,30,44] as well as a higher incidence of nonunion.[27-30] However, our study suggests that humeral fractures associated with grade III soft-tissue injuries should have bone grafting during the initial hospitalization.

## Summary

During a seven-year prospective study, 158 humeral shaft fractures in 157 patients were treated with closed intramedullary nailing. Only humeral fractures not responsive to closed reduction and immobilization and those in noncompliant patients were eligible. No immobilization was used postoperatively. Seven patients were lost to follow-up. A total of 148 fractures healed; there were three nonunions. The average time to clinical union was 7.2 weeks. There were no infections or malunions. Eight of 11 preoperative and three postoperative radial nerve palsies were lesions in continuity and healed spontaneously. The remaining three had been severed by missiles and needed further attention. Nail withdrawal occurred in eight patients; five of these needed nail revision. Final range of motion for the elbow averaged 132 degrees and shoulder abduction-external rotation averaged 168 degrees.

## Conclusions

From this study the following conclusions can be drawn: (1) Closed flexible intramedullary nailing of humeral shaft fractures can be performed safely. (2) The implants restore humeral architecture and postoperative immobilization is not necessary. (3) Fracture healing is not retarded by the use of these implants and a healing rate similar to that in conservatively treated fractures was documented. (4) Postoperative motion in the elbow and shoulder is not jeopardized and the arc of motion approaches normal. (5) Preoperative radial nerve palsy is not a contraindication to this procedure. All radial nerve palsies involving a lesion in continuity healed spontaneously.

## References

1. Rush LV: *Atlas of Rush Pin Techniques,* ed 2. Meridian, Mississippi, The Berivon Co, 1976, pp 112–133.
2. Künstcher GB: The Künstcher method of intramedullary fixation. *J Bone Joint Surg* 1958;40A:17–26.
3. Künstcher GB: Intramedullary surgical technique and its place in orthopaedic surgery. *J Bone Joint Surg* 1965;47A:809–818.
4. Ender HG: Treatment of pertrochanteric and subtrochanteric fractures of the femur with Ender pins, in *The Hip: Proceedings of the Sixth Open Scientific Meeting of the Hip Society.* St Louis, CV Mosby, 1978, pp 187–206.
5. Pankovich AM, Goldflies ML, Pearson RL: Closed Ender nailing of femoral-shaft fractures. *J Bone Joint Surg* 1979;61A:222–231.
6. Pankovich AM, Tarabishy I, Yelda S: Flexible intramedullary nailing of tibial-shaft fractures. *Clin Orthop* 1981;160:185–195.
7. Fenyo F: On fractures of the shaft of the humerus. *Acta Chir Scand* 1971;137:221–226.
8. Foster RJ, Dixon GL, Bach AW, et al: Internal fixation of humeral shaft lesions: Indications and results. *Orthop Trans* 1983;7:69.
9. Johansson O: Complications and failures of surgery in various fractures of the humerus. *Acta Chir Scand* 1961;120:469–478.
10. Kennedy JC, Wyatt JK: An evaluation of the management of fractures through the middle third of the humerus. *Can J Surg* 1957;1:26–33.
11. Lauretzen GK: Medullary nailing. *Acta Chir Scand* 1949;147(suppl):68–81.

12. Mann RJ, Neal EG: Fractures of the shaft of the humerus in adults. *South Med J* 1965;58:264–268.

13. Naiman PT, Schein AJ, Siffert RS: Use of ASIF compression plates in selected shaft fractures of the upper extremity. *Clin Orthop* 1970;71:208–216.

14. Stern PJ, Mattingly DA, Pomeroy DL, et al: Intramedullary fixation of humeral shaft fractures. *J Bone Joint Surg* 1984;66A:639–646.

15. Weseley MS, Barenfield PA, Einstein AL: Rush pin intramedullary fixation for fractures of the proximal humerus. *J Trauma* 1977;17:29–37.

16. Widen A: Fractures of the upper end of the humerus with great displacement treated by marrow nailing. *Acta Chir Scand* 1948;49:439–441.

17. Epps CH: Fractures of the shaft of the humerus, in Rockwood CA, Green DP (eds): *Fractures in Adults*. Philadelphia, JB Lippincott, 1984, vol 1, pp 653–674.

18. Balfour GW, Mooney V, Ashley ME: Diaphyseal fractures of the humerus treated with a ready-made fracture brace. *J Bone Joint Surg* 1982;64A:11–13.

19. Caldwell JA: Treatment of fractures of the shaft of the humerus by hanging cast. *Surg Gynecol Obstet* 1940;421–425.

20. Christensen S: Humeral shaft fractures: Operative and conservative treatment. *Acta Chir Scand* 1967;133:455–460.

21. Cubbins WR, Scuderi CS: Fractures of the humerus. *JAMA* 1933;100:1576–1579.

22. Eve D, Daniel RA: Treatment of fractures of the shaft of the humerus. *South Med J* 1941;34:311–315.

23. Holm CL: Management of humeral shaft fractures: Fundamental nonoperative techniques. *Clin Orthop* 1970;71:132–139.

24. Hunter SG: The closed treatment of fractures of the humeral shaft. *Clin Orthop* 1982;164:192–198.

25. Sarmiento A, Kinman PS, Galvin EG, et al: Functional bracing of fractures of the shaft of the humerus. *J Bone Joint Surg* 1977;59A:596–601.

26. Winfield JM, Miller H, LaFerte AD: Evaluation of the "hanging cast" as a method of treating fractures of the humerus. *Am J Surg* 1942;55:228–249.

27. Böhler L: Conservative treatment of fresh closed fractures of the shaft of the humerus. *J Trauma* 1965;5:464–468.

28. Campbell WC: Un-united fractures of the shaft of the humerus. *Ann Surg* 1937;105:135–149.

29. Loomer R, Kokan P: Nonunion in fractures of the humeral shaft. *Injury* 1975;7:274–278.

30. Scientific Research Committee, Pennsylvania Orthopaedic Society: Fresh midshaft fractures of the humerus in adults: Evaluation of treatment in Pennsylvania during 1952–56. *Pa Med J* 1959;62:848–850.

31. Elstrom JA, Pankovich AM, Egwele R: Extra-articular low-velocity gunshot fractures of the radius and ulna. *J Bone Joint Surg* 1978;60A:335–341.

32. Pankovich AM: Adjunctive fixation in flexible intramedullary nailing of femoral fractures: A study of twenty-six cases. *Clin Orthop* 1981;157:301–309.

33. Cartner MJ: Immobilization of fractures of the shaft of the humerus. *Injury* 1973;5:175–179.

34. Klenerman L: Fractures of the shaft of the humerus. *J Bone Joint Surg* 1966;48B:105–111.

35. Vichare NA: Fractures of the humeral shaft associated with multiple injuries. *Injury* 1973;5:279–282.

36. Chapman MW, Hansen ST: Current concepts in the management of open fractures, in Rockwood CA, Green DC (eds): *Fractures in Adults*. Philadelphia, JB Lippincott, 1984, vol 1, pp 199–218.

37. Chacha PB: Compression plating without bone grafts for delayed and nonunions of the humeral shaft fracture. *Injury* 1973;5:283–290.

38. Carroll SE: A study of the nutrient foramina of the humeral diaphysis. *J Bone Joint Surg* 1963;45B:176–181.

39. Mast JW, Spiegel PG, Harvey JP, et al: Fractures of the humeral shaft. *Clin Orthop* 1975;112:254–262.

40. Bateman JE: *Trauma to Nerves in Limbs*. Philadelphia, WB Saunders, 1962, p 386.

41. Fenton RL: Radial nerve transplant and internal fixation in cases of humerus fractures with radial nerve injury. *Bull Hosp Joint Dis* 1964;25:71.

42. Garcia A, Maeck BY: Radial nerve injuries in fractures of the shaft of the humerus. *Am J Surg* 1960;99:625–627.

43. Holstein A, Lewis GM: Fractures of the humerus with radial-nerve paralysis. *J Bone Joint Surg* 1963;45A:1382–1388.

44. Müller ME, Allgöwer M, Schneider R, et al: Fractures of the humerus, in Müller ME, Allgöwer M, Willenegger (eds): *Manual of Internal Fixation*. Heidelberg, New York, Springer-Verlag, 1970, pp 114–121.

45. Packer JW, Foster RR, Garcia A, et al: The humeral fracture with radial nerve palsy: Is exploration warranted? *Clin Orthop* 1972;88:34–38.

46. Pollock FH, Drake D, Brill EG, et al: Treatment of radial neuropathy associated with fractures of the humerus. *J Bone Joint Surg* 1981;63A:239–243.

47. Spak I: Humeral shaft fractures. *Acta Orthop Scand* 1978;49:234–239.

# Current Concepts in the Management of Open Fractures

Ramon B. Gustilo, MD

## Introduction

The three goals in the treatment of open fractures are preventing wound sepsis, obtaining fracture healing, and achieving a return to normal function.

Open fractures can be divided into three types. **Type I** is an open fracture with a clean wound less than 1 cm long (Fig. 21–1). **Type II** is an open fracture with a laceration more than 1 cm long without extensive soft-tissue damage, flaps, or avulsions (Fig. 21–2). **Type III** is an open segmental fracture, an open fracture with extensive soft-tissue damage, or a traumatic amputation. Special categories within type III include subtype III-A, gunshot injuries (adequate soft-tissue coverage of the fractured bone despite extensive soft-tissue lacerations, flaps, or high-energy trauma regardless of the size of the wound as shown in Fig. 21–3); subtype III-B, farm injuries (extensive soft-tissue injury with periosteal stripping and bony exposure, usually associated with massive contamination as shown in Fig. 21–4); and subtype III-C, an open fracture with associated vascular damage requiring repair (Fig. 21–5).

## Management of Open Fractures

The first step is immediate debridement and irrigation. This includes thorough and meticulous removal of devitalized tissues and copious irrigation (5,000 to 10,000 ml of normal saline solution and 2,000 ml of an antibiotic solution). Debridement and irrigation should be repeated within 24 to 48 hours for type III open fractures. Any large free bone fragments should be retained for stability.

Antibiotic therapy for type I and type II open fractures consists of 2 g of cefazolin sodium on admission and 1 g every eight hours for three days. For type III open fractures the cefazolin dosage should be doubled. Treatment should also include 3 to 5 mg/kg/day of aminoglycosides and 10 to 12 million units of penicillin for farm injuries. (Double antibiotic treatment should be continued for three days only.) The administration of antibiotics should be repeated during wound closure, internal fixation, and bone grafting.

It is important to achieve fracture stability because it preserves soft-tissue integrity, diminishes wound sepsis, facilitates the care of soft-tissue injuries, and allows early joint and muscle function.

External fixation should be used for all type III fractures fractures and unstable type II fractures of the tibia and other long bones.

Pins, screws, and plates should be used for articular and metaphyseal fractures. Primary nailing with reaming is contraindicated in open fractures because it leads to increased wound sepsis. Casts and splints can be used for stable type I and type II open fractures.

The goal of wound coverage is soft-tissue coverage in five to ten days. Delayed primary closure should be used for type I and type II open fractures. Delayed primary closure or skin graft should be used for subtypes III-A and III-C fractures and local flaps (gastrocnemius or soleus muscles) or microvascular transfer (latissimus dorsi muscle, for example) should be used for subtypes III-B and III-C open fractures.

Early cancellous bone grafting is desirable during delayed wound closure for comminuted or segmental fractures or if there is bone loss. Bone grafting should be delayed four to six weeks in cases in which local flaps or free muscle microvascular transfers were used. Bone grafting should be repeated in three months if radiographs demonstrate an absence of collars or if there is gross motion clinically.

Early amputation may be performed in cases with complete neurovascular loss, massive soft-tissue injury that offers little chance of functional recovery, or combined soft-tissue and bone loss.

## Discussion

There are four factors in type III open fractures that predispose to complications (infection, delayed union or nonunion, and amputation). These factors, which can occur individually or in combinations, are (1) massive soft-tissue damage, with resultant problems in bony coverage, (2) severe wound contamination, (3) compromised vascularity, and (4) fracture instability. These problems are most likely to occur in cases of high-energy trauma, typically involving the tibia and resulting in a comminuted or segmental fracture.

Severe soft-tissue loss with periosteal stripping and bony exposure, massive wound contamination, and

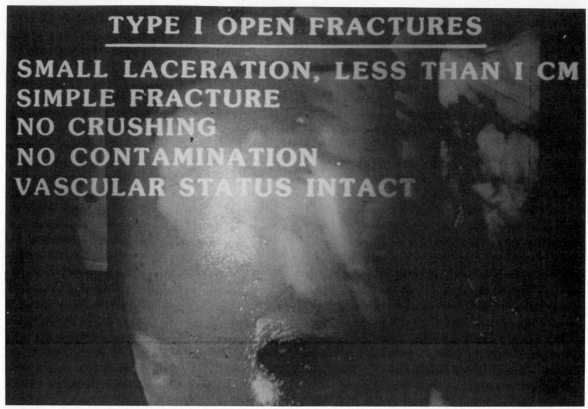

**Fig. 21–1** Type I open fracture.

arterial injury are the major determinants of outcome, rather than fracture configuration (Table 21–1). Thus, open segmental fractures usually heal without complication if there is no accompanying soft-tissue loss or compromise of the vasculature.

In their classification schema of open fractures, Rittmann and associates[1,2] described type III open fractures as external trauma involving vessels and nerves or entire muscle groups so that a functional deficit occurs. They reported that osteomyelitis developed in 15 of 200 patients but did not specify how many had type III open fractures. Gustilo and Anderson[3] classified open fractures on the basis of the extent of soft-tissue damage and defined type III open fractures as those with extensive soft-tissue involvement and other special features such as traumatic amputation, segmental open fracture, open fracture with arterial nerve injury, farm injury, and high-velocity gunshot wounds. Reported wound sepsis in type III open fractures with internal fixation ranges from 10% to 50%.[2-6] Hasenhuttl[6] reported a 17.4% incidence of delayed soft-tissue healing but only a 4.4% incidence of deep infection with osteomyelitis in 178 open fractures treated by flexible medullary wires. His complication rate compared favorably with those of others.[3,7,8] However, a critical analysis of various clinical reports of wound sepsis and of various methods of internal fixation indicates that the

**Table 21–1**
**Results at the Hennepin County Medical Center, 1955–1984**

| | | Incidence of Sepsis in 1,846 Open Fractures | | | |
| Years | Study | Overall | Type I | Type II | Type III |
| --- | --- | --- | --- | --- | --- |
| 1955–1960 | Gustilo and associates[11] | 11.8 | — | — | — |
| 1961–1968 | Gustilo and associates[11] | 5.2 | — | — | 44.0 |
| 1969–1975 | Gustilo and Anderson[3] | 2.4 | 0 | 0 | 10.2 |
| 1976–1979 | Gustilo, Mendoza, and Williams[9] | 10.1 | 0 | 1.8 | 23.0 |
| 1980–1984 | Present study | 4.4 | 0 | 2.5 | 13.7 |

incidence of wound sepsis depends on the category of type III open fracture involved (Table 21–2). Therefore, a simple type III categorization of open fractures is too inclusive because of the range of severity and the different prognoses of the injuries. Type III open fractures should be divided in order of worsening prognosis into three subtypes, subtypes III-A, III-B, and III-C.[9] The increased incidence of wound sepsis and amputation in subtypes III-B and III-C is statistically significant. Any analysis of treatment of type III open fractures is meaningless unless these subtypes are taken into consideration, particularly when the incidences of wound infection, amputation, and delayed union are considered.

Achieving fracture stability in type III open frac-ture is essential to meet three goals: (1) To improve treatment in cases of multiple trauma. One third of patients with open fractures have injuries of more

**Table 21–2**
**Wound sepsis and amputation in type III open fractures, 1980–1984**

| Clinical Data | Type III Open Fractures | | |
|---|---|---|---|
| | III-A | III-B | III-C |
| No. of cases | 40 | 18 | 22 |
| Infections | 2 | 8 | 1 |
| Delayed amputation | 0 | 1 | 3* |
| Early amputation because of vascular insufficiency | 0 | 0 | 5 |

*Two of the three were infected.

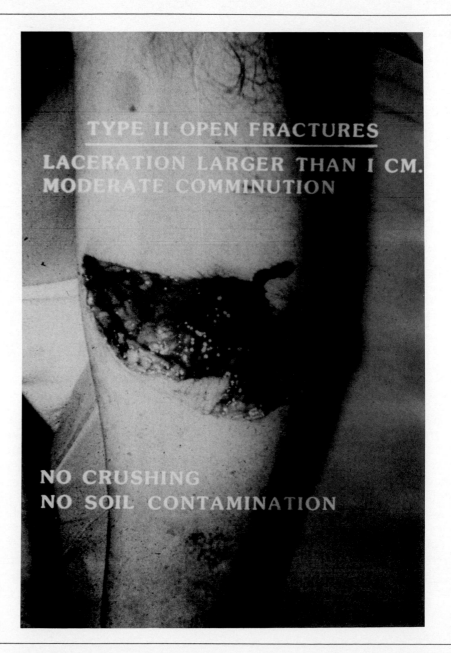

**Fig. 21–2** Type II open fracture.

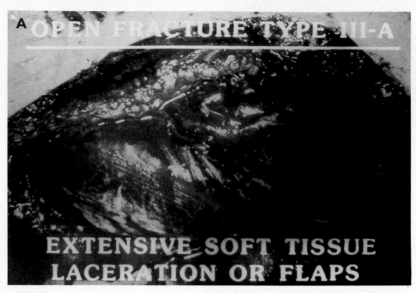

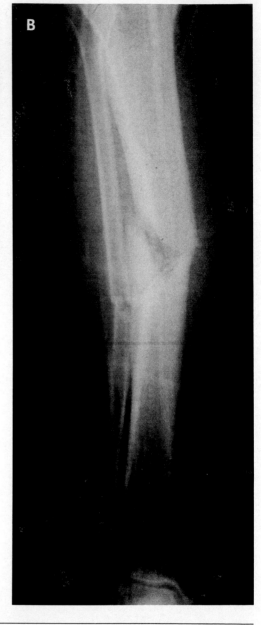

**Fig. 21–3**    Subtype III-A. **A:** Open fracture. **B:** Open fracture of the tibia.

than one system. It is imperative that these patients be mobilized early to avoid cardiorespiratory problems. (2) To minimize discomfort in the patient despite massive soft-tissue injury. These patients require repeated debridement and dressing changes in the operating room. This can be accomplished with minimal discomfort to the patient when the fractures are well stabilized. (3) To achieve fracture alignment and early joint motion in patients with multiple fractures of one extremity involving both sides of the joint. Patients who have an ipsilateral open fracture of the femur and tibia, for example, must have their fractures stabilized.

The choice of fixation device depends on the type and location of the fracture and the severity of soft-tissue damage and subsequent soft-tissue coverage requirements. In general, the author uses external fixation, in conjunction with screws and occasionally a plate, to achieve fracture stability in massive soft-tissue injury of the tibia. The use of half pins on a unilateral plane is often adequate, allowing good access for wound care and subsequent soft-tissue coverage, either by skin grafting or local flaps. External fixation is discontinued as soon as soft-tissue healing is obtained, and immobilization is continued either by cast or delayed intramedullary nailing for shaft fractures.

Occasionally the author uses plate fixation in type

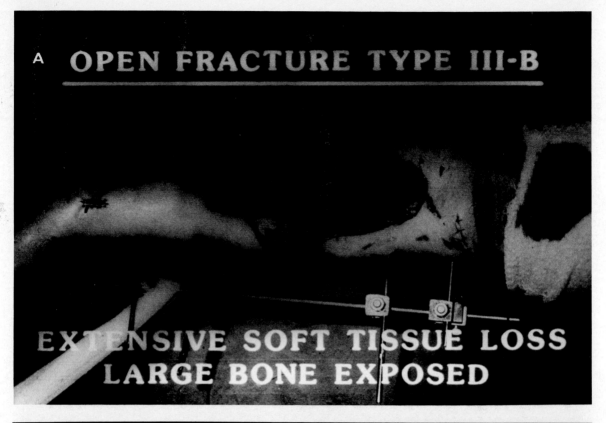

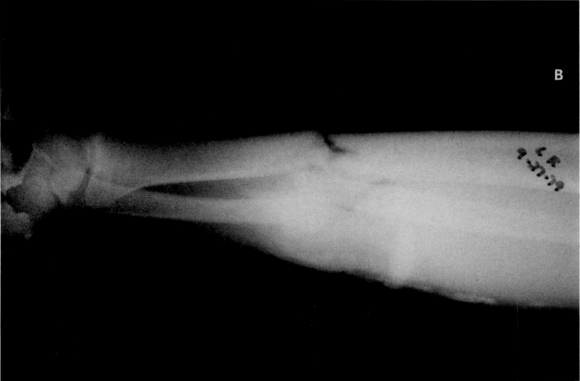

**Fig. 21–4**  Subtype III-B. **A:** Open fracture. **B:** Open fracture with comminuted fracture midshaft of the tibia and fibula.

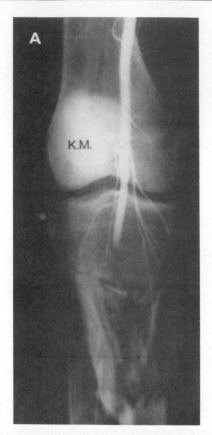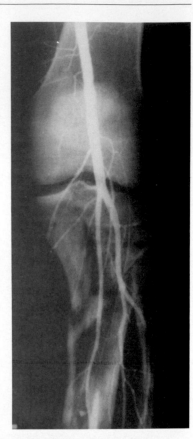

**Fig. 21–5** Subtype III-C. **A:** Arteriogram shows interruption of right popliteal artery in open fracture. **B:** Open fracture with arterial injury.

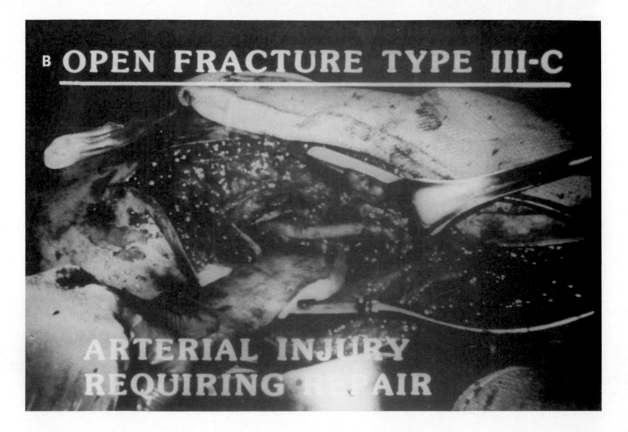

III open fractures with articular or combined articular-metaphyseal involvement and in those with extensive laceration or flaps in which no or minimal additional skin incision is required for plate application. It is ideal but not essential to cover the plate with soft tissue after its application.

## What Follows External Fixation?

For unstable type I and type II open tibial fractures primarily stabilized by external fixators, there are two avenues of treatment: (1) cast or brace treatment and early weightbearing (Sarmiento method), or (2) delayed intramedullary nailing five to seven days after removal of the external fixator. During this preoperative time period, the patient is given oral cephalosporins, 3 to 4 g/day. One to two hours before surgery the patient is given 2 g of cefazolin sodium, and then 1 g every eight hours for 24 hours.

For type III open fractures, the external fixator should be removed when the wound has healed and a long-leg cast should be applied. Oral antibiotics and cephalosporins should be given for about seven to ten days and closed intramedullary nailing should be delayed for at least that length of time. If an external fixator has been applied for six weeks or more, then internal fixation, intramedullary nailing, or plating should be delayed for another three to six weeks. Early internal fixation after removal of the internal fixator increases the incidence of wound sepsis.

The author's previous study showed that the absence of callus on radiographs three months after injury in type III open fracture indicated eventual failure to heal despite continued prolonged immobilization.[10] In the current study, all type III open fractures with marked comminution or bone loss or extensive periosteal stripping underwent cancellous bone grafting as early as three to six weeks after injury if radiographs showed no evidence of early callus formation or the fracture was clinically unstable. Grafting would certainly be undertaken by 12 weeks in such circumstances.

A number of other practical points require emphasis. It is imperative that farm or crash injuries or any injury in which there is vascular disruption be redebrided after 24 hours, as tissue necrosis unrecognized during the initial surgery is frequently found. The timing of intramedullary nailing for fracture stabilization is also worthy of comment. In the author's experience such nailing should be deferred in type III open fractures until after the second week because of the danger of infection. This is particularly true when there is extensive soft-tissue injury or accompanying vascular injury. The incidence of de-layed union or nonunion was significantly higher in patients with markedly displaced fractures.

Although soft-tissue infection in the current series was high, chronic osteomyelitis developed in only 2% of patients. However, at the latest follow-up (nonunion one year after treatment of chronic osteomyelitis), all cases have been resolved (no drainage and fracture united). This can be attributed to early diagnosis, immediate and repeated surgical debridement, and vigorous antibiotic therapy initiated from the onset. (Four patients eventually underwent amputation because of infection: two of the four had compromised vascularity [see Table 21–2].)

All patients with open fractures are regarded as being infected. Antibiotic therapy is initiated promptly and routinely continued for three days. Longer courses are used when deep-seated infection is established. Brief courses of antibiotics are repeated at the time of skin closure, bone grafting, and internal fixation.

In the last several years, the bacterial flora of wound infections have become predominantly gram-negative. In the author's latest series, 77% of organisms isolated were gram-negative compared with 24% in an earlier series. This change prompted a new antibiotic approach. Instead of using a cephalosporin alone, a cephalosporin combined with an aminoglycoside is now used. The advent of the third-generation cephalosporins may permit the use of a single drug, thus avoiding potential aminoglycoside toxicity. However, this decision depends on local factors. The use of tobramycin antibiotic beads deserves serious consideration in the treatment of infected open fractures and also in Type III open fractures.

## Summary of Treatment of Open Fractures

The following guidelines can be used in the treatment of open fractures:

Continue cefazolin sodium alone for type I and type II fractures. Use cephalosporin and aminoglycosides for type III fractures. Use tobramycin beads for packing type III wounds.

External fixation is the preferred method for securing fracture stability. Delayed nailing with reaming for type I and type II fractures may be done in ten to 21 days (after wound closure); for type III it may be done after wound healing in four to six weeks and at least ten days after removal of external fixation and seven days of oral antibiotic therapy.

In type III open fractures, wound closure should be attempted within five to ten days using direct wound closure, skin grafts, or flaps.

Early cancellous bone grafting should be used for

bone loss, severe comminution, and subtype III-B fractures. Bone grafting should be done four to six weeks after flap coverage.

## References

1. Rittmann WW, Perren SM: *Corticale Knochenheilung nach Osteosynthese und Infektion biomechanik und biologic.* Berlin-Heidelberg-New York, Springer, 1974.
2. Rittmann WW, Schibli M, Matter P, et al: Open fractures: Long-term results in 200 consecutive cases. *Clin Orthop* 1979;138:132–140.
3. Gustilo RB, Anderson JT: Prevention of infection in the treatment of one thousand and twenty-five open fractures of long bones: Retrospective and prospective analysis. *J Bone Joint Surg* 1976;58A:453–458.
4. Chapman MW, Mahoney M: The role of early internal fixation in the management of open fractures. *Clin Orthop* 1979;138:120–131.
5. Clancey GJ, Hansen ST Jr: Open fractures of the tibia: A review of 102 cases. *J Bone Joint Surg* 1978;60A:118.
6. Hasenhuttl K: The treatment of unstable fractures of the tibia and fibula with flexible medullary wires. *J Bone Joint Surg* 1981;63A:921–931.
7. Nicoll EA: Fractures of the tibial shaft: A survey of 705 cases. *J Bone Joint Surg* 1964;46B:373–387.
8. Rosenthal RE, MacPhail JA, Ortiz JE: Non-union in open tibial fractures: Analysis of reasons for failure of treatment. *J Bone Joint Surg* 1977;59A:244–248.
9. Gustilo RB, Mendoza RM, Williams DM: Problems in management of type III open fractures: A new classification of Type III open fractures. *J Trauma* 1984;24:742–746.
10. Anderson JT, Gustilo RB: Immediate internal fixation in open fractures. *Orthop Clin North Am* 1980;11:569–577.
11. Gustilo RB, Simpson L, Nixon R, et al: Analysis of 511 open fractures. *Clin Orthop* 1969;66:148–154.

# Management of Open Fracture Wounds

Michael J. Patzakis, MD

## Introduction

The importance of local host defense mechanisms in preventing infection is well recognized. However, an open fracture wound with devitalized tissue, ischemia, and soft-tissue swelling often alters the ability of local host defense mechanisms to resist infection. The importance of surgical debridement and irrigation of all open fracture wounds is a well accepted principle among surgeons.

The presence of infection often leads to prolonged hospitalization, jeopardizes the overall functional result, and is generally associated with higher complication and morbidity rates. The cardinal objectives in the treatment of open fractures are the prevention of infection and the restoration of function. To attain these goals, the principles of open fracture management must be considered. They include the taking of appropriate cultures, the institution of immediate appropriate systemic antibiotic therapy, surgical irrigation and debridement, wound management, proper stabilization of the fracture, and early bone grafting when indicated.

With the exception of low-velocity gunshot wounds, which can be treated with systemic antibiotics alone because of their low contamination and infection rates, it is imperative that every open fracture, regardless of the severity of the soft-tissue wound incurred, undergo surgical irrigation and debridement in an operating room.

## Cultures

It is important to consider open fracture wounds as contaminated wounds that are susceptible to infection. In more than 1,100 open fracture wounds treated in prospective studies at the Los Angeles County/University of Southern California Medical Center, the contamination rate was approximately 64%. Thus, treating surgeons must recognize that the antibiotics used are administered for the treatment of contamination and not for prophylaxis.

Because of the high contamination rate, it is important that cultures be taken before both wound care and antibiotic therapy begin. In the author's experience, the culture taken before any treatment is the one that gives the highest return of positive cultures in the sequence of cultures taken. In addition to pretreatment cultures, tissue cultures should also be taken of the debridement material as well as after irrigation and debridement. Because organisms isolated have included both gram-positive and gram-negative species, as well as aerobic and anaerobic organisms, both aerobic and anaerobic cultures should be taken.

The correlation between organisms isolated in the initial wound cultures and the organisms causing subsequent infection is approximately 66%. Thus, the cultures play an important role in alerting the treating surgeon as to the most probable infecting organism in the early postfracture period when infection is present.

Quantitative tissue cultures are not valuable in the initial treatment of open fracture wounds but are useful during secondary soft-tissue coverage of open fracture wounds.

## Antibiotic Therapy

The efficacy of antibiotics in open fracture wounds has been demonstrated in many reported studies.[1–8] A prospective study by Patzakis and associates[5] reported infection rates of 13.9% (11 of 79 wounds) in patients receiving no antibiotics, 9.8% (nine of 92 wounds) in patients with open fractures receiving penicillin and streptomycin, and 2.4% (two of 84 wounds) in patients receiving cephalothin. The antibiotic selected to treat contamination in open fracture wounds should be an antimicrobial agent effective against both gram-positive and gram-negative organisms. More than 85% of the *Staphylococcus aureus* coagulase-positive organisms isolated from open fracture wounds have been resistant to penicillin. Before the use of systemic antibiotic therapy in the treatment of open fracture wounds, the most commonly reported organism causing infection was coagulase-positive *S. aureus*.[3–5,7]

The extensive use of cephalosporins as antimicrobial agents in open fracture wounds has caused an increase in gram-negative infections. The probable explanation is that the routine use of cephalosporins effectively treated gram-positive organisms, but gram-negative organisms resistant to the cephalosporins then began to cause the majority of the infections.

The main decisions related to antibiotic therapy are

selecting the antibiotic or antibiotics to use, the dosage, and the length of systemic therapy.

A reasonable combination of antibiotics would be a cephalosporin in combination with an aminoglycoside (e.g., tobramycin or gentamicin). Experience with a first-generation cephalosporin and cefamandole, a second-generation cephalosporin, indicates that they are more effective than third-generation cephalosporins because the latter do not provide gram-positive coverage as effective as that of first- or second-generation cephalosporins. Another effective combination of antibiotics would include a synthetic penicillin with an aminoglycoside. The usual dosage for synthetic penicillins and cephalosporins (cephalothin, cephapirin, and cefamandole) is 100 to 200 mg/kg of lean body weight per day in divided doses with most adults receiving 1 to 2 g every four hours intravenously. The maximum dosage of either a cephalosporin or synthetic penicillin in any one patient is 12 g/day. Another frequently used first-generation cephalosporin is cefazolin sodium because of its longer duration of action. It usually is given every six to eight hours. The usual dosage for an aminoglycoside such as tobramycin or gentamicin is 3 to 5 mg/kg of lean body weight per day with most patients receiving 80 mg every eight hours. Patients who have open fracture wounds with a high propensity for clostridial myonecrosis, such as injuries occurring around farms and stables and fractures associated with vascular injuries, should also receive penicillin. Adults receive 10 million units/day in divided doses, and children receive 100,000 units/kg/day intravenously in divided doses. The period during which systemic antibiotics should be administered is an arbitrary decision, but three days is sufficient for the presence or absence of infection to be determined. In addition, the culture report is usually available and, if infection is present or if the wound is suspect, specific antibiotic therapy can be continued. Prolonged administration of antibiotic therapy (five to ten days) is not a significant factor in reducing the infection rate. In addition, the longer the antibiotic therapy is continued, the higher the incidence of antibiotic toxicity. The rate of antibiotic side effects is 3% in patients receiving antibiotics for ten days, 1% in those treated for five days, and less than 1% in those treated for three days or less.

When is it appropriate to use a single antimicrobial agent? Although both Chapman[9] and Gustilo[10] reported an infection rate of 1% or less in patients receiving a cephalosporin alone for type I open fracture wounds, the author believes that to protect against infection by both gram-positive and gram-negative organisms an aminoglycoside should be added to the cephalosporin. Although the soft-tissue wound in a type I injury is small, the amount of energy expended in some open fracture wounds is great and, therefore, untreated contamination can lead to serious and catastrophic infection. In addition, many type I and type II wounds occur around dirt and playgrounds containing gram-negative organisms, including *Pseudomonas*, and thus failure to treat for these organisms can lead to infection.

The toxicity rate in patients who receive a short course of an aminoglycoside is negligible if there is no preexisting renal disease. Thus, combined treatment with both a cephalosporin and an aminoglycoside should be used in all open fracture wounds.

Those patients who will undergo a secondary procedure such as internal fixation or muscle or soft-tissue coverage should receive systemic antibiotics for 72 hours.

## Wound Coverage

The management of open fracture wounds has been a controversial subject. There have been conflicting reports in the literature. Investigators recommending leaving open fracture wounds open include Witschi and Omer,[11] Trueta,[12] Brown and Kinman,[13] Burkhalter,[14] and Clancey and Hansen.[15] However, the value of primary closure has also been reported by several investigators.[16,17]

Benson and associates[1] concluded that a relatively uncontaminated open fracture may be closed primarily after adequate debridement without increasing the risk of infection provided that the patient is given antimicrobial therapy. They also found that a five-day delay in the closure of the wound in an open fracture after adequate debridement did not increase the risk of infection. A number of investigators believe that it is important to convert open fracture wounds to closed ones by delayed primary closure to provide a better environment for fracture healing and to prevent delayed secondary infection.[2,3,18,19]

Prospective studies at the author's institution found no difference in the infection rates for patients whose wounds were left open and for those who underwent primary closure as long as appropriate systemic antibiotics were administered. The main disadvantage of primary closure is a higher risk of clostridial myonecrosis or "gas gangrene," as reported by Brown and Kinman.[13] Patzakis and associates[5] reported two cases of clostridial myonecrosis in patients with open tibial fractures treated by primary closure but no antibiotics.

Also, experimental studies using laboratory animals showed a definite increase in the incidence of clostridial myonecrosis in animals that underwent primary closure of open fracture wounds contaminated with clostridial organisms in the presence of ischemic muscle.[20]

Patzakis and associates[8] reported an infection rate of 4.5% in 109 open tibias treated with partial closure in type I and type II open fracture wounds and with delayed primary closure in all type III wounds.

What is meant by leaving an open fracture wound "open" has not been well defined in the literature. The author's definition is taken from military surgeons, who advocate leaving a wound wide open and placing no sutures in the wound. Placement of suture material within the wound, even if the skin is left open, constitutes a partial closure of the wound.

## Type I and Type II Open Fracture Wounds

For type I and type II open fracture wounds, the author uses partial closure. Partial closure is defined as leaving the original wound open and closing the extension of the surgical wound made by the surgeon to facilitate surgical debridement. When the laceration is over the bone fracture ends, it is closed and the wound is left open on one or both sides of the fracture site. In essence, all of the wounds are left open. Smaller wounds can heal without further treatment; in a larger wound, delayed primary skin closure or split-thickness skin grafting can be used.

## Type III Open Fracture Wounds

These wounds often require a "second look" debridement 24 to 48 hours after the initial debridement. A second debridement is recommended for all type III wounds. Once the wounds are clean, it is imperative that the wound be closed within the first three to seven days after injury. The incidence of major complications was markedly increased as reported in studies by Byrd and associates,[21] Cierny and associates,[22] and Kojima and associates.[23] If exposed bone is not covered within this period, even if the wound is infection-free, a secondary infection often develops along with desiccation of the bone, and the infection rate markedly increases.

Quantitative tissue cultures are useful before delayed primary closure or soft-tissue or muscle-flap coverage. There should be fewer than $10^5$ organisms present. In addition, the Gram stain should be negative and the tissues to be covered should be clean. If these criteria are not met, the incidence of infection and failure greatly increases.

Exposed bone can be covered with a local muscle flap, a myocutaneous flap, or a free vascularized flap. In wounds involving the tibia, local muscle flaps can be used except for the distal third where a free vascularized muscle flap is often necessary. In wounds with no bone exposed and exposure of only soft tissue and muscle, split-thickness skin grafting can be used. Many wounds with good granulation tissue heal spontaneously when epithelialization proceeds from the periphery to cover the exposed tissues. In wounds with adequate skin at the time of delayed primary closure, direct skin closure can be done.

## References

1. Benson DR, Riggins RS, Lawrence RM, et al: Treatment of open fractures: A prospective study. *J Trauma* 1983;23:25.
2. Chapman MW, Mahoney M: The role of early internal fixation in the management of open fractures. *Clin Orthop* 1979;138:120–131.
3. Gustilo RB, Anderson JT: Prevention of infection in the treatment of one thousand and twenty-five open fractures of the long bones. *J Bone Joint Surg* 1976;58A:453.
4. Patzakis MJ: The use of antibiotics in open fractures. *Surg Clin North Am* 1975;55:1439.
5. Patzakis MJ, Harvey JP, Ivler D: The role of antibiotics in the management of open fractures. *J Bone Joint Surg* 1974;56A:532.
6. Patzakis MJ, Ivler D: Antibiotic and bacteriologic considerations in open fractures. *South Med J* 1977;70(suppl):46.
7. Patzakis MJ, Wilkins J, Moore TM: Use of antibiotics in open tibial fractures. *Clin Orthop* 1983;178:31.
8. Patzakis MJ, Wilkins J, Moore TM: Considerations in reducing the infection rate in open tibial fractures. *Clin Orthop* 1983;178:36.
9. Chapman MW: Current concepts in open fracture management. Read before the 53rd Annual Meeting of the American Academy of Orthopaedic Surgeons, New Orleans, February 21, 1986.
10. Gustilo RB: Current concepts in management of open fractures, in American Academy of Orthopaedic Surgeons *Instructional Course Lectures, XXXVI.* Park Ridge, American Academy of Orthopaedic Surgeons, pp 359-366.
11. Witschi TH, Omer GE: The treatment of open tibial shaft fractures from Vietnam War. *J Trauma* 1970;10:105.
12. Trueta J: "Closed" treatment of war fractures. *Lancet* 1939;1:1462.
13. Brown PW, Kinman PB: Gas gangrene in a metropolitan community. *J Bone Joint Surg* 1974;56A:1445.
14. Burkhalter WE: Open injuries of the lower extremity. *Surg Clin North Am* 1973;53:1439.
15. Clancey GJ, Hansen ST Jr: Open fractures of the tibia: A review of one hundred and two cases. *J Bone Joint Surg* 1978;60A:118.
16. Davis AG: Primary closure of compound-fracture wounds: With immediate internal fixation, immediate skin-grafts, and compression dressings. *J Bone Joint Surg* 1948;30A:405.
17. Reckling FW, Roberts MD: Primary closure of open fractures of the tibia and fibula by fibular fixation and relaxing incisions. *J Trauma* 1970;10:853.
18. Rosenthal RE, MacPhail JA, Ortiz JE: Non-union in open tibial fractures. *J Bone Joint Surg* 1977;59A:244.
19. Saad MD: The problems of traumatic skin loss of the lower limbs, especially when associated with skeletal injury. *Br J Surg* 1970;57:601.
20. Patzakis MJ, Dorr LD, Hammond W, et al: The effect of antibiotics, primary and secondary closure on clostridial contaminated open fracture wounds in rats. *J Trauma* 1978;18:34.
21. Byrd HS, Cierny G III, Tebbetts JB: The management of open tibias with associated soft tissue loss: External pin fixation with early flap coverage. *Plast Reconstr Surg* 1981;68:73.
22. Cierny G III, Byrd HS, Jones RE: Primary versus delayed soft tissue coverage for severe open tibial fractures: A comparison of results. *Clin Orthop* 1983;178:54.
23. Kojima T, Kohno T, Ito T: Muscle flap with simultaneous mesh skin graft for skin defects of the lower leg. *J Trauma* 1979;19:724.

# Functional Fracture Bracing: An Update

Augusto Sarmiento, MD

## Introduction

Certain surgical methods of fracture fixation, such as intramedullary nailing of femoral shaft fractures, have made possible a dramatic reduction in the cost of medical care. The shorter hospitalization required with these methods, along with lower morbidity, speak for the role of surgery. Traction and prolonged, costly hospitalization are difficult to justify in light of surgical advances. The same is not true for many other diaphyseal fractures for which nonsurgical treatment is often safer and does not require hospitalization.

Functional fracture bracing has undergone significant changes since this technique was first introduced in 1963.[1] During these years the author has modified his original philosophy. Before 1963 it was universally accepted that the cast used in the treatment of tibial fractures had to immobilize the knee and ankle joints. The author originally thought that the below-the-knee functional cast (PTB) developed for the treatment of diaphyseal tibial fractures could maintain limb length and fracture stability by the successful transfer of weightbearing stresses from the ground to the patellar tendon and tibial condylar flares through the critical molding of those anatomic areas.[1,2] However, additional clinical and laboratory studies demonstrated that the effectiveness of such a cast depended not on the successful transfer of stresses proximally but on stiffening of the distal extremity through compression of the soft tissues and the creation of a pseudohydraulic environment capable of maintaining alignment and fracture stability.[3]

It also became clear that the ankle joint did not have to be immobilized. Leaving that joint free produced the first functional brace,[4] one that with some modifications has been found useful by the orthopaedic surgeon. It constitutes a clearly defined alternative method of managing certain diaphyseal fractures.

The initial work with bracing of tibial fractures led to the development of similar functional braces for the treatment of other fractures.[5-14] It is important to recognize that braces used in the treatment of diaphyseal fractures do not prevent shortening of the fractured extremity. They simply assist in maintaining the shortening present immediately after the initial injury or that achieved after stable reduction. Clinical and laboratory data have shown that in closed diaphyseal fractures the initial shortening remains essentially unchanged after the gradual introduction of function and weightbearing. The amount of soft-tissue damage dictates the degree of initial and subsequent shortening. Additional overriding is not probable since the remaining intact soft tissues attached to the fracture fragments provide an elastic tethering that prevents further shortening. The pain associated with function and ambulation during the early stages of healing precludes the amount of weightbearing that would produce greater soft-tissue damage.[15-18] Therefore, the main role of a functional brace is to provide alignment stability. In open diaphyseal fractures it is often difficult to determine the true initial shortening with precision, and, therefore, the ultimate shortening cannot be predicted accurately. Damage to the soft-tissue envelope compromises the hydraulic environment created in closed fractures.

Injured tissues heal at a predictable pace determined by biologic factors not yet clearly understood. It appears, however, that the environment under which fractured extremities are maintained influences the speed of fracture consolidation and the mechanical properties of the healing callus. Rigidly immobilized long bone fractures demonstrate an absence of peripheral callus but a rapid reconstitution of medullary blood supply. This "primary callus" is mechanically weak and for a considerable period the fixation devices (plates or external fixators) provide stability.[19,20] When this primary callus eventually matures, it provides sufficient support so that the plate or external fixators are no longer necessary. Conversely, the peripheral callus that forms in the presence of motion at the fracture site, as in fractures treated with functional casts or braces, has strong mechanical properties and provides fracture stability at an earlier date. This callus eventually makes the fractured bone at the level of the fracture stronger than it was before the injury.[17-21] The author believes that this callus should be referred to as "peripheral" rather than "periosteal" callus since it is possible that the periosteum plays a relatively minor role in the production of callus in adults. This peripheral callus is probably produced by the surrounding soft tissues through a vascular invasion that is ultimately responsible for the appearance of osteogenic cells.

Clinical and laboratory studies strongly suggest that physiologically controlled motion at the fracture site produces environmental changes conducive to osteogenesis. The motion that occurs at the fracture site when the injured extremity is maintained in a physiologic environment is elastic, intermittent, and controlled by pain. Such motion produces thermic, mechanical, electrical, chemical, and vascular changes that are probably conducive to osteogenesis.[17,18] The rapid healing of fractures of the ribs and clavicle, which defy rigid immobilization and which are subjected to constant intermittent motion, demonstrates the benefits of physiologically controlled motion at a fracture site.

The capillary invasion occurs in response to the irritation produced by the moving fragments during weightbearing and function. It is scientifically important to know whether or not perithelial or endothelial cells on the walls of the invading capillaries or circulating cells undergo osteoblastic metaplasia, but from the clinical standpoint, the more capillaries at the fracture site, the greater the osteogenic activity. More endoplastic reticulum is seen in the osteoblasts formed in the presence of functional activity, strongly suggesting that the environment plays a major role in fracture repair.[17,18]

Closed, oblique, comminuted, or spiral fractures treated with functional braces develop peripheral callus and intrinsic stability sooner than nondisplaced or anatomically reduced transverse fractures. Overriding, unreduced transverse fractures also develop callus and intrinsic stability sooner.

Patients with reduced transverse fractures seem to have pain at the fracture site for longer periods than those with oblique or spiral fractures. These observations suggest that pistoning associated with rotational motion between the fragments is the type of motion most likely to encourage rapid osteogenesis. The thermic and electrical changes that take place under such conditions may cause the increased osteogenic activity.

During weightbearing the fractured extremity shortens further but returns to the initial amount of shortening during the swing phase of gait and rest. During weightbearing, the anatomically reduced transverse fracture allows the development of motion between the fragments, but this motion is only of the bending type. It may be detrimental to fracture healing. The compression between the fragments, once considered to be beneficial to osteogenesis, has value only when the mechanically weak primary callus is desired or anticipated, as in rigidly immobilized fractures treated with plates or fixators.

## Indications

Experience with functional treatment of long-bone fractures has shown that bracing has limitations and contraindications as well as indications. Elsewhere in this volume, others will place in proper prospective the indications and contraindications of this technique. They will also report their own wide clinical experiences. The following paragraphs summarize the author's own views of certain important aspects of functional fracture bracing. These views may conflict slightly with those expressed by others, but all of us share the same basic philosophy.

## Functional Bracing of Tibial Fractures

Diaphyseal tibial fractures were the first to be treated with functional braces.[1,2,4,10] The clinical results have been rewarding. Almost all of the fractures treated by the author healed (nonunion rate, 2.5%). The degree of final varus angulatory deformity was less than 5 degrees in 80.9% of the patients; 92.5% of the patients had less than 8 degrees of varus angulation. Final shortening was 1 cm or less in 91.2% of patients.[22]

There is little doubt that functional bracing of tibial fractures produces the best results in closed fractures, particularly those resulting from relatively low-energy injuries. In such fractures, the amounts of initial and final shortening ranges from 0.5 to 1 cm.

Control of major angulatory deformities in these fractures is usually possible. The brace itself often corrects deformities seen in the initial cast, particularly deformities of the valgus type.

Open fractures are less likely to give the same clinical results. These fractures are, in fact, problems related to soft-tissue abnormalities, not to the bone itself. The author usually refers to them as "incomplete, partial amputations" rather than as fractures. Greater shortening, angulation, and instability are common initially and, in many instances, necessitate additional corrective measures. The external fixator is, at this time, probably the safest and most popular method of treating many open fractures. However, internal fixation with Ender or reamed nailing has gained increased acceptance. A severe open fracture, one with a maximum amount of soft-tissue damage, is not well suited to intramedullary fixation of the reamed type because of the high incidence of infections.

The rigid immobilization provided by an external fixator is probably conducive to delayed unions and nonunions. Therefore, it is desirable to remove the fixators after a relatively short period. They must remain in place, however, long enough for soft-tissue intrinsic stability to develop about the fracture site. Once this occurs, it is often possible to create a more physiologic environment, such as that provided by the functional brace. However, it must be recognized that when soft-tissue damage is extensive and associated with initial severe shortening, removing the fixator may result in a recurrence of shortening or angulatory deformities. Three to six weeks are usual.

In severe open fractures of the tibia associated with fibular fractures, the fibular fracture may heal while the tibial fracture fails to develop callus. Varus angulatory deformity may develop after removal of the fixator and the introduction of weightbearing ambulation. It is for this reason that intramedullary fixation of those fractures may be the treatment of choice, particularly with type I and type II open fractures.

Fractures of the tibia when the fibula is intact may develop varus angulatory deformities, particularly if treated with weightbearing casts or braces. If maintained within 5 degrees, this deformity is cosmetically and physiologically acceptable.[17] Fractures with marked tibial angulation at the time of the injury have a tendency to angulate further, and it may be best to treat them by means of intramedullary fixation or by osteotomy of the fibula at a level approximately 2 inches above or below the tibial fracture. When a tibial fracture is not associated with a fibular fracture, the shorter tibial fragment tends to angulate toward the fibula. Proximal-third tibial fractures with intact fibula are most likely to develop severe angulatory deformities. This complication is also more likely to occur if the fracture is comminuted or has a geometric form that permits the unopposed displacement of the short fragment toward the fibula.[17] When isolated tibial fractures demonstrate shortening, a dislocated proximal fibula must be suspected. This complication should always be suspected whenever the isolated tibial fracture angulates in valgus rather than in varus. The anatomic reduction of the tibial fracture often results in spontaneous reduction of the dislocated fibula. If the reduction is unstable, surgery is recommended to restore stability and to prevent undesirable and painful sequelae.

Most closed diaphyseal tibial fractures resulting from relatively low-energy trauma can be braced within the first two weeks after injury. The absence of marked pain and significant swelling at the fracture site should dictate whether or not the brace can be applied. The application of the brace when the limb is painful and swollen is undesirable since the patient experiences additional discomfort. A toe-to-groin cast with the knee in a few degrees of flexion and with the ankle held at neutral attitude is recommended as the initial immobilization device.[4] Early activity while the patient is in this cast seems to shorten the time needed between injury and bracing. An equinus position of the ankle must be avoided if at all possible since immobilization of that joint after a fracture results in stiffness within a short period. The sudden freedom of the stiff ankle forces the patient to bear weight on the forefoot, creating a recurvatum deformity of the fracture site.[17]

Ambulation after the application of the brace should always be assisted with crutches or a walker. The degree of weightbearing should be dictated by the severity of symptoms. Patients should be instructed to bear significant weight on the extremity only if and when this can be done without pain.

Prefabricated braces, which the author has used for the last ten years, can be removed temporarily for hygienic purposes but should be reapplied snugly.[22] It is best not to remove the braces too often soon after they are applied. The brace should be discontinued if angulatory deformities reach an unacceptable degree of shortening. The author believes that 1 cm of shortening is always acceptable because this produces no limp and is not associated with undesirable late sequelae. In many instances shortening of almost 2 cm leaves patients unaware of the discrepancy and without a limp. Whether shortening of more than 1 cm is acceptable must be individually determined. If it is unacceptable, other measures must be used.

Angulation of less than 5 degrees in any plane or combination of planes is cosmetically acceptable in almost all instances. Visual recognition of deformities of less than 5 degrees is unlikely.[17] Although the author has looked for patients with osteoarthritis of the knee or ankle who could trace their disorders to old extra-articular diaphyseal fractures of the tibia that healed with less than 8 degrees of angulatory deformity, he has not, as yet, found such an individual. It is, therefore, very unlikely that minor angulatory deformities produce late osteoarthritic changes.

Wagner and associates[23] conducted laboratory studies in cadaver specimens by creating angulatory deformities of various types and measuring the stress resulting from those deformities on the tibiotalar joint. These studies suggested that minimal changes in the distribution of the stresses at the talotibial joint develop, probably as a result of the compensatory motion of the adjacent subtalar joints. For varus or valgus angulation at the fracture site to be acceptable, the subtalar joint must be normal. A fused or significantly limited subtalar joint before the injury prevents the necessary compensatory motion required for normal weightbearing by the foot.

In the author's opinion, tibial functional fracture braces should have extensions over the femoral condyles and proximal tibia to provide the greatest possible degree of angulatory and rotatory stability. This is particularly desirable in patients treated with the braces soon after injury and especially in those whose fractures are located in the proximal third of the tibia.

A disadvantage of prefabricated functional braces is that patients can loosen the fastening straps or remove them prematurely, with resulting loss of fracture alignment.

## Functional Bracing of Humeral Fractures

Prefabricated functional bracing of humeral fractures has provided satisfactory results.[14] The proper application of the brace results in consistent fracture healing. In the author's experience, the nonunion rate has been less than 2%. The compression of the soft tissues by the circular sleeve produces a "stiffness" of the upper arm that, when accompanied by early introduction of gravity and muscle activity, tends to correct major angulatory deformities.[14,17]

Most of the fractures treated by the author healed with less than 15 degrees of varus angulatory deformity. A mild varus angulation—the most common deformity—is often difficult to recognize clinically, particularly in an adult with muscular or flabby extremities.

Varus at the fracture site is usually produced at the time the functional sleeve is applied if the collar and cuff are attached while the shoulder is held in a shrugged attitude. When the shoulder is relaxed with the arm still held in a sling, a varus deformity could occur. It is essential, therefore, that the collar and cuff be placed around the patient's neck and elbow with the shoulder in a completely relaxed attitude.[17]

Open or closed humeral diaphyseal fractures with significant soft-tissue damage may demonstrate distraction between the fragments when the arm is stabilized in a cast initially and in a functional sleeve later. This suggests severe intrinsic soft-tissue abnormalities and, therefore, the possibility of delayed union or nonunion must be considered.

Most rotary deformities—usually of the external type—can be eliminated by the early introduction of active and passive exercises. There are patients, however, who permanently lose the last few degrees of external rotation of the shoulder. Such loss may result from mild rotation at the fracture site or from capsular contractures that develop during the painful stages of the disease process.

The level of the humeral fracture does not seem to affect the usefulness of the functional brace. Distal extra-articular fractures, particularly those with comminution, are probably the most rewarding. The presence of an associated radial palsy does not preclude the use of the functional brace. Nerve recovery has been almost universal when the fracture was closed and the nerve deficit developed immediately after the injury. Extending the elbow as early as the first or second week after the initial injury prevents the development of a flexion-contracture of the wrist. Thus, "cock-up splints" are seldom needed.

A long arm cast with a shoulder sling is the preferred initial treatment for diaphyseal humeral fractures. This cast prevents excessive motion at the fracture site and controls swelling of the elbow and forearm. Patients are more comfortable when treated in this manner for approximately one week.

When the brace is applied after the disappearance of pain and swelling, a collar and cuff should always accompany the brace. It is at this time that an iatrogenic varus deformity must be avoided. The collar and cuff should be discontinued for short times during the day so that elbow extension is gradually regained. As soon as full extension can be achieved, the cuff is discarded during ambulation and used only when the patient is lying down. The brace must be tightened regularly by the patient to maintain snugness and to prevent distal sliding that might impair or limit flexion of the elbow.

Active shoulder flexion and abduction exercises should be delayed until strong fracture stability has developed. Their early introduction predisposes to the development of angulatory deformities. Pendulum and circumduction exercises are the only exercises necessary during the first few weeks after the injury.

## Functional Bracing of Forearm Fractures

### The Isolated Ulnar Fracture

Results have been satisfactory in isolated ulnar fractures treated with functional sleeves that permit flexion and extension of the elbow and minimal limitation of pronosupination of the forearm. Nonunion rates with this method of treatment are less than 2%.[13,14,17,19] Angulatory deformity—especially ulnar angulation toward the radius—are common but usually do not exceed 5 degrees. This degree of deformity is associated with minimal or no loss of pronosupination.[6]

A functional sleeve may be applied as soon as the acute symptoms subside. In the author's experience, these sleeves are applied within one week of the initial insult. The sleeves are later removed for hygienic purposes.

Early radiographs frequently suggest development of a nonunion as the gap between the fragments seems to increase, but peripheral callus eventually bridges the fracture and closes the defect with osseous tissues.

The functional sleeve allows unencumbered use of all joints. Pain prevents complete pronosupination of the forearm during the early stages. With continued use of the extremity, complete or almost complete recovery of motion eventually takes place.

### Isolated Radial Fractures

Functional bracing has a limited role in isolated radial fractures. Most such fractures are the result of falls on the outstretched hand and are therefore associated with distal radioulnar abnormalities. Restoration and maintenance of length of the radius is necessary to avoid painful, unstable radioulnar articulation. At the present time, surgery and internal fixation are the best treatment.

However, in some instances the injury occurs directly over the radius, producing a fracture with no associated radioulnar abnormality. If the fragments are in a reasonably good alignment and interlocked, such fractures may be treated with functional braces to prevent pronosupination of the forearm while permitting flexion and extension of the wrist and limited elbow motion.[11,17]

## Functional Bracing of Both Bones of the Forearm

It has been accepted for some time that fractures of both bones of the forearm are best treated by means of plate fixation because of the technical difficulty of obtaining or maintaining closed reduction. However, plate fixation is not always free of complications and undesirable sequelae can occur. Infections, nonunions, delayed unions, failure of fixation, and refractures after plate removal are not uncommon. Even under the best of circumstances, plated forearms usually have a residual permanent limitation of pronosupination. This limitation ordinarily measures only a few degrees and often is not recognized by the patient who inconspicuously compensates by shoulder flexion and rotation.

Although the initial results were encouraging,[11,17] it became apparent that consistent achievement was technically demanding.

The author believes that functional bracing is a viable alternative in the treatment of some diaphyseal fractures of both bones of the forearm. Braces are not applied until soft-tissue stability has been obtained. Approximately three weeks of cast immobilization is required. With this nonsurgical method nonunions are extremely rare and although anatomic reduction is seldom achieved or maintained, the residual malalignment is within physiologic levels.

Other investigators have conducted studies to determine the effects of angulatory deformities in forearm pronosupination and have found, in cadavers at least, that 10 degrees of angulatory deformity creates minimal limitation of pronosupination of the forearm. Patients with fractures that healed with less than 10 degrees of angulatory deformity had limitations of motion less significant than those found in laboratory studies.[6,17,24]

Failure to obtain or maintain reduction in a cast, or later in a brace, calls for surgical intervention, which may then be more difficult.

## Functional Bracing of Femoral Shaft Fractures

Considerable progress has been made in the surgical treatment of femoral shaft fractures. Closed intramedullary and interlocking closed nailing have been so successful that other methods are rapidly becoming obsolete. Long ago, the author recognized that functional bracing of femoral fractures was associated with a high incidence of angulatory deformities, particularly in fractures located in the proximal or middle thirds of the diaphysis.[10,17]

Bracing produces satisfactory results when used in the treatment of diaphyseal fractures located in the distal third. Angulatory deformities have been minimal.[10,17] In many distal diaphyseal fractures, particularly in an elderly patient with osteoporosis, functional bracing may be the treatment of choice. A short period of recumbency followed by the application of the brace and the introduction of weightbearing ambulation eliminates complications such as infections, loss of implant fixation, and prolonged knee stiffness.

## References

1. Sarmiento A, Sinclair WF: Application of prosthetic-orthotic principles of orthopaedics. *Artif Limbs* 1967;11:28-32.
2. Sarmiento A: A functional below-knee cast for tibial fractures. *J Bone Joint Surg* 1967;59A:5.
3. Sarmiento A, Latta L, Zilioli A, et al: The role of soft tissues in the stabilization of tibial fractures. *Clin Orthop* 1974;105:116–129.
4. Sarmiento A: A functional below-knee brace for tibial fractures. *J Bone Joint Surg* 1970;52A:295–311.
5. Connolly JF, Dehne E, LaFollette B: Closed reduction and early cast-brace ambulation in the treatment of femoral fractures: Part II. Results in 143 fractures. *J Bone Joint Surg* 1973;55A:1581–1599.
6. Hack B, Brys D, Tarr RR, et al: The effects of angular deformities of the radius and ulna on pronosupination of the forearm. Presented at the 53rd Annual Meeting of the American Academy of Orthopaedic Surgeons, New Orleans, Feb. 25, 1986.
7. Crotwell WA III: The thigh-lacer: Ambulatory nonoperative treatment of femoral shaft fractures. *J Bone Joint Surg* 1978;60A:112–117.
8. DeLee JC: Ipsilateral fracture of the femur and tibia treated in quadrilateral cast-brace. *Clin Orthop* 1979;142:115-122.
9. Mooney V, Nickel VL, Harvey JP Jr, et al: Cast-brace treatment for fractures of the distal part of the femur: A prospective controlled study of 150 patients. *J Bone Joint Surg* 1970;52A:1563–1578.
10. Sarmiento A: Functional bracing of tibial and femoral shaft fractures. *Clin Orthop* 1972;82:2–13.
11. Sarmiento A, Cooper JS, Sinclair WF: Forearm fractures, early functional bracing: A preliminary report. *J Bone Joint Surg* 1975;57A:297–394.
12. Sarmiento A, Pratt GW, Berry NC, et al: Colles' fractures: Functional bracing in supination. *J Bone Joint Surg* 1975;57A:311–317.
13. Sarmiento A, Kinman PB, Murphy RB, et al: Treatment of

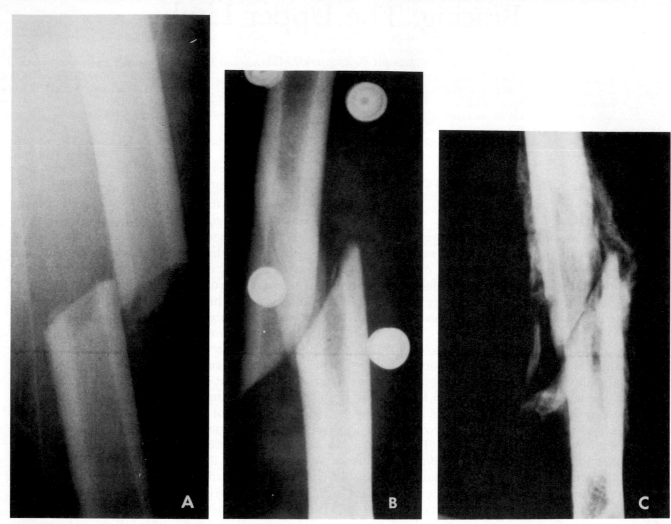

**Fig. 24–1** **A:** In stage I fracture healing, acute symptoms restrict functional activity and fracture site displacement is determined by the initial disruption of the soft tissues at the time of injury. On the day of injury, the radiograph shows only the disruption of bone. (Reproduced with permission from Sarmiento A, Latta LL, Tarr RR: The effects of function in fracture healing and stability. American Academy of Orthopaedic Surgeons *Instructional Course Lectures, XXXIII.* St Louis, CV Mosby, 1984, pp 83–106.) **B:** The fragments are free to displace to the point where intact soft tissues tether their position and resist further motion, as in this humerus fracture on the day of injury in the fracture brace. **C:** After the muscle spasms relax, there is less overriding because the fracture site motion is elastic. The fragments healed in the relaxed position, where callus formed. The radiolucent area indicates where the fragments had displaced in early callus formation.

animals as well as humans, refractures in this stage of fracture healing commonly occur adjacent to the original fracture site and not through the peripheral callus formation. Thus, because the early bridging is the most peripheral portion of the callus, a radiolucent line may persist at the original fracture site for a long period of time after strength has been regained in the bone structure during stage III callus formation.

The fourth and fifth stages of fracture healing are of radiographic significance but not of great clinical significance. If function has been present since early healing, stress has been present on the tissues formed in the callus. And if functional recovery of the patient has been otherwise uneventful, fracture line consoli-

dation, stage IV, simply demonstrates calcification of an endochondral nature, which obliterates the original fracture line on radiographs. During stage IV, however, only a minor alteration of callus mechanical properties is evident (Fig. 24–6). The final stage of fracture healing, stage V, may last for many years. It is the remodeling of the callus structure to reconstitute the normal diaphyseal bone and its medullary canal. Remodeling provides an impressive change on radiographs that is usually associated with no change in clinical symptoms or functional activity of the patient (Fig. 24–7).

### Fracture Stability

In the first two stages of fracture repair, the limb

must be mechanically stabilized to achieve comfortable functioning and to maintain alignment of the fragments. Fracture braces provide this stability through soft-tissue compression, which provides stiffness to the limb and mechanical support to maintain levels of tissue strain within the limits allowable for healing of tissue during functional activity.[6,7,12] In stage I, soft-tissue compression must supply all of the support to the limb as no intrinsic stability has been achieved by early soft-tissue healing in this immediate post-injury state. In this stage of healing, compression greatly enhances rigidity of the limb to support the relatively compliant soft-tissue coupling between the bone ends during functional activity. Soft-tissue compression is therefore necessary to reach relatively normal levels of activity after edema has subsided and pain becomes minimal.

The cylindrical shape of a fracture brace provides mechanical stability in the early stages of fracture healing. The cylindrical shape provides structural rigidity as the cylinder compresses the soft tissues. The cylinder's material need not be very rigid because the structural rigidity of a cylinder encompassing and compressing the soft tissues depends only slightly upon the material properties of the brace. It depends mainly upon the size and shape of the brace.

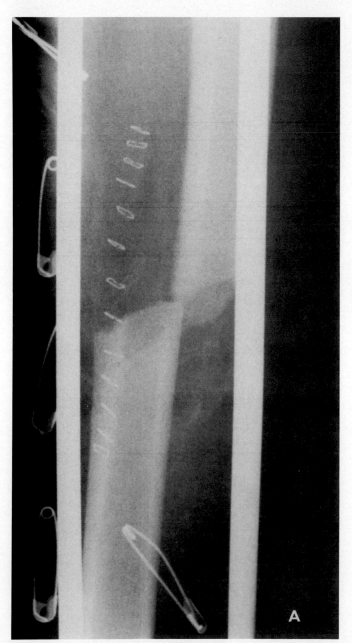

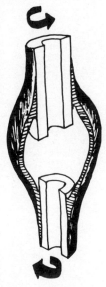
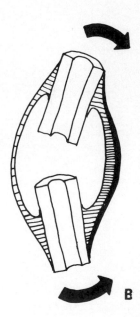

**Fig. 24–2  A:** The femur fracture shown was taken to surgery 2.5 weeks following injury for delayed open medullary fixation, at which time abundant callus was found to consist of soft tissues and provide a rubbery, elastic connection between the fragments. **B:** In this early stage of healing, a new soft-tissue coupling has formed between the bone ends, which are compliant enough to allow for rotation, bending and some translation at the fracture site. These motions are well controlled by the elastic soft tissues, which return the fragments to the position they were in when the soft tissue coupling formed.

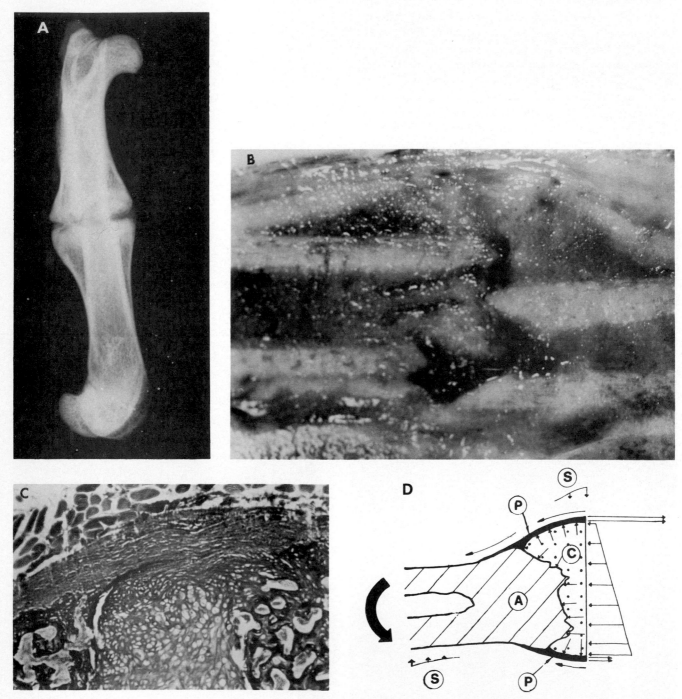

**Fig. 24–3** **A:** Stage II soft-callus formation in the rat. The radiograph shows new bone formation in the subperiosteal region, but radiolucent materials still bridge the fracture site. **B:** In a gross longitudinal section of the callus at two weeks, the fracture site shows hematoma capped by a dense fibrous tissue layer in the peripheral bridging region, which appears as a new thickened periosteum across the callus. **C:** Histologically, the well oriented collagen fibers can be appreciated in this newly formed periosteum bridging the fracture site between the subperiosteal regions of new bone formation covering the early cartilage formation. **D:** A diagram of a callus structure illustrates the mechanical role of the soft tissues bridging the fracture site. The dense collagenous material in the peripheral portion, P, provides good resistance in tension while the cartilage and fibrous tissue in the central bridging region, C, provides excellent compressive resistance. Thus, the two regions act in concert much like the anulus fibrosus and nucleus pulposus coupling the vertebral bodies by providing the needed tensile and compressive resistance to the stresses of bending and torsion. Since the callus is still compliant, relative motion between the fragments can occur and resistance to bending can be assisted by the compression of the surrounding soft tissues, S, in this early phase of fracture healing.

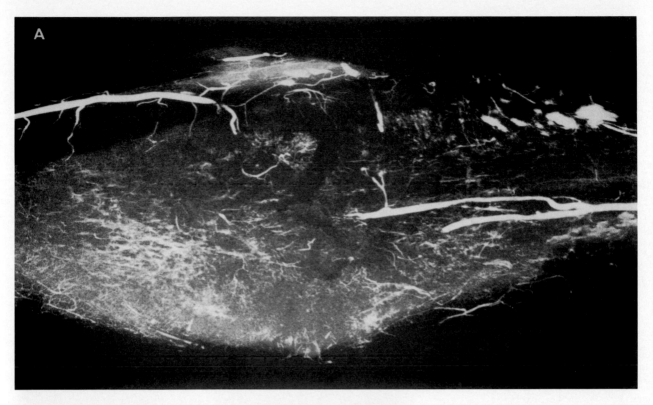

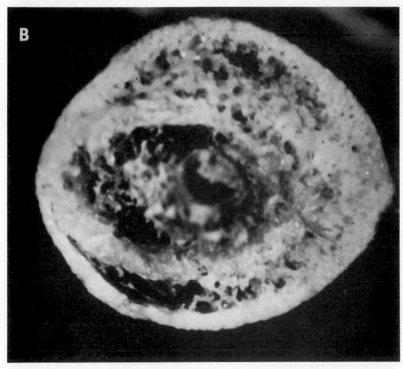

**Fig. 24–4  A:** Medullary circulation is almost always disrupted at a fracture site, and early vascular invasion comes from the peripheral soft tissues, stimulated by muscle function (upper left). **B:** The first blood supply to the bridging tissues comes from the periphery; thus the first calcification of tissue bridging the fracture site occurs in the periphery. Consequently, the most well remodeled bridging tissue is in the periphery of the callus, as shown in this refracture surface of rat callus with cartilage covering the ends of the original diaphyseal bone. (Reproduced with permission from Sarmiento A, Latta LL: *Closed Functional Treatment of Fractures*. New York, Springer-Verlag, 1981.)

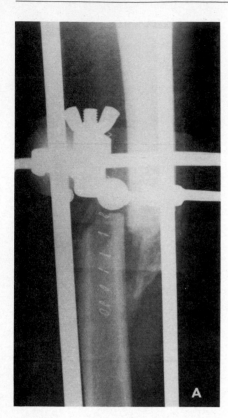

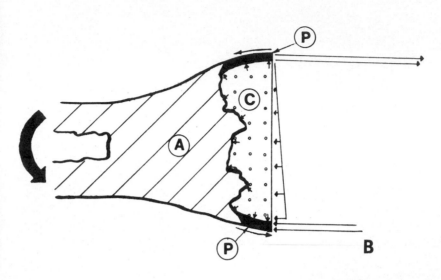

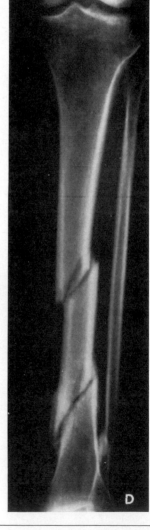

**Fig. 24–5  A:** With peripheral calcification and persistence of soft tissue in the central portion of the bridging callus, an outline of the peripheral callus appears on radiograph, but radiolucency persists in the central portion, as shown in this same femur fracture six weeks following injury. **B:** At this point, the callus is rigid because the peripheral bone formation bridging the fracture site can resist both in tension and compression, which relieves a great deal of the compressive stress on the central portion of the callus, providing rigidity termed "hard callus," or stage III fracture healing. This peripheral bone has a significant mechanical advantage because of the size of the callus. Thus, while radiolucency persists in the radiograph of the callus, the callus often is stronger than the surrounding bone. **C:** This fact has been demonstrated in healing rat fractures five weeks following fracture. **D:** It has been demonstrated in the human by this patient who sustained a refracture in the midshaft of his tibia while the distal spiral fracture of his tibia was in stage III fracture repair. (Reproduced with permission from Sarmiento A, Latta LL: *Closed Functional Treatment of Fractures.* New York, Springer-Verlag, 1981.)

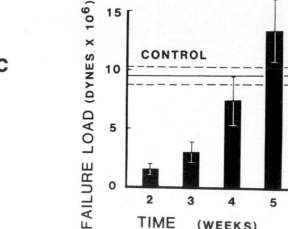

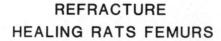

**C**

To illustrate, a piece of meat was wrapped around a hinge and the rigidity of the system measured under a combination of compression and bending loading similar to the typical loading on a broken limb during functional activities. Wrapping brown paper around the meat to confine and compress it increased the rigidity of the system nearly 100 times (Fig. 24–8). Wrapping the same piece of meat with a sheet of Orthoplast and compressing the soft tissue increased the rigidity of the system only two times over the rigidity provided by the brown paper. This simple model illustrates the relative importance of soft-tissue compression compared with material rigidity of the brace. Orthoplast is at least 100 times more rigid than the brown paper.

Soft tissues confined in a cylinder that provides compression have a mechanical advantage in three-point resistance to angulation of the confined bone fragments (Fig. 24–8). Rotational and length stability,

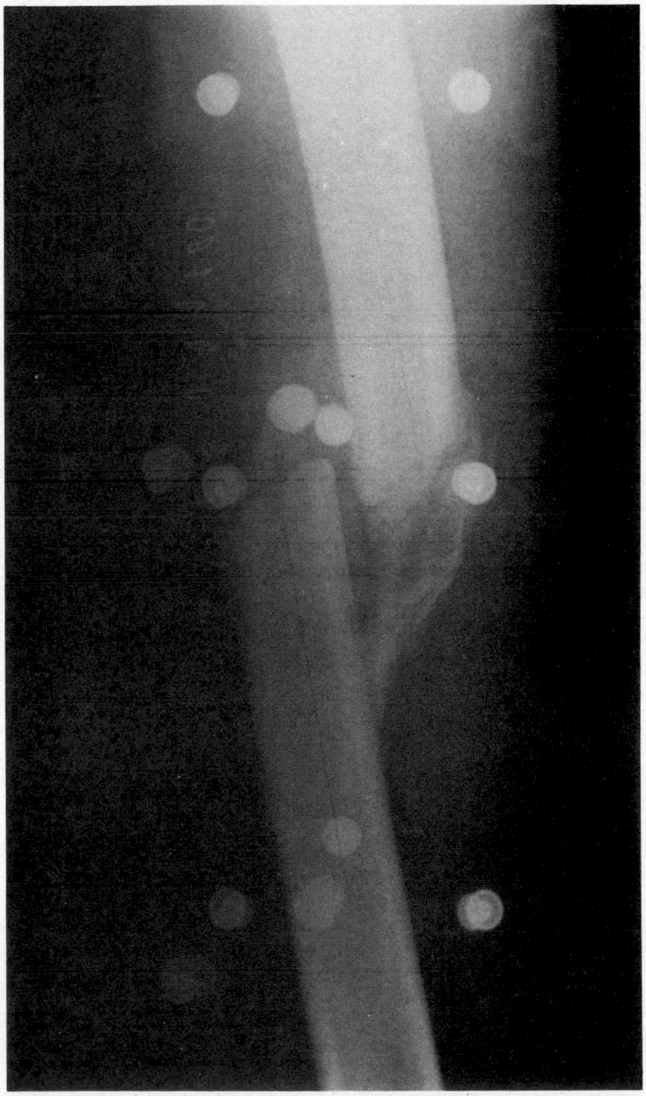

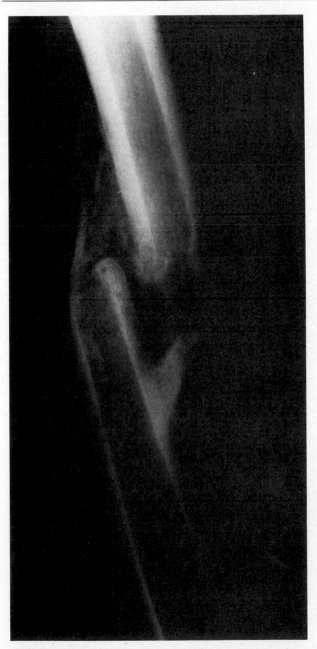

**Fig. 24–7** Stage V fracture healing involves remodeling of the total callus structure, as the biologic system attempts to regenerate diaphyseal bone. In the same femur fracture 41 weeks following injury, a late phase of this remodeling is demonstrated by major shrinkage of the periosteal callus and smoothing of the bone ends.

**Fig. 24–6** Stage IV fracture healing does not significantly improve the mechanical strength of the healing bone but is a radiographically distinct stage in fracture healing. Endochondral ossification obliterates the central radiolucent zone and the fracture line consolidates, as in this same femur fracture eight weeks following injury. (Reproduced with permission from Sarmiento A, Latta LL, Tarr RR: The effects of function in fracture healing and stability. American Academy of Orthopaedic Surgeons *Instructional Course Lectures, XXXIII*. St Louis, CV Mosby, 1984, pp 83–106.)

however, is significantly poorer than angulatory stability. By the time the callus has reached stage II fracture healing, the soft tissue in the callus provides sufficient inherent stability to resist rotation and pistoning of the fragments. Early functional activity can take place with minimal discomfort as long as the limb is stabilized through soft-tissue compression against angulation. Under these conditions, near-normal functional activity can be resumed prior to reaching stage III.

## Humeral Shaft Fractures

### Introduction

Closed methods have been successful in managing humeral shaft fractures because of the high rate of union[14-27] and achievement of acceptable levels of cosmesis and function without anatomic reduction.[14-17,19,22-26,28] Historically, the most common methods of nonoperative treatment have been coaptation splints, hanging casts, and Velpeau band-

**Fig. 24–8  A:** This simple model of an unstable limb consists of a hinge wrapped with a piece of meat and bent by an eccentric compression load. **B:** Soft-tissue compression accomplished by a very weak and compliant brown paper enhanced the rigidity of the system nearly 100 times. **C:** Soft-tissue compression with an Orthoplast sleeve increased the rigidity only by another twofold. Thus, the soft-tissue compression of the cylindrical encasement and not the rigidity of the material in the sleeve was the major factor providing rigidity to the system.

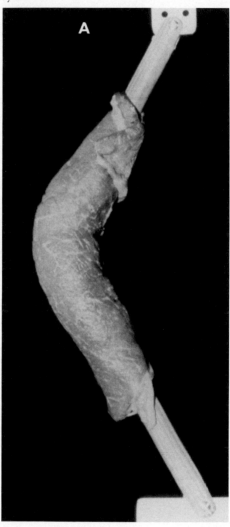
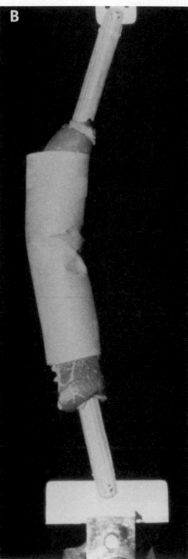
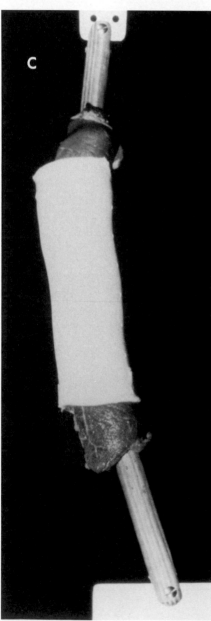

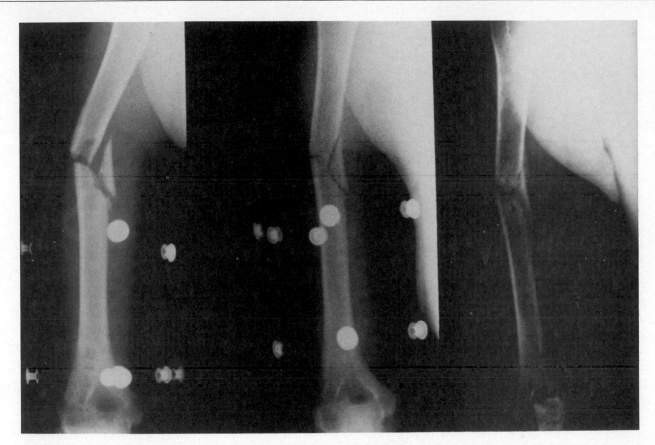

**Fig. 24–9** Fracture bracing of the humerus takes advantage of the inherent instability of the upper arm. The typical varus and internal rotation deformity produced by positioning the arm in a sling can be reduced by early gravity alignment of the extremity. The elbow can be straightened and passive exercises can begin while the fracture site is still unstable. Continuing this early function and natural gravity alignment encourages an acceptable alignment at final healing.

ages.[14,16,18,19,24–26,29,30] However, many problems have been associated with these methods, including (1) adhesive capsulitis of the shoulder, (2) elbow stiffness after device removal, (3) transient inferior shoulder subluxation caused by disuse atrophy, and (4) lengthy periods of rehabilitation following immobilization.

In the mid-1970s, Sarmiento[31,32] demonstrated that in the lower extremity early motion and early function eliminated many of the problems associated with prolonged immobilization. Applying these concepts to the humerus, he and his co-workers successfully treated humeral fractures with custom-fitted fracture braces.[22] Despite rewarding results, it became obvious that the application of custom-fitted devices had significant disadvantages. The technique was time-consuming, expensive, and required the services of an experienced orthotist. As bracing became more popular, problems arose with inconsistent quality of application, limited durability of materials, poor adjustability of the custom braces, and overall poor delivery of service to the patients.[27,33] A satisfactory, standardized, prefabricated brace was needed that would be easy to apply, low in cost, comfortable, and removable for hygienic purposes while still permitting early function and clinical efficacy.[34,35]

## Design Considerations

The humerus is in an inherently unstable limb segment, with only one bone surrounded by a thick layer of soft tissue and often a thick layer of adipose tissue. It is therefore not uncommon to see internal rotation and varus angulation deformities in patients initially treated with a hanging cast. Fracture bracing management is designed to take advantage of the early instability in the arm by achieving elbow extension as early as possible, which provides gravity alignment of the arm and early functional activity, with a natural realignment of the fragments (Fig. 24–9). Patients treated with a sling commonly experience an early varus and internal rotation deformity. With fracture bracing, these patients achieve realignment of the fragments, with early functional activity and gravity alignment. This situation is the only one in the authors' experience in which improved alignment of the fracture fragments contained within a fracture brace can be anticipated.

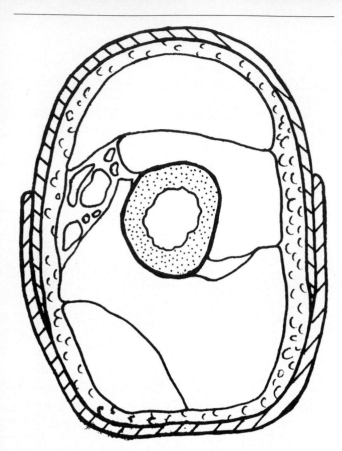

**Fig. 24–10** The cross section of the interlocking shells maintains the natural curvature of the biceps and flattening of the triceps during circumferential adjustments.

Another main objective in brace design and application is the achievement of early motion of the elbow joint and arm, which naturally activates the musculature surrounding the fracture site. As stated previously, this muscle activation in the fracture area may be important for maintaining the optimal milieu for fracture healing in a stressful environment where motion occurs at the fracture site.

Custom brace designs accomplished these mechanical goals by developing the proper clinical protocol. Because of the perceived minor role of the brace, development of prefabricated designs seemed easy. The earliest prefabricated device developed by Sarmiento consisted of a one-piece, wrap-around polypropylene sleeve. Although polypropylene is rigid and durable, material properties are not critical to brace function. Therefore, the authors chose low-density polyethylene, which has adequate durability, but is more compliant than polypropylene. Thus, comfort can be achieved without sacrificing structural rigidity. Capps and Sarmiento[35] simultaneously came to similar conclusions.

Patients with wrap-around sleeves reviewed by the authors at the University of Miami had an increased number of angulatory deformities.[27] In the authors' experience, then, the optimal design of a humerus fracture brace provides adjustability by means of anterior and posterior interlocking shells (Fig. 24–10). The anterior components should have a bicipital contour to maintain suspension, while the posterior component should be flat to mold the triceps. Velcro straps allowing for adjustability during the various phases of fracture healing maintain soft-tissue compression (Fig. 24–11).[17] Braces with suspension straps are awkward and unnecessary. Designs that have an over-the-shoulder extension are to be avoided, as they prohibit full range of motion of the shoulder and frequently cause limitation of shoulder motion after brace removal. Designs that do not completely encompass the soft tissues of the extremity should also be avoided, as they violate the basic principle of soft-tissue encasement[8,9] and, therefore, cannot provide adequate soft-tissue compression and fracture stability.

### Indications and Contraindications

Fracture bracing is indicated for fractures of the humeral diaphysis. The contraindications here are essentially the same as the general contraindications for fracture bracing: (1) massive soft-tissue or bony loss in the extremity, (2) unreliable or uncooperative patients, and (3) inability to obtain or maintain acceptable alignment.

### Treatment Protocol

In managing humeral shaft fractures, fracture bracing requires the same meticulous attention to detail as does operative reduction and internal fixation. A prefabricated orthotic device will lead to excellent results if early function and early motion are encouraged. In the authors' initial applications to the humerus, bracing was a secondary means of management. Since 1983, however, the authors have applied fracture braces primarily on the day of injury.

The present protocol developed at the University of Miami consists of (1) alignment of the fracture, (2) application of the prefabricated device over cast padding, and (3) application of a sling on the initial day of injury (Fig. 24–12A). The patient is seen the following day for reevaluation of neurovascular status and edema. The patient is then seen approximately one week after injury, at which time the cast padding is removed and a double layer of cotton stockinette is applied to the extremity. The brace is reapplied and a radiograph is obtained to check for satisfactory alignment (Fig. 24–12, B and C). The patient is then instructed by the occupational therapist to begin pendulum exercises of the shoulder, passive flexion of the upper extremity, and active function of the hand, wrist, and elbow within the brace. At this point, the brace can be removed for hygienic purposes only, and the patient is supplied with an extra cotton stockinette for cleaning and changing. During the second week after injury, alignment within the brace is checked radiographically (with the patient in the upright position), and active use of the hand, wrist, elbow, and shoulder are encouraged.

The patient is then seen at intervals of three or four weeks. At each visit, the extremity is evaluated radiographically and clinically. Function and range of motion are regularly evaluated. When evidence of union is confirmed both clinically and radiographically, brace use is discontinued (Figs. 24–12, D and E, and 24–13). The patient is evaluated on a long-term basis thereafter.

For open fractures, initial treatment consists of operative irrigation, exploration and debridement, and intravenous antibiotic therapy; the wounds are left open. Fracture bracing is used at the time of the first dressing change.

### Results and Discussion

At the University of Miami's Special Fracture Clinic, 337 humeral shaft fractures have been treated, with 208 patients evaluated at follow-up. The average age of the patients was 36 years with a range of 15 to 90 years. The mean time until union for closed fractures was 9.5 weeks and for open fractures 13.6 weeks. The mean time until union for the entire group was 10.6 weeks with a range of five to 20 weeks.

**Anatomy** Fractures were evaluated with reference to angulation, rotation, and shortening. The average varus-valgus angulation was 5 degrees. The average anterior-posterior angulation was 3 degrees. Eighty-nine percent of the patients had 8 degrees or less of varus or valgus angulation; 86% had 8 degrees or less of anterior or posterior angulation. It has generally been agreed that in the humerus minor angulatory deformities are clinically insignificant[16,22,25,27,28] and the authors' experience confirms the findings of others. No clinically significant rotational deformities were detected.

Shortening was evaluated by radiograph. The mean radiographic shortening was 4 mm with a range of 1 to 15 mm. In this series, no patient with humeral shortening demonstrated any clinically significant functional or cosmetic problems. Indeed, humeral shortening of up to 5 cm has been shown to be clinically insignificant.[36]

**Function** Function was evaluated in terms of shoulder and elbow range of motion and performance of daily activities. Ninety-three percent of the authors' patients achieved an excellent functional result, demonstrating nearly full range of motion of the extremity. Five percent of the patients achieved a good functional result, lacking up to 15 degrees of terminal forward flexion of the shoulder or up to 5 degrees of terminal extension at the elbow. Two percent of the patients achieved a poor result secondary to nonunion of the fracture. The overwhelming majority of patients required formal physical or occupational therapy only in the first few weeks of their injury during brace wear. Only a few patients required post-treatment rehabilitation of the extremity.

**Complications** Complications following this technique were minimal. Four patients (2%) developed nonunion. These patients had open reduction and internal fixation with bone grafting and subsequently healed with good functional results. Two patients (1%) had problems with skin maceration. These pa-

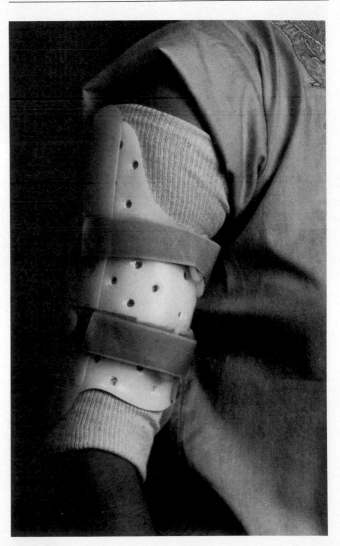

**Fig. 24–11** The humerus fracture brace developed at the University of Miami Special Fracture Clinic provides encasement for the soft tissues in the mid-section of the arm, relief for a complete range of motion of the elbow and shoulder, and just enough molding of the biceps to maintain suspension with soft-tissue compression.

## Conclusions

Patients with isolated ulnar shaft fractures can be treated with prefabricated fracture braces with excellent to good results in more than 90% of the cases. The high union rate can probably be attributed to allowing early extremity function with its resultant known beneficial effects on fracture healing. The best anatomic and functional outcome is seen in distal-third fractures with less than 10 degrees of angulation at the time of brace application.

Fractures in the proximal two-thirds must be braced with caution because unacceptable angulation may ensue. If angulation is greater than 10 degrees, then two options exist: (1) perform a closed reduction and immobilize in plaster for two additional weeks and then brace; or (2) perform an open reduction and rigid internal fixation.

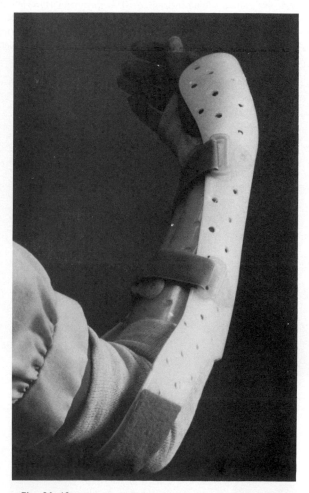

**Fig. 24–18**   The Colles' fracture brace developed at the University of Miami Special Fracture Clinic holds the forearm in a position of relaxed supination. The wrist is blocked in dorsiflexion and radial deviation, and the elbow is blocked from full extension in order to maintain the supination position of the forearm and to maintain suspension of the device. Otherwise, elbow flexion, wrist volar flexion and finger function are unrestricted.

## Colles' Fractures

### Introduction

Historically, the management of Colles' fracture has been controversial.[16,53–72] Numerous methods have been advocated in the treatment of these injuries; the efficacy of bracing Colles' fractures may be questioned. The authors had the opportunity to evaluate several patients who had been treated with external fixation, internal fixation, and closed cast immobilization. On critical analysis, a significant number of these patients had major complications and problems associated with these methods of treatment.

In 1975, Sarmiento and associates[62] reported on the use of fracture braces for fractures of the distal radius. Their conclusion was that functional bracing in supination was a reliable, effective method of treatment for Colles' fractures. A basic principle in brace treatment was to position the forearm in supination. The reasons for treatment in supination are the following: (1) inactivation of brachioradialis[62]; (2) reduction of dorsal-ulnar dislocations[66]; (3) improved leverage on radial collateral ligament (to hold radial length)[66]; (4) parallel position of forearm bones facilitates[66] evaluation of reduction and effective immobilization; (5) facilitates rehabilitation (pronation naturally regained)[66]; (6) loss of pronation compensated for by shoulder abduction[66]; (7) scapholunate dislocation[74] is earlier and more easily recognized, while late complications can be prevented; and (8) flexor muscle mechanical advantage[74] maintains volar compression and minimizes extensor deforming forces.

The question of supination versus pronation has certainly not been resolved.[16,58,59,62,65,66,68–72] In a prospective study by the senior author, a group of patients with fractures of the distal radius braced in supination had anatomic and functional results superior to those braced in pronation.[65,72] Historically, however, functional bracing for Colles' fractures has not been popular or practical. One of the major limitations was the necessity to apply a custom device. This process had inherent problems: (1) loss of reduction by the orthotist at the time of brace application; (2) expense; (3) time; (4) inconvenience of application; and (5) inconsistent and unreliable brace designs and materials. For these reasons, the use of a prefabricated brace has definite advantages over a custom brace.

### Design Considerations

The brace preferred by the authors is composed of a dorsal and volar component. The dorsal component maintains the wrist in ulnar deviation and prevents extension by blocking it at 30 degrees of volar flexion (Fig. 24–18). Full wrist flexion is allowed

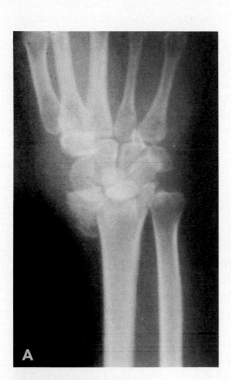

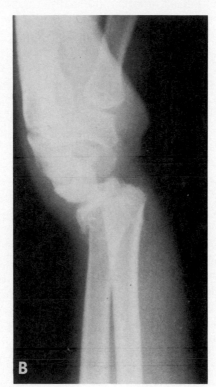

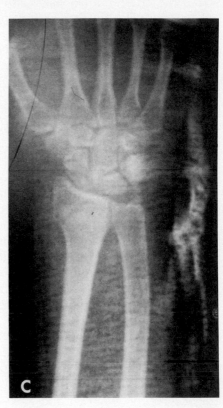

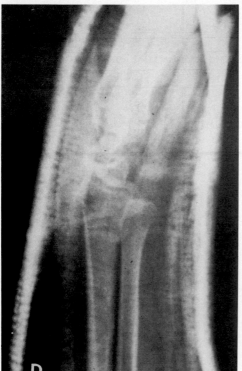

**Fig. 24–19** **A and B:** Type IV badly displaced Colles' fracture. **C and D:** It was reduced on the day of injury and placed in a long-arm cast in relaxed supination with the wrist in volar flexion and the hand in ulnar deviation.

within the brace, but extension and radial deviation are blocked. The forearm is in supination. A volar shell compresses the volar forearm surface to control rotation and maintain a snug fit. There is a supra-condylar elbow extension that prevents rotation and also helps with suspension by preventing slippage of the brace distally. Velcro straps are used to maintain fit. The braces are constructed of low-density poly-ethylene and have vent holes to allow for comfort.[73]

### Treatment Protocol

On the initial day of injury, patients with Colles' fractures are seen in the emergency department, where a closed reduction is performed (Fig. 24–19). It is of utmost importance to have adequate anesthesia for the reduction. In the authors' experience, intrahematoma infiltration with lidocaine is usually insufficient to achieve anatomic restoration by manipulation. The preferred method of anesthesia is intravenous regional block with lidocaine. If, however, this method is impossible or ineffective, then either axillary block or general anesthesia should be used. After anesthesia is administered, the patient is placed in Chinese finger trap suspension with 15 to 20 lb of countertraction for 10 to 15 minutes. The countertraction is then removed and a closed manipulation performed. Anatomic restoration should be sought. A long-arm cast or sugar-tongs plaster is applied in supination with the wrist in 30 degrees of flexion and maximum ulnar deviation. The importance of achieving an anatomic reduction cannot be overemphasized, as the initial reduction will determine the anatomic end result. On the day following reduction, the patient is seen for a neurovascular status and edema. One week after injury, the patient is reevaluated. Alignment is assessed radiographically and a one-week follow-up is arranged.

The second week after injury alignment is evaluated radiographically. If the alignment is satisfactory and the edema has subsided, the plaster is removed and a Colles' prefabricated fracture brace is applied over a double cotton stockinette (Fig. 24–20, A and B). The double stockinette assists in controlling edema. Another radiograph is then obtained to assess alignment with the brace applied.

The patient is then instructed to use the hand, wrist, and elbow, to keep the arm elevated at night, and not to remove the brace. The patient is seen in follow-up on the third week after injury. During this interval, the patient is usually scheduled for occupational therapy for continued range of motion of the hand, wrist, and elbow in the brace. At the third week after injury, an additional radiograph is obtained and, if the results are satisfactory, the patient may be instructed to remove the brace after bathing for hygienic purposes only. The brace should never be removed for more than one or two minutes during a stockinette change. If healing is not progressing normally, the brace should not be removed.

At the sixth week after injury, the fracture brace is removed, radiographs are obtained, function is evaluated and encouraged, and a follow-up is arranged in three to four weeks (Fig. 24–20, C and D). At subsequent visits, evaluation of range of motion and function are performed (Fig. 24–21). Physical or occupational therapy may be prescribed if necessary and further follow-ups are arranged for long-term evaluation.

### Clinical Results

Between 1980 and 1985 at the University of Miami Special Fracture Clinic, 470 patients with displaced Colles' fractures, types II and IV, were examined. Of this number, 106 were excluded or had inadequate follow-up, while 364 patients with 372 fractures were evaluated and treated on a long-term basis. The average follow-up was 10.5 months with a range of three to 31 months. The average time in a plaster cast was 12 days; the average time in the brace was 32 days; the average time to union was 44 days.

All fractures were classified by type as described by Sarmiento and associates[62] in 1975: type I is nondisplaced and extra-articular; type II is displaced and extra-articular; type III is nondisplaced and intra-articular; and type IV is displaced and intra-articular. Anatomic results were evaluated with regard to volar tilt, radial deviation, and radial length. Normal average values are as follows: volar tilt, 11 degrees; radial deviation, 24 degrees; radial length, 12 mm.[65] The results were then evaluated based on the criteria described by Lidstrom[74] in 1959. Based on these criteria, 84% achieved excellent or good anatomic results. Functional results were evaluated based on the criteria of Gartland and Werley[59] in 1951. Using their criteria, 90% achieved excellent or good functional results.

### Complications

The most common complications associated with Colles' fractures are loss of reduction, reflex sympathetic dystrophy, severe edema, and median nerve palsy.

**Reflex Sympathetic Dystrophy** Reflex sympathetic dystrophy (RSD) is frequently associated with a certain patient personality type. The hysterical or uncooperative patient who is excessively apprehensive or unwilling to perform early finger and wrist motion during the course of treatment may develop this syndrome. Prevention is, therefore, stressed and patients with the personality traits associated with RSD should be referred for immediate occupational therapy. An additional preventative measure is to encourage metacarpophalangeal joint flexion early in the course of treatment to prevent stiffness of the fingers and to insure a good functional result. Once the syndrome develops, extensive therapy and splinting for a long period are necessary. Fortunately, with fracture bracing techniques, RSD is uncommon.

**Dependent Edema** Dependent edema may develop in extremities that are not elevated sufficiently or that are braced very early. During the first week, edema usually resolves with frequent elevation of the extremity on pillows and encouragement of function and finger pumping exercises. Edema usually subsides by the third week if these measures are instituted.

**Median Nerve Palsy** In this series, median nerve palsy was usually related to poor initial casting technique. Very frequently the wrist was placed in excessive volar flexion (greater than 30 degrees) or the cast was too tight. The authors' preferred treatment of median nerve palsy involves removal of the initial cast or immobilization device, application of sugar-tongs plaster, and hospitalization of the patient for elevation and observation. In the overwhelming majority of cases, the median nerve palsy will resolve spontaneously. However, if a median nerve palsy is associated with a large volar fracture fragment displaced into the carpal tunnel and spontaneous improvement

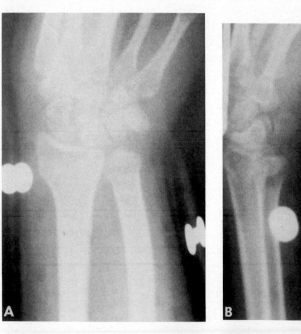

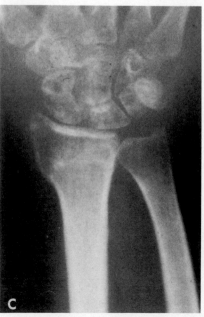

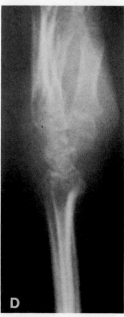

**Fig. 24–20  A and B:** Ten days following injury, the patient was placed in a fracture brace. **C and D:** The reduction was maintained until brace removal eight weeks following injury.

does not occur within the first week, then surgical exploration may be indicated. If the carpal tunnel is released during surgical exploration, the fracture should be stabilized either internally or with an external fixator to maintain fracture position. This procedure allows the wrist to be placed in the neutral position, which is preferable for postoperative carpal tunnel exploration, but which is contraindicated for Colles' fracture management.

**Loss of Reduction**  In the authors' experience, loss of reduction appears to be related to the quality of the initial reduction. If an unsatisfactory initial reduction is accepted, progressive collapse is generally the rule. Very frequently, however, with the use of functional bracing techniques the patient may still achieve a satisfactory functional result despite loss of reduction and unsatisfactory anatomic results. If, however, loss of reduction and malunion are associated with a poor functional result or are unacceptable for any reason, then operative intervention may be indicated.

Mechanical, anatomic, and physiologic factors may contribute to loss of reduction of the fracture. Since maintenance of reduction may depend on these factors, they should be considered in order to insure a satisfactory outcome.

In the normal anatomy, the axial forces across the wrist and forearm fall within the volar half (compression side) of the radius. What the authors have called "the volar axial force line," therefore, can be drawn on a lateral radiograph (Fig. 24–22A) by drawing the central longitudinal axis of the radial shaft (line A) and extending it through the distal radial joint. Next, the midpoint of the radiolunate joint is identified (point B) and a line parallel to the longitudinal axial line is drawn (line B-C). If this line (volar axial force line) falls volar to the longitudinal axis line, then the forces are properly distributed across the wrist. If the line falls dorsal to the longitudinal line, the forces across the wrist are dorsal and fracture collapse may occur or progress. (See Fig. 24–22B.)

The fracture configuration is a significant anatomic factor in determining stability. The most significant factor is the presence of volar cortical comminution.[73] In the typical Colles' fracture, the dorsal cortex tends to be comminuted, while the volar cortex is usually noncomminuted. However, in some cases, the volar cortex will also be comminuted. It has been the authors' experience that volar cortical comminution is associated with instability. If the fracture is under-reduced, dorsal collapse may be expected. Similarly, if the fracture is overreduced and the volar cortices of the proximal and distal fragments do not abut, collapse may also occur.

Muscular forces are the physiologic factors that determine stability. The forces of the extensor carpi radialis brevis and longus, extensor digitorum communis, and brachioradialis muscles have a role in fracture stability. Ideally, an effort should be made to maximize volar forces across the wrist and minimize extensor forces. Since the comminuted side tends to be the tension side (the extensor surface), the stresses on the compressive (volar) side of the bone must be

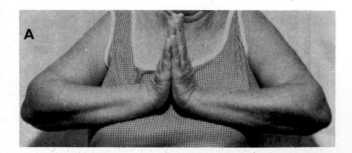
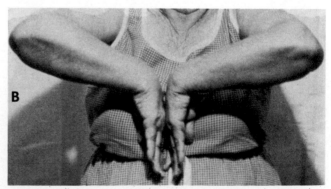
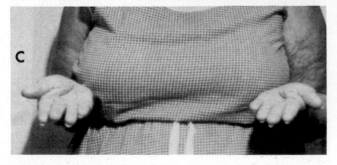
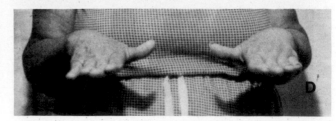

**Fig. 24–21**  **A and B:** One month following brace removal, the patient demonstrates near-normal range of wrist flexion and extension. **C and D:** Forearm rotation is also nearly normal.

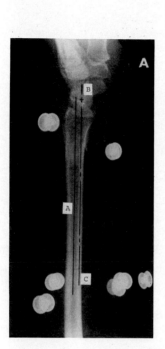
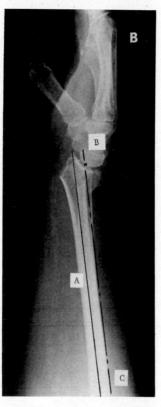
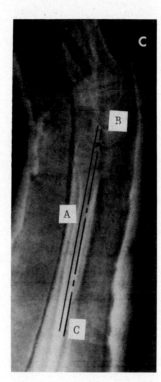
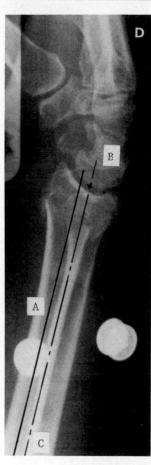

**Fig. 24–22**  **A:** The central longitudinal axis of the radial shaft is extended through the distal radial joint, A. Through the midpoint of the radiolunate joint, B, a parallel line, B-C, should fall volar to A. **B:** Initial radiograph of injury demonstrates dorsal displacement with typical dorsal position of axial joint line, B-C. **C:** Post reduction radiograph with arm in plaster cast demonstrates inadequate alignment of fracture as manifested by persistent dorsal position of axial joint line, B-C. **D:** Radiograph of arm in the fracture brace demonstrating progressive dorsal collapse and dorsal displacement of axial joint line, B-C. Dorsal collapse was seen in the majority of the cases that were reduced without proper reestablishment of the axial joint line.

maximized. Positioning the forearm in supination, as compared with pronation, provides a mechanical advantage to the flexor muscles and simultaneously minimizes the pull of the extensors.[62,65,73] In addition, the force of the brachioradialis is minimized in supination.[67]

## Conclusions

When properly applied in the carefully selected patient, the use of a prefabricated brace for Colles' fracture management is a reliable method of treatment. Its effectiveness in controlling fracture position while allowing early function and motion of the hand and wrist has been proven.[62,65] The complications and problems associated with invasive techniques are uncommon with bracing, and prolonged therapy after treatment is less common than with many other methods of management. The advantages, therefore, also include the benefit of cost effectiveness as well as

minimizing stiffness and the need for rehabilitation associated with Colles' fractures.

## References

1. Sarmiento A, Latta LL, Zilioli A, et al: The role of soft tissues in stabilization of tibial fracture. *Clin Orthop* 1974;105:116.
2. Lippert FG, Hirsch C: The three-dimensional measurement of tibial fracture motion by photogrammetry. *Clin Orthop* 1974;105:130.
3. Yamagishi M, Yoshimura Y: The biomechanics of fracture healing. *J Bone Joint Surg* 1955;37A:1035–1068.
4. Sarmiento A, Schaeffer J, Beckerman L, et al: Fracture healing in rat femora as affected by functional weight-bearing. *J Bone Joint Surg* 1977;59A:369.
5. Latta LL, Sarmiento A, Tarr RR: The rationale of functional bracing of fractures. *Clin Orthop* 1980;146:28.
6. Sarmiento A, Latta LL, Tarr RR: Principles of fracture healing: Part II. The effects of function in fracture healing and stability. American Academy of Orthopaedic Surgeons *Instructional Course Lectures, XXXIII.* St Louis, CV Mosby Co, 1984, pp 83–106.

7. Latta LL, Sarmiento A: Periosteal fracture callus mechanics, in *Symposium on Trauma to the Leg and its Sequela.* St Louis, CV Mosby Co, 1980.

8. Zych GA, Zagorski JB, Latta LL: Current concepts in fracture bracing: Part I. Upper extremity. *Orthopaedic Surgery Update.* Princeton, New Jersey, Continuing Professional Education Center, 1986, vol 4, lesson 18.

9. Sarmiento A, Latta LL: *Closed Functional Treatment of Fractures.* New York, Springer-Verlag, 1981.

10. Connolly JF, Dehne E, LaFollette B: Closed reduction and early cast-brace ambulation in the treatment of femoral fractures: Part II. Results in one hundred and forty-three fractures. *J Bone Joint Surg* 1973;55A:1581.

11. Kruse RL, Kelly PJ: Acceleration of fracture healing distal to a venous tourniquet. *J Bone Joint Surg* 1974;56A:730.

12. Perren SM: Physical and biological aspects of fracture healing with special reference to internal fixation. *Clin Orthop* 1979;138:175.

13. White AA, Panjabi MM, Crelin ES, et al: A quantitative biomechanical study of fracture repair. Kappa Delta Award Paper 3, Presented at the 43rd Annual Meeting of the American Academy of Orthopaedic Surgeons, New Orleans, 1976.

14. Böhler L: *The Treatment of Fractures,* suppl vol. New York, Grune & Stratton, 1966.

15. Cave EA: *Fractures and Their Injuries.* Chicago, Year Book Publishers, 1958.

16. Charnley, J: *The Closed Treatment of Common Fractures.* Baltimore, Williams & Wilkins, 1961.

17. Christensen S: Humeral shaft fractures, operative and conservative treatment. *Acta Chir Scand* 1967;133:455.

18. DePalma AF: *The Management of Fractures and Dislocations.* Philadelphia, WB Saunders, 1970.

19. LaFerte AD, Nutter PD: The treatment of fractures of the humerus by means of hanging plaster cast—"Hanging cast." *Ann Surg* 1941;114:919.

20. McMaster WC, Tivnon MC, Waugh TR: Cast brace for the upper extremity. *Clin Orthop* 1975;109:126–129.

21. Parrish FF, Murray JA: Surgical treatment for secondary neoplastic fractures: A retrospective study of 96 patients. *J Bone Joint Surg* 1970;52A:655–686.

22. Sarmiento A, Kinman PB, Galvin EG, et al: Functional bracing of fractures of the shaft of the humerus. *J Bone Joint Surg* 1977;59A:596.

23. Scientific Research Committee, Pennsylvania Orthopaedic Society: Fresh midshaft fractures of the humerus in adults. *Pa Med J* 1959;62:848.

24. Stewart MJ, Hundley JM: Fractures of the humerus: A comparative study in methods of treatment. *J Bone Joint Surg* 1955;37A:681–692.

25. Stewart MJ: Fractures of the humeral shaft, in Adams JP (ed): *Current Practice in Orthopaedic Surgery.* St Louis, CV Mosby Co, 1964.

26. Winfield JM, Miller H, LaFerte AD: Evaluation of the "hanging cast" as a method of treating fractures of humerus. *Am J Surg* 1942;55:228.

27. Zagorski JB, Schenkman JH: The management of humerus fractures with prefabricated braces. *Orthop Trans* 1983;7:516.

28. Hudson RT: The use of the hanging cast in treatment of fractures of the humerus. *South Surgeon* 1941;10:132.

29. Klenerman L: Fractures of the shaft of the humerus. *J Bone Joint Surg* 1966;48B:105.

30. Holm CL: Management of humeral shaft fractures: Fundamentals of nonoperative techniques. *Clin Orthop* 1970;71:132.

31. Sarmiento A: A functional below-the-knee brace for tibial fractures. *J Bone Joint Surg* 1967;49A:855.

32. Sarmiento A: A functional below-the-knee brace for tibial fractures. *J Bone Joint Surg* 1970;52A:295.

33. Zagorski JB, Schenkman JH: The use of prefabricated functional orthoses for fractures of the tibia, humerus and distal radius. *Orthop Trans* 1982;6:88.

34. Balfour GW, Mooney V, Ashby ME: Diaphyseal fractures of the humerus treated with a ready-made fracture brace. *J Bone Joint Surg* 1982;64A:11.

35. Capps CC, Sarmiento A: Prefabricated fracture brace for humeral shaft fractures. Presented at the 52nd Annual Meeting of the American Academy of Orthopaedic Surgeons, Las Vegas, Nevada, January 1985, p 101.

36. Burhalter WE: Personal communication.

37. Rockwood CA, Green, DP: *Fractures in Adults.* Philadelphia, JB Lippincott, 1984.

38. Holstein A, Lewis GB: Fractures of the humerus with radial-nerve paralysis. *J Bone Joint Surg* 1963;45A:1382.

39. Garcia A Jr, Maeck BH: Radial nerve injuries in fractures of the shaft of the humerus. *Am J Surg* 1960;99:625.

40. Kettlekemp DB, Alexander H: Clinical review of radial nerve injury. *J Trauma* 1967;7:424.

41. Shah JJ, Bhatti NA: Fracture of humerus and radial nerve paralysis. *Orthop Trans* 1982;6:455.

42. Szalay EA, Rockwood CA: Fractured humerus with radial nerve palsy. *Orthop Trans* 1982;6:455.

43. Altner PC, Hartman JT: Isolated fractures of the ulnar shaft in the adult. *Surg Clin North Am* 1972;52:155–170.

44. Anderson LD: Fractures of the shafts of the radius and ulna, in Rockwood CA, Green DP (eds): *Fractures,* ed 2. Philadelphia, JB Lippincott Co, 1984, vol 1, pp 541–542.

45. Anderson LD, Sisk TD, Tooms RE, et al: Compression plate fixation in acute diaphyseal fractures of the radius and ulna. *J Bone Joint Surg* 1975;57A:287–296.

46. de Buren N: Causes and treatment of non-union in fractures of the radius and ulna. *J Bone Joint Surg* 1962;44B:614–625.

47. Hooper G: Isolated fractures of the shaft of the ulna. *Injury* 1974;6:180–184.

48. Pollock FH, Pankovich AM, Prieto JJ, et al: The isolated fracture of the ulnar shaft: Treatment without immobilization. *J Bone Joint Surg* 1983;65A:339–342.

49. Sarmiento A, Cooper JS, Sinclair WF: Forearm fractures: Early functional bracing—A preliminary report. *J Bone Joint Surg* 1975;57A:297.

50. Sarmiento A, Kinman PB, Murphy RB, et al: Treatment of ulnar fractures by functional bracing. *J Bone Joint Surg* 1976;58A:1104.

51. Grace TG, Witmer BJ: Isolated fractures of the ulnar shaft. *Orthop Trans* 1980;4:299.

52. Zych GA, Zagorski JB, Latta LL: Treatment of isolated ulnar fractures with prefabricated fracture braces. *Clin Orthop* 1987;219:88–94.

53. Böhler L, in Graves EWH (ed): *The Treatment of Fractures.* William Ward & Co, 1935, pp 227–234.

54. Brady LP: Double pin fixation of severely comminuted fractures of the distal radius and ulna. *South Med J* 1963;56:307–311.

55. Cassebaum WH: Colles' fractures: A study of end results. *JAMA* 1950;143:963–966.

56. Cole JM, Obletz BE: Comminuted fractures of the distal end of the radius treated by skeletal transfixion in plaster cast. *J Bone Joint Surg* 1966;48A:931–945.

57. DePalma AF: Comminuted fractures of the distal end of the radius treated by ulnar pinning. *J Bone Joint Surg* 1952;34A:651–662.

58. Dowling JJ, Sawyer B Jr: Comminuted Colles' fractures: Evolution of a method of treatment. *J Bone Joint Surg* 1961;43A:657–668.

59. Gartland JJ, Werley CW: Evaluation of healed Colles' fractures. *J Bone Joint Surg* 1951;33A:895–907.

60. Green DP: Pins and plaster treatment of comminuted fractures of the distal end of the radius. *J Bone Joint Surg* 1975;57A:304.

61. Older TM, Stabler EV, Cassebaum WH: Colles' fracture: Evaluation and selection of therapy. *J Trauma* 1965;5:469–476.

62. Sarmiento A, Pratt GW, Berry NC, et al: Colles' fractures: Functional bracing in supination. *J Bone Joint Surg* 1975;57A:311.

63. Scheck M: Long-term follow-up of treatment of comminuted fractures of the distal end of the radius by transfixation with Kirschner wires and cast. *J Bone Joint Surg* 1962;44A:337–351.

64. Clancy GJ: Percutaneous Kirschner wire fixation of Colles' fractures: A prospective study of thirty cases. *J Bone Joint Surg* 1984;66A:1008–1014.

65. Sarmiento A, Zagorski JB, Sinclair WF: Functional bracing of Colles' fractures: A prospective study of immobilization in supination vs. pronation. *Clin Orthop* 1980;146:175.

66. Raisbeck CC, Ungersma JA: Paradoxical reduction of Colles' fracture. *J Bone Joint Surg* 1967;49A:1246.

67. Sarmiento A: The brachioradialis as a deforming force in Colles' fractures. *Clin Orthop* 1965;38:86.

68. Mason K: The management of Colles' fractures. *Med Illustrated* 1954;8:837–842.

69. Unger B, Lund S, Rasmussen P: Early results after Colles' fracture: Functional bracing in supination vs. dorsal plaster immobilization. *Acta Orthop Trauma Surg* 1984;103(4):251–256.

70. Stewart HD, Innes AR, Burke FD: Functional cast-bracing for Colles' fractures: A comparison between cast-bracing and conventional plaster casts. *J Bone Joint Surg* 1984;66B:749–753.

71. Wilson C, Veneer RM: Colles' fracture: Immobilization in pronation or supination. *J R Coll Surg Edinb* 1984;29(2):109–111.

72. Zagorski JB: Functional bracing of Colles' fractures: A prospective study of immobilization in supination vs pronation. *Orthop Trans* 1979;3:62.

73. Zagorski JB, Zych G, Latta L, et al: Colles' fracture management using prefabricated braces. *Orthop Trans* 1986;10:471–472.

74. Lidstrom A: Fractures of the distal end of the radius: A clinical and statistical study of end results. *Acta Orthop Scand* 1959, suppl 41.

# Modern Concepts in Functional Fracture Bracing: The Lower Limb

Gregory A. Zych, DO

Joseph B. Zagorski, MD

Loren L. Latta, PE, PhD

Newton C. McCollough III, MD

## The Role of Soft-Tissue Mechanics in Lower Limb Bracing

In the lower limb, motion at the fracture site can be extensive in the early phases of fracture healing because of the high mechanical demands of weight-bearing.[1-3] As in the upper limb, controlled motion at the fracture site with early functional activity is recoverable or elastic. When controlled by soft-tissue compression, displacement of the fragments with functional activity results in zero net displacement. Fracture instability and controlled fracture site motion are, therefore, not the same. Fracture instability results in a positive net displacement. Loss of reduction and subsequent malunion is a product of instability, *not* of controlled motion at the fracture site, which affects healing by causing abundant periosteal callus formation. Motion controlled by rigid internal fixation is microscopic; it affects healing by preventing periosteal callus formation and causing direct bone formation.[4]

Fracture stability is affected by the intrinsic strength of the soft tissues or, in the case of internal fixation, the strength of fixation. In the unstable phase of fracture healing, relative immobilization of weightbearing bones is important. During stage II fracture healing, intrinsic stability is achieved by soft-tissue healing; the limb becomes stable in rotation and length but remains unstable in angulation.[5] Fracture brace support through soft-tissue compression can provide the required angulatory stability to allow for early functional activity in the second stage of fracture healing. Therefore, the authors' preferred treatment of fractured weightbearing bones involves initial immobilization in a cast or traction during the unstable phase of fracture healing, followed by functional activity in a fracture brace begun during the soft-callus phase of fracture healing.

With soft-tissue compression in a fracture brace, the hydraulic or incompressible, fluid nature of the soft tissues helps control motion at the fracture site and provides rigidity to the limb.[6] Such controlled motion at the fracture site, however, is not directly proportional to the load applied.[7] The first few millimeters of displacement occurs with a relatively small load. This motion occurs because the slack is being taken up in the system of soft tissue and fracture brace. Once this slack has been taken up, increases in load are associated with far less motion, and limb rigidity can be achieved by soft-tissue compression with the encompassing fracture brace sleeve. Thus, at relatively small loads, several millimeters of motion can be observed by cineradiography at the fracture site. At the same time, in the same fracture, weightbearing may be possible with only a few more millimeters of motion.[1,3] The rigidity of the limb with soft-tissue compression provided by the fracture brace is similar to the original stiffness of the limb once a few millimeters of motion has taken place at the fracture site (Fig. 25–1). Thus, fracture-site motion can be controlled under weightbearing conditions by the brace and progressive deformity and malunion can be prevented.

The intrinsic strength of the soft tissues provides the stability to resist progressive deformity. The amount of initial displacement of the fragments at the time of injury is proportional to the degree of soft-tissue disruption or loss of intrinsic soft-tissue strength (Fig. 25–1). Therefore, early functional activity can be resumed with the fragments in their initially displaced position with no further instability beyond that provided by the initial injury. If overriding fragments from the initial injury are reduced and early weightbearing is begun, the fragments will return to the initial overriding experienced at the time of injury. At this point the intrinsic strength of the soft tissues can stabilize against further shortening. If the initial overriding is unacceptable, however, it is impractical to attempt to reduce the fragments and begin early functional activity and weightbearing in a fracture brace. Intrinsic soft-tissue strength must develop in a reduced position to maintain that reduced position. Early soft-tissue healing can be accomplished in three to four weeks in most fractures and by six weeks in highly damaged fractures with soft-tissue loss. To maintain reduced overriding for this time period, some other form of fixation is required, such as non-weightbearing casts, external or internal fixation. After intrinsic stability is regained by soft-tissue healing, it is possible to place the patient in a fracture brace and allow weightbearing and functional activity with maintenance of limb length by the soft tissues and maintenance of angulation by the brace (Fig. 25–2). In those patients who

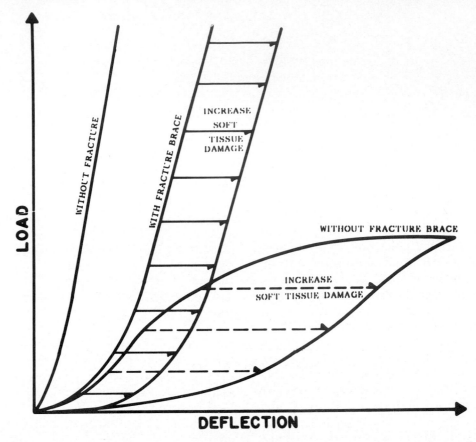

**Fig. 25–1** Axial compression applied in the laboratory to an above-knee amputation specimen produces a minor deflection between the foot and the knee when the tibia and fibula are intact, resulting in a curve with very steep slope (labeled "without fracture") demonstrating high rigidity in the leg. With production of a closed fracture, the leg shortens under the same loading condition by overriding of the fracture fragments and angulation producing a curve of much lower rigidity (labeled "without fracture brace"). Increasing the soft-tissue damage at the site of the fracture produces an increase in overriding in the fragments, which shifts the load deflection curve to the right, but does not change its basic characteristic slope (labeled "increase soft tissue damage"). By confining the limb in a fracture brace, fracture motion still occurs because of overriding of the fragments, but angulation is minimized and a great deal of the rigidity of the leg is restored (shown by the curve labeled "with fracture brace"). In the leg with soft-tissue damage, the characteristic of the curve in a fracture brace remains the same, but is shifted to the right indicating an increase in overriding of the fragments while in the fracture brace. (Reproduced with permission from Latta LL, Sarmiento A, Tarr RR: The rationale of functional bracing of fractures. *Clin Orthop* 1980;146:35.)

require a length reduction, early ambulation, however, must not begin until late stage II fracture healing. By stage III the fracture brace can be maintained simply to enhance function or protect the limb from direct trauma. In the majority of cases, the fracture brace is not necessary mechanically during stage III fracture healing and thereafter.

Angulatory stability provided by fracture braces is related to the diameter of the limb and the length of the cylinder supporting the limb through the soft tissues. With a mid-shaft fracture in a long narrow limb segment, angular stability is excellent. With limbs that are larger in diameter and contain more adipose tissue, the leverage of the fracture brace is reduced and angulatory control is less adequate. Fractures that are not in the mid-shaft region and that come close to the ends of the cylindrical portion

of the fracture brace also have very poor leverage through the soft tissues, with the short fragment becoming very difficult to control by a fracture brace. In these instances, an alternative treatment method, or longer periods of immobilization in a cast, or supplementary fixation may be necessary to achieve early stage III healing before a fracture brace is applied in the weightbearing limb.[6,8]

## Femoral Shaft Fractures

### Introduction

Fractures of the long bones, particularly femoral fractures, are being seen with increasing frequency by the orthopaedist because of the increase in high-energy trauma, especially from motor vehicle acci-

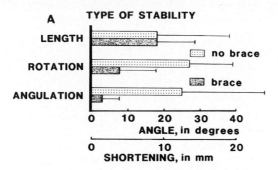

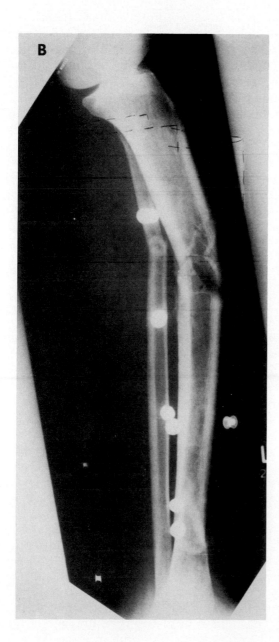

**Fig. 25–2** **A:** Closed fractures created in above-knee amputation specimens were tested with compression load, axial torsion, and bending moments. The position of the bone fragments after load had been applied and relaxed is the net displacement indicated by the bars on the graph. The motion at the fracture site that occurred when load was applied, but recovered with relaxation of load, is indicated by the bracket extending from the bar. The most significant stability and control of motion at the fracture site provided by the brace is in angulation. Angulatory stability is the last to be achieved clinically. Thus, patients functioning early in the brace who have sufficient length and rotation stability in stage II fracture healing are still unstable in angulation. **B:** Angular instability is demonstrated by this patient who did not maintain snugness of the fracture brace with early weightbearing five weeks following injury, which allowed the fracture to angulate as the interlocking shells of the brace separated (outlined proximally). **C:** After retightening the brace and resuming ambulation, the ease with which the brace corrected and stabilized the angulation is further demonstrated by this radiograph.

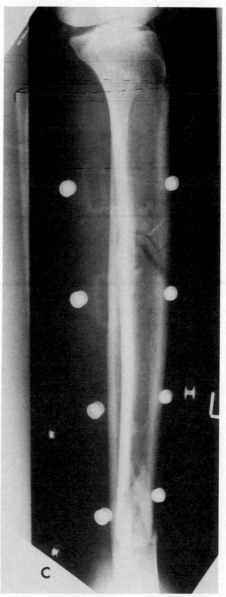

dents. Clearly, for most femoral shaft fractures the current treatment of choice is closed intramedullary nailing, because of its low morbidity, high union rate, and the physiologic advantages to the multiply injured patient.[9] In certain situations, however, closed intramedullary nailing may not be feasible or practical, such as when the necessary equipment or technical proficiency is lacking to perform the procedure successfully.

Skeletal traction, therefore, remains an important method for the management of femoral shaft fractures. The traction is usually maintained for a period of four to six weeks, at which time several options exist until fracture union can be demonstrated clinically. Spica cast immobilization for several weeks is an alternative, but it is cumbersome, not well accepted by patients, and often results in prolonged rehabilitation. Cast bracing has been advocated to allow active return to function and weightbearing, and the clinical results have been well documented.[2,9-13] In the authors' experience some disadvantages exist with the use of cast braces. Wound access is limited, and proper hygiene is difficult. Angulatory deformities can be corrected by wedging of the cast brace, but often this procedure is complicated and may require a complete change of the cast brace. A cast brace also makes it difficult to accommodate volume changes in the thigh secondary to swelling or atrophy.

A plastic fracture brace has several advantages over a cast brace[14,15]: (1) Ability to remove a fracture brace readily permits wound access and good skin hygiene; (2) an adjustable thigh section adapts easily to swelling or atrophy; (3) patient acceptance is high; and (4) the fracture brace has sufficient durability to withstand the normal or prolonged treatment course.

In 1972, Sarmiento published the results of his study in which 70 femoral fractures were treated with a custom-fabricated Orthoplast brace with metal knee hinges and uprights attached to the shoe.[14] Fracture union was achieved in an average of 15 weeks without a nonunion. Fractures of the middle or proximal thirds of the femur had the most angulation and shortening. Limitation of knee motion was encountered often, and the author concluded that the optimal treatment of femur fractures was probably surgical.

### Design Considerations

Because the femur is a single bone surrounded by a bulky layer of soft tissues, the thigh is an unstable limb segment (Fig. 25–3). Heavy mechanical demands are placed upon the femur, most notably, varus moments in the proximal region. Because fractures in the proximal portion of the femur have very poor leverage in this soft tissue mass and the bone has a great deal of mobility through the soft tissue, it is extremely difficult to control varus angulation

through the soft tissues with a fracture brace. The soft tissue surrounding the distal femur is much less bulky and tends to have less adipose tissue surrounding it. This anatomic difference coupled with the added leverage of the long proximal fragment makes the distal fracture in the femur more inherently stable than the proximal fracture and more controllable with fracture bracing methods.

Double upright knee joints provide added mediolateral stability (Fig. 25–4). These joints are coupled to the leg by a component very similar to the tibial fracture brace. A footpiece is essential for maintaining suspension of the brace. Since mediolateral instability is the most common problem in the femur, the closure of the proximal sleeve is mediolateral, with medial and lateral interlocking shells (Fig. 25–3C and 25–4). Thus, by maintaining the tightness of the sleeve, the mediolateral dimension reduces maximally to maintain the angular control in this plane.

Active motion of the knee should be achieved as soon as possible in order to activate the muscles surrounding the fracture site and thus maintain function during early phases of fracture repair. Since activation of the knee joint places stress on the bone and the callus forming at the fracture site, and since there is inherent angular instability in the femur, late stage II or stage III fracture healing must be achieved prior to application of a fracture brace and weightbearing.

### Indications and Contraindications

While the authors use closed intramedullary nailing to treat most femoral shaft fractures, a prefabricated, low-density, polyethylene fracture brace has been used for certain selected fractures (Fig. 25–4). The indications for the femoral fracture brace include closed or open distal-third shaft fractures. Fractures with nondisplaced intra-articular extension may be braced, with weightbearing delayed an appropriate length of time to allow early healing of the articular surfaces. Some degree of fracture stability should be present prior to applying the femoral fracture brace. This stability can be achieved by an initial four- to six-week period in skeletal traction to develop early callus. The fracture brace may be applied when the fracture is said to be "sticky" or "rubbery" and has no fracture tenderness and only slight angulatory motion to stress.

The fracture reduction must be satisfactory at the time of brace application, since the femoral brace will only maintain the reduction, and not obtain it. Depending on multiple factors, such as the age of the patient, the type of fracture, and anticipated functional goals, up to 7 degrees of valgus, 5 degrees of varus, and 10 degrees of anterior or posterior angulation is acceptable. Shortening is evaluated based on the above-mentioned factors; 10 to 15 mm is consid-

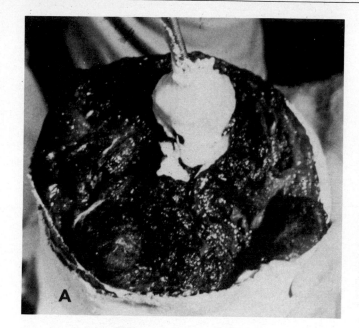

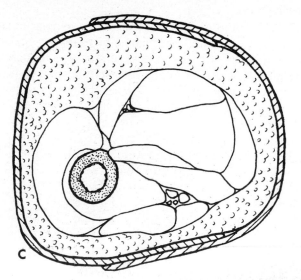

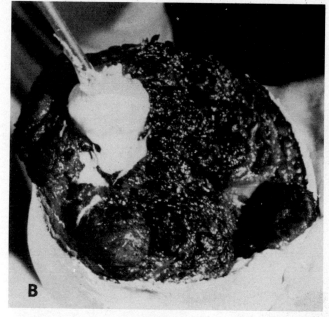

**Fig. 25–3** This above-knee amputation in the mid-thigh region with a long-leg cast applied up to the proximal border of the soft tissues has a rod cemented in the femur for application of load to the limb. Hand application of a minimal valgus moment (**A**) and a varus moment (**B**) demonstrates the mobility of the femur in the surrounding mass of soft tissue even with the confinement of the cylindrical cast. (Reproduced with permission from Sarmiento A, Latta LL: *Closed Functional Treatment of Fractures*. New York, Springer-Verlag 1981, p 53.) **C:** Since the varus moment on the femur is the most difficult to control through the soft tissues, the cross section of the brace is shaped to flatten the lateral soft-tissue mass and provide for maximal mediolateral adjustment, as the brace is tightened to accommodate changes in swelling and muscle atrophy without altering the shape of the brace's cross section.

ered acceptable for most patients. Malrotation is poorly tolerated by the patient, may cause difficulty with gait and should not be accepted.

Contraindications to femoral fracture bracing include (1) insufficient fracture stability prior to brace application; (2) most fractures located in the middle and proximal thirds of the femoral shaft; (3) displaced, intra-articular fractures; (4) patients with obese thighs; and (5) patients with neurovascular impairment or inability to cooperate with the protocol.

## Protocol

A strict protocol must be followed if fracture brace treatment is elected. After initial resuscitation, patients are placed in skeletal traction with a proximal tibial pin (Fig. 25–5). Four to six weeks of traction are required, depending on the individual fracture. Traction is discontinued when the fracture is nontender to stress and radiographs show some early callus. The tibial pin is removed and the femoral fracture brace is applied on the day traction is discontinued. The patient begins partial weightbearing ambulation and active motion exercises of the extremity (Fig. 25–6, A and B). The fracture-brace thigh portion must be adjusted often to accommodate for volume changes. A weightbearing radiograph of the femur in the brace is obtained to confirm that fracture reduction is maintained. Generally, the patient should be scheduled for outpatient follow-up within two weeks.

One to two weeks after discharge, the brace must be checked for proper fit and a radiograph in the brace must be obtained to check alignment. (If alignment is or becomes unsatisfactory, alternative treatment techniques such as ORIF may be necessary. Poor alignment will not improve by itself in the brace, and may become worse.) Range of motion is checked. Progressive weightbearing is encouraged. Patients are then followed at monthly intervals until clinical fracture union is achieved. Alignment is checked radiographically and range of motion and function are tested at each visit. Clinical union is defined as full, painless weightbearing, in addition to bridging

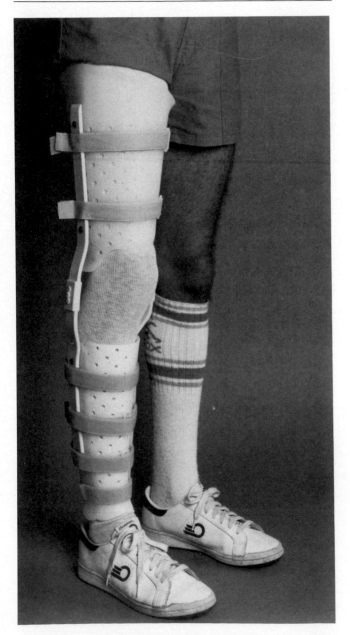

**Fig. 25–4**   The femoral fracture brace developed at the University of Miami Special Fracture Clinic consists of medial and lateral interlocking shells with a thigh section connected by double upright polycentric knee hinges to a tibial section, with a footpiece to maintain suspension.

and remodeling callus as demonstrated on radiographs (Fig. 25–6, C and D). Rehabilitation should be continued until joint motion and muscle strength are maximized.

### Results

Femoral fracture braces were applied to 17 patients at the University of Miami's Special Fracture Clinic. All fractures were located in the distal third of the femur and were comminuted. Eight fractures were open, mostly because of low-velocity gunshots. The mean time of skeletal traction before brace application was 5.8 weeks. The mean time to clinical fracture union and full unsupported weightbearing was 14 weeks. All fractures healed. Mean angulation was 6 degrees of valgus. At follow-up, 14 of 17 patients (82%) had 90 degrees or more of knee flexion, but only two patients regained normal knee motion. Shortening was less than 15 mm in all patients in this group (Tables 25–1 and 25–2).

### Complications

Complications of femoral fracture bracing are usually secondary to noncompliance or to inappropriate prescription of the brace. Loss of fracture reduction is related to insufficient fracture stability at the time of brace application or to use of the brace for proximal fractures. Distal edema in the foot and ankle may be caused by wearing the brace too tightly or by improper elevation of the extremity when not walking. Decreased joint motion is avoidable by early institution of extremity function.

### Conclusions

Femoral fracture bracing is a suitable management alternative for selected fractures of the distal third of

**Table 25–1**
**Femoral fractures**

| Clinical Data | Mean | Maximum |
| --- | --- | --- |
| Angulation (degrees) | | |
| Anteroposterior | 5 | 14 |
| Mediolateral | 3 | 10 |
| Shortening (mm) | 10 | 24 |
| Knee motion (degrees) | 94 | 140 |
| Time to union (wks) | 14 | 22 |

**Table 25–2**
**Femoral fracture complications**

| Complication | No. | % of Total |
| --- | --- | --- |
| Nonunion | 0 | 0 |
| Malunion* | 4 | 24 |
| Knee motion < 90° | 2 | 12 |

*Anteroposterior angulation > 10°; mediolateral angulation > 7°; *or* > 10 mm of shortening.

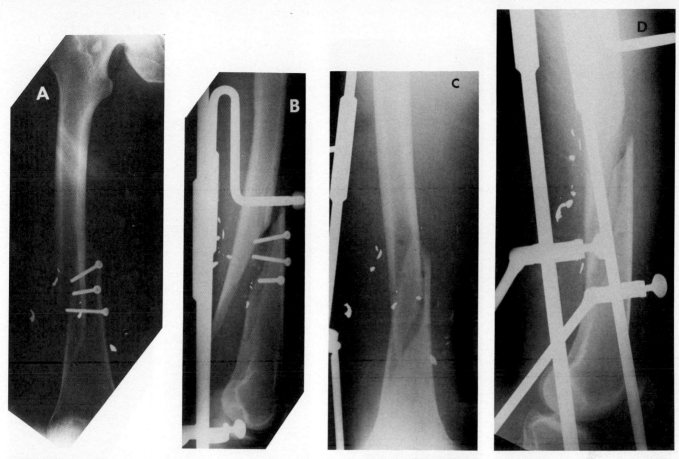

**Fig. 25–5   A and B:** This distal femoral fracture secondary to a gunshot wound was initially treated at another institution; the patient arrived a few days after injury with failed internal fixation. **C and D:** His femur was placed in traction for four weeks.

the femoral shaft. Patients must be able to tolerate four to six weeks of skeletal traction, and the fracture reduction must be satisfactory prior to brace application. Some angulation and shortening are to be expected, depending on fracture type and the degree of comminution. Functional results are satisfactory in most patients, but are not equivalent to those obtained with closed intramedullary nailing.

## Tibial Shaft Fractures

### Introduction

The successful use of fracture bracing in the treatment of tibial shaft fractures has been well documented.[6,14,16–19] Over the past two decades, the work of Sarmiento and others has produced successful results using this technique in selected fractures of the tibia. Over the past several years at the University of Miami Department of Orthopaedics and Rehabilitation, the authors have carefully evaluated the results of using fracture bracing in the treatment of tibial fractures and have refined the indications in an effort to improve results.

### Design Considerations

The limb segment of which the tibia is a part is inherently stable. It consists of the tibia and fibula connected by an interosseous membrane surrounded by very muscular soft tissue and is well-suited to soft-tissue control with fracture braces. Studies have indicated that the loads placed on the limb transfer primarily through the soft tissues in the early phase of fracture healing; only about 15% of the load transfers through the brace.[6] Thus, the primary role of the fracture brace is to control angulation. Rotational and length stability must be achieved prior to bracing.[19]

The cylindrical portion of the fracture brace provides the major share of mechanical stabilization to the limb. Laboratory tests were performed on fresh above-knee amputation specimens with closed fractures of the tibia and fibula created to simulate early stage I fracture healing. Casts and braces were applied to provide stabilization and soft-tissue compression to control fracture site motion.[6,19] Portions of the casts and braces were selectively, progressively removed to determine their mechanical role under the

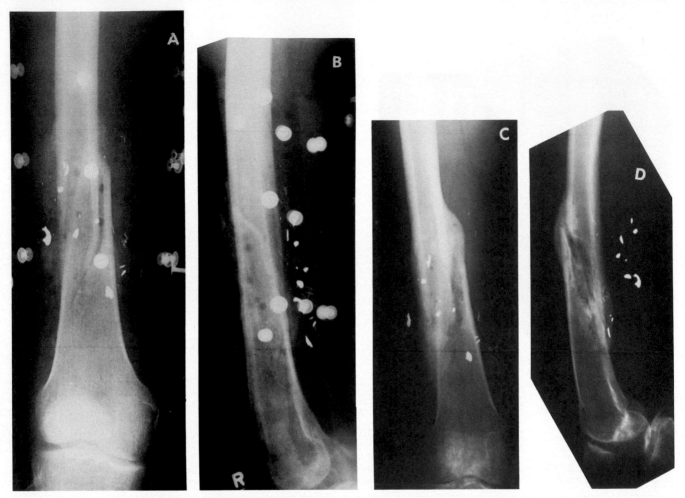

**Fig. 25–6    A and B:** He was transferred to a brace with early callus almost five weeks following injury. **C and D:** The fracture maintained alignment with weightbearing in the brace and healed uneventfully.

isolated load conditions of compression, bending, and rotation. Under these conditions of fracture-site instability in severe mid-shaft fractures of the tibia and fibula, the footpiece and the condylar extensions of the devices demonstrated a negligible role in controlling angulation, rotation, or shortening of the limb (Fig. 25–7).

Prior to 1980, during the years when the authors were using custom-applied Orthoplast braces of the PTB design, a number of patients removed the supracondylar components of their tibial fracture brace. There was no detectable difference in outcome between these patients and those braced with the PTB design. This finding stimulated an investigation of 30 patients with short-leg, custom-applied braces that did not extend above the tibial tubercle. The results observed in these 30 patients were not significantly different from the results observed in patients with the PTB brace design. This clinical experience supported the laboratory evidence that the supracondylar component of the PTB design device was

unnecessary. Limited trials with a prefabricated tibial fracture brace using the PTB design provided similar support for these clinical and laboratory findings. The authors, therefore, began using a prefabricated tibial brace that did not extend proximal to the tibial tubercle nor distal to the supramalleolar area of the leg.

In studies using instrumented fracture braces,[6] it was demonstrated that approximately 80% of the loads are borne in the proximal half of the fracture brace. This finding has been corroborated clinically by patients who feel the strongest evidence of load transfer in the brace in the bulky calf muscles of the proximal half of the limb. Although it is impractical to mold an interosseous groove in the leg as in the forearm, the natural triangular shape of the leg can be molded by the proximal portion of the sleeve of the tibial brace. In custom application of fracture braces, maintenance of this wedge anteriorly and the flattening of the posterior musculature has produced good clinical results.[5,6] To maintain this soft-tissue molding in the proximal half of the brace during circumferential adjustment of the device, an interlocking shell design was developed that maintains its triangular cross section with circumferential adjustments (Fig. 25–8). Using this design in a prefabricated brace, it is possible to maintain the basic principle of soft-tissue molding and soft-tissue compression that has proved clinically effective in custom fracture brace applications. A simple heel cup is sufficient to suspend the brace. The preferred material for the brace is low-density polyethylene because of its material property of flexibility. Thus, the brace has structural rigidity stemming from its cylindrical design as well as flexibility (Fig. 25–9).

It is critical to free the motion of the joint immediately distal to the fracture site in order to activate the muscles surrounding the fracture site. Thus, ankle motion must be available to the patient as soon as pain-free weightbearing has been demonstrated in the functional short-leg cast. Measurements taken on normal individuals, with casts and braces applied to their legs, demonstrate that it is possible to obtain a near-normal electromyographic (EMG) profile for the plantar flexors and dorsiflexors in a fracture brace (Fig. 25–10). Immobilization of the ankle joint in a short-leg functional cast significantly decreases the activity of the dorsiflexors and reduces activity of the plantar flexors. Similar electromyographic studies

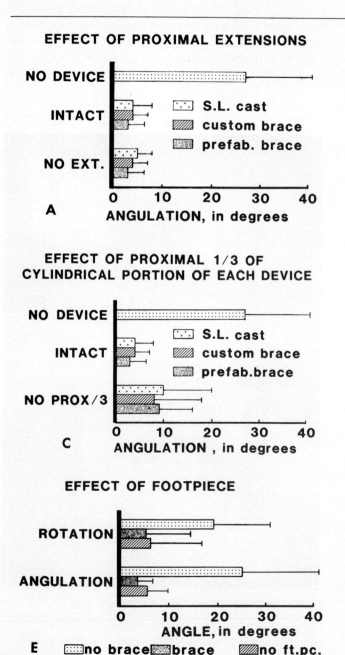

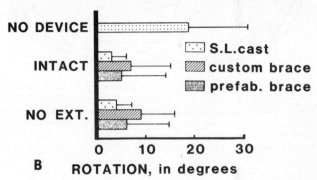

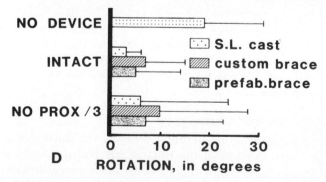

**Fig. 25–7**  In laboratory studies, fracture stability was measured and is displayed in graphic form similar to that described in Fig. 25–2A. Progressive removal of the condylar extensions on tibial short-leg casts, custom and prefabricated braces had minimal effect in controlling angulation (**A**) and rotation (**B**). In the same legs, removal of the proximal third of the cylindrical portion of the same short-leg casts, custom and prefabricated braces produced a major change in angulatory stability (**C**) and rotation (**D**). **E:** Removal of just the footpiece from the brace also had only a minor effect on rotational and angulatory stability under the same loading conditions.

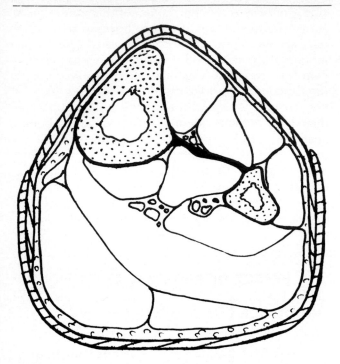

**Fig. 25–8**  The cross section of the proximal half of the lower leg is somewhat triangular. This shape can be emphasized by flattening the bulky posterior soft tissues with anterior and posterior interlocking shells so that the shape can be maintained with tightening of the brace. Compression of the soft tissues aids in load transfer and maintenance of angular stability, and the triangulation of the soft tissues helps in controlling rotation.

of patients with fractures four to six weeks following injury demonstrate that on the day of brace application these muscles do not regain normal activity. However, within a week or two of brace application, with normal unsupported weightbearing, relatively normal EMG patterns have been demonstrated. Thus, ankle motion with weightbearing does enhance functional activity.

### Indications and Contraindications

The indication currently used by the authors for fracture bracing of the tibia is any fracture considered to be diaphyseal. The contraindications include patients who are uncooperative, extremities in which there is neurologic or vascular impairment, limbs with excessive angulation or shortening, inadequate fracture stability, unstable segmental fractures, and extremities with massive soft-tissue or bone loss. Additionally, relative contraindications include extremities with loss of reduction or malalignment, and tibiae with very distal short oblique or very proximal oblique fractures.

### Protocol

Patients are initially seen in the emergency department where a reduction of the fracture is performed.

If an adequate reduction cannot be accomplished, patients should be taken to the operating room for a closed reduction under general anesthesia. A long-leg, well-padded cast is initially applied and the patient is given a cast boot. All patients with tibial fractures are hospitalized for 48 hours for limb elevation and observation of the neurovascular status. Physical therapy to achieve partial weightbearing is begun with crutches as tolerated on the third day following reduction, and patients are encouraged to advance to full weightbearing as soon as possible. Alignment is checked radiographically. Follow-up is arranged for one to two weeks after discharge.

On the third week after reduction, if the fracture is stable, the long-leg cast is replaced by a short-leg functional cast, a snug-fitting cast identical to the Sarmiento PTB cast[20] except that it does not have a supracondylar extension, nor does it have the patellar tendon indentation (Fig. 25–11). After the cast has been applied, new radiographs are obtained to check

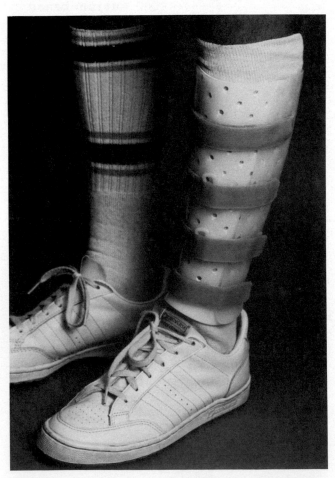

**Fig. 25–9**  The prefabricated tibial fracture brace developed at the University of Miami Special Fracture Clinic consists of anterior and posterior interlocking shells suspended by a simple posterior upright footpiece that allows for full range of motion of the ankle and knee.

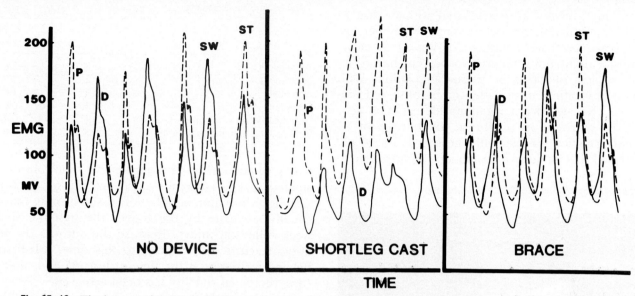

**Fig. 25–10**   The integrated EMG signals from the plantar flexor group (P) and the dorsal flexor group (D) were significantly altered in both the stance (ST) and swing (SW) phases of gait with ankle immobilization in a short-leg cast. With the application of a brace, which allowed normal ankle motion, the same subject demonstrated near normal return of EMG activity. Thus, ankle motion does stimulate more normal muscle activity around a tibial fracture site.

alignment. A physical therapist should see the patient to provide further instruction on full weightbearing using crutches. The patient is given an appointment for the fifth week following reduction.

On the fifth week after reduction, alignment is checked radiographically. If satisfactory, the short-leg functional cast is removed and a prefabricated tibial fracture brace is applied. Radiographs are then obtained. If satisfactory, patients are again encouraged to engage in full weightbearing using a canvas shoe. Patients with closed fractures should be instructed not to remove the brace. For open fractures, patients are allowed to remove the brace as necessary for dressing changes. Patients are scheduled for follow-up one week later.

If on the fifth week after reduction, alignment is unsatisfactory or has changed, the brace is removed and a new short-leg cast is applied for four weeks to correct the alignment. In some cases, alternative treatment techniques (ORIF) may be necessary. In the authors' experience, however, changes in alignment with the brace are uncommon.

On the fifth to seventh week after injury, alignment should be checked radiographically. If the alignment is satisfactory, patients are instructed in removal of the brace for hygienic purposes only. Weightbearing is not permitted out of the brace. For open fractures, patients are allowed to remove the brace for dressing changes, as necessary. Full weightbearing is continued and patients are seen at monthly intervals. Radiographs are obtained at each follow-up and the range of motion and function are evaluated. Once union is confirmed clinically and radiographically, the brace is discontinued (Figs. 25–12 through 25–14 illustrate this protocol).

## Results

Between July 1980 and January 1986 a study was performed at the University of Miami Jackson Memorial Medical Center; 753 patients with 773 tibial shaft fractures were seen. One hundred eighty patients had inadequate follow-up, and 92 patients were excluded from the study because they required treatment in addition to fracture bracing and could not follow the protocol described here. Thus, 481 patients with 501 fractures were included. The average time to union for closed injuries was 15.5 weeks; the average time to union for open fractures was 23 weeks (Table 25–3).

**Table 25–3**
**Tibial fractures**

| Clinical Data | Results | | % With Excellent or Good Results* (No. = 501) |
|---|---|---|---|
| | Mean | Maximum | |
| Angulation (degrees) | | | |
|   Anteroposterior | 2.9 | 14 | 90 (≤ 5°) |
|   Mediolateral | 2.6 | 13 | 92 (≤ 5°) |
| Rotation (degrees)† | 3.8 | 9 | — |
| Shortening (mm) | 8.0 | 35 | 95 (≤ 15 mm) |
| Time to union (wks) | | | |
|   Closed fractures | 15.5 | — | — |
|   Open fractures | 23.0 | — | — |
| Range of motion | — | — | 96 (full) |
| Function | — | — | 98 (no limp) |

*Definitions of excellent or good results appear in parentheses.
†Measured only in 25 randomly selected patients.

## Anatomy

Anatomic results were evaluated with respect to rotation, angulation, and shortening. Ninety percent of the patients had 5 degrees or less of anterior-posterior angulation. Ninety-two percent had 5 degrees or less of varus or valgus angulation. With respect to rotation, most patients were observed subjectively. No significant rotational deformities were observed to occur in the brace. In a series of 25 patients, rotation was carefully measured. This study confirmed that subjective evaluation was adequate to

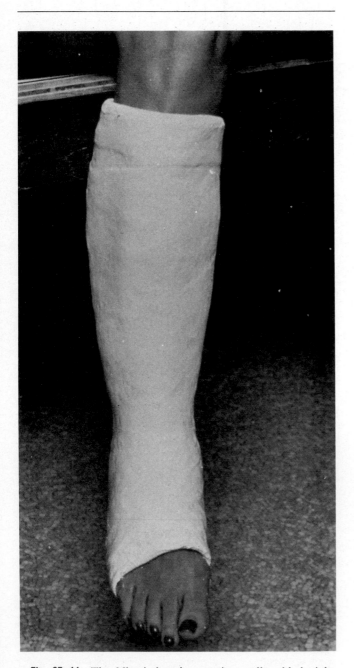

**Fig. 25–11**  The Miami short-leg cast is a well-molded, tight-fitting ambulatory cast without the proximal condylar extensions applied in the same manner as the Sarmiento PTB cast.

**Table 25–4**
**Tibial fracture complications**

| Complication | No. | % of Total |
| --- | --- | --- |
| Angulation > 12° | 18 | 3.6 |
| Shortening > 2.5 cm | 6 | 1.2 |
| Nonunion | 8 | 1.6 |
| Refracture | 3 | 0.6 |
| Skin maceration | 2 | 0.4 |
| Total patients with complications | 23 | 4.6 |

assess rotation. The authors believe that rotational stability is the first stability achieved during fracture healing. It is maintained by soft-tissue healing that is usually adequate by the fourth through the sixth week following injury. Because the authors do not apply fracture braces prior to this time, soft-tissue healing is present at the time of bracing and, therefore, rotational stability has been achieved.

On radiograph, the average shortening was 8 mm. This length was consistent regardless of fracture location with the exception of segmental fractures, which averaged 14 mm. Ninety-five percent of all fractures shortened less than 1.5 cm (Table 25–3). Because of the excessive shortening of segmental fractures, the authors no longer use closed fracture bracing technique alone for routine segmental fractures.

### Function

Functional results were assessed with respect to ankle and knee range of motion and gait pattern. Ninety-six percent of the patients had a full, normal range of motion. Two percent of the patients had a mild limp that was corrected with a shoe lift.

### Complications

Complications following this method were minimal compared to other techniques. They included angulation of greater than 12 degrees in 18 cases (3.6%); shortening of 2.5 cm or more in six cases (1.2%); nonunion in eight cases (1.6%); refracture in three cases (0.6%); and skin maceration in two cases (0.4%) (Table 25-4). (Many of these patients were the same, representing a total of 23 extremities or 4.6% in this overlapping group.)

### Angulatory Deformities

Angulatory deformities are usually related to casting technique, poor initial reduction, or poor patient compliance. The majority in whom this complication occurred had had either an inadequate initial reduction with unacceptable angulation (> 5 degrees) initially, had not returned for their appointments, had removed their braces prematurely, or had reapplied them improperly. The fracture brace must fit snugly about the leg in order to maintain soft-tissue stability

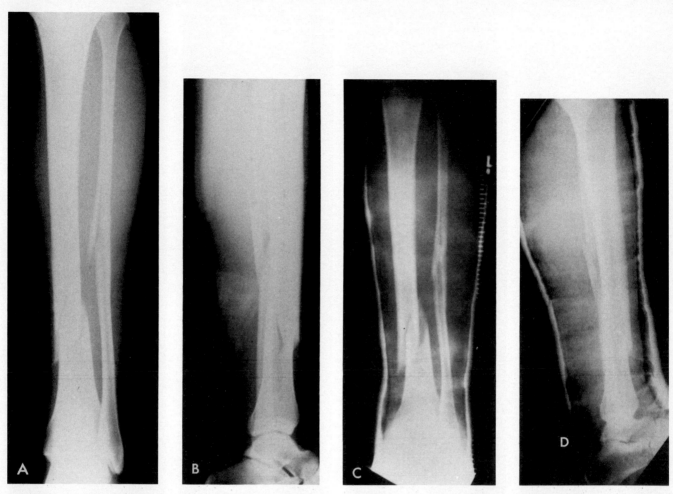

**Fig. 25–12    A and B:** This closed, distal-third, spiral oblique fracture of the tibia with an associated fibular fracture was placed in a long-leg cast with the initial overriding of the fragments accepted. **C and D:** At two weeks, partial weightbearing was accomplished and the patient was transferred to a short-leg, well-fitted cast.

and alignment. A loose-fitting brace or cast will allow angulatory deformities to occur or progress.

Minor angulatory deformities are, however, clinically and functionally insignificant.[6,14–24] Up to 5 degrees of angulation in any plane usually does not present a problem. Valgus, however, and anterior bowing tend to be less cosmetically acceptable than varus or recurvatum. Functionally, however, there are no conclusive data to demonstrate that minor angulatory deformities have any long-term effect on the knee or ankle.

### Shortening

Shortening is a reality that must be accepted with nonoperative techniques using fracture bracing or other weightbearing methods. Minor length discrepancies tend not to be a problem.[6,14–22,24–27] Discrepancies of 1.5 cm or more may require a shoe lift in order to prevent gait abnormalities or other related complaints. The most frequently asked question regarding tibial shortening is "How much shortening is acceptable?" The answer depends on such variables as the patient's sex, age, and occupation, the nature of the fracture, associated injuries, the skill of the surgeon, and the goals of the patient. Clearly, shortening acceptable in an elderly, sedentary patient might be unacceptable in a young athlete.

### Skin Maceration

A few patients who did not follow hygienic instructions and who did not change their stockinette developed skin rashes or maceration. These conditions are easily treatable with brace removal, cleansing of the extremity, application of drying lotion, and stockinette change. Skin problems may be prevented by patient instruction on proper cleansing techniques.

### Nonunion

A certain percentage of patients will experience nonunion. Occasionally, this situation seems to be related to the delayed onset of weightbearing (after six weeks). It has been the authors' experience as well

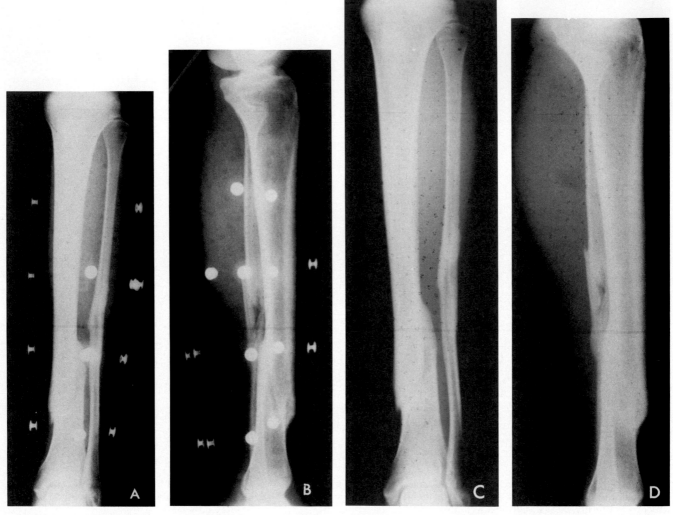

**Fig. 25–13 A and B:** The patient progressed to full weightbearing within two weeks and was placed in a tibial fracture brace, where he maintained good alignment with continued full weightbearing. **C and D:** At 14 weeks, the fracture was healed and the brace was removed.

as the experience of others that the initiation of weightbearing after the first six weeks of injury is associated with a higher incidence of nonunion.[6,14–19,25,27–29] The authors' preferred management once nonunion is established is open reduction and internal fixation with bone grafting.

## Conclusions

When properly utilized, the use of prefabricated braces for tibial shaft fractures has been shown to be effective in the majority of patients. Strict attention to detail, however, is essential if satisfactory results are to be achieved. Changes in protocol, expansion of recommended indications, or improper use may have serious consequences. When properly used, however, the overwhelming majority of patients will have excellent motion, early return to normal activities, and minimal limb atrophy, in addition to satisfactory anatomic and cosmetic results.

## Special Indications for Fracture Bracing

### Introduction

Until recently, fracture bracing was utilized as a component of nonsurgical treatment of certain long-bone fractures. Fracture braces provide soft-tissue compression and angular stability to the fracture, and also play a minor role in load transfer.

Clinical observations have also suggested that other effects may be attributable to the fracture brace. For example, patients have demonstrated enhanced extremity function while in the brace as measured by muscle force estimates (Fig. 25–15) and corroborated by subjective reports. Also, it has been believed for many years that patients feel more psychologically secure while using the brace.[30] The exact mechanism for these effects is unknown, but the authors have postulated that soft-tissue compression from the brace improves proprioceptive feedback, which may alter muscle forces. These known and theoretical effects have been used to develop several "special" indications for fracture bracing.

### Biomechanical Considerations

A small amount of motion occurs at the fracture site at a relatively low level of load with soft-tissue control using a cast or fracture brace. In fact, soft-tissue support of the limb with a fracture brace cannot be achieved until some motion has occurred at

the fracture site. A high degree of rigidity is achieved at the fracture site by internal fixation. Thus, there is a basic conflict in concept between fracture bracing and internal fixation. The amount of motion that must occur at the fracture site to effect soft-tissue compression through a fracture brace and thus provide stiffness to the limb would generally constitute a failure of most internal fixation methods. Thus, a fracture brace would not, on theoretical grounds, help support internal fixation.

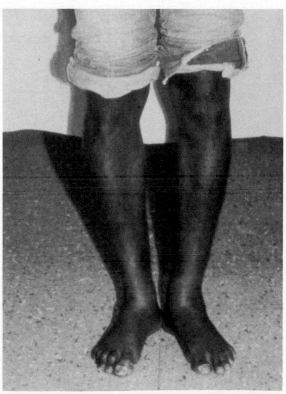

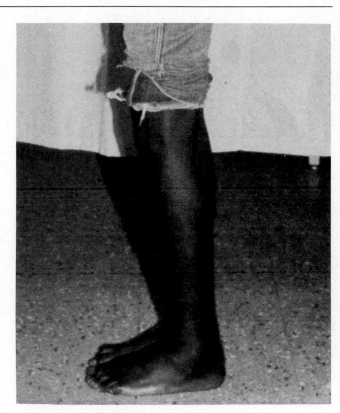

Fig. 25–14 The patient demonstrated near-normal range of motion of the knee and ankle.

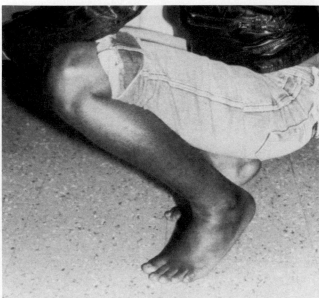

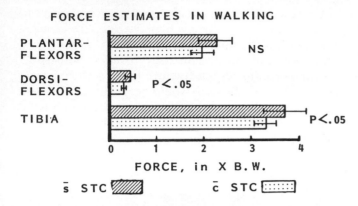

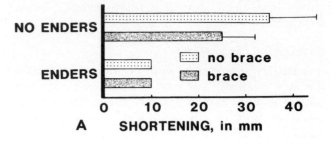

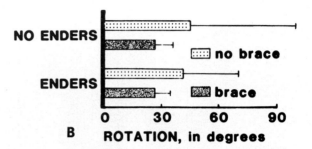

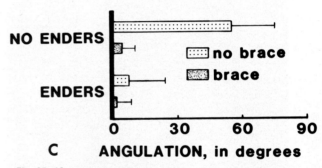

**Fig. 25–15** By "calibrating" the EMG values for known torques about the ankle joint measured on a Cybex machine, it is possible to estimate the muscle forces proportional to EMG patterns. With the same electrode placements, EMG recordings of a patient ambulating with soft-tissue compression (STC) in a tibial fracture brace were compared with EMG recordings for the same individual ambulating without the fracture brace. The estimated force of the plantar flexors and dorsiflexors was slightly reduced with soft-tissue compression, which produced a statistically significant drop in estimated force on the tibia.

As mentioned previously, external fixation or traction can be used to maintain limb length until soft-tissue healing can provide the intrinsic strength necessary for the maintenance of length under functional activity with fracture bracing. Thus, fracture bracing can be applied secondarily after removal of external fixator or traction. Alternative means of maintaining length include nonrigid types of fixation that maintain length but not rotation nor angulation. Fracture bracing can easily provide the angulatory and rotational stability once length has been stabilized through loose medullary fixation. It is anticipated that motion will still take place at the fracture site and abundant periosteal callus will form under these conditions. These events are not incompatible; they supplement each other. Laboratory studies have demonstrated that the brace can play a major role in limb support with medullary fixation, but a relatively minor role with rigid internal fixation.[31] Under similar laboratory conditions, loose Ender nails were placed in a tibia with a very unstable fracture created in an above-knee amputation specimen. The relatively loose fixation with two Ender nails demonstrated poor rotational and angulatory stability but good length stability (Fig. 25–16). Application of a fracture brace to the limb enhanced angulatory stability significantly and increased the rotational resilience. This study showed the feasibility of applying fracture braces during stage II healing to control angulation and aid in rotation while the fracture is maintained by nonrigid medullary fixation. This treatment would disturb normal fracture healing minimally.

With the rigidity maintained by fixation or the

**Fig. 25–16** Unstable fractures of the tibia and fibula were tested under the same conditions and reported graphically in the same manner as described in Fig. 25–2A. These tests demonstrated the effectiveness of Ender nails and the ineffectiveness of the fracture brace in stabilizing against overriding of the fracture fragments (A). Two Ender nails loosely applied in the medullary canal were much less effective than the fracture brace in controlling rotation (B) and angulation (C). But the combination of Ender nails and braces provided adequate stability in all degrees of freedom.

rigidity that occurs in stage III fracture healing, the fracture brace and soft-tissue compression would seemingly play little role in mechanical protection of the limb. However, in laboratory simulations of stress concentration in bone surrounded by soft tissue, soft-tissue compression increased the compressive, bending, and torsional loads required to fracture the bone at a defect. This increase in load was 15% to 20%, statistically significant but still relatively minor.

The forces in the agonist and antagonist muscles of patients with soft-tissue compression applied by a fracture brace were measured by electromyogram. These forces were then measured without the brace. From these measurements, it was possible to calculate the potential reduction in load on the bone for a given functional activity (Fig. 25–15). This reduction

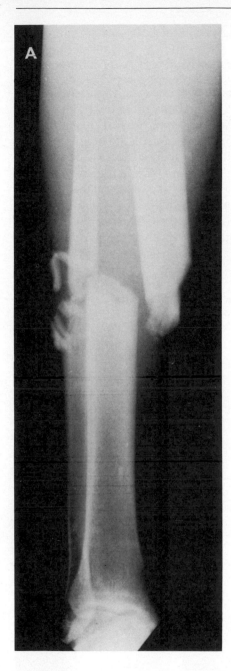

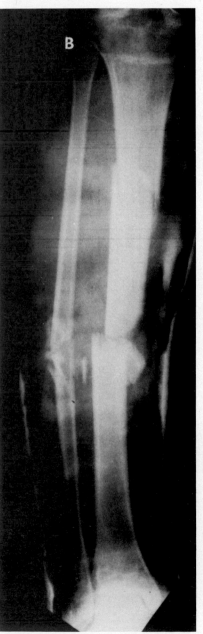

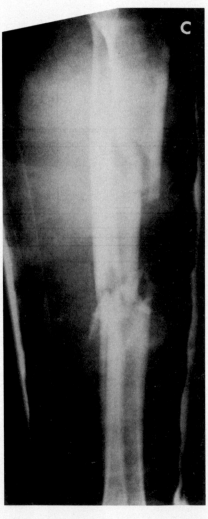

**Fig. 25–17  A:** This open, displaced, comminuted, segmental fracture was initially debrided. **B and C:** Delayed internal fixation with two Ender nails was performed five days following injury.

is apparently caused by a reduced need for antagonist muscle activity to control the function about the activated joint. With soft-tissue compression, the reduction in antagonist activity is accompanied by a minor reduction in the agonist activity, which results in a significant difference in the estimated load on the bone. Combining these active and passive affects, a significant degree of mechanical protection might be provided to a limb that has suboptimal internal fixation or a bony defect that subjects the bone to mechanical failure with early functional activity. Thus, brace application and soft-tissue compression may enable patients to resume early functional activity with a reduced risk of mechanical failure and without the need for prolonged immobilization.

## Indications and Contraindications

Fracture bracing can be used (1) as an adjunct to internal fixation; (2) secondary to external fixation; (3) for stress protection; and (4) in cases of nonunion.

**Adjunct to Internal Fixation** In certain fractures, fracture bracing and internal fixation have been used concomitantly. The authors have used this approach in 40 cases. Internal fixation using flexible intramedullary Ender or Rush nails does not often provide sufficient fracture stability without the use of some type of external support. Likewise, certain fractures cannot be adequately stabilized by fracture braces alone. However, combining the two techniques allows the surgeon to combine the advantages of both.[32]

**Fig. 25-18**   **A and B:** After two weeks in a short-leg cast with partial weightbearing, the patient was transferred to a brace. Note that the pins are not tightly packed in the medullary canal and are not carefully fitted into the malleoli to control rotation and angulation; the brace provides that. **C and D:** With continued function, the patient healed without further shortening.

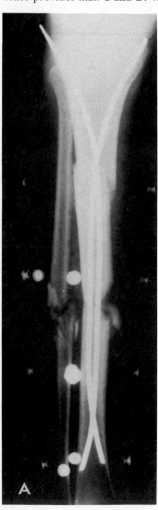
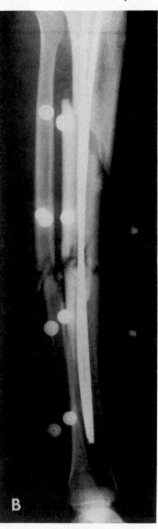
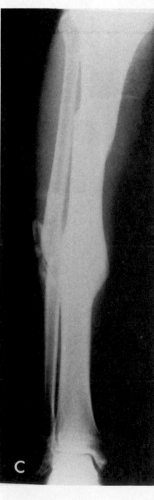
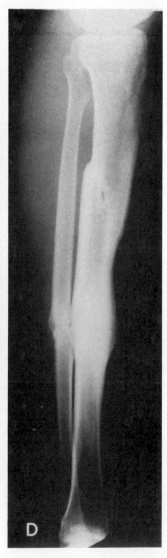

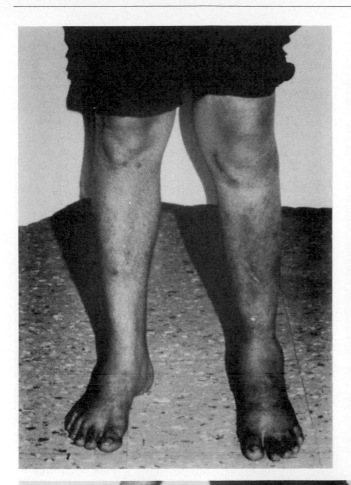

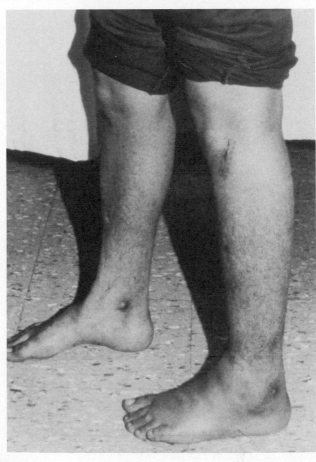

**Fig. 25–19**  He demonstrated a good range of motion eight months following injury.

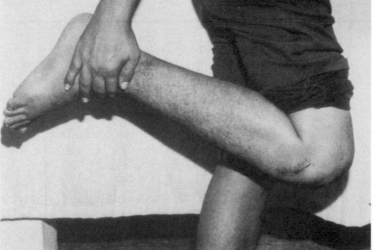

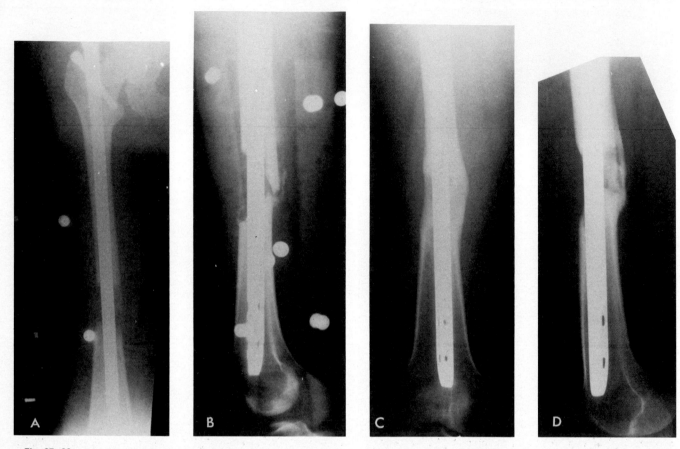

**Fig. 25–20    A and B:** This open, comminuted femoral fracture was treated with a closed intramedullary locking nail, but distal locking was not performed. The patient was placed in a fracture brace and began partial weightbearing three weeks following injury. **C and D:** At six months, the fracture healed without further shortening or angulation.

This approach has been used clinically in the treatment of segmental tibial shaft fractures. In the authors' experience, segmental fractures frequently shorten excessively when only fracture braces are used. Therefore, the authors prefer to stabilize segmental fractures by closed flexible intramedullary nails, usually two placed in an antegrade manner through proximal metaphyseal portals. Postoperatively, the patient is placed in a short-leg functional cast, with weightbearing, until most of the swelling and pain subside (Figs. 25–17 to 25–19). At approximately two weeks, the cast is discontinued and a standard prefabricated tibial fracture brace applied. The usual protocol for the use of a tibial fracture brace is then followed until complete union is achieved. The anatomic and functional results using the combined brace and internal fixation are equal to those obtained with nonsegmental fractures.

This method has also been helpful in the management of unstable, single transverse or short oblique fractures of the tibia with excessive initial shortening. Some humeral shaft fractures have also been treated successfully with this technique. The major role of the fracture brace is to improve angulatory stability; it plays a lesser role in promoting length and rotational stability. In certain femoral shaft fractures that exhibit rotational instability after intramedullary nailing, femoral fracture braces have been utilized for three to six weeks postoperatively to provide supplemental rotational control until early intrinsic fracture stability is obtained. With this type of brace, knee motion is not limited, as it may be in a long-leg cast.

**Secondary Bracing After External Fixation** Because of improvements in design and materials, external fixation has become an important mode of treatment of severe fractures of the extremities. External fixation is usually employed to manage the soft-tissue injury associated with open fractures and is discontinued after several weeks when the soft tissues have healed. At this stage, however, the fracture is usually not yet healed and requires some type of external support until complete union occurs. There is also a small but finite risk of fracture through the stress risers created by pin removal. The authors have used fracture braces after external fixator removal with the advantages of supplying some mechanical support to the bone while permitting adjacent joint motion. The fracture brace is continued until clinical fracture union occurs (Figs. 25–20 to 25–22).

Some patients are treated with external fixation as the sole method to achieve fracture union. In these cases, however, when the external fixation is removed, fracture remodeling is incomplete and the risk of stress risers from pin removal is still present. Several authors have recently recommended that an orthosis be used to protect the bone for periods as long as a few months.[33,34] The authors have had limited but favorable experience with use of a fracture brace.

**Stress Protection** Stress risers in bone may be produced by removal of internal fixation plates, surgical biopsy, or penetrating missile injury. Regardless of the cause, the potential complication is fracture through the stress risers, often prolonging the rehabilitation period and the return of the patient to normal activity. If the bone can be protected until bone remodeling is complete, this complication could be eliminated.

The authors have used fracture braces for bone protection after plate removal in both the upper and lower extremities. In the humerus and femur, the appropriate brace is worn for eight to ten weeks. For fractures of the femur and tibia, the authors recommend it be worn a minimum of 12 weeks with partial weightbearing for the first eight weeks, depending upon the condition of the bone and muscles. The braces are comfortable and do not interfere with function. The authors have not seen a fracture after plate removal following this protocol. Of course, the period of brace wear should be adjusted according to the timing of plate removal and the bone quality.

**Nonunion** Patients with established long-bone nonunions frequently require surgical repair of non-

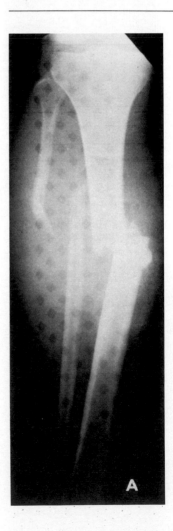
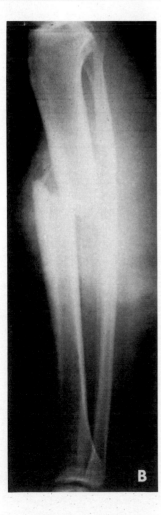
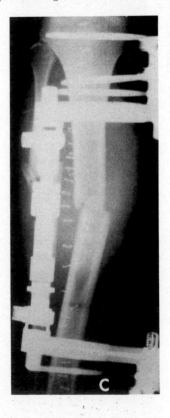
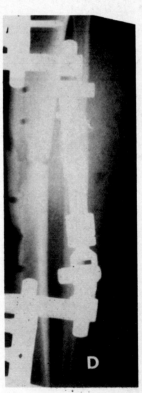

**Fig. 25–21 A and B:** This open, displaced, comminuted fracture of the tibia and fibula was initially debrided. **C and D:** External fixation was used to maintain length until soft-tissue healing could provide length and rotational stability.

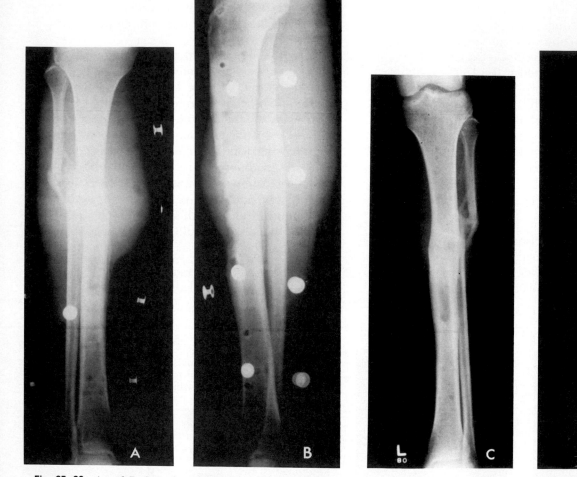

**Fig. 25–22** **A and B:** Length and rotational stability were sufficient to apply the brace at five weeks to maintain angulation during weightbearing. **C and D:** Six months following injury, the fractures were healed.

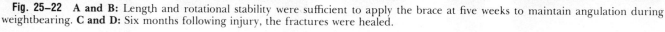

union. The soft-tissue envelope surrounding the non-union is often in suboptimal condition for operation, because of muscle atrophy and poor skin hygiene from prolonged cast immobilization. Additionally, the bone is osteoporotic from disuse and lack of weightbearing. A fracture brace can be used preoperatively until the nonunion can be repaired surgically.[6] Stabilizing the nonunion with the brace will encourage the patient to use the extremity as much as possible, thus decreasing muscle and bone atrophy and mobilizing stiff joints. The brace may also be removed as often as necessary to care for the skin.

## Conclusions

The special indications for fracture bracing are continuing to be developed and refined as the authors' clinical experience grows. Using braces for these indications has reduced patient morbidity, particularly when fractures are caused by stress risers and incompletely healed fractures. After brace application, patients function better than those immobi-lized in casts. The combination of flexible internal fixation and fracture bracing holds great promise for many applications.

### References

1. Sarmiento A, Latta LL, Zilioli A, et al: The role of soft tissues in stabilization of tibial fracture. *Clin Orthop* 1974;105:116.
2. Connolly JF, Dehne E, LaFollette B: Closed reduction and early cast-brace ambulation in the treatment of femoral fractures: Part II. Results in one hundred and forty-three fractures. *J Bone Joint Surg* 1973;55A:1581.
3. Lippert FG, Hirsch C: The three-dimensional measurement of tibial fracture motion by photogrammetry. *Clin Orthop* 1974;105:130.
4. Perren SM: Physical and biological aspects of fracture healing with special reference to internal fixation. *Clin Orthop* 1979;138:175.
5. Latta LL, Sarmiento A: Mechanical behavior of tibial fractures, in *Symposium on Trauma to the Leg and Its Sequelae*. St Louis, CV Mosby Co, 1980.
6. Sarmiento A, Latta LL: *Closed Functional Treatment of Fractures*. New York, Springer-Verlag, 1981.

7. Latta LL, Sarmiento A, Tarr RR: The rationale of functional bracing of fractures. *Clin Orthop* 1980;146:28.

8. Sarmiento A, Kinman PB, Latta LL: Fractures of the proximal tibia and tibial condyles: A clinical and laboratory comparative study. *Clin Orthop* 1979;145:136.

9. Miller CW, Anderson L, Grossman J, et al: Comparison of three treatments for fractures of the diaphysis of the femur. *Surg Gynecol Obstet* 1978;146:572–576.

10. Bailey JD, Hackethorn JC, Dunley J, et al: Cast-brace treatment of femoral fractures. *Contemp Surg* 1976;8:32.

11. Hardy AE, White P, Williams J: The treatment of femoral fractures by cast-brace and early walking: A review of seventy-nine patients. *J Bone Joint Surg* 1979;61B:151–154.

12. Crotwell WA III: The thigh-lacer: Ambulatory non-operative treatment of femoral shaft fractures. *J Bone Joint Surg* 1978;60A:112.

13. Mooney V, Nickel VL, Harvey JP, et al: Cast-brace treatment for fractures of the distal part of the femur. *J Bone Joint Surg* 1970;52A:1563.

14. Sarmiento A: Functional bracing of tibial and femoral shaft fractures. *Clin Orthop* 1972;82:2.

15. Zych GA, Zagorski JB, Latta LL: Current concepts in fracture bracing: Part II. Lower extremity. *Orthop Surg* 1986;5:18.

16. Sarmiento A: A functional below-the-knee brace for tibial fractures. *J Bone Joint Surg* 1970;52A:295.

17. Sarmiento A, Sobol PA, Sew Hoy Al, et al: Prefabricated functional braces for the treatment of fractures of the tibial diaphysis. *J Bone Joint Surg* 1984;66A:1328–1339.

18. Zagorski JB, Schenkman JH, Latta LL, et al: Prefabricated brace treatment for diaphyseal tibial fractures. *Orthop Trans* 1985;8.

19. Zagorski JB, Latta LL, Finnieston A: Comparative tibial fracture stability in casts, custom and pre-fabricated braces. *Orthop Trans* 1984;7:332.

20. Sarmiento A: A functional below-the-knee cast for tibial fractures. *J Bone Joint Surg* 1967;49A:855.

21. Rockwood CA, Green DP: *Fractures in Adults.* Philadelphia, JB Lippincott, 1984, p 1298.

22. Nicoll EA: Fractures of the tibial shaft: A survey of 705 cases. *J Bone Joint Surg* 1964;46B:373.

23. Haines JF, et al: Is conservative treatment of diaphyseal tibial shaft fractures justified? *J Bone Joint Surg* 1984;66B:84.

24. Charnley J: *The Closed Treatment of Common Fractures*, ed. 3. Baltimore, Williams & Wilkins Co, 1968.

25. Brown PW, Urban JG: The early weight-bearing treatment of open fractures of the tibia: An end-result study of sixty-three cases. *J Bone Joint Surg* 1969;51A:59.

26. Weissman SL, Herold HZ, Engelberg M: Fractures of the middle two-thirds of the tibial shaft: Results of treatment without internal fixation. *J Bone Joint Surg* 1966;45A:257.

27. Dehne E: Treatment of fractures of the tibial shaft. *Clin Orthop* 1969;66:159.

28. Connolly JF: Common avoidable problems in nonunions. *Clin Orthop* 1985;194:226.

29. Heppenstall RB, et al: Prognostic factors in nonunion of the tibia. *J Trauma* 1984;24:790.

30. Mooney V: Current Concepts in Fracture Management, unpublished AAOS postgraduate course, Miami Beach, Florida, 1977.

31. Neustein P, Tarr R, Bashner B, et al: Strain patterns in the tibial fracture brace: A comparison of alternative management protocol. *Trans 29th ORS* 1983;8:368.

32. Wiss DA, Merritt J, Thalgott J, et al: Flexible medullary nailing of tibial shaft fractures. *Orthop Trans* 1985;9:431.

33. Bucholtz R, et al: Sequential dismantling of external fixation devices in the treatment of segmental defects of the tibia. Presented at the 11th International Conference on Hoffmann External Fixation, 1985.

34. Rorabeck CH: Treatment of tibial shaft fractures with combined external and minimal internal fixation. Presented at the 11th International Conference on Hoffmann External Fixation, 1985.

# Fractures of the Distal Femur

## Introduction

Vert Mooney, MD

A fracture of the distal femur is an extremely complex fracture with which to deal. In the past, the percentage of treatment failures was significant. Ideal care still remains somewhat controversial. The lack of consensus is based on two factors: the epidemiology of the fracture and the training and experience of the surgeon.

This fracture occurs in two separate types of populations. The first group is made up of young persons who have experienced significant trauma. Thus, the fracture may be open and associated with several other injuries, including other fractures in the same limb. In general, this individual will present with significant comminution, but with bone of reasonably good quality. The second group of individuals sustains this fracture because the distal femoral cortex has thinned out as it broadens to the metaphysis of the distal femur, causing a weak link in the bone. As bone quality diminishes with age or the femur is affected by metastatic disease, this weak link is prone to fracture with only moderate to minimal trauma. In these cases, comminution is caused not so much by the force of the injury, but rather by the brittle osteoporotic bone.

Another factor influencing the care of these fractures is the experience and training of the surgeon. Surgeons who train at centers of fracture brace care tend to believe that the majority of fractures can be managed by closed reduction and early cast-brace immobilization. On the other hand, surgeons whose training and experience are acquired at trauma centers are most skilled in the surgical treatment of distal femoral fractures.

In the discussions that follow, each author will present his particular point of view and methods of treatment, based on the principles outlined in his initial sections. Each method is complex, difficult to learn, and has notable potential pitfalls. Each author will provide technical details to allow the reader sufficient information on which to decide which method is most appropriate to care for the distal femur fracture, given such variables as patient age and circumstances of the injury.

Connolly points out the pitfalls of surgical care based largely on technical failures. Thus, the conservative, limited, approach is advocated. To what degree those fractures treated by closed care deviate from return to normal anatomy—length, angulation and rotation—has not been established. Nearly all results of closed care are at least minor failures when normal anatomy is considered the acceptable result. Although Connolly suggests that when failures of conservative care are recognized, they can proceed to operative care, it should be noted that a fracture treated several weeks following trauma—perhaps with a percutaneous traction pin serving as a source of minor infection—cannot be compared in simplicity to surgical treatment provided at the time of injury.

Johnson emphasizes recent advances in surgical care as a means of reducing hospital stays as well as providing better knee motion. He also emphasizes that no technique can be appropriate for all fractures. A wide array of implants are discussed. The most recent implant in common use is the interlocking nail, which seems superior to all other methods if bone stock is sufficient to tolerate the distal fixation. The series of patients from the Parkland study certainly compares favorably to all others.

Zickel bases his discussion on experience with the innovative appliance of his design. He frankly admits that it is more appropriate for older patients (two thirds of the patients in his series). His overall results were excellent—with only a small incidence of knee pain caused by technical failures occurring in the repair of intra-articular fractures. Many of the fractures required auxiliary support systems, such as a cast-brace. In addition, nearly a fifth of the patients in his series had to have devices removed because of pain and tenderness related to failure of solid fixation in the individual with osteoporosis. Overall, however, it is an ideal instrument for situations in which the alternative fixation systems are unworthy, and prolonged traction and cast-bracing seem to cause complications.

Thus, choice of treatment depends on epidemiology and surgical experience. There is no correct or incorrect approach. To a certain extent, therefore, what is best for the patient also depends on what the surgeon perceives as best based on skill and experience.

# Closed Management of Distal Femoral Fractures

## John F. Connolly, MD

The author has made the following observations about distal femoral fractures: closed management remains the treatment of choice; these fractures are second only to open tibial fractures as a source of nonunion and other serious complications; furthermore, distal femoral fractures appear to be unique in the frequency with which nonunion follows inadequate surgical fixation. Such complications are generally avoidable since 85% are stable injuries that can be managed by closed reduction and early cast-brace immobilization.

Closed reduction requires technical skills and clinical judgment. Fracture deformity in the distal femur is best judged clinically rather than radiographically. Usually, deformities to be anticipated and avoided with closed treatment are torsional ones that are not adequately assessed by radiographs. Torsional or varus internal rotational deformities can be prevented by early application of the cast-brace and by allowing knee motion before the fracture becomes fixed in a malrotated position.

Operative fixation should be extremely selective for specific fractures in this area. The best indications for operative fixation are displaced fractures in the elderly, bedridden patient who cannot tolerate cast-bracing. "Floating knee" problems such as fractures of the distal femur and proximal tibia as well as nonunions are other common indications for internal fixation. Such fractures are most effectively treated by intramedullary devices that do not distract fracture fragments or enlarge the fracture gap.

## Problems and Solutions

A number of healing problems in the distal femur result from solutions imposed on fracture healing, either by attempted operative fixation or by prolonged nonoperative treatment in traction. In a recent review of 100 nonunions[1] evaluated over a six-year period, 13 occurred in the distal femur and all but one followed plate or attempted external fixator immobilization of the fracture. Two specific contributing factors identified as avoidable are bone gap produced by overvigorous surgical debridement and bone resorption induced by plate fixation.

### Bone Gap From Surgical Debridement

Fractures in the distal femur are frequently associated with comminution of the femoral condyles and metaphysis. Surgeons inexperienced in the treatment of these injuries tend to remove loose bone fragments

considered to be devitalized and potential sequestra. Paradoxically, however, these same fragments must then be replaced by equally devascularized autologous bone grafts in order to fill the gap produced by bone excision. In the interim, such gaps lead to hematomas and infection. The best ultimate outcome then is an arthrodesis (Fig. 26–1). The error of assuming that bone fragments must be excised is made apparent by contrasting the results of excision to those of autoclaving large extruded condylar or diaphyseal fragments and then reinserting them into the fracture site (Fig. 26–2). Such extruded fragments, aided by autologous grafting, can heal with adequate preservation of function.

Bone graft and bone fragments serve three important functions: they provide a source of osteogenic cells, despite the lack of direct blood supply to the fragments; they induce bone formation from surrounding soft tissues; and they fill spaces and thereby diminish hematoma and scar formation, filling in the fracture gap. Consequently, bone fragments should be preserved and guarded.

### Bone Gap From Load-Absorbing Fixation

In 25% of cases, attempted plate fixation of distal femoral fractures fails to achieve the desired goals and results in serious complications.[2-6] These data contradict findings of recent studies from several centers demonstrating that by using meticulous technique and bone grafting, excellent results can be achieved with plate fixation of the distal femur.[7,8] However, competent surgeons who only occasionally attempt this fixation procedure experience unacceptably high rates of failure. In a review of avoidable causes of nonunion, plate fixation of the distal femur was second only to prolonged external fixation of the tibia as a source of fracture healing problems.[1] The usual reason for this situation is that plate loosening occurs before fracture union. The load-absorbing effect of the plate then encourages osteoclastic resorption of fracture fragments and widening of the fracture gap (Fig. 26–3). This subsequent unsatisfactory biomechanical state prevents fracture impaction, which would ordinarily occur with load-sharing devices such as the Zickel or other intramedullary nails. The result, then, is persistent pain at the fracture gap until the fixation device finally fails.

### Management Based on Mechanisms of Injury and Mechanics of Knee Function

Consistently, distal femoral fractures result from direct trauma.[4,9] In most cases, an elderly woman falls on her flexed knee, producing the typical supracondylar fracture with posterior displacement of the condyles. Alternatively, the automobile occupant or motorcyclist sustains a direct blow to the anterolateral

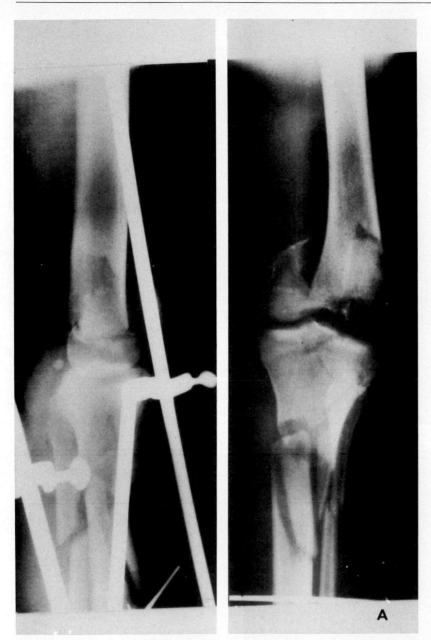

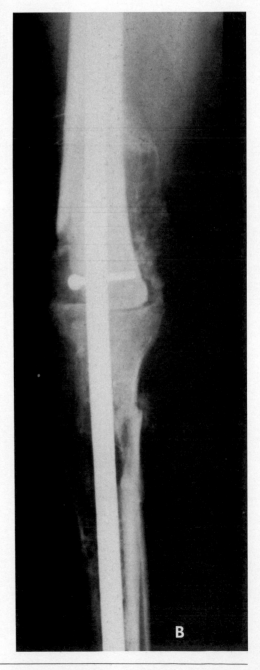

**Fig. 26-1  A:** Radiographs of this 21-year-old motorcyclist demonstrate comminuted open fractures of his distal femur and proximal tibia one month following injury. Operative reports indicated that bone fragments totalling 62 g had been removed during surgical debridement. **B:** Radiograph of the eventual outcome, with arthrodesis caused by infection in the surgically induced bone gap.

**Fig. 26–2 A and B:** A-P and lateral radiographs showing an open distal femur fracture similar to the comminution shown in Fig. 26–1. The patient came to the emergency room with the entire lateral femoral condyle extruded out of the wound. After the wound was debrided, the extruded, devascularized condyle was autoclaved and reimplanted into the wound. One month later when the wound had healed, bone grafting was performed by bone marrow injection. **C and D:** A-P and lateral radiographs four months following injury show satisfactory healing of the shaft to the devitalized condylar fragment when the cast-brace was removed.

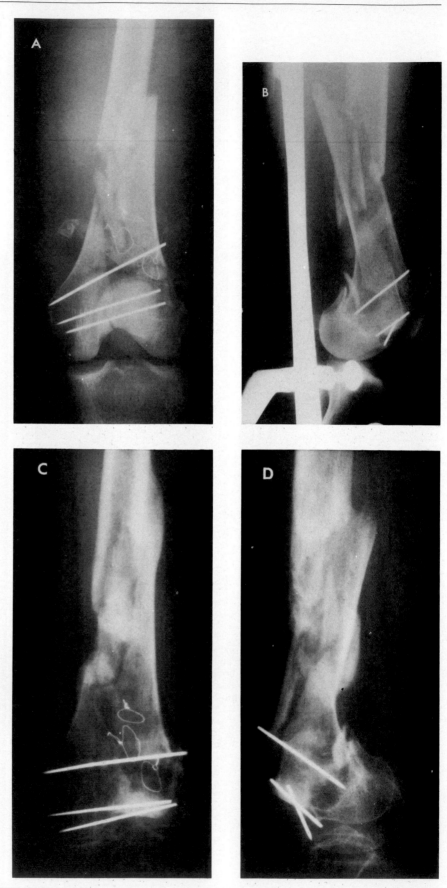

or anteromedial aspect of the distal femur, which comminutes the metaphysis and displaces the distal fragment in the direction of the applied load. It is the direction of applied load and not any muscle pull that consistently deforms the fracture and that must be overcome to achieve reduction. The objective of reduction is not to align all the fracture fragments anatomically but to restore the knee joint axis to its normal relationship with the axes of the hip and ankle. The technique of cast-bracing depends on early reduction before fracture deformities develop and uses knee motion to align the axis of the knee and hip.[10] Such an approach is analogous to treatment of phalangeal and metacarpal fractures by "buddy-taping," which permits joint motion and prevents torsional malalignment of the finger.

Treatment of distal femoral fractures should encourage rather than inhibit formation of external callus. External callus ordinarily forms early in this well-vascularized region, except when impeded by "rigid" fracture immobilization. In most instances, the objectives of functional restoration and prompt union can be achieved readily by closed reduction and ambulation in a cast-brace.[11-13]

## Techniques of Closed Reduction and Cast-Brace Treatment

Closed reduction and early cast-brace application prevents most complications but does require that close attention be paid to both the mechanics and details of application.[9] Since most distal femoral fractures are stable, the cast-brace should be applied as early as possible (usually within the first week). The stability of the distal femoral fracture, as evidenced by electrogoniometric and cineroentgenographic techniques to measure motion, has been demonstrated.[12,14] Because most supracondylar fractures, particularly in the elderly, are produced by a fall on the flexed knee, the reduction is readily accomplished by extending the knee fully. The cast-brace is then applied with the knee held extended, externally rotated, and in slight valgus (Fig. 26–4). This eliminates the most common deforming tendency, varus of the knee, which in the past was associated with prolonged traction that internally rotated the distal fracture fragment and, therefore, the knee joint[4,9] (Fig. 26–5).

The thigh cast should be molded firmly down around the femoral condyles to provide fracture

**Fig. 26–3  A and B:** Lateral radiographs of a distal femoral fracture treated by blade plate fixation show progressive bone resorption over a six-month period caused by loosening of the plate and osteoclastic resorption. **C:** The nonunion was ultimately treated by intramedullary Zickel nail and bone grafting, which allowed fracture impaction and satisfactory union.

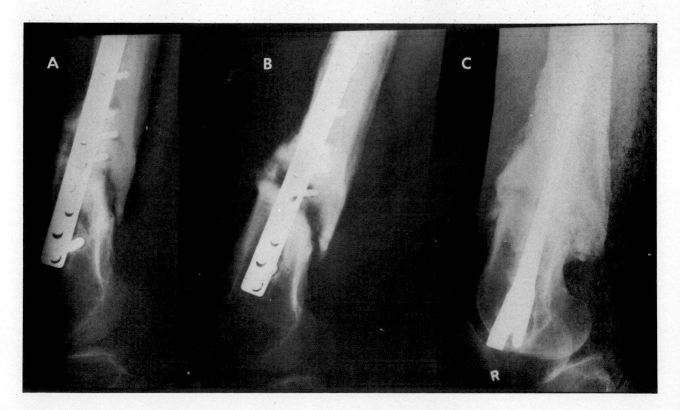

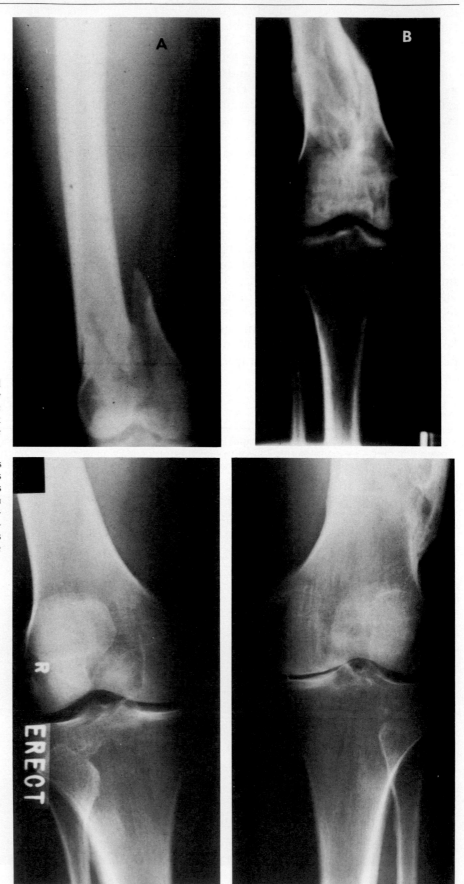

**Fig. 26–4** **A:** A-P radiograph of a typical supracondylar fracture, which commonly results from a fall on a flexed knee. **B:** Radiograph shows healing with abundant callus by 14 weeks after early cast-brace application and mobilization of the patient.

**Fig. 26–5** A-P radiographs as well as clinical evaluation of the patient six years after distal femoral fracture indicate varus internal rotation of the knee caused when the distal fragment was being rotated internally in traction, while the proximal fragment was rotated externally. The result was the wearing down of the medial joint space illustrated here.

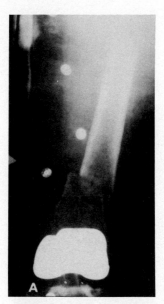
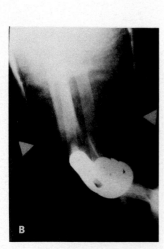
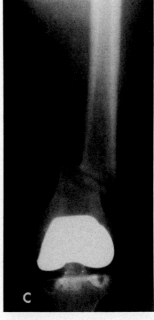
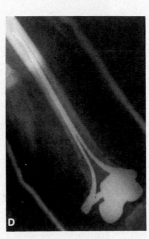

**Fig. 26–6    A and B:** A-P and lateral radiographs show a cast-brace applied too high (arrows) above the supracondylar fracture associated with the total knee prosthesis. Overconcern about maintaining knee motion led to failure to support the fracture. The result was eventual nonunion. **C and D:** A-P radiographs showing nonunion at six months, requiring fixation with a Zickel nail.

stability. Particular care should be taken to include the fracture site within the cast. A thigh cast that ends too high above the knee allows shearing displacement of the fracture and nonunion (Fig. 26–6).

A further common mechanical problem in reducing distal femoral fractures that result from direct blows to the anterior distal thigh is posterior fracture angulation. This is frequently only accentuated by tibial traction, which tightens the quadriceps and bowstrings over the fracture. The deformity can be corrected using distal femoral traction to pull the distal fragment anteriorly, thereby countering the usual displacement forces (Fig. 26–7).

A final concern is to maintain congruity of the femoral condyles with the tibial surfaces. If the supracondylar fracture has split the condyles, the fracture can be reduced and held by percutaneous Steinmann pins (Fig. 26–7) or Knowles pins (Fig. 26–8) supplemented by cast-brace support. The shaft fragment is allowed to impact into the condyles and heal with pronounced external callus. Shortening of 1 to 2 cm is quite consistent with excellent function (Fig. 26–9).

### Indications for Open Reduction

The arguments for internal fixation of distal femoral fractures based on economic considerations or

DRG mandates do not apply if early closed reduction and cast-bracing are used effectively. The cast-brace should permit mobilization as rapidly as does operative treatment, but without the inherent problems of the latter. Unfortunately, the enthusiasm for operating on distal femur fractures seems difficult to resist. Indeed, although the majority of distal femoral fractures can be treated by closed cast-brace technique, minimizing complications, a few require prompt internal fixation. These include the supracondylar fracture sustained by elderly, immobile patients being transferred from bed to chair (Fig. 26–10). These elderly, bedfast patients with osteoporosis do not heal well with cast treatment but can be managed quite effectively by load-sharing devices such as the Zickel nail. Similarly, the unstable "floating knee"[15] or fractures associated with multiple injuries frequently require internal stabilization, again with load-sharing intramedullary nail devices.[16,17] Finally, nonunions subsequent to failure of plate fixation have responded well to bone grafting and Zickel nail fixation.[17] However, more recent experience with interlocking nails in managing these nonunions has encouraged the more frequent utilization of this method.

A final recurring problem is the supracondylar fracture above a total knee prosthesis. The general consensus at this time, both from the literature and from the author's experience, is that most of these

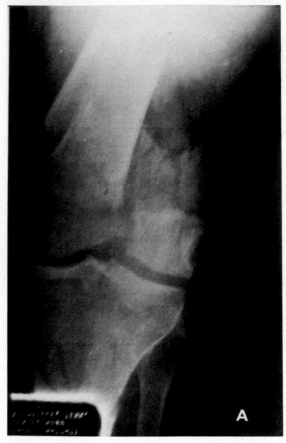

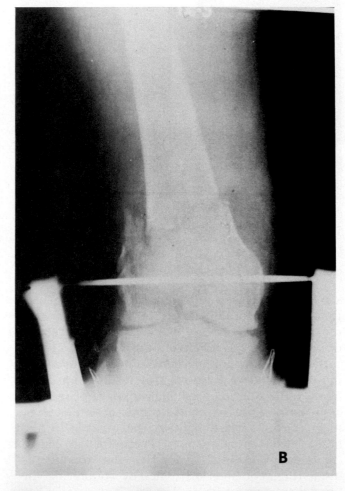

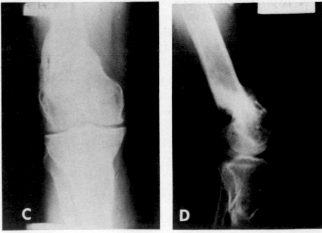

**Fig. 26–7   A:** A-P radiographs showing a comminuted supracondylar fracture associated with an undisplaced proximal tibial fracture. **B:** The fracture of the femur was reduced with distal femoral traction. **C and D:** A-P radiographs show prompt healing at 16 weeks, subsequent to closed reduction with distal femoral traction and early cast-brace application.

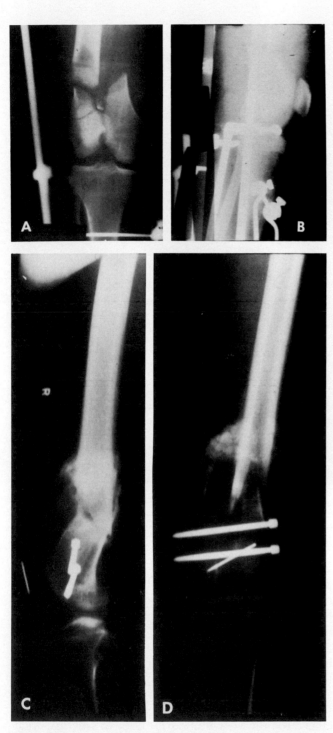

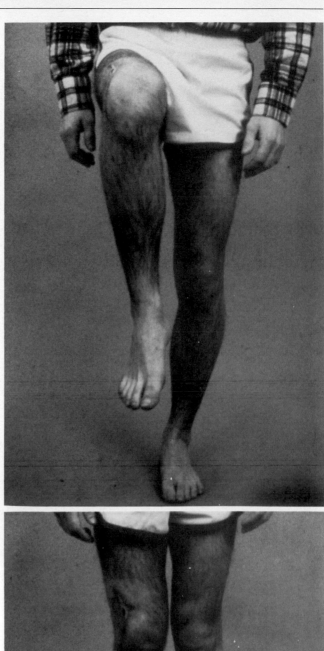

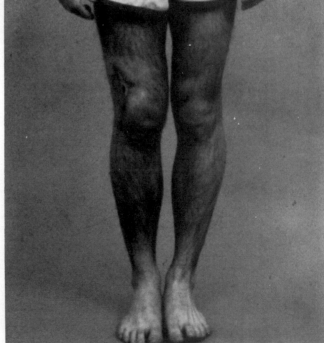

**Fig. 26–8  A and B:** Lateral and A-P radiographs show a comminuted open femoral fracture in which the condyles could not be reduced by traction. **C and D:** A-P and lateral radiographs at 12 weeks show reduction of the condyles with percutaneous Knowles pins, and prompt healing of the condylar fracture fragment with external callus. This patient was mobilized in the cast-brace by the second week after injury.

**Fig. 26–9** Clinical photographs of patient showing active range of knee motion shortly after cast brace removal at 12 weeks.

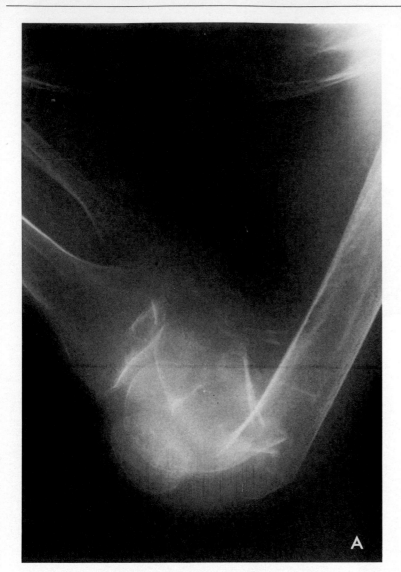
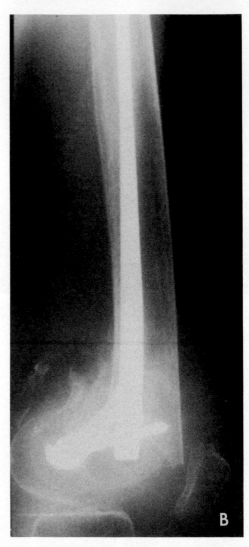

**Fig. 26–10** **A:** Lateral radiograph shows a typical displaced supracondylar fracture in a bedridden patient with osteoporosis who sustained the fracture when being transferred to a chair. **B:** Lateral radiograph shows fixation with a supracondylar Zickel nail, considered the ideal treatment to stabilize what was essentially a pathologic fracture.

can be treated by closed methods.[18-20] However, adequate reduction and stabilization are essential (Fig. 26–6). If the fracture is not immobilized adequately by cast-brace, prompt operative intervention is indicated, again with a load-sharing device.

## Summary

Since closed treatment is effective in 80% to 85% of distal femoral fractures, operative intervention is not recommended. Unnecessary surgery produces unwarranted complications.

The cast-brace technique should be used in the first week or two after injury to prevent deformities commonly associated with distal femoral fractures. The thigh cast should be carefully molded well over the femoral condyles. Distal femoral traction is preferred to proximal tibial traction to correct fracture deformities.

If the closed reduction technique is not satisfactory in the early period after injury, operative intervention can still be readily accomplished.

Percutaneous pin fixation of the condyles or intramedullary load-sharing devices are the treatment of choice for the very limited number of fractures that require open reduction and internal fixation.

### References

1. Connolly J: Common avoidable problems in nonunions. *Clin Orthop* 1985;194:226–235.

2. Fisher WD, Hamblen DL: Problems and pitfalls of compression fixation of long bone fractures: A review of results and complications. *Injury* 1978;10:99.

3. Loomer RL, Meek R, DeSommer F: Plating of femoral shaft fractures: The Vancouver experience. *J Trauma* 1980;20:1038.

4. Neer CS, Grantham SA, Shelton ML: Supracondylar fracture of the adult femur. *J Bone Joint Surg* 1967;49A;591.

5. Roberts JB: Management of fractures and fracture complications of the femoral shaft using the ASIF compression plate. *J Trauma* 1977;17:20.

6. Schatzker J, Lambert DC: Supracondylar fractures of the femur. *Clin Orthop* 1979;138:77.

7. Giles JB, DeLee JC, Heckman JD, et al: Supracondylar-intercondylar fractures of the femur treated with a supracondylar plate and lag screw. *J Bone Joint Surg* 1982;64A:864–870.

8. Mize RD, Bucholz RW, Grogan DP: Surgical treatment of displaced, comminuted fractures of the distal end of the femur. *J Bone Joint Surg* 1982;64A:871.

9. Connolly JF: (DePalma's) *The Management of Fractures and Dislocations, An Atlas.* Philadelphia, WB Saunders, 1981, p 1460.

10. Connolly JF: Torsional fractures and the third dimension of fracture management. *South Med J* 1980;73:884.

11. Borgen D, Sprague BL: Treatment of distal femoral fractures with early weight-bearing. *Clin Orthop* 1975;3:156–162.

12. Connolly JF, Dehne E, Lafollette B: Closed reduction and early cast-brace ambulation in the treatment of femoral fractures: II. Results in one hundred and forty-three fractures. *J Bone Joint Surg* 1973;55A:1581.

13. Mooney V, Nickel VL, Harvey JP, et al: Cast-brace treatment for fractures of the distal part of the femur. *J Bone Joint Surg* 1970;52A:1563.

14. Connolly JF, King P: Closed reduction and early cast-brace ambulation in the treatment of femoral fractures: I. An *in vivo* quantitative analysis of immobilization in skeletal traction and a cast-brace. *J Bone Joint Surg* 1973;55A:1559.

15. Fraser RD, Hunter GA, Waddell JP: Ipsilateral fracture of the femur and tibia. *J Bone Joint Surg* 1978;60B:510.

16. Shelbourne DK, Brueckmann FR: Rush-pin fixation of supracondylar and intercondylar fractures of the femur. *J Bone Joint Surg* 1982;64A:161.

17. Zickel RE, Fietti VG, Lawsing JF, et al: A new intramedullary fixation device for the distal third of the femur. *Clin Orthop* 1977;125:185.

18. Short WH, Hootnick DR, Murray DG: Ipsilateral supracondylar femur fractures following knee arthroplasty. *Clin Orthop* 1981;158:111.

19. Delport PH, Van Audekercke R, Martens M, et al: Conservative treatment of ipsilateral supracondylar femoral fracture after total knee arthroplasty. *J Trauma* 1984;24:846-849.

20. Merkel KD, Johnson EW: Supracondylar fracture of the femur after total knee arthroplasty. *J Bone Joint Surg* 1986;68A:29.

## P A R T  C

# Internal Fixation of Distal Femoral Fractures

### Kenneth D. Johnson, MD

The surgical treatment of fractures of the distal third of the femur is a demanding and difficult undertaking. The topic has been controversial until the past ten years.[1-3] Relatively recent advances have improved the overall results of the surgical treatment of distal third femoral fractures. These advances include improved surgical instrumentation, more extensive surgical experience, better intramedullary nailing techniques, and new methods of rehabilitation. We now have a better understanding of the basic principles of surgical fracture management, the mechanics of individual implants, and which fracture patterns are better treated by one surgical technique than another. Postoperative fracture rehabilitation now includes early range-of-motion exercises utilizing continuous passive motion machines.

The combined "personality" of the injury[4] should dictate whether the patient will benefit from surgical treatment of the fracture. Surgical treatment should be both possible and advantageous. Certain variables, such as the presence of intra-articular fractures, ipsilateral injuries ("floating knee"), or the soft-tissue status (open fracture or vascular injury), make surgical treatment almost imperative. The surgeon must interpret the fracture pattern correctly, understand the basic principles of surgical fracture treatment and the mechanics of the implants, and possess the practical experience and skill needed to handle potential surgical complications. Finally, the surgical procedure itself cannot be successful unless both the surgeon and the patient clearly understand the principles of postoperative fracture rehabilitation. The patient must be able to comply with the postoperative demands of surgical fracture management.

There have been several attempts to classify likenesses and differences among distal femoral fractures.[2,5,6] Distal femoral fractures generally share certain common features: (1) they are unstable and often comminuted; (2) they often have an intra-articular component; (3) they are often associated with other ipsilateral injuries ("floating knee"); and (4) they tend to occur either in patients with multiple injuries or in elderly patients. All of these factors make it difficult to achieve rigid internal fixation that will permit early postoperative functional rehabilitation.

The primary aim of treatment by open reduction and internal fixation is to restore the anatomic alignment of the femur and to return the patient to normal function at the earliest possible date. At Parkland Memorial Hospital, more experience with the surgical treatment of distal third femoral fractures allowed the development of both absolute and relative indications for and contraindications to surgical intervention and anatomic reconstruction of the distal third femoral fracture. Some of these contraindications might indicate the need for another surgical procedure such as arthrodesis or amputation. Absolute indications for surgical reconstruction include intra-articular fractures, acute open fractures, fractures with associated vascular injury, ipsilateral lower extremity fractures, fractures in patients with multiple injuries, and fractures that cannot be reduced. Relative indications for surgical reconstruction include isolated extra-articular fractures amenable to traction or cast-bracing and fractures in osteoporotic bone of an elderly patient. Contraindications to surgical reconstruction include fractures with preexisting infection, fractures with severe soft-tissue damage or loss, and any fracture in a patient with multiple injuries whose condition is still unstable.

The timing of surgical reconstruction is an important factor. The surgery should be performed as soon as possible when necessary equipment and experienced assistance are available. Open fractures are emergency procedures, as are displaced intra-articular fractures and fractures in the patient with multiple injuries. These fractures should be treated surgically within 24 hours (sooner in open fractures to prevent colonization of the wound).

## Surgical Technique

Open reduction and internal fixation of intra-articular distal femoral fractures requires a rather long extensile incision (Fig. 26–11). This incision is based along the lateral aspect of the femoral shaft, extending proximally as far as necessary. The incision curves anteriorly at the level of the lateral femoral condyle to lie 1 cm lateral to the tibial tubercle. The incision then extends distally along the proximal shaft of the tibia, 1 cm lateral to the anterior crest of the tibia as far distally as necessary. This incision gives adequate exposure to the anterior and lateral aspect of the distal femur but occasionally interferes with the ability to reach the medial aspect of the distal femur. If this is necessary, an osteotomy of the tibial tubercle can be performed to elevate the extensor mechanism, allowing access to the medial aspect of the distal femur. The tibial tubercle should be drilled and tapped before the osteotomy. Occasionally, when the proximal tibia also has a comminuted fracture, a Z-plasty of the patellar tendon should be performed to elevate the extensor mechanism proximally.

After adequate surgical exposure of the fracture site, the femoral condyles are reapproximated and provisionally stabilized with smooth Kirschner wires. Next, interfragmentary lag screws are used to reapproximate the articular surface of the distal femur.

**Fig. 26–11** **A:** Skin incision for ORIF distal femoral fracture. **B:** Osteotomy of tibial tubercle.

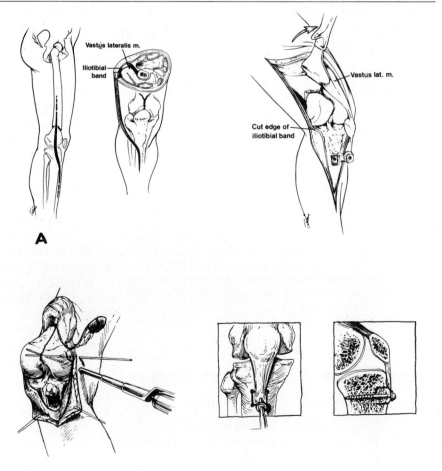

**A**

**B**

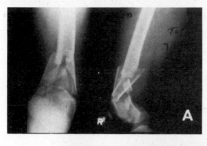
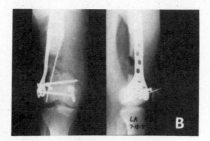
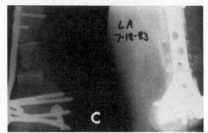

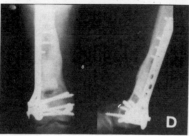
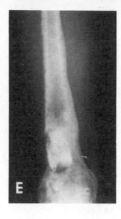

**Fig. 26–12**  ORIF distal femoral fracture using synthetic bone graft material. **A:** Closed comminuted intra-articular fracture of distal femur in a 22-year-old female. **B:** Intraoperative radiograph for assurance of alignment. Large defect present caused by excision of devitalized fragments of bone (no soft-tissue attachments). **C:** Postoperative radiograph demonstrating synthetic bone graft and cancellous bone filling defect. **D:** Solid union five months following injury. **E:** Hardware removal.

**Fig. 26–13**  Medial plate used for excessive medial comminution in conjunction with lateral angle blade plate. Note tibial tubercle osteotomy for exposure.

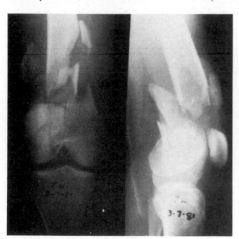
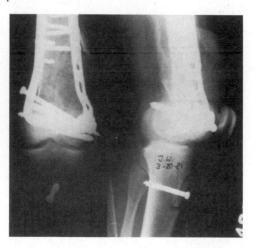

Positioning of these individual lag screws should be based on the implant to be used. Specific implants will be discussed later.

Whether or not a bone graft is necessary in these fractures has been widely discussed. The author recommends the liberal use of cancellous graft obtained from either the iliac crest or the greater trochanter. Bone grafting should always be done when there is comminution in the transition area between the femoral diaphysis and the distal metaphysis. Cancellous bone grafting should also be placed where a medial cortical defect or comminution is present opposite a plate. Recently, synthetic bone grafting materials have been used to fill large dead

spaces. These have not been used alone but in conjunction with ample cancellous bone graft or bone marrow aspirate (Fig. 26–12).

There has been some question as to whether an additional medial plate is necessary when medial comminution is a problem (Fig. 26–13). Several investigators consider it to be useful. In the author's opinion, this additional plate is not of major benefit in most cases. It is a local irritant to medial soft tissues and impedes optimal postoperative motion. It adds little additional stability to a well-reconstructed distal femoral fracture. It requires additional soft-tissue dissection that may jeopardize or devitalize fracture fragments. If medial comminution is a problem or a

**Table 26–1**
**Distal femoral fractures\* in young and elderly patients**

| Clinical Data | Young Patient | Elderly Patient |
|---|---|---|
| Energy | High | Low |
| Soft-tissue damage | Greater | Lesser |
| Comminution | Yes | No |
| Open | Yes | No |
| Articular extension | Yes | No |
| Bone stock | Good | Osteoporotic |
| Ipsilateral | Yes | No |
| Injuries | Multiple | Isolated |
| Choice of fixation | | |
| 1. | Condylar buttress plate | Zickel device |
| 2. | Supracondylar compression screw | Condylar buttress plate |
| 3. | Angle screw blade | Supracondylar compression screw |
| 4. | Interlocking nail | Traction and cast-brace |

\*With open reduction and internal fixation.

medial defect occurs, the author recommends using ample cancellous bone grafting along the medial aspect of the femur.

Among the surgeon's aids in reconstructing these difficult fractures is the femoral distractor, which can assist in maintaining length and alignment during the initial stage of provisional stabilization (Fig. 26–14). Occasionally, these fractures require a large amount of longitudinal traction. This can be provided by an assistant or by a femoral distractor. Bone graft substitutes are useful for large defects. These are never used alone but in conjunction with cancellous bone graft or bone marrow aspirate. These substitutes may play an increasing role in the future when dealing with large bone defects, particularly in the area of metaphyseal bone. Radiographs should be taken frequently or an image intensifier used throughout the surgical procedure. Each definitive step should be verified by radiographic evaluation or image intensification before the next stage of the surgical procedure begins.

## Preferred Implants

The choice of an appropriate implant is critical in the surgical reconstruction of fractures of the distal femur. The author has found that no one device is appropriate for every fracture. The implant chosen for fixation of a distal femoral fracture in a young patient may differ distinctly from that chosen for an elderly patient (Table 26–1). Fractures in younger patients generally require more energy; this, in turn, produces more soft-tissue damage. They are more apt to be comminuted and open, and often have an intra-articular extension. Conversely, fractures in elderly patients often involve soft osteoporotic bone. The energy expended is much lower, producing less soft-tissue damage, and intra-articular extension is less common. The author uses intramedullary devices whenever possible in elderly osteoporotic bone.

## Screw Plate Devices

The displaced intra-articular fracture, which requires extensive dissection for reconstruction of the joint surface, should be fixed with a plate-like device. The implants to be considered include a condylar buttress plate, a 95-degree compression screw, and an angle blade plate. Each implant has advantages or disadvantages that must be considered.

The condylar buttress plate is specifically designed to lie along the distal lateral aspect of the femur (Fig. 26–15) and it is not meant to be used in any other area. The flare of the distal aspect of the device is designed for either a right or left femur fracture; therefore, both right-leg and left-leg devices must be stocked. The implant allows multiple cancellous screws to be placed across the distal metaphysis of the femur, which is helpful when there are several longitudinal splits through the articular surface. This plate is useful when comminution is extensive or osteoporosis is severe. In osteoporosis, the extra screws in the plate may provide support if one or two screws become loose. The device produces excellent alignment and stability when inserted correctly. The lateral flare of the condylar buttress plate should lie directly over the flare of the lateral condyle. If placed proximally or distally, it may lead to a varus or valgus alignment. This is sometimes a problem if comminution is extensive.

The device is quite simple to insert and does not require driving a nail or a large screw across a tenuously fixed articular fracture. Unfortunately, the device is not as strong as an angle blade plate or a compression hip screw, and if loaded early it may bend and fail. It is an excellent implant to use in intra-articular fractures in either a young patient with significant comminution or in an elderly patient with osteoporosis and an intra-articular extension of the fracture, if the patient can be relied on not to load the device until early fracture healing has occurred.

The 95-degree angle blade plate guarantees the best fracture alignment and offers excellent stability when used by an experienced surgeon[3,6–11] (Fig. 26–16). Its disadvantages are that it is technically difficult to apply and that it requires accurate place-

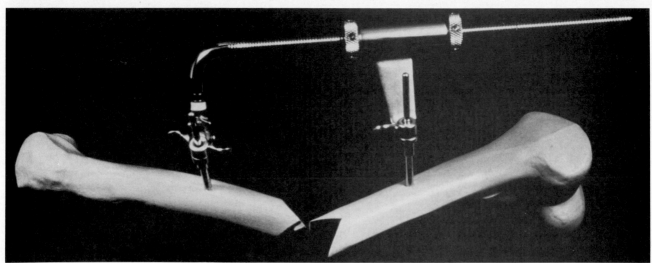

**Fig. 26–14**  Femoral distractor.

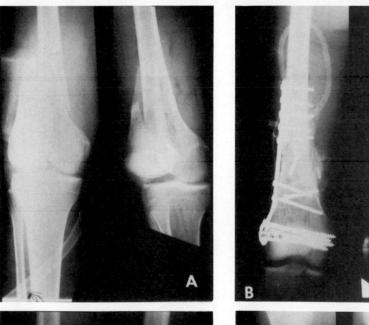

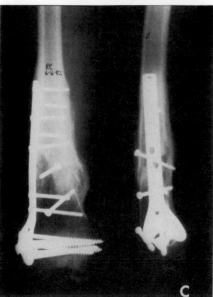

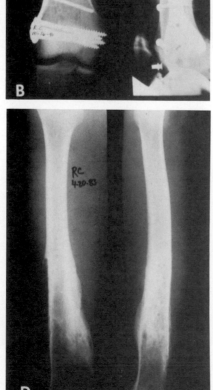

**Fig. 26–15**  ORIF distal femoral fracture utilizing condylar buttress plate. **A:** Closed comminuted intra-articular fracture in an 18-year-old male. **B:** Postoperative radiograph demonstrating alignment. Note medial bone graft. **C:** Solid union at eight months following fracture. **D:** Plate removal 18 months following fracture.

ment in all three planes. It is not always feasible in fractures with severe intra-articular comminution. Also, it is driven across comminuted fractures like a nail.

Compression screw plate systems are gaining in popularity[5] (Fig. 26–17). They are particularly useful when used for internal fixation of hip fractures. The supracondylar compression screw device used for the distal femur also has a 95-degree angle between the plate and barrel for the screw. The advantages of this implant are that it offers excellent fracture alignment and stability; it may allow some compression of the metaphyseal component of the fracture with the diaphyseal component of the fracture; and it is easier

to insert than the angle blade plate. The device requires excellent alignment in two planes but allows a degree of freedom in the third plane in that the screw can easily be turned into or out of the bone for better alignment of the plate with the screw. The device has the disadvantage of being rather large, requiring the removal of a significant amount of bone in the femoral condyles. Earlier devices had a bulky shoulder at the 95-degree angle bend, which can interfere with the iliotibial band during knee flexion, making postoperative range-of-motion exercises difficult.

The device should always be keyed or in the locked mode. This may be either by the design of the screw's

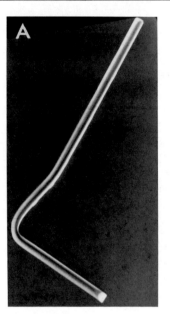
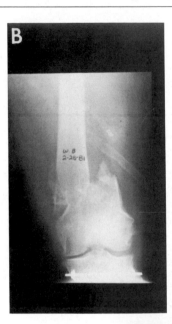
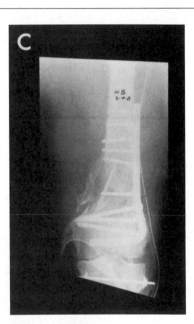
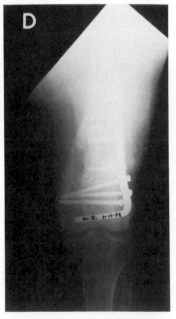

**Fig. 26–16** ORIF distal femoral fracture utilizing angle blade plate. **A:** Photograph of 95-degree angle blade plate. **B:** Comminuted distal femoral fracture in a 62-year-old female (previous ORIF tibial plateau fracture). **C:** ORIF with angle blade plate. Note medial bone graft. Bolt removal from proximal tibia prior to wound closure. **D:** Solid union one year following injury.

articulation in the barrel of the plate or by locking the distal fragment to the plate with an extra metaphyseal screw. If it is not keyed, the distal fragment may pivot on the screw in the condyles with flexion and extension of the knee. The device should also have oval holes that allow some angulation of screws across the plate to improve interfragmentary compression. Newer designs now available may make this device even more attractive.

Occasionally, a straight, broad, dynamic compression plate is the only implant long enough to be used. This implant is appropriate when comminution is not severe in the intra-articular area and the fracture line is long, extending for a good distance up the femoral shaft as in a spiral fracture. After provisional stabilization, the plate can be bent to fit the contour of the distal femur.

### Intramedullary Devices

Intramedullary devices include the Zickel device, locked intramedullary nails, antegrade Ender nails, and Rush rods.

The Zickel supracondylar device has proven to be useful in extra-articular or nondisplaced intra-articular fractures. The device is most useful in elderly osteoporotic bone and seldom requires the additional use of a brace. The surgical procedure is usually done by exposing the fracture site to obtain an easy, gentle reduction during insertion of the intramedullary nail. The device is easy to insert. The author has not used this device in comminuted or displaced intra-articular fractures in younger patients.

The locked intramedullary nail is gaining popularity for use in comminuted femoral and tibial shaft fractures (Fig. 26–18). The device is basically an intramedullary nail with accommodation for cross fixation of bolts through the nail, both above and below the fracture. This cross fixation uses bolts or blades. In distal femoral shaft fractures, the device has the advantage of being a load-sharing device that may allow earlier weightbearing. The device is inserted in the proximal rather than the distal femur utilizing a closed technique. It may, however, require some open surgery for insertion of bolts as a distal locking mechanism. The disadvantages are that it requires some intact distal bone length (at least 6 to 8 cm) and good general bone quality. It is not useful for displaced intra-articular fractures; however, it has been used with nondisplaced intra-articular fractures that can be treated with percutaneous lag screws prior to the insertion of the nail (Fig. 26–19). The device, which usually requires no postoperative brace, will permit excellent knee motion.

One must be cautious about using this device in

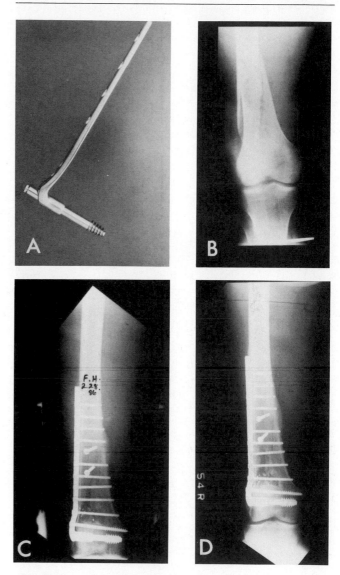

**Fig. 26–17** ORIF distal femoral fracture utilizing supracondylar compression screw. **A:** Photograph of 95-degree supracondylar compression screw. **B:** Comminuted distal femoral fracture in a 23-year-old male. **C:** ORIF. Note use of postoperative hinged orthosis. **D:** Early union eight months following fracture.

distal third femoral fractures. If a relatively small intramedullary nail (12 or 13 mm) is used and the patient is allowed to bear full weight immediately, the nail may fracture at the most proximal bolt site (Fig. 26–20). If this particular device is chosen for a distal extra-articular fracture of the femur, weightbearing must be avoided for six to eight weeks until early fracture healing has occurred. Use of a larger nail (14 to 16 mm) should also be considered.

Intramedullary devices require less dissection of the fracture site, allow earlier weightbearing, and are load-sharing; therefore, they are stressed to a lesser degree than eccentrically placed screw-plate devices. Their disadvantages are that they are useful only for extra-articular or intra-articular nondisplaced fractures, and they require some length of bone (generally 6 to 8 cm).

Antegrade Ender nailing, a technique described by Browner and associates,[12] involves placing several Ender nails from proximally to distally with the tip of the nails curving into the medial and lateral femoral condyles. The technique is used for only infraisthmic or extra-articular fractures, often requires a cast-brace, and offers no major advantages over other intramedullary devices. It does not control rotation quite as well as other devices.

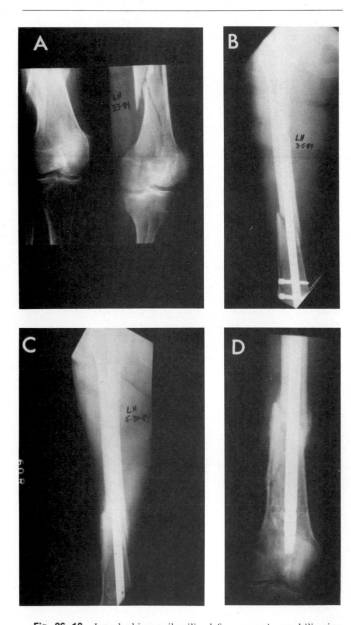

**Fig. 26–18** Interlocking nail utilized for operative stabilization of distal femoral fracture. **A:** Closed, spiral, distal femoral fracture in a 68-year-old female, no intra-articular extension. **B:** Closed insertion of static locked intramedullary nail. **C:** Early union three months following injury allowing removal of distal bolts from nail. **D:** Solid union five months following injury.

Rush rods are similar in application to the Zickel device. They should be used with a screw to prevent the nail from backing out with knee motion. Rush rods offer no advantage over the Zickel implant.

## External Fixation

External fixation can be used for distal femoral fractures. It may be used in conjunction with internal fixation, as with several screws to fix intra-articular extensions. The device is useful only for those fractures with preexisting infection or severe soft-tissue damage. Generally speaking, the device is really useful only in a limb-salvage procedure and should be reserved for that purpose alone. The Wagner leg-lengthening device is an excellent external fixator that uses large 6-mm pins (Fig. 26–21). It is rigid and stable. Other external fixators, such as the AO or Hoffmann external fixator, can be used with several 5-mm pins and stacked bars or tubes placed in a unilateral or half-frame fashion and extending from the lateral aspect of the femur. The device has limited application to only the most severe circumstances.

## Postoperative Management

After closure of the wound, the patient should be placed either in the 90/90 position on a Böhler-Braun frame (Fig. 26–22) for four to six days or in a continuous passive motion machine to assist in maintaining active range of motion of the knee (Fig. 26–23). Suction drainage should be applied for approximately 36 to 48 hours postoperatively. Physical therapy should be instituted beginning on the first postoperative day with major emphasis on isometric muscle training and supportive mobilization of the knee. If the continuous passive motion machine is used, emphasis shifts from mobilization of the knee to muscle-strengthening exercises. A cast-brace or functional bracing with a custom-molded orthosis is occasionally necessary, particularly with comminuted or osteoporotic fractures. These braces may be used even after open reduction and internal fixation because they can improve long-term results. Foot-flat ambulation (partial weightbearing, approximately 10 to 15 lb) is begun as soon as it can be tolerated. The patient must avoid heavy weightbearing exercise until early fracture healing has occurred. The author recommends increasing partial weightbearing, beginning at approximately the sixth postoperative week, at increments of 10 to 15 lb per week until full body weight can be borne. Crutches are used until the patient is confident about full weightbearing ambulation. The implant should not be removed for at least 12 months after open reduction and internal fixation. In general, load-sharing devices such as intramedul-

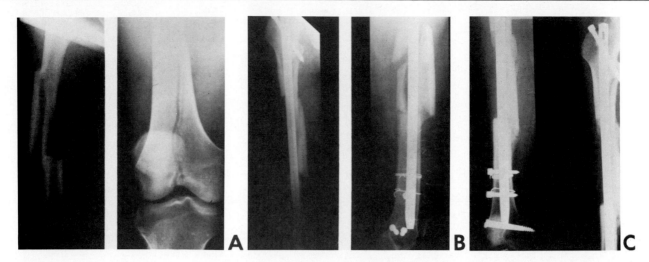

**Fig. 26–19** Locked nail used for distal femoral fracture in presence of nondisplaced intra-articular fracture extension. **A:** Comminuted femoral shaft fracture in a 28-year-old male with nondisplaced intra-articular extension into the knee. **B:** Postoperative radiograph demonstrating internal fixation with static locked intramedullary nail and two interfragmentary compression screws. Cerclage wires used to maintain reduction during nail insertion. **C:** Solid union present three months following injury.

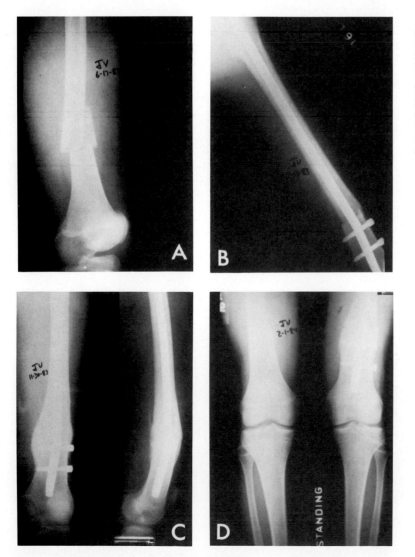

**Fig. 26–20** Fracture of 12-mm intramedullary nail at proximal-most distal bolt hole when full weight-bearing was allowed immediately following fracture fixation. **A:** Comminuted extra-articular distal femur fracture in a 17-year-old male. **B:** Treatment with 12-mm distal dynamic locked intramedullary nail. Weightbearing ambulation allowed immediately following surgery. Fracture of nail noted at proximal-most distal bolt hole one month following fracture. **C:** Fracture healed uneventfully five months following fracture. **D:** Normal knee motion and alignment seven months following fracture.

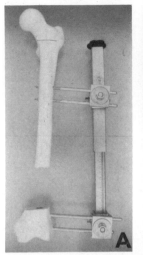
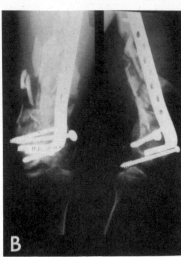
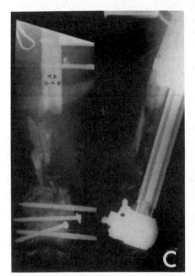
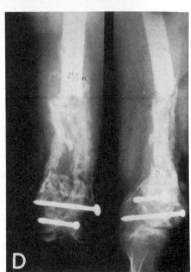

**Fig. 26–21** External fixation used as a salvage procedure for distal femoral fracture. **A:** Photograph demonstrating application of Wagner external fixator to distal femur. **B:** Comminuted intra-articular fracture in a 25-year-old female treated elsewhere by ORIF utilizing angle blade plate and bone graft. **C:** Massive infection four weeks following surgery necessitating debridement of bone and hardware with application of external fixation. **D:** Early union five months after fracture following bone graft. Knee range of motion 10 to 80 degrees of flexion.

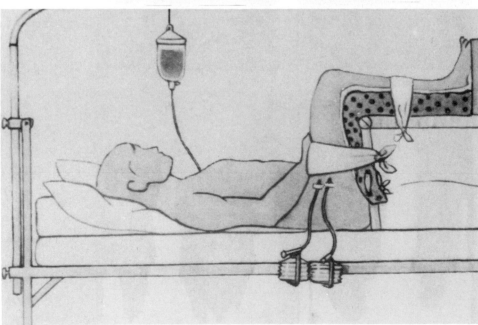

**Fig. 26–22** Patient with fractured leg on a frame with the hip flexed 90 degrees and the knee flexed 90 degrees (the 90/90 position).

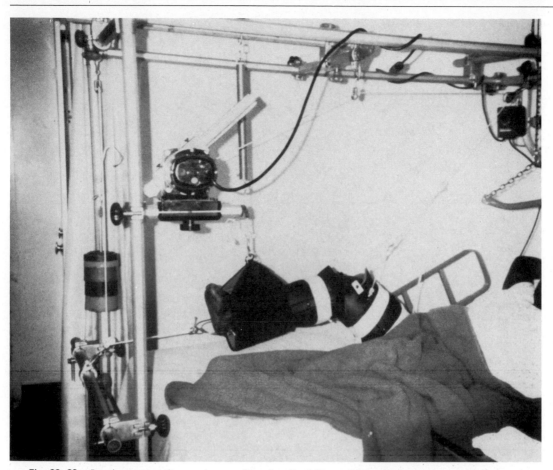

**Fig. 26–23**  Continuous passive motion machine for distal femoral fractures.

lary nails may be removed sooner than plates, which are load-bearing devices. Plates generally should not be removed until 18 to 24 months after fracture fixation. Again, caution is needed when interlocking nails are used for distal femoral fractures. Full weightbearing should be avoided until early fracture union is radiographically apparent (six to eight weeks).

### Discussion

Satisfactory results using open reduction and internal fixation have been increasing as opposed to treatment of distal femoral fractures with traction or a cast-brace (Table 26–2). Technological improvements in implants and improved surgical techniques have made the surgical fixation of distal femoral fractures increasingly possible. The technique demands great skill and sound judgment on the part of the surgeon. The patient's history and life style, as well as fracture pattern and bone density, must be reviewed carefully if the correct implant is to be selected. No one implant produces excellent results in every case.

Complications with distal femoral fractures have been reported. Major complications include nonunion, delayed union, infection, implant failure, loss of knee motion, and other associated medical problems (decubitus ulcers, urinary tract infections, pneumonia, or thromboembolic diseases). The major drawback to surgical management of supracondylar fractures of the femur has been the real or potential threat of infection. Because of the increased incidence of open fractures, the extensive surgical dissection required, and the prolonged operating time that is often necessary, the threat of infection has been a major concern. Older studies from the 1960s reported postoperative infection rates of almost 20%.[2,13] In more recent reports, infection rates ranging from 0% to 5.8% have been more common.[5,7,8,14] Meticulous surgical technique, broad-spectrum antibiotics, and rigid internal fixation seem to deter infection. Open wounds are returned to the operating room after five to seven days for delayed wound closure or skin grafting.

At Parkland Memorial Hospital, where almost all distal femoral fractures are treated surgically, patients obtain more consistent fracture alignment, range of motion of the knee, and better healing. These surgical procedures require fewer hospital

**Table 26–2**
**Comparison of results in various studies**

| Year | Study | Treatment* | No. of Cases | Results (% Good, Fair, or Excellent) | Infection (%) | Nonunion (%) |
|------|-------|-----------|--------------|--------------------------------------|---------------|--------------|
| 1966 | Stewart et al[13] | ORIF | 69 | 54 | 6 | 14 |
|      |                   | T & C | 144 | 67 | 0 | 6 |
| 1967 | Neer et al[2] | ORIF | 29 | 31 | 28 | 17 |
|      |               | T & C | 48 | 42 | 4 | 2 |
| 1971 | Slatis et al[11] | ORIF | 20 | 94 | 5 | 0 |
| 1972 | Olerud[3] | ORIF | 15 | 60 | 25 | 7 |
| 1973 | Connolly et al[15] | T & C | 39 | 82 | 0 | 2 |
| 1974 | Chiron et al[1] | ORIF | 72 | 75 | 2 | 0 |
| 1974 | Shelton et al[9] | ORIF | 14 | 71 | 0 | 0 |
| 1974 | Schatzker et al[8] | ORIF | 24 | 88 | 0 | 0 |
|      |                    | T & C | 39 | 46 | 3 | 13 |
| 1979 | Schatzker and Lambert[7] | ORIF | 35 | 74 | 0 | 6 |
| 1982 | Giles et al[5] | ORIF | 26 | 89 | 0 | 1 |
| 1982 | Mize et al[10] | ORIF | 30 | 97 | 2 | 0 |
| 1983 | Healy and Brooker[14] | ORIF | 47 | 87 | 1 | 2 |
|      |                       | T & C | 21 | 71 | ? | 1 |

*ORIF, open reduction with internal fixation; T & C, traction and cast.

days than closed treatment. This ultimately results in better function for the patient and marked savings. Nonunion rates with surgical fracture treatment should be less than 4%, which is similar to those reported with traction and cast-brace treatment.[15] This has been true in several recently reported series.[5,7,14] The incidence of delayed union or nonunion can be decreased by the generous use of primary autogenous bone grafting, anatomic reduction, and stable fixation. Medical complications are markedly decreased by early mobilization, which is made possible by stable internal fixation of fractures. Loss of knee motion is decreased by stable fracture fixation, which lessens pain, and the early institution of range-of-motion exercises through the use of physical therapy, or the use of a continuous passive motion machine (Fig. 26–22). When knee motion is near normal, there is considerably less stress on the surgical implants. Range of motion should be lost only when it is impossible to reconstruct the intra-articular aspect of the distal femur anatomically. Range of motion after internal fixation must be at least 0 to 110 degrees to be considered acceptable. Malunion secondary to shortening of more than 2 cm or a malalignment of more than 5 degrees is not acceptable.

## References

1. Chiron HS, Tremoulet J, Casey P, et al: Fractures of the distal third of the femur treated by internal fixation. *Clin Orthop* 1974;100:160.
2. Neer CS II, Grantham SA, Shelton ML: Supracondylar fracture of the adult femur. *J Bone Joint Surg* 1967;49A:591.
3. Olerud S: Operative treatments of supracondylar-condylar fractures of the femur. *J Bone Joint Surg* 1972;54A:1015.
4. Tile M: *Fractures of the Pelvis and Acetabulum.* Baltimore, Williams and Wilkins, 1984.
5. Giles JB, DeLee JC, Heckman JD, et al: Supracondylar–intercondylar fractures of the femur treated with a supracondylar plate and lag screw. *J Bone Joint Surg* 1982;64A:864.
6. Müller ME, Allgower M, Schneider R, et al: *Manual of Internal Fixation.* New York, Springer–Verlag, 1979.
7. Schatzker J, Lambert DC: Supracondylar fractures of the femur. *Clin Orthop* 1979;138:77.
8. Schatzker J, Horne G, Waddell J: The Toronto experience with the supracondylar fracture of the femur, 1966–1972. *Injury* 1974;6:113–128.
9. Shelton ML, Grantham SA, Neer CS II, et al: A new fixation device for supracondylar and low femoral shaft fractures. *J Trauma* 1974;14:821–835.
10. Mize RD, Bucholz RW, Grogan DP: Surgical treatment of displaced, comminuted fractures of the distal end of the femur. *J Bone Joint Surg* 1982;64A:871.
11. Slatis P, Ryoppy S, Huihinen VM: AOI osteosynthesis of fractures of the distal one third of the femur. *Acta Orthop Scand* 1971;42:162.
12. Browner BD, Burgess AR, Robertson RJ, et al: Immediate closed antegrade Ender nailing of femoral fractures in polytrauma patients. *J Trauma* 1984;24:921–927.
13. Stewart MJ, Sisk TD, Wallace SL Jr: Fractures of the distal third of the femur. *J Bone Joint Surg* 1966;48A:784.
14. Healy WL, Brooker AF: Distal femoral fractures: Comparison of open and closed methods of treatment. *Clin Orthop* 1983;174:166.
15. Connolly JF, Dehne E, LaFollette B: Closed reduction and early cast-brace ambulation in the treatment of femoral fractures: Results in one hundred and forty-three fractures. *J Bone Joint Surg* 1973;55A:1581.

# P A R T D

# Supracondylar Fractures: A Method of Fixation

### Robert E. Zickel, MD

Supracondylar fractures and fractures of the distal femoral shaft are difficult to treat. Poor bone stock, proximity to the knee joint, and a truncated shaft make this area of the femur less suitable for internal fixation than other areas. Because of the technical problems of open reduction and internal fixation, many surgeons prefer to treat these fractures conservatively.[1] Traction, casts, and cast-braces are acceptable conservative approaches. In elderly patients or patients with multiple injuries, who should be mobilized early, these methods can prolong hospitalization and confinement to bed.

Most fixation devices for the distal femur have been modified bone plates that conform to the distal femur, with screws, bolts, or nails used for fixation in the intracondylar area.[2-4] These devices are not ideal for severely comminuted fractures or in elderly patients with cortical thinning resulting from osteopenia. Intramedullary rods, designed for the middle third of the shaft, often do not provide adequate control of the distal femur. Interlocking nails, which have recently gained popularity, may be applicable to fractures at the junction of the middle and distal thirds of the shaft (infraisthmic fractures), but do not afford adequate fixation for fractures of the lower shaft and supracondylar areas. Flexible nails, such as those designed by Rush, have been used for several decades. Stability is achieved with these devices by three-point fixation, creating a spring-like effect in the intramedullary canal. The three points of fixation are the point of insertion in the condyle, the point of deflection off the opposite cortex, and the point of return to the cortex on the side of the original insertion. Difficulties with Rush pins may be caused by intraoperative bending modifications of the nail before insertion. The Rush pin technique was used extensively at the author's institution before 1969. With this method, there were problems of cutting out, backing out, or deformation of the appliance after insertion (Fig. 26–24).

Ender nails, which were initially designed for fractures of the proximal femur, have been used by some surgeons in the manner of Rush pins. Browner and associates[5] inserted the pins in an antegrade fashion through the trochanteric notch of the femur, drove them distally through the femoral isthmus, and permitted them to splay out in the distal femoral canal. An unacceptable failure rate, caused by backing out of the nails, has curtailed this method of treatment.[6] Kolmert and associates[7] reported success with Ender nails in 34 cases when they inserted them through the femoral condyle, much like Rush nails, but transfixed them with screws at the condylar end, after slightly modifying the Ender appliance.

In 1970, a special intramedullary fixation device for the distal femur was designed at St. Luke's Hospital in New York City. This stainless steel nail had a flexible stem with a ski-shaped tip and a rigid curved condylar end to match the femoral canal of the distal femur. Inserted like the Rush nail, it differed signifi-

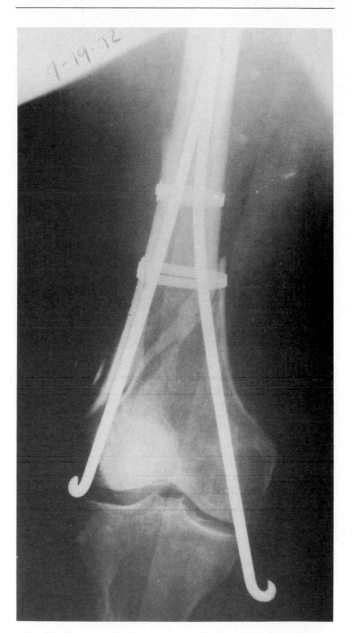

**Fig. 26–24** Complications with the double Rush pin technique, with pins cutting and backing out.

cantly in its design, as it could be anchored by a transfixion screw at its condylar base. The stem of the appliance was rectangular rather than round in cross section (unlike the Rush and Ender appliances). It was flexible in only one plane—that necessary to permit tracking from the condyle up through the proximal canal. The distal or condylar end of the appliance was large (11 mm sq in cross section), and curved to match the medullary canal condyle. This part was cannulated to receive a 0.25-inch buttress thread compression lag screw.

The present design includes six intramedullary rods, three for the medial condyle and three for the lateral condyle. The three in each group differ

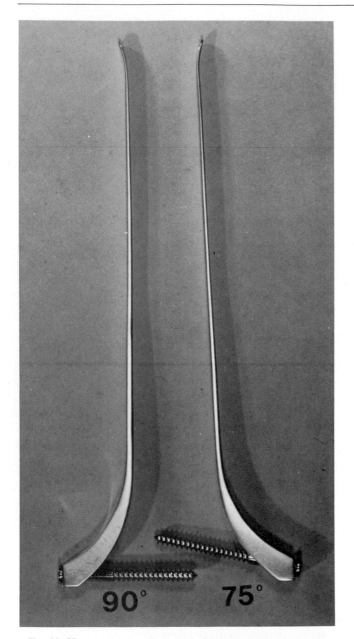

**Fig. 26–25** Anteroposterior view of intramedullary supracondylar device with anchoring compression screw. Lateral nail screw angle, 90 degrees; medial nail screw angle, 75 degrees.

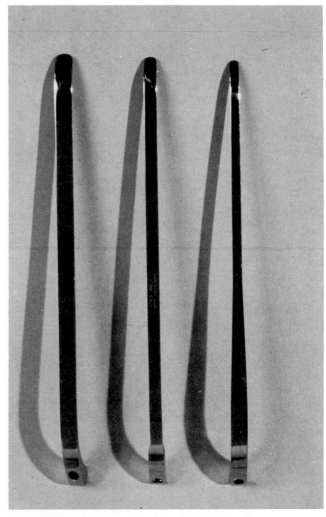

**Fig. 26–26** Three widths of intramedullary nail: 11 mm, 7.5 mm, and 4 mm.

among themselves only in the width of the stems (4 mm, 7.5 mm, and 11 mm). The medial and lateral rods differ in the angulation of the tunnel, with the lateral rod subtending a tunnel angle of 90 degrees with the stem and the medial rod subtending a tunnel angle of 75 degrees with the stem. This design difference was necessary because of the distal posture of the medial femoral condyle (to prevent encroachment into the intracondylar notch by the compression lag screw). Although the thickness of the metal is the same in all nails, the width of the stem can be significant, because the wider stems are stiffer than the narrower stems. This can be a consideration in an

osteopenic bone when a thinner stem with increased flexibility should be used to avoid intraoperative fracture. The 0.25-inch compression lag screw with buttress threads has a snap ring in its shank to engage a groove in the tunnel of the nail. This was designed to keep the screw from backing out in poor bone stock (Figs. 26–25 and 26–26)

## Method

The supracondylar nails may be inserted by a closed or an open method, depending on the morphologic features of the fracture and whether or not an acceptable closed reduction can be achieved. Many fractures can be reduced and fixed without exposing the fracture site. However, if significant comminution and displacement are present, both open reduction and additional fixation may be necessary.

In a closed nailing, after reduction, two small incisions are made longitudinally in the area of the medial and lateral condyle. The adductor tubercle and the patella provide landmarks for location of the incision. An image intensifier allows metallic markers to be used on the skin to determine the proper level for the incision. The author performs most closed nailings with the patient's leg draped freely on an operating table equipped with a radiotransparent image board. If the surgeon prefers, a fracture table can be used to achieve reduction before insertion of the nails (Fig. 26–27).

The entrance point for the nails should be in the anterior two thirds of the condyles and as distal as possible without violating the articular cartilage of the condyle. A curved awl is used for preparing a channel in each condyle; insertion of the awl is monitored on the image intensifier. The two channels should be in different planes. Usually, the channel in the lateral condyle is anterior to that in the medial condyle. This permits the nails to cross in separate planes rather than deflecting each other. In addition, the anchoring screws when inserted should not abut on the opposite nail. Reaming the medullary canal may be necessary in young patients in whom the trabecular bone is still quite dense. It is rarely necessary in elderly patients, once the channels in the condyles have been prepared. If reaming is required, flexible intramedullary reamers should be used. Once the femur has been prepared, two nails are selected for insertion, one medial and one lateral. Each is marked appropriately but they really differ only in the angle of the tunnel in the large condylar portion of the rod. The selection of the width of the stem is influenced by the size of the medullary canal and the quality of the bone stock. In a femur in a younger patient with a wide canal, a 7.5- or 11-mm nail may be selected. In an elderly patient with osteopenia, the thinner, 4-mm nail may be selected because of its increased flexibility (Fig. 26–28, A and B).

The two nails may be the same or different in width (e.g., a 4-mm and a 7.5-mm nail; a 4-mm and an 11-mm nail; two 7.5-mm nails). Once the two nails have been selected, they can be inserted manually under image monitoring through the wide channels in the femoral condyle. Once both cross the fracture and appear in the medullary canal on biplane imaging, they should be driven with alternate short advances until the condylar end of each nail is completely seated, either flush with the cortex or slightly beneath the cortex of the condyle. The 0.25-inch compression anchoring screws are passed through

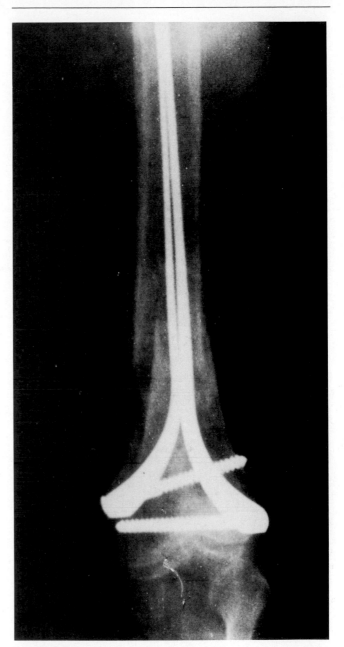

**Fig. 26–27** Closed nailing in slightly displaced transverse fracture in an elderly patient. The patient was able to sit in a chair on the first postoperative day.

the tunnel after it is predrilled with a 3/16-inch drill. A lock-ring in the smooth shank of the lag screw engages a circular groove in the tunnel of the nail.

### Open Reduction

Open reduction is necessary in some fractures because satisfactory reduction cannot be achieved or because additional fixation is needed to stabilize oblique fractures or comminuted fragments. In such cases, a major incision is made, usually through an anterolateral approach. An attempt should be made

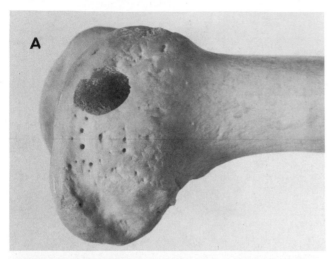

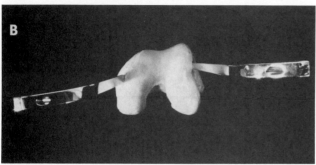

**Fig. 26-28 A:** The entrance point for channel in condyle should be as distal as possible and in the anterior two thirds of the condyle. **B:** Coronal view shows placement of nails in two different planes. Lateral nail is anterior to medial nail.

to stay just anterior to the iliotibial band and to dissect the vastus lateralis muscle from the central slip of the rectus femoris muscle. The vastus intermedius, encountered next, can be bluntly separated over the fracture site. The author prefers this approach to a full lateral approach because it gives better anterior access to the entire condylar area. If the surgeon so desires, the major incision may be medial with the plane just posterior to the vastus medialis. This approach actually provides a better plane than the anterolateral approach, but risks encountering the femoral or the medial genicular artery. These structures must be identified and avoided. When an open approach is used, periosteal stripping should be kept to a minimum and accessory fixation used as indicated. Stainless steel 18-gauge cerclage wires provide the necessary accessory fixation in most cases (Fig. 26–29, A, B, and C).

Supracondylar fractures with intracondylar fracture extensions are the most difficult technically. Exposure of the knee joint is almost always necessary so that the condyles can be reduced anatomically before insertion of the appliance. Kirschner wires have been used to stabilize these condyles before

insertion of the appliance. However, compression lag screws are preferable, as they help prevent separation of the condyles during insertion of the intramedullary nails.

After surgery, the knee and leg are partially immobilized with bulky dressings and a knee immobilizer. A posterior plaster splint (or, rarely, a cylinder case) may be used at the discretion of the surgeon. Early in the author's series, casts or cast-braces were often used but they are now used only occasionally in unstable fractures. Nonweightbearing standing and ambulation may begin when the patient is comfortable and able to use a walker or crutches. In very elderly or senile patients, early ambulation should not begin until fracture healing is clinically evident, but the patient may be transferred to a chair in the immediate postoperative period.

## Clinical Series

Of 82 femurs treated with this appliance before April 1984, 69 had fractures and 13 involved arthritic knees undergoing supracondylar osteotomies. Fifty-five of the patients were 60 years old or older. The youngest patient was 17 years old and the oldest was 104 years old. Fifty-three were women and 27 were men. Two patients had bilateral operations. Sixty-three fractures and 13 osteotomies were followed to union. Six patients were lost to follow-up or died before healing could be determined. All but one fracture united primarily, but five of the osteotomies failed to unite after one operation and required additional surgery.

Fractures were classified as follows: high transverse, low transverse, long oblique, low oblique, and "T" or "Y" fractures. There were two pathologic fractures, and one femur was stabilized because of a lytic lesion with impending fracture. Additional fixation with 18-gauge cerclage wire was used in 22 femurs; in four, a third intramedullary nail was inserted in antegrade fashion from the proximal femur.

Ten of 11 high transverse fractures united and one did not. Five had the additional support of cast-braces and three limbs had ipsilateral tibial fractures ("floating knees"). All of these femurs united.

A third intramedullary rod was inserted in four high transverse or infraisthmic fractures. With this technique, the third rod is introduced into the piriform fossa, in a manner similar to that used for other intramedullary rods for the femur, and nested with two previously inserted supracondylar nails. The Street nail was particularly useful for this procedure because of its diamond shape.

There were nine low transverse fractures. One patient died two months after surgery, but in the others the fractures united at an average of 15 weeks. Accessory fixation was not necessary in this group. Five received additional support from cast-braces.

Of 13 long oblique fractures, one was lost to follow-up, leaving 12 for evaluation. Two of the pathologic fractures were in this group; one of these united. The second patient died before union was achieved. Two fractures required accessory fixation and five received external support from casts or cast-braces. All nonpathologic low oblique fractures in this group healed.

Of 21 low oblique fractures, three were lost to follow-up but the remainder of this group united uneventfully. Fifteen required additional fixation with cerclage wires and six were supported with cast-braces for six weeks postoperatively.

There were 15 "T" or "Y" fractures or supracondylar fractures with a vertical extension into the intracondylar area. Threaded pins or screws were used to maintain reduction in eight of these before insertion of the supracondylar nail. Twelve of the 15 were protected by casts or cast-braces immediately after surgery. Four of these fractures, although united, later caused knee pain and restriction of motion.

A review of intraoperative and postoperative radiographs showed that four were not adequately reduced.

## Supracondylar Osteotomies

Supracondylar nails were used to stabilize varus supracondylar osteotomies done for lateral compartment arthritis in 13 knees. Five of these failed to unite primarily and required reoperation. Salvage procedures included the use of bone grafts and, often, wider nails than those used initially. Four eventually healed with the second procedure and one did not.

## Knee Motion

Range of knee motion was recorded in 57 patients one to seven years after surgery. Forty-two knees had ranges of more than 90 degrees, five had ranges of less than 60 degrees, and ten had ranges between 60 and 90 degrees. The "T" and "Y" fractures had the poorest range of motion; only 45% achieved 90 degrees of motion or more.

**Fig. 26–29   A:** Comminuted fracture of the distal third of the femur in a 66-year-old woman. **B:** Open reduction with internal fixation including cerclage wire technique. **C:** Healed fracture four months after surgery. Note proximal plate from hip nailing done several years previously.

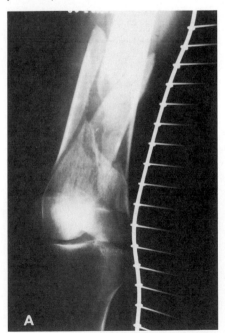
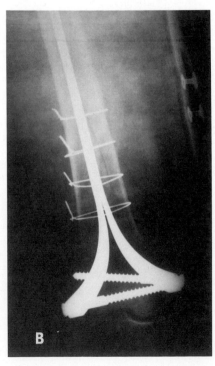
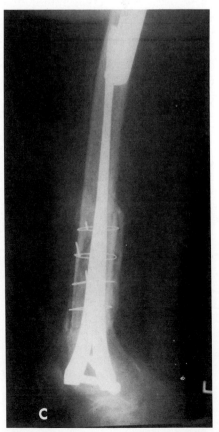

## Complications

Four infections developed, one deep and three superficial. The femur with a deep infection had Paget's disease with a bowed deformity. The infection was treated with wound care and antibiotics, with the nails left in place until fracture healing eventually occurred. The fracture united 18 weeks later and the nails were then removed. Some drainage persisted for several months, but this eventually resolved. Three years postoperatively, there had been no recurrence of the infection. The three superficial infections responded to wound care and antibiotics and healed uneventfully. Thirteen appliances were removed because of tenderness in the condylar region. This was caused in part by screws backing out before the lock-ring modification that was later incorporated into the system. A special extractor was designed to facilitate extraction and there were no refractures during or after extraction of the appliances.

## Discussion

Since the first report on this appliance in 1977, a total of 82 femurs have undergone surgery through April 1984.[8] Modifications of the appliance and surgical techniques have decreased intraoperative and postoperative complications. Although the appliances have been used in patients of many ages, two thirds of the patients were more than 60 years old.

In recent years, more of these procedures have been closed nailings and fewer legs have been immobilized postoperatively in casts or cast-braces. This has significantly decreased postoperative morbidity and improved knee motion. The use of a third intramedullary rod, nested with the two supracondylar rods in high transverse or infraisthmic fractures has been particularly encouraging. As might be expected, the "T" or "Y" supra-intracondylar fracture group had the poorest knee motion and were the most difficult to treat. Careful reduction and transcondylar fixation of the condyles must be performed before insertion of the appliance.

The high initial nonunion rate in the osteotomy group remains an enigma. Most of these procedures were performed through an anterolateral approach with a oscillating power saw. The question arises as to whether bone necrosis from the saw and a small contact surface, permitting rotational motion, contributed to the failures. The use of wider nails to provide better rotational stability, as was done in some of the salvage procedures, may be a better choice in the osteotomy group.

The high rate of union in the fracture group was particularly encouraging. It seems that this method of fixation can be helpful in many of these difficult fractures.

## References

1. Neer CS II, Grantham SA, Shelton ML: Supracondylar fracture of the adult femur. *J Bone Joint Surg* 1967;49A:591.
2. Boronni M, Botteli GC: The treatment of severe fractures of the lower end of the femur with Judet's screwplate. *Ital J Orthop Trauma* 1975;1:99.
3. Brown A, D'Arcy JC: Internal fixation for supracondylar fractures of the femur in the elderly patient. *J Bone Joint Surg* 1971;53B:420.
4. Elliott RB: Fractures of the femoral condyles: Experiences with a new design femoral condylar blade plate. *South Med J* 1959;52:80.
5. Browner BD, Burgess AR, Robertson RJ, et al: Immediate closed antegrade Ender nailing of femoral fractures in polytrauma patients. *J Trauma* 1984;24:921–927.
6. Browner BD: Personal communication, 1982.
7. Kolmert L, Egund N, Persson BD: Internal fixation of supracondylar and bicondylar fractures using a new semi-elastic device. *Clin Orthop* 1983;181:204.
8. Zickel RE, Hobeika P, Robbins DS: Zickel supracondylar nails for fracture of the distal end of the femur. *Clin Orthop* 1986;212:79–88.

# External Fixation of the Upper Extremity

William P. Cooney III, MD

Douglas K. Smith, MD

## Introduction

Fractures of the upper extremity can be difficult management problems. While not subjected to the same weightbearing forces and repetitive stress as the lower extremities, the upper extremities can sustain severe bone and soft-tissue damage that requires aggressive treatment. Various forms of external fixation are often needed to restore the limb to full functional capacity. This discussion will define the specific indications for and applications of external fixation, review equipment options, and present results of treatment of significant upper-extremity fractures and soft-tissue injuries.

The application of "external splints" to the upper extremity is not a new concept in fracture treatment; in fact, it is a rebirth of techniques and principles well-recognized by our orthopaedic forefathers. What is new in this field is the application of biomechanical and biomaterial principles and techniques to make external "fixators" both efficient and practical.[1] Since 1907,[2-4] enthusiasm for external fixation has varied. Ingenuity of design along with trial and error methods were evident in early discussions of the subject.[5-7] Recent enthusiasm for external fixation is based on the success of past techniques along with progress made in developing lighter metals,[8] more biologically tolerated pins and bone screws, as well as fixator designs that allow for compression, distraction, or alternative load sharing between the fixator and bone. In contrast to internal fixation of fractures, less foreign material is present within the wound and fewer complications from wound sepsis are encountered with external fixation. It incorporates improved biomechanical techniques as well as important biologic principles to provide a reliable fracture treatment alternative.

This discussion will review the authors' experience with upper limb external fixation, which extends over ten years and reflects experience with a wide range of injuries treatable with external fixation. The principles in treatment of hand injuries; unstable fractures of the distal radius; and severe bone and soft-tissue injuries of the forearm, arm, elbows, and shoulder involving high-energy stress and multiple soft-tissue loss will be presented. The rationale given for selecting specific equipment as well as a discussion of equipment options will provide the surgeon reason-able choices for each specific clinical problem. The limitations of these techniques as well as the contraindications will also be discussed.

## Hand Injuries

Hand fractures that are open, complicated by segmental fracture or bone loss, or involve the joint articular surface are primary indications for external fixation.[9,10] More specifically, we believe that all open fractures of the metacarpals and phalanges with skin loss or obvious sepsis should probably be treated by external fixation techniques.[11,12] Similarly, intra-articular joint damage with or without sepsis may be treated best by external fixation to achieve fracture reduction (by ligamentotaxis) or, if indicated, by primary arthrodesis.[13] Septic nonunions that require excision of the nonunion site can be resolved by interposition bone grafting and external fixation. Lastly, bone loss associated with segmental fractures can often be best stabilized or lengthened by applying a distraction-lengthening external fixation frame.[12]

With proper external fixation, soft-tissue and skeletal injuries of the hand and wrist can be stabilized, wound debridement performed, and reconstruction of tendons, nerves, and vessels achieved without compromising plates, screws, or internal fixation wires. External fixation can be continued until bone union is achieved or it can be removed for either cast or late open treatment of the bone injury.[12]

### Equipment

The Hoffmann mini-exoskeletal fixator has revolutionized the application of small frames to the hand and serves as an excellent alternative to larger, less versatile devices such as the Roger Anderson frame or Hoffmann C-series devices. It is definitely superior to pins and plaster. Made with the precision of a fine watch, this device originated with Henri Jaquet in Switzerland.[11,13] The versatility of the equipment allows either half-frame or double-frame systems to be chosen, depending on the fracture stability required (Fig. 27–1). With most phalangeal fractures, for example (Fig. 27–2A), the half frame is sufficient (Fig. 27–2B). Two pins inserted proximal and two pins inserted distal to the fracture provide excellent stability and control when secured to the mini-frame (Fig. 27–2, C and D) and primary fracture healing can be anticipated (Fig. 27–2E) with excellent return of function (Fig. 27–2F). In addition, the sliding swivel clamps of this frame can rotate up to 90 degrees to adapt to individual fracture location and either compression or distraction forces can be exerted through the sliding swivel clamps. Overcompression should be avoided, however, to prevent fracture angulation.

The double frame consists of two support rods, two connecting-pin holders, and two sliding swivel clamps (Fig. 27–1). It provides greater stability than the half frame since it employs continuous threaded Bonnel-type pins. It has been used primarily for very comminuted thumb and metacarpal fractures or for fractures of the distal radius (both open and closed).[12,14] In addition, the system can maintain bone length secondary to bone loss or a segmental fracture. We have had success with fractures near the joint, for which we have applied both half frames and full frames in an effort to maintain early motion. The joint can be moved actively or passively while the fracture is held rigid with the external pins and frame.

For fractures of phalanges or metacarpals that also enter the joint and in which reconstruction of the joint articular surface would be difficult or in which sepsis is present, a combination of joint fusion and fracture immobilization has been performed by combining one mini-frame with an extension unit from another.

**Technique**

With unstable or comminuted fractures of the phalanges or metacarpals, the fracture must be reduced before applying the Hoffmann mini-fixator. Brachial block or Bier block anesthesia is preferred, although occasionally local anesthesia will suffice. Finger traps are used to achieve fracture reduction. Once reduction has been obtained by traction or manipulation, the mini-pin insertion guide is applied to direct the predrilling (1.5-mm drill) and subsequent pin insertion (2-mm pins). The latter requires a special hand chuck. The pins are inserted through the pin insertion guide, which provides alignment for two pins inserted above and two below the fracture or fusion site. The pin guide is essential to measure the depth of pin insertion and to prevent angulation (Fig.

**Fig. 27–1** The external mini-fixation device (Jacquet) demonstrating the double frame (upper left) and single frame (upper right) assemblage. Special pin guides (HM1), hand chuck (HM2), socket wrench (HM4), wrenches (HM24, HM55), and pin point breachers (HM3) assist pin insertion and frame. Either 2-mm or 3-mm threaded or smooth pins (HM65, HM60) or Bonnell pins (HM70) can be used with simple or sliding swiveling clamps.

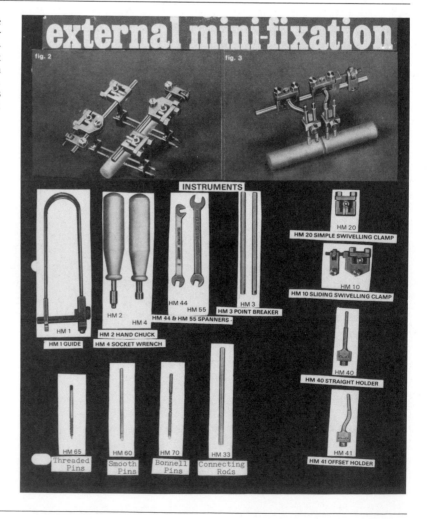

27–1). Once the pins are properly positioned, the exoskeletal frame is secured to the pins, utilizing offset pin holders to keep the frame away from the skin. When tightening the screws, finger-tip compression is symmetrically applied (the pins are a bit delicate and will fracture if excessive or asymmetric torque is applied).

## Complications

Problems associated with external fixation of the hand occur when initial fracture reduction is not obtained, when the location of important soft tissue is ignored, or when incorrect pin insertion leads to inadequate fixation at the pin-bone interface. Pins must be placed laterally using the prescribed pin

**Fig. 27–2    A:** Mini-fixation of phalanx fracture. Incomplete finger amputation with open fracture of the proximal phalanx. **B:** Skeletal model of Jacquet mini-fixateur applied with 2-mm continuously threaded pins connected to a single swiveling clamp (proximal) and sliding swiveling clamp (distal). **C and D:** Single frame applied; compression achieved through the sliding swiveling clamp. Anatomic alignment in both anteroposterior and lateral radiographs. **E:** Fracture union achieved by eight weeks. **F:** Excellent finger motion preserved.

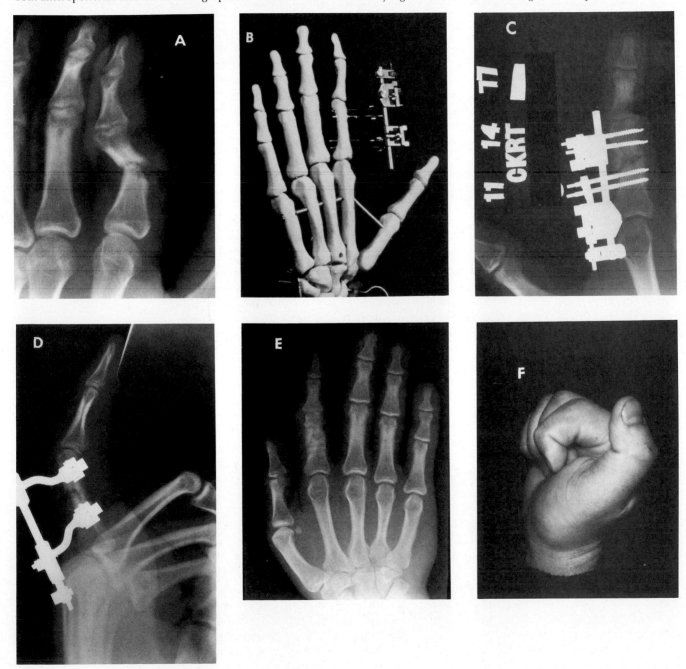

guide to avoid the volar neurovascular structures and the dorsal extensor tendon system. With midshaft phalangeal fractures, lateral pin placement is not a problem because a soft-tissue free interval exists. However, at the proximal interphalangeal (PIP) and metacarpophalangeal (MCP) joints, pins may pass through important tendon structures that could restrict joint motion or cause tissue injury. Open pin insertion may be indicated in these situations.

Pin insertion may be particularly difficult in unstable metacarpal fractures in which open pin insertion is necessary to identify the extensor tendons, the dorsal venous structures, and the radial artery. Predrilling of pin sites is necessary so that the threaded pins can be inserted by hand, avoiding local thermal necrosis.

### Results

In a series of 20 hand and carpal fractures treated with the Hoffmann mini-fixation frame, Riggs and Cooney were able to obtain primary union in each fracture (100%).[12] In addition, union was not delayed and extremely injured digits and hands were salvaged. There were no cases of sepsis or amputation of the injured part. Joint motion after hand fractures was 5 degrees to 80 degrees of flexion-extension (mean) at the MCP joint and 10 degrees to 65 degrees of flexion-extension at the PIP joint. Grip strength averaged more than 60% of the uninjured side. In most of these injuries, associated tendon injuries or intra-articular fractures accounted, in part, for the loss of finger motion and hand strength.

The mini-external fixator was also used for joint fusion and treatment of delayed union. In one hand, simultaneous PIP joint fusion and proximal phalangeal fracture fixation was achieved and the result was excellent. Two other patients had delayed union associated with cross K-wire fixation that failed, but they were successfully treated by external fixation with the Jaquet Mini-Fixateur.[12]

Intra-articular fractures of the distal radius in small-boned patients were also well managed by the Hoffmann mini-fixator: primary bone union was achieved in 12 cases.[15] In many of these intra-articular fractures, the fracture alone was transfixed, and the radiocarpal joint was mobilized to provide early joint motion.

### Conclusion

External fixation is a practical solution to complex hand, finger and wrist fractures, nonunions, and segmental loss of bone from injury or disease. It provides the optimal environment for both soft-tissue and bone healing. The adaptability of the Hoffmann mini-frame allows for a wide variety of angles and positions for pin placement so that soft tissues can be avoided and hand function is not compromised. The mini-Hoffmann half frame or full frame gives rigid stability with up to 90 degrees of adaptability. Complications can be avoided by careful attention to the details of predrilling, careful pin insertion, and frame application. An effort should be made to avoid fracture distraction. Compression can be applied and increased during the treatment period. We recommend exoskeletal fixation for open, comminuted, or segmental fractures of the hand and wrist when more traditional techniques of pinning, tension band wiring, or plate fixation would fail or compromise soft-tissue healing or function.

## Wrist Fractures

Intra-articular fractures of the distal radius are currently the most common indication for external fixation in the upper extremity.[16] The principle of "fracture reduction maintained by fixed traction" is not new, having been stated by Böhler almost 60 years ago.[7] It remains a sound concept for effective treatment of fractures about the wrist. Those who disfavor external fixation for fractures of the distal radius have misinterpreted the concept. Unstable fractures of the distal radius that involve the wrist joint were previously ignored simply because there was no effective way of holding the many comminuted, often osteoporotic fragments in place.[17] Casting has proved inadequate because the multiple fragments cannot stabilize each other; open reduction has been condemned as foolish because neither pins nor plates can provide stability.

External fixation has emerged as the definitive treatment of the unstable distal radius fracture, and it is now clear that intra-articular fractures of the distal radius should be distinguished from the general grouping of injuries labeled Colles' fracture.

### Principles of Treatment

The French have developed the principle upon which the use of external fixation is based; it is called ligamentotaxis—the ability to maintain fracture reduction by traction on the carpal ligaments and joint capsule.[1,18,19] This principle is applied in the cast treatment of distal radius fractures in which the wrist is flexed and the ulnar deviated to tighten the capsule and periosteum of the distal radius. With external fixation, however, more longitudinal traction is applied to obtain fracture reduction. As a result, extreme positions of joint flexion and carpal tunnel compression can be avoided. By trial and error, we have learned that about 3 to 5 kg (up to 10 lb) of traction will maintain most distal radius fractures in a reduced position and not produce excessive joint stiffness.[16,20]

In the treatment of distal radius fractures, the following points are most important and need special emphasis (Fig. 27–3): (1) obtain fracture reduction prior to external fixation; (2) use longitudinal traction and a gentle compression or manipulation to reduce the fracture and avoid extreme hyperflexion and extension maneuvers; (3) maintain external fixation for eight weeks to prevent secondary collapse or shortening; (4) use a quadrilateral frame for biplanar fracture support (unilateral frames are adequate but limited in achieving radioulnar stability); (5) apply pins close to, not farther away from, the fracture site to increase fracture rigidity; (6) mobilize soft tissues early, especially by finger flexion and extension; (7) prevent pin loosening by careful pin insertion. (Predrilling is best and a self-tapping, self-drilling pin is superior to a smooth pin. The pin-bone interface is the weakest link in the external fixation system.[8])

### Technique of External Fixation

The technique of external fixation common to all forms of external fixation of the distal radius follows a prescribed protocol of fracture reduction and subsequent fracture stabilization.[11,15,16,20,21] The following procedure is recommended: (1) axillary block or Bier block anesthesia; (2) finger-trap traction with 3 to 5 kg of countertraction; (3) fracture reduction during distraction by gentle compression of the fracture fragments; (4) external frame application by first inserting the distal pins in the base of the second and third metacarpals, then centering the external fixateur over the wrist and forearm, and, finally, placing proximal pins in the distal third of the radius; (5) application of supportive splints to maintain forearm supination (preferred position for ulnar styloid fractures or triangular fibrocartilage tears).

Pin insertion must be carefully performed by using a low-torque, low-speed drill or preferably a predrilled system and hand chuck. Overdrilling, producing heat, is the leading cause of pin-site drainage and the sequestrum formation of osteomyelitis.[21] Threaded pins are superior to smooth pins and a predrilled pin system is best. In addition, the frame should be as close to the skeleton as soft-tissue swelling will allow, and the pins should be inserted closer to, not farther from, the fracture site. Both factors minimize pin bending, improve fracture stability, and should help prevent loss of fracture reduction.

External fixation is maintained for eight weeks and is usually followed by two to three weeks of supportive splinting. Early removal of the frame has resulted in loss of reduction. In the senior author's experience,[15,20] fracture settling was most frequent if removal occurred before seven weeks or when small,

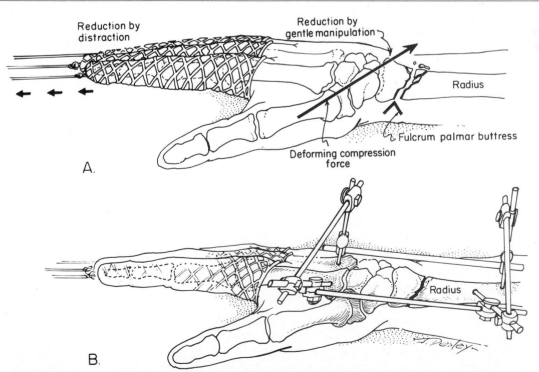

**Fig. 27–3  A:** Principles of treatment of distal radius fractures. Reduction by distraction; gentle manipulation and correction of deformity utilizing a fulcrum buttressed on the palmar cortex. **B:** Reduction maintained by a quadrilateral frame external fixation; 3-mm threaded pins are inserted into the metaphysis of metacarpals II and III, and into both cortices of the distal radius where the mid third and distal third join. (Reproduced with permission from Cooney WP, Linscheid RL, Dobyns JH: External pin fixation of unstable Colles' fractures. *J Bone Joint Surg* 1979;61A:840–845.)

smooth pins or K-wires were used rather than threaded 3-mm pins. During postfixation splinting, a physical therapy program is initiated to help recover hand and wrist motion and strength.

## Complications

Complications related to external fixation of the distal radius are similar to the complications associated with other treatment methods for the Colles' fracture.[21,22] Drainage and loosening at the pin site occurred in 25% of the patients studied by the senior author,[16] but they were considered minor problems that rarely affected the total treatment program. With improved pin insertion, these problems have occurred less frequently. Major complications occurred in 13% of the patients, the incidence being unrelated to the type of frame employed. These complications affected the eventual treatment outcome, with some having severely compromised extremity function. Upper limb dystrophy (shoulder-hand-finger syndrome) is the most serious of these complications.[17,21] It is associated with a painful pin site (tendon or nerve irritation) or is related to persistent but untreated carpal tunnel syndrome. In some patients, the very presence of the frame produces such fear that they will not use the extremity; this reaction requires prompt frame removal. Recognition of early upper limb dystrophy, early treatment with active hand, elbow, and shoulder motion, and pain control by stellate blocks are essential to prevent the serious sequelae of this condition.

## Results

The results of external fixation of intra-articular fractures of the distal radius have generally been excellent. A number of series now demonstrate that 90% good-to-excellent results, both clinical and radiologic, can be anticipated.[11,12,14,16,20,21,23-25] The anatomic results and the clinical results correlated well and are related to maintaining fracture length and preventing excessive dorsal angulation (Fig. 27–4). Limitation of wrist motion caused by ligament and capsule stiffness occurs early, but our studies show that this will usually resolve by seven to nine months following injury. As a result, early motion using "hinged" wrist external fixator units does not appear to be necessary. The results of a study in which wrist motion using fixation of just the fracture site (mini-external system) was compared with transcarpal fixation using ligamentotaxis frames clearly demonstrated that final range-of–motion differences were not significant.[16] Also of interest, the results following primary external fixation versus secondary external fixation have been similar, showing that a delay in treatment, if casting fails, is not detrimental to the patient. In our early series,[20] poor results occurred in only 4% of patients, and most of these had upper limb dystrophy

associated with repeated manipulations and very late external fixation. In our combined series,[11,16] motion of the wrist averaged 48 degrees of extension, 47 degrees of flexion, and 37 degrees of radioulnar deviation (Fig. 27–5). Grip strength was 54% to 60% that of the uninjured side, supination was 67 degrees, and pronation was 62 degrees (Fig. 27–6). Long-term radiographic assessment (Fig. 27–7) has demonstrated only a slight loss of length or anatomic alignment of the distal radius and distal radioulnar joint should be anticipated.

The results using external fixation are superior to those achieved with pins and plaster or with various forms of plaster immobilization of the distal radius. Comparing previous series using conventional treatment[17] with modern application of external fixation clearly demonstrates the advantages of this technique in its ability to maintain fracture alignment, produce a normal-looking wrist, and, above all, improve the long-term functional results for the patient.

## Conclusion

External fixation of fractures of the distal radius has provided a new method of treating a difficult and common fracture, especially one associated with significant comminution and a large degree of fracture displacement. Improved hand and wrist function has resulted. Obtaining an accurate reduction first and then applying the frame to maintain the reduction requires re-emphasis. Only newer frames[26] are designed to assist in reduction. With the various quadrilateral frames, loss of reduction will be unusual. Wrist stiffness, present early following external fixation, gradually resolves and wrist motion returns to approximately 80% of normal.

## External Fixation of the Forearm and Arm

High-energy injuries sustained as a result of today's mechanized society have increased the need for external fixation of upper extremity injuries involving the arm and forearm.[27,28] Besides the obvious bony injury, significant soft-tissue damage with associated nerve and vessel injury[29] has made treatment of these injuries difficult and a challenge to the orthopaedic surgeon. For many of these problems, external fixation has re-emerged as an ideal fracture management system, since it provides the needed fracture and soft-tissue stabilization, and, if properly applied, promotes progression to primary bone healing.[1,30,31]

The very nature of many of these injuries predisposes the limb to delayed fracture healing so that extensive reconstruction with bone grafts, local or distant pedicle flaps (including free flaps), and late tendon and nerve reconstruction is needed.[32,33] Salvage of upper extremity injuries that would previously have resulted in amputation is now possible.

**Fig. 27–4**   External fixation of the wrist. **A:** A comminuted fracture of the distal radius (Frykman VII). **B:** Reduction achieved with longitudinal traction and gentle fracture reduction results in near anatomic alignment on anteroposterior radiographs. **C:** Lateral radiographs showing near anatomic alignment with longitudinal traction and gentle fracture reduction. **D:** Low-profile (Ace-Colles) frame. Early hand function is encouraged by hand, forearm rotation, and shoulder elevation. **E:** Final radiographic result shows faint fracture line, perfectly restored radiocarpal and radioulnar articulations. Functional result mirrored the radiographic excellence.

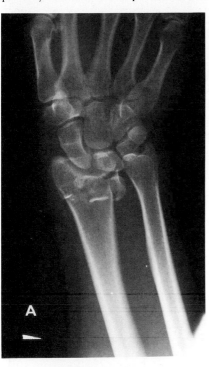

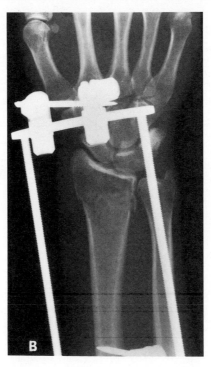

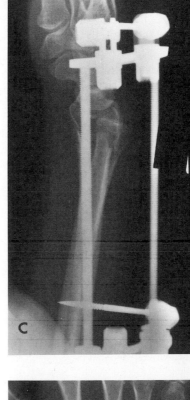

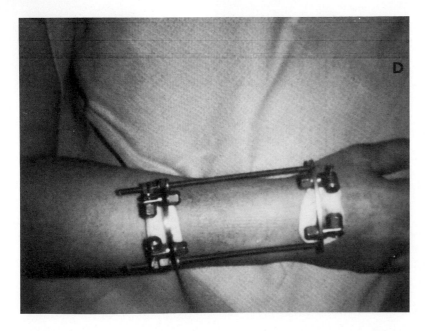

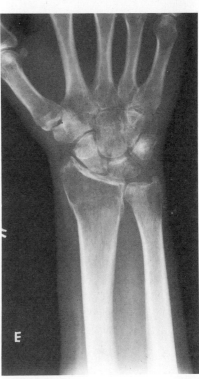

**Fig. 27–5** External fixation of distal radius fractures. Results (left) wrist extension (48 degrees) and wrist flexion (47 degrees) with range of motion (shaded). Results (right) wrist radial deviation (11 degrees) and wrist ulnar deviation (26 degrees) with range of motion (shaded).

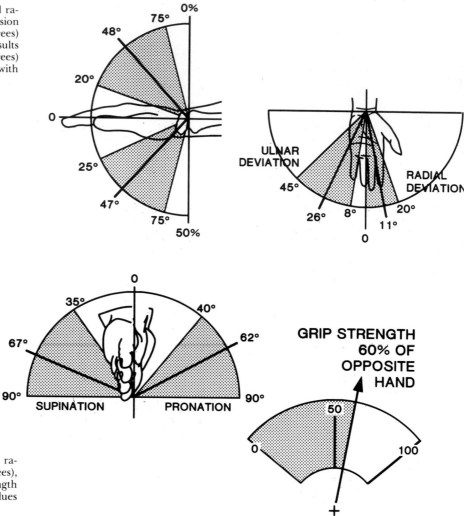

**Fig. 27–6** External fixation of distal radius fractures. Supination (67 degrees), pronation (62 degrees), and grip strength 60% that of opposite hand (mean values from combined series of cases).

## Principles

To achieve a functional limb with bone and soft-tissue integrity, specific principles of treatment must be followed. The first of these is to achieve a satisfactory wound environment by wound debridement and excision of avascular compromised tissue.[34] Quantitative wound cultures can be helpful in determining the extent of wound contamination.[35] When there are more than $10^5$ organisms/cc of wound tissue, then a significant wound infection has been shown to be present.[35] In our view, external fixation is indicated in such an extremity. Vascular reconstruction,[36–38] when indicated, can proceed under a stable skeleton with appropriate vein grafts to major vessels as needed. Wounds are packed open, or split-thickness skin grafts can be temporarily applied. We prefer additional debridement at 48 hours and continued debridement until the wound looks clinically clean and cultures demonstrate less than $10^3$ organisms/cc.[1] Delayed primary wound closure is then performed, often with skin grafts or pedicle flaps.

Because of the nature of the injuries for which external fixation is used in the upper extremity, delayed bone grafting is often required.[27,39] If the fracture is unstable, bone grafting in combination with internal fixation should be considered, usually ten to 14 days after removal of the external fixation.[32] Cabanela and Cooney[40] recommend this approach ten weeks or longer after treatment, if fracture healing has not progressed and if there is suggested fracture instability. In our experience, primary bone healing can be achieved in 60% of upper extremity fractures, with the remainder requiring bone grafting to achieve fracture union. For many diaphyseal humerus and forearm fractures in which fracture healing is delayed, internal fixation may be necessary for fracture union and often provides a better setting for eventual tendon or nerve reconstruction. Joint mobilization, particularly if the frame impedes reconstructive efforts, may be improved after internal fixation.

In open wounds with soft-tissue contamination, the decision to use internal versus external fixation is difficult.[36,41] Internal fixation is preferred when the injury is closed or minimally contaminated (Gustilo type I: quantitative culture shows fewer than $10^2$ organisms/cc of skin).[34,42] Internal fixation may be used for selected cases of moderately contaminated wounds (Gustilo type II; moderate contamination, cultures show $10^3$ organisms/cc), but the wound must be left open. In the authors' opinion, however, external fixation is generally preferred in this setting.

External fixation is preferred whenever the wound is grossly contaminated (quantitative cultures demonstrate more than $10^5$ organisms/cc) or if there are open, comminuted fractures, especially with loss of bone stock (Gustilo type III). If the fracture is adjacent to joints where firm fixation with plates would be difficult, external fixation again appears best. Lastly, there are many fractures ordinarily suitable for internal fixation, but because they have excessive soft-tissue loss, external fixation is the best treatment.

The Gustilo classification[42] of soft-tissue injury is a most helpful method of determining the best treatment for extremity trauma. Grade I wounds have minimal soft-tissue injury, a small skin wound, and little or no soft tissue stripping. Grade II wounds have moderate skin and muscle injury with moderate wound contamination. Grade III wounds have severe soft-tissue injury with devitalized skin muscle and neurovascular injury that threaten limb survival. The majority of Gustilo grade II and III extremity injuries should be treated by primary external fixation.

### Indications

The indications for upper limb external fixation are related to the nature of the original injury and the alternative treatments available.[1,23,27,40] External fixation is indicated when there are (1) open fractures (Gustilo types II or III); (2) segmental fractures associated with bone loss; (3) fractures about the elbow or shoulder joint, or open joint fracture-dislocations (Galeazzi or Monteggia fracture-dis-

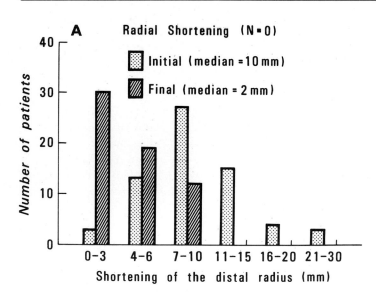

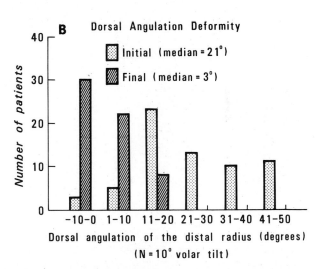

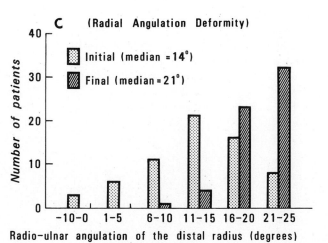

**Fig. 27–7** Radiographic results. **A:** Comparison of pre-reduction and post-reduction measurements of radial shortening (N = normal). **B:** Dorsal angulation deformity. **C:** Radial angulation deformity. (Reproduced with permission from Cooney WP, Linscheid RL, Dobyns JH: External pin fixation of unstable Colles' fractures. *J Bone Joint Surg* 1979;61A:840–845.)

locations); or (4) infected nonunions of long bones. Extensive wound contamination alone is often the strongest reason to consider external fracture fixation as the primary method of limb stabilization.

In forearm injuries, external fixation is preferred in open, both-bone forearm fractures.[5,23,24] Treatment decisions should be based on each fracture independently. That is, external fixation either of the radius, ulna, or both should be determined by the type of soft-tissue coverage over each bone. If the radius fracture is closed but the ulna fracture open with adjacent soft-tissue injury, the radius can be treated by internal fixation and the ulna with external fixation. With external fixation, a minimum of soft-tissue dissection is required and little foreign material is left in the wound (Fig. 27–8). In forearm fracture-dislocations, separate treatment of both the fracture and joint injury is required and includes open debridement and joint stabilization with K-wires. The advantages of external fixation in such injuries are rigid stabilization, biplanar immobilization, open wound observation and debridement, and segmental skeletal fixation when there are ipsilateral extremity injuries.

For fractures and dislocations around the elbow,[32,43] external fixation (Figs. 27–9 and 27–10) is indicated for open comminuted intra-articular fractures, nonunion or delayed union of supracondylar fractures, and soft-tissue interposition arthroplasty. The posterior approach to the elbow can be used for open pin insertion and direct bone grafting of the fracture site. In elderly patients with intercondylar fractures who have osteoporosis, external pin fixation of the intra-articular fracture can be performed, and additional segments of the external fixation frame applied to provide additional support, proximal and distal to the elbow joint.

For fractures of the humerus, the main indication for external fixation is a midshaft fracture associated with soft-tissue injury, particularly compound wounds with extensive contamination.[27,39,44] In our experience, this injury occurs most frequently in farm-implement accidents that produce complete or nearly complete limb amputation. Open fractures from motor vehicle accidents or work-related injuries[41] may also require external fixation of the fracture depending upon the extent of the soft-tissue injury. Severe fracture comminution, nerve or vessel injury alone or in association with other soft-tissue damage, as well as ipsilateral extremity injuries (forearm and humerus combined) are additional reasons for primary external fixation.[29] Most humeral fractures should be treated by closed reduction, and we have not recommended or applied external fixation as a primary treatment for closed injuries despite its clinical use by others for these types of injuries.[45,46]

## Equipment

Through experience, we have found that a wide variety of equipment options exist for the surgeon treating massive upper limb trauma. Pins and a hanging cast or pins and methacrylate cement can be used in external fixation, but specifically designed external fixation systems appear to provide better stability and adaptability. Prior to frame application, the first step is to obtain anatomic fracture reduction. The single-sided frames (Hoffmann C-series and Wagner frame) offer less stability than do biplanar half-frame systems (Ace-Fisher, Roger Anderson, or ASIF units). However, the Hoffmann quadrilateral frame is ideally suited for humerus fractures when it is applied with half pins positioned 90 degrees to each other (Fig. 27–10A). The lateral and posterior pin placements provide the least potential for nerve or vessel injury, and elbow motion can be initiated even with pins placed through the triceps aponeurosis. The Ace-Fisher frame is similarly adaptable to the humerus with half-pin fixation. The semicircular frame can be positioned to conform to a number of soft-tissue injuries, allowing access for wound care, skin grafting, and local or distant pedicle flaps.

## Technique

Once a decision has been made to proceed with external fixation of the upper extremity, we recommend the following treatment program: (1) thorough wound debridement of all necrotic or avascular tissue (a Water Pik provides a jet pulse lavage and assists debridement); (2) quantitative wound cultures[35] using an aliquot of tissue measuring 1 cc, homogenized and diluted, are performed (one bacterium/hpf indicates contamination to at least $10^5$); (3) vascular reconstruction of brachial or radial/ulnar arteries and appropriate veins; (4) open wound treatment (wound closure is acceptable if the wound can be debrided clean and if quantitative cultures are less than $10^3$).

The external fixation frame is inserted once wound debridement has been completed and usually before vascular reconstruction. Open pin insertion is usually necessary in the proximal forearm and both distal and proximal arm to avoid vessel or nerve damage.[22] In the forearm, the radius and ulna should be treated independently by placing fixation pins (three pins preferred) proximal and distal to the fracture site. The Hoffmann C-series has been most commonly used; a cross-bar can be added to prevent forearm rotation. The Roger Anderson frame is more versatile in placement but is less rigid than the Hoffmann frame. The Ace-Fisher frame can be adapted to the radius and ulna, but 3-mm pins should be used in place of the standard 4-mm pins.

External fixation about the elbow for supracondylar and transcondylar fractures is performed by

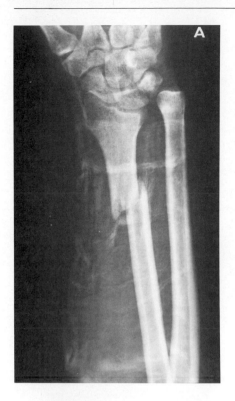

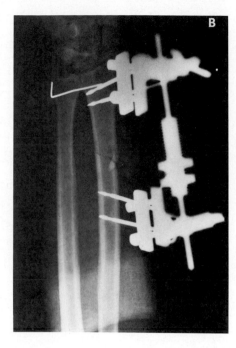

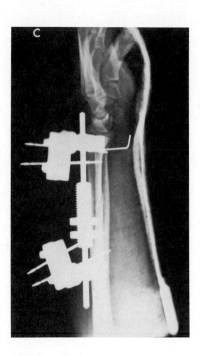

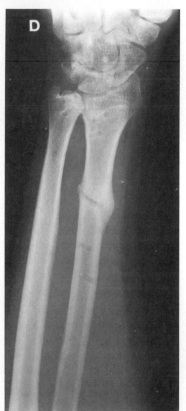

**Fig. 27–8    A:** External fixation of fractures of the forearm. Both fracture site and ulnar head dislocation are open fractures (Galeazzi fracture-dislocation). **B and C:** External fixation with two pins proximal and two distal to radius fracture. Repair of the triangular fibrocartilage and joint K-wire fixation with forearm in supination (the position of joint reduction). **D:** United fracture of distal third of the radius and reduced distal radioulnar joint.

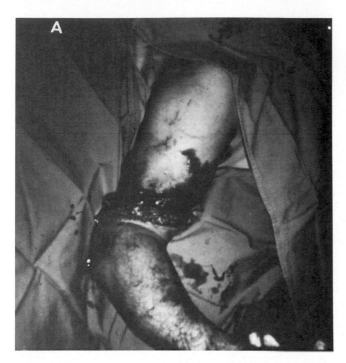

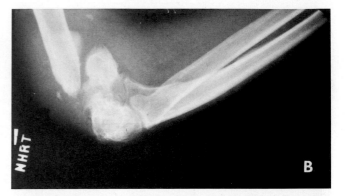

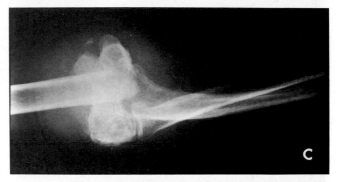

**Fig. 27–9** **A:** External fixation of distal humerus. Incomplete amputation through the distal humerus. Extensive soft-tissue damage with radial and median nerves destroyed and the brachial artery disrupted. **B and C:** Comminuted distal humerus fracture with foreshortening and posterior angulation. **D:** With open reduction, humerus length was restored and external fixation performed with three pins proximal and three pins distal to fracture site.

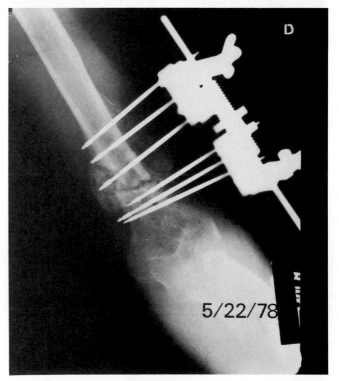

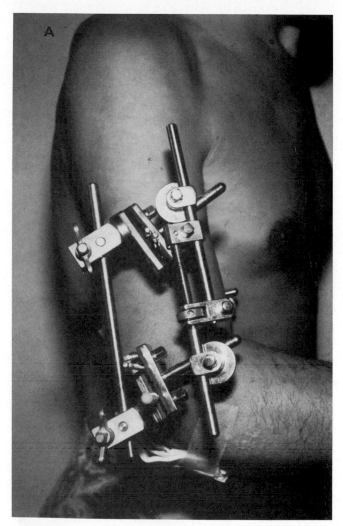

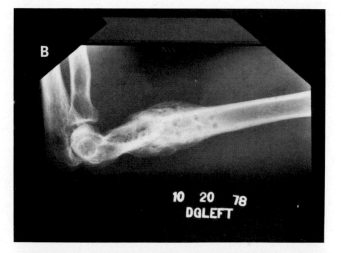

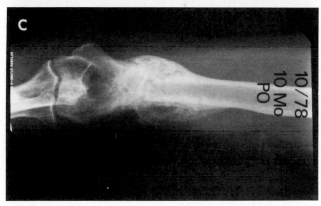

**Fig. 27–10    A:** Quadrilateral frame (Hoffmann) connected to supporting threaded pins. Lateral placement of frame allowed early elbow motion. **B and C:** Fracture union ten months following injury. Neurovascular continuity restored. A good result achieved despite severe soft-tissue and bone injury.

open techniques through a posterior approach (Van Gorder or triceps splitting). Reduction of the articular surface is performed and a Bonnel-type pin used to hold the fragments in place. Under direct visualization, pins are placed proximal to the fracture with retractors protecting the ulnar and radial nerves. Distally, pins are placed transcondylar to avoid the joint, or if joint distraction is necessary, a hinged distractor is applied with distal pins in the proximal ulna. Early elbow-joint motion can be considered in such cases. Supracondylar fractures or nonunions are treated a bit differently by using a half-pin system. The pins are placed posteriorly and laterally, preferably at a 90-degree angle to one another. The posterior pins can be placed through the triceps aponeurosis without harmful effects, and the lateral pins placed carefully to avoid the radial nerve. More recently, we

have avoided medial incisions by using the image intensifier to determine the position of pins and the depth of placement.

External fixation of the humeral shaft and neck is performed with similar techniques of open pin insertion using the image intensifier to avoid the medial neurovascular structures. With a quadrilateral frame, only the lateral approach to pin placement is used, but with the two half-pin systems (Ace-Fisher and ASIF) pins are applied laterally and posteriorly. To avoid angulation at the fracture site, care must be taken not to apply excess compression through the frame. Shortening of the humerus should be considered only for primary nerve repair or vessel repair, and, in most circumstances, artery and nerve grafts are preferred.

Secondary bone grafting has been necessary in

over 40% of our humeral and forearm injury cases, but it should be performed no sooner than eight weeks following injury when the wounds are closed and soft-tissue healing has occurred. Cancellous iliac crest graft can be used alone or in combination with an internal fixation plate. For delayed union or nonunion of the humerus, we have had success with a proximal tibia onlay cortical bone graft placed anteriorly on the humerus. If internal fixation is contemplated, the external fixation frame should be removed one week in advance of open fracture treatment.

## Results

In 40 high-energy fractures of the upper extremity (hand and wrist excluded) reviewed at the Mayo Clinic (unpublished data), good-to-excellent results (limb salvage, fracture union, and function 75% of normal) were achieved in 30 patients (75%). Poor results followed three failed limb replantations (two from overwhelming sepsis). Fair results in seven patients (17.5%) were associated with delayed nerve reconstruction, secondary surgery to secure bone union, and less than 50% of normal limb function. Traumatic wounds of the forearm (78% of the series) fared slightly better than humeral (midarm) fractures (20% of the series). The presence of comminution (88%), open wounds (93%), and associated muscle and neurovascular damage (45%) accounted in part for the less successful cases.

Orthopaedic treatment goals for these severe injuries were limb salvage, fracture healing, and optimization of patient satisfaction and function. External fixation was able to meet these goals in 75% of our patients. Concern about delayed union, pin-tract drainage, and pin loosening is frequent, but these complications did not affect the final outcome in this series. These findings are similar to those reported by Rich and associates (1971),[36] who compared internal versus external fixation of extremity wounds and found a higher amputation and device-related complication rate with internally fixed fractures. Jackson and associates (1978),[30] Bennett (1981),[27] and Edwards and associates (1982)[29] also reported increased limb salvage with external fixation. Bennett[27] reported on 25 complex open fractures; complete limb salvage was achieved despite 17 major nerve injuries and five major vascular injuries. Primary bone union was delayed in 60% of cases and all required secondary bone grafting.

Studies from Finland,[43] Belgium,[44,46] and France[19] share principles of treatment similar to our experience in the United States and recommend external fixation for high-energy trauma. Only a few surgeons suggest external pin support for less complicated forearm or humeral fractures.[45] The broad range of complications found in earlier reports appears to reflect the severity of the injuries, but as technical advances and surgical experience have increased, these problems appear to have lessened. Careful pin insertion, good frame construction, early bone grafting, and occasional supplemental internal fixation are lessons learned from this experience.

## Summary

External fixation of forearm and arm fractures is an excellent treatment option, particularly in compound, comminuted fractures that result from high-energy trauma. Limb salvage and good function have been achieved in 75% of cases by applying the principles outlined. Problems with delayed bone union have been recognized and emphasize the importance of supplemental bone grafting. A number of external fixation systems are applicable to these upper limb fractures, and the authors have not found one system superior to the others. Open pin insertion is preferred, and pins (three proximal and three distal) are ideally placed near the fracture site for optimal stability.

## References

1. Brooker AF, Cooney WP, Chao EY: *Principles of External Fixation.* Baltimore, Williams and Wilkins, 1983, pp 5–23, 165–199.
2. Haynes HA: Treating fractures by skeletal fixation of individual bones. *South Med J* 1939;32:720.
3. Hoffmann R: Rotule à os pour la réduction dirigée, non sanglante, des fractures (ostéotaxis). *Helv Med Acta* 1938;6:844–850.
4. Lambotte A: *L'intervention operatoire dans les fractures.* Brussels, Lambertin, 1907.
5. Anderson R: Fractures of the radius and ulna: A new anatomical method of treatment. *J Bone Joint Surg* 1934;16:379.
6. Anderson R: Fracture of the humerus: A functional method of treatment. *Surg Gynecol Obstet* 1937;64:919–926.
7. Böhler L: *The Treatment of Fractures.* New York, Grune and Stratton, 1929.
8. Chao EYS: Biomechanics of external fixation, in Brooker AF, Cooney WP, Chao EY: *Principles of External Fixation.* Baltimore, Williams and Wilkins, 1983, pp 165–199.
9. Asche G, Haas HG, Klemm K: The external mini-fixator: Applications and indications in hand surgery, in Brooker AF, Edwards CC (eds): *External Fixation: The Current State of the Art.* Baltimore, Williams and Wilkins, 1979, pp 105–110.
10. Asche G, Burny F: Indikation für die Anwendung des Minifixateur externe: Eine statistische Analyse. *Aktuel Traumatol* 1982;12:103–110.
11. Cooney WP: External mini-fixators clinical applications and techniques, in Johnston RM (ed): *Advances in External Fixation.* Chicago, Year Book Medical Publishers, 1980, pp 155–172.
12. Riggs SA, Cooney WP: External fixation of complex hand and wrist fractures. *J Trauma* 1983;23:332–336.
13. Burny F, Andrianne Y: The external minifixator, in *Manual of Application.* Geneva, Orthopaedic and Trauma Service, University Clinic of Brussels, Hospital Erasme, University of Brussels and Jaquet Orthopedic, 1983.
14. Forgon M, Mammel E: The external fixateur in the manage-

ment of unstable Colles' fractures. *Int Orthop* 1981;5:9–14.

15. Cooney WP: Current management of fractures of the distal radius and forearm: Experience with external pin fixation, in Brooker AF Jr, Edwards CC (eds): *External Fixation. The Current State of the Art.* Baltimore, Williams and Wilkins, 1979, pp 83–105.

16. Cooney WP: External fixation of distal radius fractures. *Clin Orthop* 1983;180:44.

17. Frykman G: Fracture of the distal radius including sequelae—shoulder-hand-finger syndrome: Disturbance of the distal radio-ulnar joint and impairment of nerve function. A clinical and experimental study. *Acta Orthop Scand* 1967;(suppl 108):1–154.

18. Santavirta S, Karaharju E, Ko-Kola O: The use of osteotaxis as a limb salvage procedure in compound injuries of the upper extremity. *Orthopedics* 1984;4:642–648.

19. Vidal J, Rabischong P, Bonnel F, et al: Étude bioméchanique du fixateur externe d'Hoffman dans les fractures de jambe. *Montpellier Chir* 1970;1:43–52.

20. Cooney WP, Linscheid RL, Dobyns JH: External pin fixation of unstable Colles' fractures. *J Bone Joint Surg* 1979;61A:840–845.

21. Cooney WP: Complications of Colles' fractures. *J Bone Joint Surg* 1980;62A:613.

22. Green SA: *Complications of External Fixation: Atlas of External Fixator Pin Placement.* Springfield, Charles C Thomas, 1981, pp 56–72.

23. Andrianne Y, Hinsenkamp M, Burny F: Hoffmann external fixation of fractures of the radius and ulna. *Orthopedics* 1984;7(5):845–850.

24. DeLee JC: External fixation of the forearm and wrist. *Orthop Rev* 1981;6:43.

25. Riccardi L, Diquergiovanne W: The external fixation treatment of distal articular fractures of the radius. *Orthopedics* 1984;7:637–641.

26. DeBastiani G, Aldeghess R, RenziBrivio L: The treatment of fractures with a dynamic axial fixator. *J Bone Joint Surg* 1984;66B:538–544.

27. Bennett JB: External fixation of complex open injuries of the upper extremity. *Orthop Trans* 1982;6:403.

28. Bohler J: External fixation of fractures. *Surgical Rounds* 1981;9:69–89.

29. Edwards CC, Robertson RJ, Browne BD, et al: The use of external skeletal fixation in the upper extremity. *Orthop Trans* 1982;6:403.

30. Jackson RP, Jacobs RR, Neff JR: External skeletal fixation in severe limb trauma. *J Trauma* 1978;18:201–205.

31. Sisk TD: General principles and techniques of external skeletal fixation. *Clin Orthop* 1983;180:96–100.

32. Stein H, Horer D, Horesh Z: The use of external fixators in the treatment and rehabilitation of compound limb injuries. *Orthopedics* 1984;7(4):707–710.

33. Stern RE, et al: The Wagner external fixator: For skeletal stabilization in devascularizing injuries to the upper and lower extremities. *Orthop Rev* 1984;13(12):693–700.

34. Gustilo RB, Anderson JT: Prevention of infection in the treatment of one thousand and twenty-five open fractures of long bones. *J Bone Joint Surg* 1976;58A:453–458.

35. Fitzgerald RH, Cooney WP, Washington JA, et al: Bacterial colonization of mutilating hand injuries and its treatment. *J Hand Surg* 1977;2:85–89.

36. Rich NM, et al: Internal versus external fixation of fractures with concomitant vascular injuries in Vietnam. *J Trauma* 1971;11(6):463–473.

37. Spencer FC, Grove RV: The management of arterial spasm in battle casualties. *Ann Surg* 1955;141:304–308.

38. Weiland A, Robinson H, Futrell JW: External fixation of a replanted upper extremity: Case report. *J Trauma* 1976;16:239–241.

39. Fischer D, Behrens F, Johnston R: Symposium: External fixation of fractures. *Contemp Orthop* 1983;6(5):113–132.

40. Cabanela ME, Cooney WP: External fixation of the upper limb. Proceedings of the Scandanavian Orthopaedic Association, Esbo, Finland, Sept 26–29, 1982, pp 104–105.

41. Kamhin M, Michaelson M, Waisbrod H: The use of external fixation in the treatment of fractures of the humeral shaft. *Injury* 1979;9:245–248.

42. Gustilo RB: *Management of Open Fractures and Their Complications.* Philadelphia, WB Saunders, 1982.

43. Kaukonen JP, Karaharju E: External fixation of severe fractures of the distal antebrachium. Proceedings of the Scandanavian Orthopaedic Association, Esbo, Finland, Sept 26–29, 1982, pp 194–198.

44. Hinsenkamp M, et al: External fixation of the fracture of the humerus. *Orthopedics* 1984;7(8):1309–1314.

45. Burny F, Hinsenkamp M, Donkerwolcke M: External fixation of the fractures of the humerus: Analysis of 100 cases, in Vidal J (ed): *The Hoffmann External Fixation.* Montpellier, 1979, pp 191–202.

46. Burny F, Demolder V, Hinsenkamp M, et al: Traitement des fractures d'humerus par fixateur externe: Etude de 62 cas. *Acta Orthop Belg* 1979;45:47–56.

# The Cervical Spine

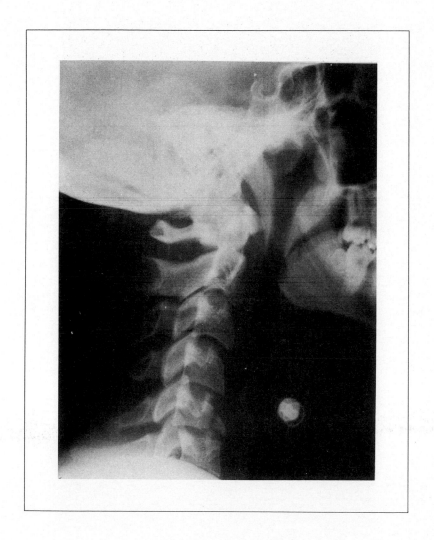

# Radiographic Evaluation of Patients With Cervical Spine Injury

George Alker, MD

## Introduction

The initial radiographic examination of patients with suspected cervical spine injury is of far-reaching importance in terms of management and outcome. It is a team effort, and the radiologist is an important member of the team. The author is a neuroradiologist who works in close cooperation with orthopaedic surgeons, emergency room physicians, and others in a large trauma center and spinal cord injury unit.

The assessment of a patient with suspected neck injury must start with a careful, detailed description of the accident. An effort should be made to determine the mechanism of injury. This information is generally obtained by the referring physician, who then shares it with the radiologist. In patients with head injuries and those with multiple injuries, a significant injury to the cervical spine may be overlooked, particularly if the patient is unconscious. It is, therefore, prudent to suspect injury to the neck until it can be excluded on the basis of a thorough physical or radiographic examination. In the emergency room of the Erie County Medical Center, a large tertiary-care hospital and trauma center with a spinal cord injury unit, radiographic examination of the cervical spine is performed on everyone with head injuries or multiple injuries before any other radiographic examination is undertaken.

## Imaging Techniques

### Plain Films

The initial examination consists of a cross-table lateral view of the cervical spine with the patient in the supine position, as well as an anteroposterior and an odontoid view with the mouth open. The lateral view must include all seven cervical vertebrae and the C7-T1 interspace. The protective collar used in the transportation of the patient is left in place. A so-called swimmer's view, taken with one of the patient's arms raised over the head and the other down by the side may be required to visualize the lower cervical segments. These films are reviewed by a radiologist before other views are taken. Additional projections, particularly oblique and "pillar" views, may be necessary if the findings are in question.[1] Flexion and extension views in lateral projection may be required. These must be done under the direct supervision of a

physician and, if at all possible, with the cooperation of the patient to prevent additional injury from this maneuver. Flexion and extension must never be performed forcibly.

### Tomography

Conventional radiographic tomography is now less frequently used because of the availability of computed tomographic (CT) scanning. It is useful, however, in odontoid fractures in which the direct lateral projection may be of significant help. The transverse axial plane of the CT scan lies generally parallel to the fracture line of the dens and is thus less useful.

### CT Scanning

In recent years, CT scanning has assumed an increasingly important role in the evaluation of patients with spinal injury. It is the most helpful imaging procedure and is widely available today. One of its main advantages is the cross-sectional view that provides better visualization of the vertebral arches and articulating processes than is possible with other imaging techniques.[2] All modern CT scanners have computer programs that permit reconstruction of the transverse axial sections into images in the coronal, sagittal, or oblique planes, providing significant further information in most instances. CT scanning involves minimal patient positioning since such examinations are generally performed with the patient lying comfortably in the supine position. One of the Erie County Medical Center scanners has been modified with a pulley system to allow skeletal traction while the patient is being examined. CT requires less radiation than many other radiographic techniques, particularly polytomography. This factor may be significant in younger patients. At the Erie County Medical Center, patients are brought immediately to the CT scanner suite from the emergency room for the evaluation of spinal injuries if the initial plain film examination discloses a fracture or dislocation or if spinal injury is suspected on the basis of the physical examination. CT scanning early in the patient's examination facilitates treatment planning, an important factor in achieving the best functional result possible.

### Myelography

Conventional radiographic myelography is seldom used in acute spinal injury today. The need to place the patient in the prone position makes stabilization of the injured spine rather difficult. If indicated, CT with intrathecal water-soluble contrast material is preferable to conventional myelography. Until recently, the author used metrizamide in a concentration of 170 mg of iodine per milliliter and a dose of 5 to 8 ml with CT scanning for examination of the cervical spinal cord. With the availability of the newer contrast agents, a 5- to 10-ml dose of Iohexol-180 or Iopamidol-200 is preferable for this purpose. The main advantages of CT myelography over conventional myelography are that it requires less patient positioning, the dose of contrast material is smaller, it provides cross-sectional views, and it may be combined with the initial CT scan. The main indication for CT myelography in acute spinal injury is an incomplete cord lesion suspected of being caused by a nonosseous mass, e.g., disk herniation or hematoma in the spinal canal.

### Nuclear Magnetic Resonance Imaging (MRI)

MRI, the newest imaging technique, promises to be extremely useful in evaluating patients with compromise of the spinal cord. It permits the visualization of the cord in exquisite detail in the sagittal, coronal, and axial planes. While CT shows the size and shape of the spinal cord and its environment, particularly if intrathecal contrast enhancement is used, MRI without a contrast-enhancing agent shows, in addition, some of the internal structures of the cord and reveals intramedullary lesions such as cysts, hematomas, or edema. There are limitations, however, which at this time interfere with the routine use of MRI in acute spinal injury. The major limitation is that ferromagnetic objects cannot be placed close to the MRI scanner because of the strong magnetic field. This limitation precludes the use of respirators, oxygen tanks, and most traction devices. It will be necessary to design future appliances without using iron. Another significant limitation is that most MRI scanners are constructed so that the patient is inserted into a long tubular structure for an examination that takes an hour or more. Monitoring of a seriously injured patient inside the scanner may not be possible. No doubt many of these limitations will be overcome eventually in this fast-growing field of medical imaging.

### Cervical Spine Injuries Related to Mechanism of Injury

Most cervical spine injuries can be classified on the basis of the mechanism of injury. It is important to obtain as much information as possible about the circumstances of the accident and to pass this on to the radiologist so that the examination can be devised to obtain the maximum amount of information as expeditiously as possible. Good communication among members of the team caring for the patient is of utmost importance. If the mechanism of injury is known, a certain type of fracture or dislocation may be anticipated. Conversely, if one knows the type of injury suffered by the patient, the mechanism of injury may be reconstructed.

On the basis of mechanism of injury, the major cervical fractures or dislocations may be classified as follows: (1) Jefferson fracture; (2) odontoid fracture; (3) hangman's fracture; (4) teardrop fracture; (5) mid or low cervical dislocation; and (5) unilateral or rotatory dislocation.

Obviously, not all injuries can be classified into these six categories. Seldom, for example, is the mechanism a pure flexion or extension. Usually it is a combination of these, with one mechanism predominant.

### Jefferson Fracture

**Mechanism of Injury: Axial Load** This fracture is also called burst fracture of the atlas.[3] A common cause of injury is a fall, striking the vertex, for example during gymnastics or a steep dive into a swimming pool, or by hitting the roof of the car in a motor vehicle accident. On conventional radiographs, a Jefferson fracture is best seen in an odontoid view with mouth open (Fig. 28–1). The lateral masses of the atlas are separated, each displaced laterally, causing an overhang beyond the edge of the articulating surface of the C2 vertebra. A combined overhang on the right and left of C1 relative to C2 of more than 7 mm is said to be diagnostic of a rupture of the transverse ligament and of a burst fracture.[4] Cross-sectional CT views are the best means of evaluating the full extent of the fracture. Although frequently depicted in textbooks as fracture of the right and left side of the anterior arch and of the right and left side of the posterior arch of the atlas, a total of four fractures, this situation is seldom if ever seen in clinical practice. This was clarified by Dr. Marvin Hays, Department of Orthopedic Surgery, University of New Mexico. In his experience, as in the author's, there are usually only two fractures, one involving the anterior and the other the posterior arch of the atlas. Occasionally there is a compression fracture of a lateral mass of the atlas if the axial load is asymmetric.[5] The Jefferson fracture is difficult or impossible to diagnose by a single lateral view of the cervical spine. The fracture of the posterior arch may be seen in the lateral view, and soft-tissue swelling in the retropharyngeal space may call attention to the possibility of a fracture anteriorly.

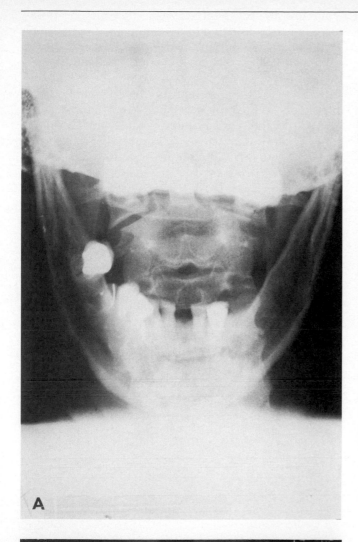

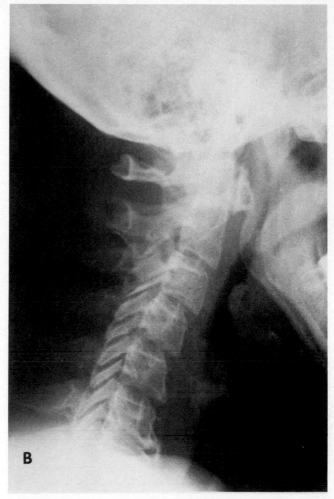

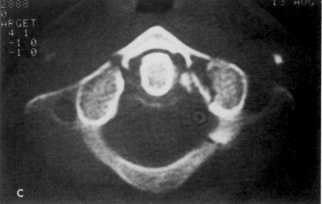

**Fig. 28–1**  Jefferson fracture in a 55-year-old woman who fell, landing on her vertex. **A:** Odontoid view with the mouth open shows the characteristic overhang of the lateral masses of the atlas in relation to C2. **B:** The lateral view shows retropharyngeal edema and fracture of the posterior arch of the atlas. **C:** CT shows an anterior and a posterior arch fracture and compression fracture of the left lateral mass.

### Odontoid Fracture

**Mechanism of Injury: Extension or Flexion** Odontoid fractures are among the most common of cervical spine fractures. Falls and motor vehicle accidents are the most frequent causes of injury. The classification proposed by Anderson and D'Alonzo as type I, type II, and type III fractures is widely accepted.[6] Of these, type I, the small avulsion fracture of the tip of the dens, is rare. Type II and type III occur with approximately equal frequency. A type II dens fracture involves the base of the odontoid process itself, while a type III fracture is somewhat more inferior in position and involves the vertebral body (Fig. 28–2). Differentiation of these two types is of prognostic significance. CT scanning is less useful in type II odontoid fracture than in any other cervical injury. The fracture line is generally parallel to the transverse-axial plane of the CT scan and the fracture may in fact be missed. Reconstruction in the sagittal or coronal plane may allow the diagnosis to be made. A type III fracture may be demonstrated on the CT scan because it involves the vertebral body.

Tomography in the lateral projection may be necessary in cases in which the diagnosis is in doubt. Occasionally, flexion and extension views are necessary to assess the instability of the fragments (Fig. 28–3). These views must be taken with the utmost caution to prevent significant displacement of the fragments and resultant spinal cord compression. Ordinarily, the cervical spinal canal at the C1 and C2 levels is large relative to the size of the spinal cord and, consequently, cord compression is uncommon in odontoid fractures.

### Hangman's Fracture

**Mechanism of Injury: Extension and Axial Load or Extension and Distraction** This injury received its intriguing name because of its similarity to that produced by judicial hanging, in which the knot of the noose is placed in the midline under the chin, and the condemned individual is dropped from a height of several feet.[7,8] Under these circumstances the mechanism of injury is hyperextension and distraction, producing fractures of the pedicles of C2 and disruption of the C2-C3

**Fig. 28–2** **A:** Type II fracture of the dens. **B:** Type III fracture of the dens. Both these patients sustained their injuries in falls.

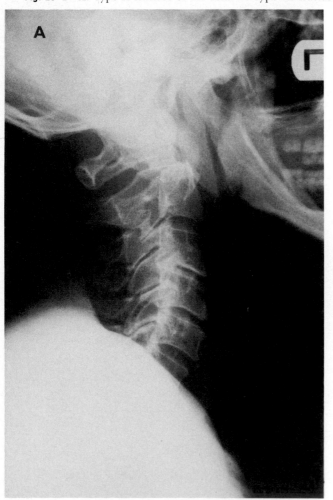

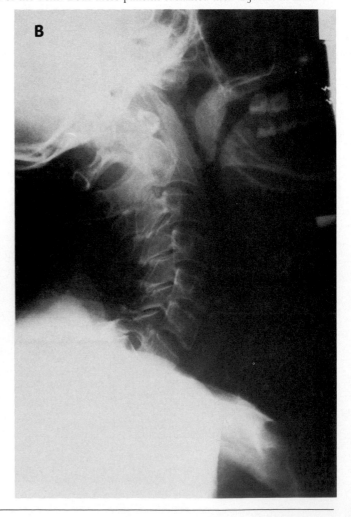

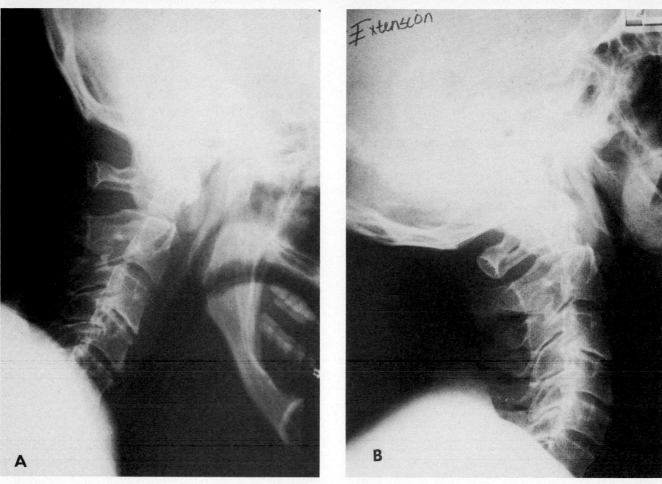

**Fig. 28–3   A:** Flexion view.  **B:** Extension view; both demonstrate the instability of this type II fracture.The fracture is almost invisible on the flexion view.

**Fig. 28–4**   "Hangman's fracture." This 16-year-old pedestrian was struck by a car from behind as he was walking along the road. **A (flexion) and B (extension):** These films and were taken post mortem. Note the marked instability of the fragments. Death was caused by transection of the spinal cord.

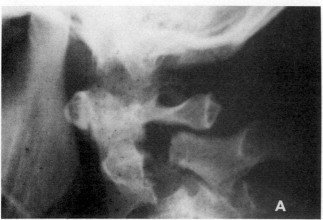

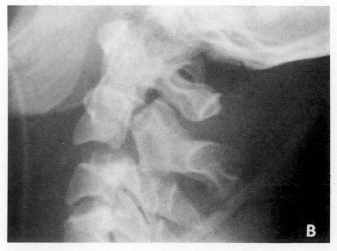

interspace with separation of the vertebrae at that level and traction on the spinal cord. A descriptive term applied to this injury is "traumatic spondylolisthesis of the axis" (Fig. 28–4). A common means of injury is a motor vehicle accident, in which the forehead of a front-seat passenger not wearing a seatbelt strikes the top portion of the windshield. This fracture also occurs when a pedestrian is struck by a motor vehicle from behind. In the first instance, the mechanism is hyperextension and axial load on the upper cervical spine; in the second instance, it is hyperextension and distraction, the inertia of the head providing the distracting force as the body is thrust forward. The resulting injury is the same regardless of which of the two mechanisms is involved. The disk space deformity is best seen on the lateral radiograph. The fractures of the pedicles are perhaps demonstrated even better on CT scanning. Because of the large size of the spinal canal relative to the spinal cord at this level, many patients with this injury are neurologically intact, although a series of radiographic investigations conducted by the author and associates on victims of fatal traffic accidents showed several "hangman's fractures" with complete dislocation of C2 that resulted in transection of the spinal cord.[9,10] When the mechanism is extension and axial load, fractures of the posterior arch of the atlas may be associated with this injury.

### Teardrop Fracture

**Mechanism of Injury: Axial Load and Flexion** The common cause of injury is diving into water that is shallower than the diver anticipated, which results in the vertex striking the bottom, with the momentum of the body causing the severe hyperflexion that follows. A similar mechanism is involved when the rider of a bicycle or motorcycle is thrown over the handlebars or when a football player executes a vigorous tackle (spearing). The resultant injury is best seen on the lateral radiograph (Fig. 28–5). The characteristic findings are anterior wedging of the involved vertebral body (almost invariably C5), a triangular fragment of the anterior aspect of the vertebral body, which gives it the name "teardrop fracture," and retropulsion of the posterior inferior aspect of the vertebral body into the spinal canal. There is also a midsagittal fracture of the involved vertebral body and often of the body of the vertebra below it. This finding is best demonstrated on CT scanning. Similarly, the best, and sometimes the only, way to see the fractures of the vertebral arch is in the cross-sectional views of the CT scan. CT also best demonstrates the encroachment of the posterior inferior aspect of the vertebral body into the spinal canal. Because of the location of the intruding fragment, damage is generally greatest in the anterior aspect of the spinal cord.[11] The

teardrop deformity is almost always at C5 with the C4 and C6 vertebrae involved much less often.

### Mid or Low Cervical Dislocation

**Mechanism of Injury: Flexion** At times there are either no fractures associated with this injury or only very minor ones. Both apophyseal joints are disrupted with frequent locking of one or both inferior articulating facets of one vertebra in front of the superior articulating facet of the vertebra below (Fig. 28–6). The result is a marked decrease in the anteroposterior diameter of the spinal canal and, since this injury occurs in the mid or low cervical level where the spinal cord has its physiologic enlargement, cord compression is very likely.[12] The common means of injury is violent whiplash in a motor vehicle accident, particularly a rear-end collison, or a fall without major axial load. The findings are best demonstrated on the lateral radiograph. CT is very helpful in identifying fractures of the vertebral arches and articulating processes. The treatment options (open reduction vs closed reduction) frequently depend on the presence or absence of fractures and ligament damage.

### Unilateral or Rotatory Dislocation

**Mechanism of Injury: Lateral Flexion and Rotation** This injury is probably the most difficult of all cervical spine injuries to detect. The findings are usually subtle and the diagnosis requires careful scrutiny of the available radiographs. In the lateral view, the characteristic finding is the lack of superimposition of the right and left articulating processes of a given vertebra on a film that appears to be a satisfactory lateral projection (Fig. 28–7). It will be noted that the articulating processes below the level of injury are nicely superimposed, whereas all of those above the injury are displaced in front of one another, resembling an oblique projection. Careful attention must be paid to the alignment of the spinous processes in the anteroposterior view. At the level of unilateral dislocation, the spinous process will be displaced toward the side of the dislocated facet joint. All the spinous processes above the level of the dislocation will be similarly displaced to the same side. On CT scanning the characteristic scalloped deformity of one facet joint will be evident while the joint on the other side remains normal in appearance. The vertebrae above the lesion are rotated to some degree. The rotation can be quantitated by imaging several adjacent vertebrae and determining the degree of rotation with a protractor. The lateral flexion apparently stresses one of the facet joints and the rotatory force then dislocates it. The common causes of injury are falls and motor vehicle accidents in which the victim is thrown against an object in the vehicle. The characteristic

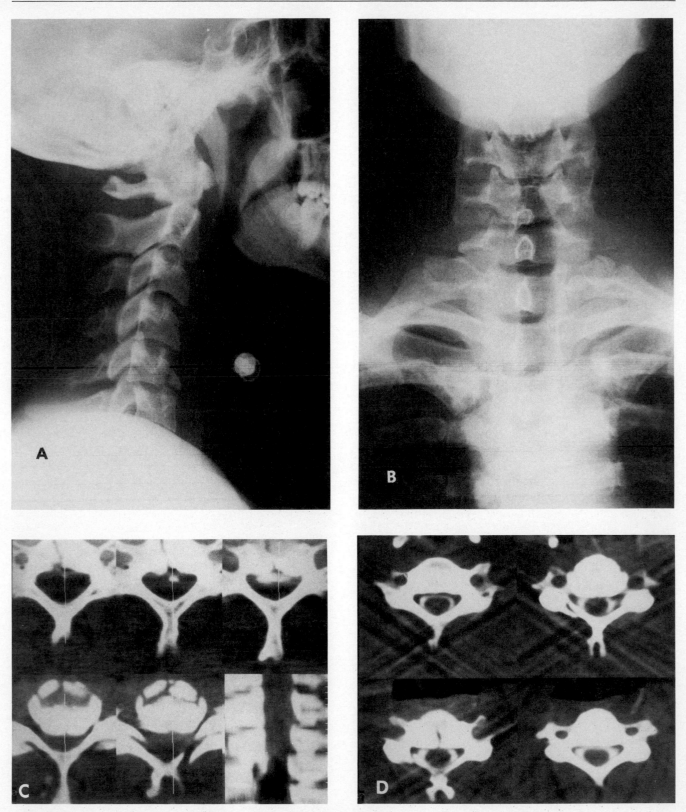

**Fig. 28–5** Teardrop fracture sustained by a 23-year-old man while diving into a swimming pool. **A:** The lateral view shows the characteristic fractures of the vertebral body. **B:** The anteroposterior view shows the midsagittal fractures. **C:** CT reveals the fractures of the vertebral arch and the intrusion of bony fragments into the spinal canal. The reformatted image in the sagittal plane is seen in the lower right corner of the composite image of several sections. **D:** CT myelography shows the enlarged, edematous cord compressed by the intrusion of fragments into the spinal canal.

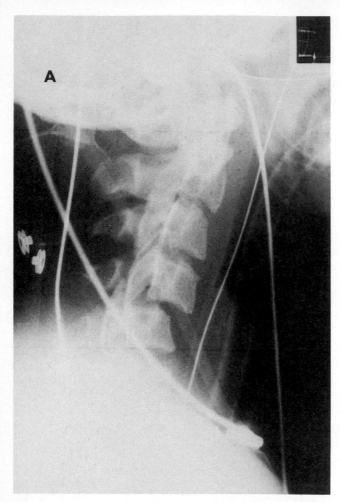

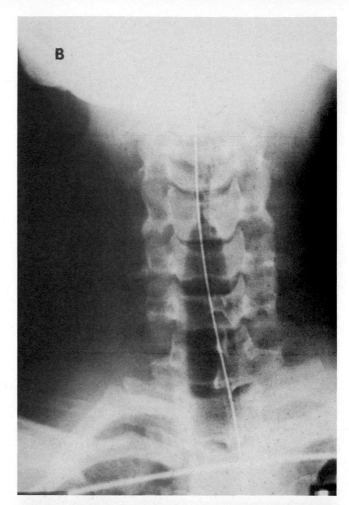

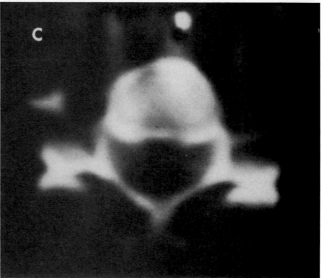

**Fig. 28–6** Anterior dislocation of C4 in relation to C5 in a 19-year-old victim of severe "whiplash." The patient, who was not wearing a seatbelt, was a front-seat passenger in a car that went out of control. He became quadriplegic. **A:** The lateral radiograph shows the dislocated, locked facets. **B:** The anteroposterior view is of little help. **C:** CT shows the characteristic double image of the articulating processes on both sides.

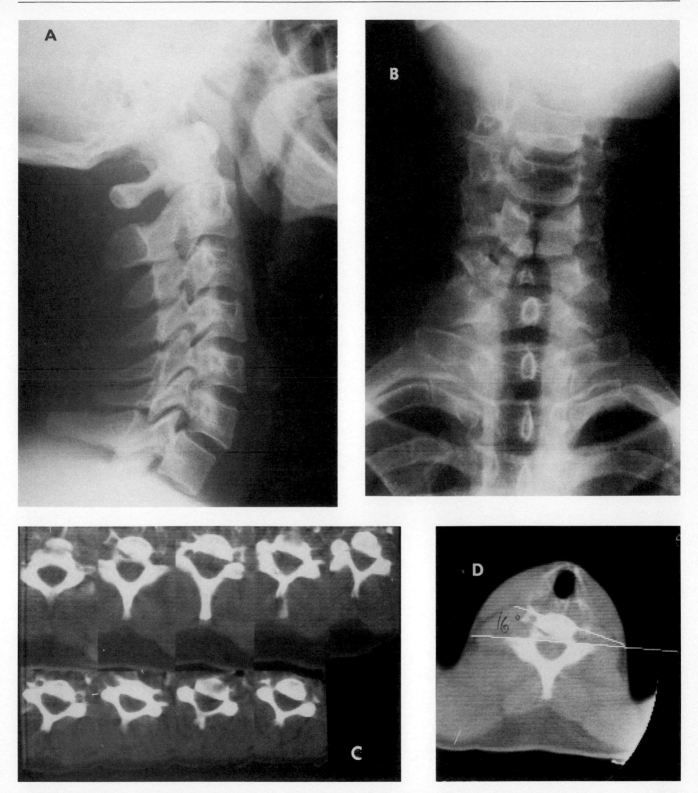

**Fig. 28–7**   Unilateral rotatory dislocation of C5 over C6 in a 37-year-old man. He was driving a car that ran off the road and overturned. The man was not wearing a seatbelt and was thrown laterally against the window. He complained of severe right arm pain. **A:** Lateral view shows the unilateral dislocation. Above the level of dislocation the facets are in front of one another.  **B:** Anteroposterior view shows the right lateral displacement of the spinous processes at and above the level of dislocation. **C:** CT shows the double image of the right articulating process and the rotation of C5 towards the left. **D:**  This slice shows the vertebral arch of C6 and the body of C5. The rotation of C5 can be measured easily.

clinical manifestation is severe radicular pain resulting from compression of the nerve root, as the rotatory dislocation reduces the size of the intervertebral foramen of the affected side.

## Summary

The radiographic evaluation of a patient with cervical spine injury should be prompt and efficient. Proper cooperation between the referring orthopaedic surgeon and the radiologist and shared knowledge of the circumstances of the accident results in rapid, accurate, and cost-effective assessment of the injury, which facilitates treatment planning.

## References

1. Abel MS: *Occult Traumatic Lesions of the Cervical Vertebrae*. St Louis, Warren H Green Inc, 1970, pp 16–17.
2. Steppe R, Bellemans M, Boven F, et al: The value of computed tomography scanning in elusive fractures of the cervical spine. *Skel Radiol* 1981;6:175–178.
3. Jefferson G: Fracture of the atlas vertebra. *Br J Surg* 1920;7:407.
4. White AA III, Panjabi MM: *Clinical Biomechanics of the Spine*. Philadelphia, JB Lippincott, 1978, pp 203–204.
5. Hays M, Alker G: *Burst Fracture of the Atlas*. In press.
6. Anderson LD, D'Alonzo RT: Fractures of the odontoid process of the axis. *J Bone Joint Surg* 1974;56A:1664.
7. Francis WR, Fielding JW: Traumatic spondylolisthesis of the axis. *Orthop Clin North Am* 1978;9:1011–1027.
8. Garfin SR, Rothman RH: Traumatic spondylolisthesis of the axis (hangman's fracture), in Bailey RW (ed): *The Cervical Spine*. Philadelphia, JB Lippincott Co, 1983, pp 223–232.
9. Alker GJ, Oh YS, Leslie EV, et al: Postmortem radiology of head and neck injuries in fatal traffic accidents. *Radiology* 1975;114:611.
10. Alker GJ, Oh YS, Leslie EV: High cervical spine and craniocervical junction injuries in fatal traffic accidents: A radiological study. *Orthop Clin North Am* 1978;9:1003–1010.
11. Schneider RC, Kahn EA: Chronic neurological sequelae of acute trauma to the spine and spinal cord. *J Bone Joint Surg* 1956;38:985.
12. Bohlman HH: Acute fractures and dislocations of the cervical spine. *J Bone Joint Surg* 1979;61A:1119.

# Injuries to the Upper Cervical Spine

J. William Fielding, MD

## Atlas Ligament Tears*

The anatomy and function of the atlantoaxial ligaments are well known.[1] The anterior stability of the first cervical vertebra relative to that of the second is maintained primarily by the transverse ligaments, supplemented by the alar and other ligaments. Posterior stability is mediated by abutment of the anterior part of the ring of the atlas against the odontoid process.

When the atlantoaxial ligaments are intact, the normal joint space between the odontoid process and anterior arch of the atlas does not exceed 3 mm in adults and is usually unchanged during flexion and extension.[2-5] Injury to these ligaments allows displacement of the axis so that the distance between the arch of the atlas and the odontoid process exceeds 3 mm.[3]

### Biomechanical Study

**Functional Anatomy** The atlantoaxial ligament complex can be considered to consist of two parts: primary and secondary stabilizing components. The primary component, the transverse ligament, is a tight band extending between tubercles on the medial sides of the lateral masses of the atlas. Passing behind the odontoid process and lying in a shallow groove on its posterior surface, the transverse ligament confines the odontoid process within the articular notch on the posterior surface of the anterior arch of the atlas.

The most important structures in the secondary or auxiliary stabilizing component are the alar ligaments, the only other ligaments with sufficient structural strength to obstruct anterior displacement of the atlas. The alar ligaments extend from either side of the apex of the odontoid process upward and laterally to the medial side of each occipital condyle. They limit rotation and provide a second line of defense against anterior atlantoaxial subluxation.

The other "auxiliary" ligaments include the apical ligament of the odontoid process, the cruciate and accessory atlantoaxial ligaments, and the capsular ligaments. These are well described in standard anatomic texts[1] (Fig. 29–1).

**Materials and Methods** Twenty fresh cadaver specimens were used to correlate ligament disruption with anterior displacement of the atlas on the axis. Each specimen included the base of the occiput and the first three cervical vertebrae and was dissected en bloc, wrapped in gauze moistened with physiologic saline, and frozen at -20C until required for testing. Before testing, the third cervical vertebra was removed and the lower half of the axis was cleaned of all soft tissue. All ligaments in the occiput-atlantoaxial complex were left intact. The lower half of the axis was then embedded in a block of aluminum epoxy compound to provide a firm support. Testing was carried out directly after thawing and embedding, the specimen being kept moist with physiologic saline throughout the entire process.

For testing, the epoxy block was bolted firmly to a support, resulting in rigid fixation of the second cervical vertebra, with the occiput and the first cervical vertebra left free for the application of test loads. Force was applied to the first cervical vertebra horizontally by means of a sling of braided wire, approximately 1 cm wide, placed around the posterior and lateral elements. The braided sling was expandable across its width, and therefore conformed to the irregular contours of the posterior part of the ring of the atlas without slipping. A force applied to this sling served to pull the first cervical vertebra and the occiput anteriorly in a slightly flexed position, while the second cervical vertebra, which was firmly embedded in the base, remained stationary (Fig. 29–2).

The anterior shift of the first cervical vertebra at the instant of rupture of the transverse ligament ranged from 3 to 5 mm. After the rupture, free movement was possible over a slightly greater range, but in no instance did the odontoid process fracture before failure of the ligament. After failure of the transverse ligament, the force necessary to produce further anterior shift, up to the end point of 12 mm, ranged from 20 to 120 kiloponds (mean, 72 kiloponds) for the entire series. The alar ligaments typically stretched but did not break during the 12-mm displacement. Some elastic recoil was present when the load was removed so that a residual anterior shift of less than 12 mm remained.

After removal of the first cervical vertebra, the force required to fracture the odontoid process alone in the 15 specimens tested ranged from 70 to 180 kiloponds, but was never significantly less than the

*This material was reprinted and adapted from: Tears of the transverse ligament of the atlas: A clinical and biomechanical study. J. William Fielding, MD, George Van B. Cochran, MD, James F. Lawsing III, MD, and Mason Hohl, M.D. *J Bone Joint Surg* 1974;56A:1683–1691.

force required to cause complete failure of all the ligaments in the same specimen. The fractures of the odontoid process did not occur through the base. The fracture line extended laterally from the base of the odontoid process through the superior articular processes so that the entire anterior third of the vertebra was displaced anteriorly.

The biomechanical data demonstrated three points: (1) In most individuals, the transverse ligament represents a strong primary defense against anterior shift of the first cervical vertebra. In some, the transverse ligament possesses very little strength despite the lack of demonstrable local or systemic disease. In one specimen (not included in the experimental series), the ligament underwent degeneration and ruptured with light finger pressure during preliminary dissection. There was no correlation between ligament strength and age in this series. (2) The acute shift of the first on the second cervical vertebra under load does not exceed 3 mm if the transverse ligament is intact. The ligament itself ruptures within a range of 3 to 5 mm, representing a very firm, inelastic band of tissue. (3) After rupture of the transverse ligament, the auxiliary ligaments, primarily the alar ligaments, are usually inadequate to prevent further significant displacement of the first on the second cervical vertebra when a force similar to that which ruptured the transverse ligament is applied. Although the alar ligaments appear thick and strong, they stretch with relative ease and permit significant displacement.

In this series, anterior displacement of the atlas on the axis ranged from 5 to 11 mm (mean, 7.2 mm), as measured between the midportion of the posterior border of the anterior arch of the atlas and the adjacent portion of the odontoid process. In two patients, the anterior displacement of the atlas was associated with excessive flexion, producing a V-shaped gap between the anterior arch and the odontoid process. In these patients the degree of anterior shift was measured at the midportion of the anterior arch of the atlas. This was believed to represent rupture of all but the lower fibers of the transverse ligament, allowing the first cervical vertebra to "hinge" forward on these intact lower fibers.

### Diagnosis

In the experimental series, results in all 20 specimens were consistent, but there was a wide variation in ligament strength. Four ligaments were unaccountably weak and required 12 to 30 kiloponds for rupture. Most of the ligaments exhibited intermediate strength (40 to 110 kiloponds) and others were exceptionally strong (135 to 180 kiloponds), some despite the advanced age of the subjects from which they came. The higher loads recorded for ligament failure during rapid loading were predictable in light of the viscoelastic property of ligaments. This property also explained the tendency of loads to diminish by stress relaxation when the full 12-mm shift was maintained.

Even at the higher loading rates the odontoid process did not fracture before rupture of the ligament. Since bone is weaker in tension, it seems logical that preloading of the odontoid process would render it more susceptible to fracture, but a light tension load applied to the odontoid process during some of these tests did not alter the result.

Spence and associates[6] studied the strength of the transverse ligament in relation to burst fractures of

---

**Fig. 29–1** Ligamentous complex at the atlantoaxial articulation.

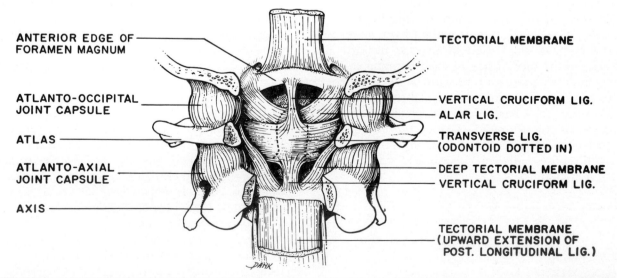

ANTERIOR EDGE OF FORAMEN MAGNUM

ATLANTO-OCCIPITAL JOINT CAPSULE

ATLAS

ATLANTO-AXIAL JOINT CAPSULE

AXIS

TECTORIAL MEMBRANE

VERTICAL CRUCIFORM LIG.

ALAR LIG.

TRANSVERSE LIG. (ODONTOID DOTTED IN)

DEEP TECTORIAL MEMBRANE

VERTICAL CRUCIFORM LIG.

TECTORIAL MEMBRANE (UPWARD EXTENSION OF POST. LONGITUDINAL LIG.)

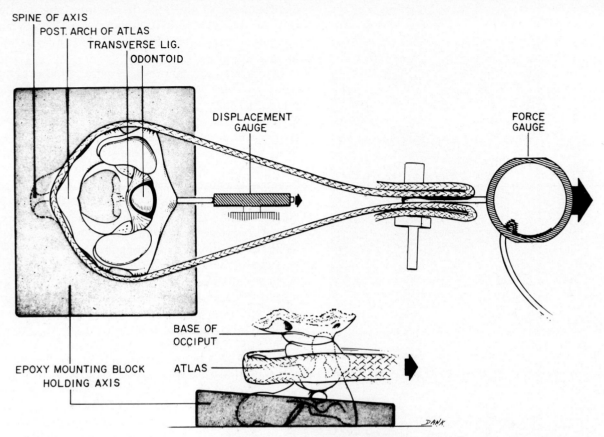

**Fig. 29–2** Diagram of test apparatus: the second cervical vertebra is mounted firmly in cast epoxy. Load is applied to the first cervical vertebra by a circumferential braided wire sling and measured by an electronic force gauge. Anterior shift of the first cervical vertebra relative to the second cervical vertebra is measured by a linear potentiometer acting as a displacement gauge. (Reproduced with permission from Fielding JW, Cochran GVB, Lawsing JF III, et al: Tears of the transverse ligament of the atlas: A clinical and biomechanical study. *J Bone Joint Surg* 1974;56A:1683–1691.)

the atlas, but they used a different technique. Steel pins, placed through the lateral masses of the atlas, were spread by a mechanical testing machine after the anterior and posterior arches had been divided. Thus, a pure tensile force was applied to the transverse ligament. In their series of ten specimens, the breaking strength was 38 to 104 kiloponds (mean, 58 kiloponds). The ligament stretched a mean of only 2.3 mm before significant resistance developed. Rupture occurred with an elongation of 4.8 to 7.6 mm (mean, 6.3 mm). Despite a different experimental technique, their results were remarkably close to those reported here.

The inference from the biomechanical data and from reports in the literature is that a displacement of 5 mm or more is evidence of disruption of the transverse ligament.[2–4,6] The patients described in these reports all had definite severe head injuries, and most complained of prolonged neck pain after injury. Those without cervical pain had neurologic symptoms that focused attention on the cervical spine and prompted radiographic examination of that re-

gion. It should be noted that these patients had more extensive displacement of the atlas (7.5 to 11 mm) than did the patients without neurologic symptoms (5 to 6.5 mm).

The extreme danger of chronic or acute atlanto-axial displacement has been well documented[6–12] (Fig. 29–3). Watson-Jones[11] pointed out the particular risk of an anterior shift of the atlas over the axis with an intact, normal odontoid process; the spinal cord is more easily damaged by crushing against the odontoid process. The situation is less dangerous if the odontoid process is atrophic or fractured and carried forward with the atlas (Fig. 29–4).

The anteroposterior diameter of the ring of the atlas is about 3 cm. The spinal cord and the odontoid process are each approximately 1 cm in diameter, about one-third the diameter of the ring. According to Steel's rule of thirds, the remaining centimeter of free space allows for some degree of pathologic displacement.[5] Therefore, anterior displacement of the atlas exceeding 1 cm (the thickness of the odontoid process) threatens the adjacent segment of cord.

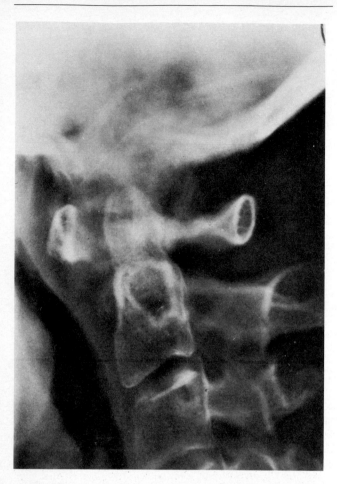

**Fig. 29–3** C1 is displaced forward by ligament deficiency.

As the cardiac and respiratory centers lie at this level, displacement of the atlas is life-threatening. If the ring of the atlas is capacious (more than 3 cm in diameter) there is less danger; if it is narrow, there is more danger.

In correlating clinical cases with a biomechanical study, we must consider the pertinence of the experimental model. In the biomechanical study, the force applied to the first cervical vertebra, displacing it on the second cervical vertebra, was from the posterior direction; also, an even greater force was necessary to fracture the odontoid process once the transverse ligament was torn. Whether a direct traumatic force so applied ever occurs in clinical situations is arguable. Certainly, fracture of the odontoid process occurs with greater frequency than does pure atlantoaxial subluxation. This suggests that an adequate experimental model for odontoid fracture remains to be developed, perhaps one including greater attention to forces transmitted through the alar ligaments. The experimental model may actually represent an unusual set of circumstances in terms of the direction of the application of force. More usual circumstances, such as cervical hyperextension or hyperflexion injuries, might apply different directional forces to the odontoid, for example, from an anterior direction. When such injuries occur, injuries to the scalp often allow one to infer the probable direction of force applied.

**Fig. 29–4** Forward dislocation and fracture-dislocation of atlas. If the odontoid is displaced forward there is less danger of cord compression. (Reproduced with permission from Trickey EL (rev): Injuries of spine, in Wilson JN (ed): *Watson-Jones Fractures and Joint Injuries.* London, Churchill Livingstone Inc, 1976, pp 789–849.)

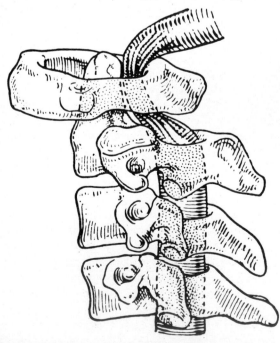
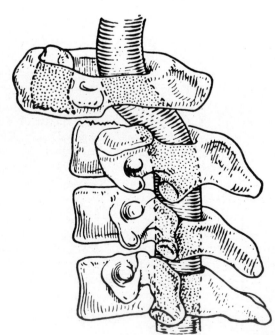

## Rotatory Fixation*

Rotatory deformities of the atlantoaxial joint may be caused by a variety of conditions and are usually short-lived and easily correctable. On rare occasions, they persist, causing torticollis resistant to treatment. Such persistent rotation was termed rotary fixation of the atlantoaxial joint by Wortzman and Dewar.[13] The term atlantoaxial rotatory fixation is preferred since the fixation of the atlas on the axis may occur with subluxation or dislocation, or when the relative positions of the atlas and axis are still within the normal range of rotation.

### Functional Anatomy

The transverse ligament, the primary stabilizer of the atlantoaxial complex, prevents excessive anterior shift of the atlas on the axis. The other supporting structures, mainly the paired alar ligaments, are secondary stabilizers preventing anterior shift.[13-17] The alar ligaments also prevent excessive rotation, the predominant motion between the atlas and the axis, with the right alar ligament limiting left rotation and vice versa.[18]

Coutts[14] noted that when the transverse ligament is intact, the atlantoaxial articulation pivots on the eccentrically placed odontoid and complete bilateral dislocation of the articular processes can occur at approximately 65 degrees of rotation, with resultant narrowing of the diameter of an average-sized canal at the level of the atlas to 7 mm—sufficient to damage the cord. Coutts also noted that when a deficiency of the transverse ligament allows 5 mm of anterior displacement of the atlas on the axis, complete unilateral dislocation can occur at 45 degrees of rotation, narrowing the diameter of the canal at the level of the atlas to 12 mm.

The vertebral arteries are located so that they are not affected by the extremes of normal rotation, even though each vessel is fixed in the foramen transversarium. However, they can be severely compromised by excessive rotation, particularly if it is combined with anterior displacement. Brain-stem and cerebellar infarction and even death have resulted from excessive head rotation that damaged these vessels.[17,19]

### Radiographic Findings

The radiographic features of rotatory fixation may be confusing because it is difficult to position the patient and interpret the roentgenograms correctly. Even the normal upper part of the cervical spine may show considerable variation because of a slight mal-alignment of the head or the radiographic beam and the many congenital and developmental anomalies that occur in this region.[13,18]

Studies of routine roentgenograms, tomograms, and cineroentgenography suggest that the following manifestations of rotation of the atlas on the axis may be present in any patient with torticollis:

**Open-mouth Anteroposterior Projection** Whichever lateral mass of the atlas has rotated forward appears to be wider and closer to the midline (medial offset) and the opposite mass appears to be narrower and farther away from the midline (lateral offset).

On the side where the atlas has rotated backward (right side on right rotation and vice versa), the joint between the lateral masses of the atlas and axis is sometimes obscured by apparent overlapping.

In most normal individuals, the spinous process of the axis does not deviate significantly from the midline until rotation of more than 50% of total normal rotation has occurred (that is, deviation to the left with right rotation and vice versa). However, if any lateral flexion (tilt) is associated with rotation of the cervical spine below the atlas, the spinous process of the axis may appear to deviate markedly from the midline (deviated to the right with left tilt and vice versa).[18] Therefore, if the spinous process of the axis, the best indicator of axial rotation, is tilting in one direction and rotated in the opposite direction, rotatory fixation or torticollis, whatever the cause, is present. The chin and the spinous process are usually on the same side of the midline (Fig. 29–5).

**Lateral Projection** If one wedge-shaped lateral mass of the atlas has rotated anteriorly to the normal location of the oval anterior arch of the atlas, measurement of the atlas-dens interval may sometimes be difficult. Lateral tomograms, however, usually resolve this problem. Because anterior displacement of the atlas may significantly constrict the spinal canal, it is important to obtain this measurement (Fig. 29–6).

**Tomography** Tomograms in the anteroposterior projection may show the two lateral masses of the atlas to be in different coronal planes, falsely suggesting that one lateral mass is absent (Fig. 29–7).

These manifestations are not diagnostic of rotatory fixation but indicate only rotation of the atlas with respect to the axis. They should lead to further investigation.

Probably the most useful procedure to demonstrate atlantoaxial rotatory fixation is cineroentgenography in the lateral projection. This procedure demonstrates that the posterior arches of the atlas and axis move as a unit during attempted neck rotation. Normally, the atlas clearly rotates independently on the relatively immobile axis.

Wortzman and Dewar[13] suggested that a persistent

---

*This material was reprinted and adapted from: Atlanto-axial rotary fixation. J. William Fielding, MD, and Richard J. Hawkins, MD. *J Bone Joint Surg* 1977;59A:37–44.

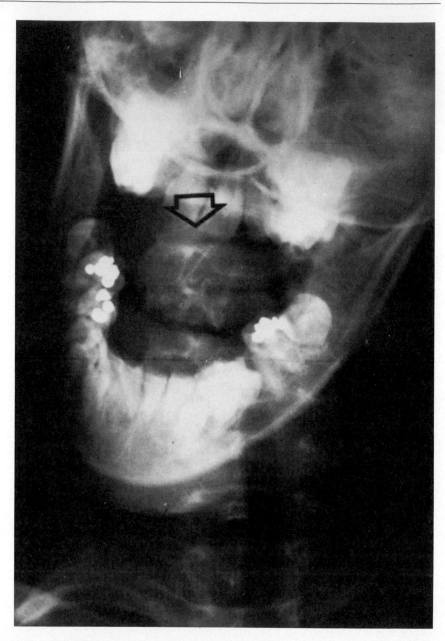

**Fig. 29–5** Anteroposterior roentgenogram showing the chin (symphysis menti) and bifid spine of the axis on the same side of the midline. (Reproduced with permission from Fielding JW, Hawkins RJ: Atlanto-axial rotary fixation. *J Bone Joint Surg* 1977;59A:37–44.

asymmetric relationship of the dens to the articular masses of the atlas, not correctable by rotation, is the basic diagnostic criterion for this condition. This asymmetry can be demonstrated by an open-mouth roentgenogram with the neck in 15 degrees of rotation to the right and to the left. Although this method of demonstrating fixation is accurate, fixation is more easily shown by cineroentgenography. If cineroentgenography is not available, the method of Wortzman and Dewar can be used.

If the rotatory fixation is complicated by rupture or deficiency of the transverse ligament, the atlas-dens interval when the neck is flexed may be greater than 3 mm in older children and adults and greater than 4 mm in younger children.[2-5] Occasionally, such pathologic anterior displacement of the atlas on the axis may produce a compensatory swan-neck deformity of the lower part of the cervical spine.

### Classification

Rotatory fixation has been classified into four types (Fig. 29–8):

**Type I** Without anterior displacement of the atlas (displacement of 3 mm or less).

This is the most common deformity, occurring within the normal range of atlantoaxial rotation where the transverse ligament is intact, so that the dens acted as the pivot.

**Type II** With anterior displacement of the atlas (displacement of 3 to 5 mm).

This is the second most common lesion. It is associated with deficiency of the transverse ligament and unilateral anterior displacement of one lateral mass of the atlas while the opposite, intact joint acted as the pivot. In these patients there is abnormal anterior displacement of the atlas on the axis and the amount of fixed rotation was in excess of normal maximum rotation.

**Type III** With anterior displacement (displacement greater than 5 mm).

This type is associated with a deficiency of both the transverse and secondary ligaments. Both lateral masses of the atlas are displaced anteriorly, one more than the other, producing the rotated position.

**Type IV** With posterior displacement.

This rare lesion occurs when a deficient dens allowed posterior shift of one or both lateral masses of the atlas, with one of them shifting more than the other so that the atlas was rotated on the axis.

This classification provides some guidance as to prognosis and treatment. Type I is the most benign because the transverse ligament is intact. Type II, with a deficient transverse ligament, is potentially dangerous. Types III and IV are extremely rare but are potentially catastrophic. It is therefore important to recognize types III and IV promptly and to initiate proper treatment.

### Etiology and Mechanism of Fixation

The cause of the fixation remains obscure, since no

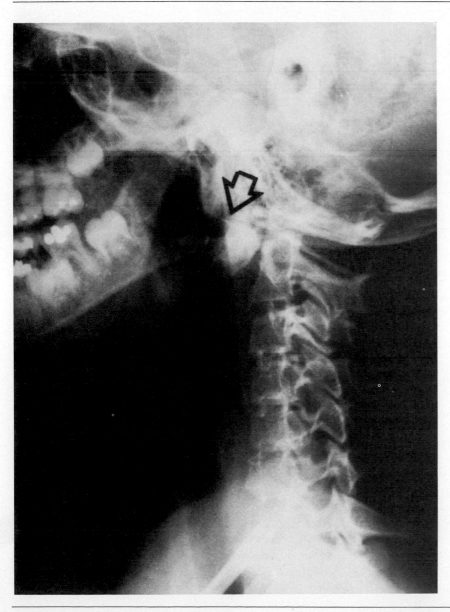

**Fig. 29–6** Lateral roentgenogram of the cervical spine showing the wedge shape of the lateral mass of the atlas that has rotated forward to occupy the position normally held by the oval anterior arch of the atlas. This projection suggests assimilation of the atlas into the occiput. The two halves of the posterior arch, although not well visualized, are not superimposed on each other because the head is tilted. (Reproduced with permission from Fielding JW, Hawkins RJ: Atlanto-axial rotary fixation. *J Bone Joint Surg* 1977;59A:37–44.)

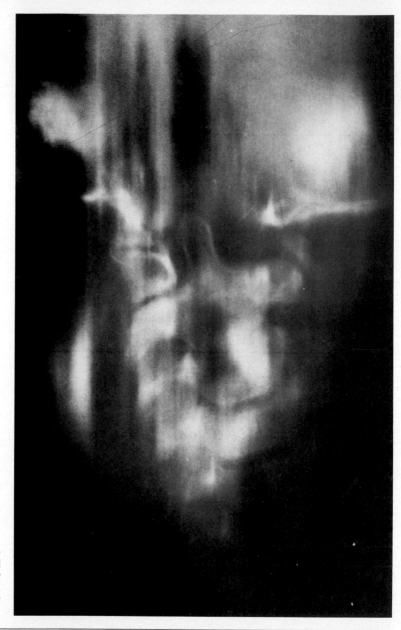

**Fig. 29–7** Anteroposterior tomogram of the atlanto-axial region erroneously suggests that one lateral atlantal mass is absent, but it has actually rotated to another plane. (Reproduced with permission from Fielding JW, Hawkins RJ: Atlanto-axial rotary fixation. *J Bone Joint Surg* 1977;59A:37–44.)

anatomic or autopsic evidence bearing on this question is available. Wittek[20] suggested that there is an effusion in the synovial joints producing stretching of the ligaments. Coutts[14] proposed the theory that synovial fringes may block reduction when inflamed or adherent, whereas Fiorranni-Gallotta and Luzzatti[21] believed that the deformity results from rupture of one or both alar ligaments and the transverse ligament. Watson-Jones[11] postulated hyperemic decalcification with loosening of the ligaments. Grisel[22] suggested that muscle contracture might follow an upper respiratory tract infection and be a factor. Hess and associates[23] concluded that a combination of factors, including muscle spasm, prevent reduction in the early stages. Wortzman and Dewar[13] postulated damage of an unknown type to the atlantoaxial

articular processes. In the early stages, reduction is probably obstructed by swollen capsular and synovial tissues and by associated muscle spasm.

If the abnormal position persists because of a failure to achieve reduction, ligament and capsular contractures develop and cause fixation.

Rotatory fixation may be associated with anterior or, rarely, posterior displacement of the atlas on the axis. With anterior displacement there must be ligamentous deficiencies, caused by either trauma or infection. The combination of rotatory and anterior displacement is easily explained but there is no explanation for the obstruction to reduction.

After fractures with rotatory fixation, the mechanism of fixation may be secondary to obvious articular damage.

### Diagnosis

To diagnose atlantoaxial rotatory fixation, one must be alert to the possibility of fixation and appreciate the anatomic and radiographic characteristics of the atlantoaxial joint. The diagnostic criteria are a resistant torticollis and fixation of the atlas on the axis demonstrated radiographically.

Unexplained persistent torticollis, particularly in younger patients, should not be dismissed lightly. The differential diagnosis includes congenital torticollis, infection of the cervical spine, cervical adenitis, congenital anomalies of the dens, syringomyelia, cerebellar tumors, bulbar palsies, and ocular problems. An important finding differentiating spasmodic torticollis or so-called wry neck from this condition is that the shortened sternocleidomastoid muscle is the deforming force and is in spasm in spasmodic torticollis, whereas in rotatory fixation the elongated sternocleidomastoid may be in spasm (especially in the early stages) as if attempting to correct the deformity.

The usual pattern is a persistent torticollis in a young person beginning spontaneously after trivial trauma or after an upper respiratory tract infection. The diagnosis of fixation may be delayed until many types of treatment have been unsuccessful.

The radiographic findings can be confusing. Plain roentgenograms and tomograms are helpful, since they often indicate that the atlas is rotated on the axis, but these findings are not pathognomonic of fixation because the same relationship may be seen in individuals who are normal or who have torticollis from other causes. If the plain roentgenograms or the tomograms show evidence of atlantoaxial rotation, further investigation, such as computed tomographic scan, is warranted. Cineroentgenography will confirm the presence of fixation. However, open-mouth projections with the neck in neutral position and in 15 degrees of rotation to the right and left of the midsagittal plane may show the fixation if cineroentgenography is not available. Flexion-extension stress radiographs will rule out any anteroposterior displacement.

### Treatment

If there is rotatory fixation, atlantoaxial stability may be compromised and even a minor injury to the neck may be catastrophic, especially when anterior displacement is present. Skeletal skull traction of some form should be applied. If the deformity is corrected, the reduction is maintained in some form of immobilization, such as continued traction or a Minerva jacket. However, since the deformity may recur after this interval, patients with long-standing fixation (more than three months) are probably best treated by fusion. Manipulation of these fixed deformities is not recommended because of the inherent dangers.

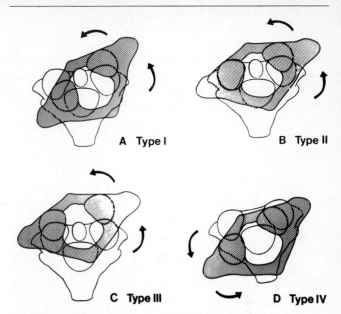

**Fig. 29–8** Four types of rotatory fixation. **A:** Type I: rotatory fixation with no anterior displacement and the odontoid acting as the pivot. **B:** Type II: rotatory fixation with anterior displacement of 3 to 5 mm and one lateral articular process acting as the pivot. **C:** Type III: rotatory fixation with anterior displacement of more than 5 mm. **D:** Type IV: rotatory fixation with posterior displacement. (Reproduced with permission from Fielding JW, Hawkins RJ: Atlanto-axial rotary fixation. *J Bone Joint Surg* 1977;59A:37–44.)

### Discussion

In one series of 17 patients with this rare deformity, the displacement was difficult or impossible to correct, and in most the deformity recurred when conservative treatment was concluded. The average delay between onset and diagnosis was 11.6 months. In most cases it was not possible to determine whether earlier diagnosis and aggressive conservative treatment would have prevented this severe form of rotatory fixation.

Although simple support or even observation is usually all that is needed for atlantoaxial rotatory displacement, the cases in which these simple measures will not prevent the development of fixed deformity cannot be differentiated from those with the common, easily resolvable rotatory displacement.

The importance of recognizing atlantoaxial rotatory fixation lies in the fact that it may indicate a compromised atlantoaxial complex leading to potential neural damage or even death.

Long-standing rotatory fixation, like long-standing torticollis for any reason, may cause facial asymmetry in younger patients.

Neural involvement, more common when both rotatory and anteroposterior displacement are present, ranges from mild nerve-root irritation causing paresthesias to gross motor involvement and even fatal cord compression.

## Traumatic Spondylolisthesis*

Traumatic spondylolisthesis of the axis involves bilateral fractures of the pedicles and may be caused by vehicular and diving accidents, or other deceleration injuries. The lesion, which has been called "hangman's fracture," is characteristically produced by hyperextension and axial loading, but has also been described as resulting from flexion and axial loading[2,18,19,24-28] (Fig. 29–9).

Hanging was used as a method of execution in the Roman Empire and in the British Isles in the early fifth century by the Jutes, Angles, and Saxons. Execution by this method was a public spectacle, and because the words of the law, "hanged by the neck until dead," gave no specific means of death, many offenders suffered slow strangulation[29-31]. In the late 18th century, efforts were made to make hanging a more certain means of execution. The length of the drop was increased, but decapitation sometimes occurred as a result of excessive drop[28,32]. A scientific approach to length of drop and placement of the knot was attempted, and Paterson[33] in 1890 published tables correlating drop distance and body weight. Marshall in 1888[34] and 1913[31] devised a hanging piece to ensure submental knot placement and consistent results.

In 1913 Wood-Jones[35] first described the bony anatomy of the lesion in the dried remains of five individuals hanged with the knot in a submental position. All specimens showed bilateral axis pedicle fractures and Wood-Jones later[36] postulated that complete disruption of the ligaments and disk between the second and third cervical vertebrae resulted in transection of the cord and instantaneous death. The mechanism of injury was hyperextension combined with sudden, violent distraction. These findings were confirmed by Vermooten[37] in 1921. In 1965 Schneider and associates[32] described a similar bony lesion in patients after vehicular accidents and other sudden deceleration injuries, and drew attention to the common association with injuries to the face or head. They used the term "hangman's fracture," but the mechanics of the two lesions are different. Hyperextension is common to both lesions, but the distraction produced by judicial hangings is absent in the other injuries and is replaced by axial loading. This probably accounts for the very different incidence of neural damage, and "traumatic spondylolisthesis of the axis" is a more appropriate term for the lesion[25].

Many investigators have reported on aspects of this fracture, which was at first thought to be a flexion

*This material was reprinted and adapted from: Traumatic spondylolisthesis of the axis. William R. Francis, MD, J. William Fielding, MD, Richard J. Hawkins, John Pepin, MD, and Robert Hensinger, MD. *J Bone Joint Surg* 1981;63B:313–318.

injury because of the forward movement of the body of the axis[38]. Others consider the injury to be caused by hyperextension. Opinions on initial treatment depend on the investigators' views of the injury's inherent stability. Cornish[39] regarded the injury as grossly unstable and recommended surgical stabilization, but others did not consider primary surgical treatment to be necessary. Many different treatment regimens have been described and the question of inherent stability of the fracture is not yet resolved.

### Discussion

On the basis of a series of 123 patients, it can be concluded that the neurologic result of bilateral fractures of the pedicle of the axis from motor vehicle accidents and other deceleration injuries differs dramatically from that of the similar fracture produced by hanging with a submental knot. This difference can be explained by the anatomy and the probable mechanism of injury. The axis vertebra is transitional between the atlas and the more uniform lower cervical spine, with rotation and lateral gliding as its main function. The upper and lower articular surfaces of the axis do not lie in the same vertical plane. This alignment creates the elongated bony bridge of the pars interarticularis, and during hyperextension and axial loading angular and shear stresses are probably maximal in this region.

Thus, the sequence of events during fracture may be that a blow on the face causes extension of the cervical spine, stretching the anterior ligamentous structures and compressing the posterior bony facets until the pars interarticularis is fractured. If extension continues, the anterior longitudinal ligament and disk fail in tension with or without an avulsion of bone from the body of C2 or C3. Continued force will separate the disk from the body of the third or, less commonly, the second cervical vertebra with rupture of the posterior longitudinal ligament and marked separation of the bones. It is at this stage that any neurologic injury probably occurs. Immediately after injury, the body of the axis moves forward on the third cervical vertebra, by a distance dependent on the extent of disruption of ligaments and disk. This forward movement is allowed by the loss of restraint resulting from fracture of the posterior element. Anterior displacement of the body of the axis enlarges the spinal canal and the intervertebral foramina, and this decompression is believed to be the reason for the low incidence of neurologic injury in the absence of any distraction. This forward movement led some early investigators to believe the primary injury to be in flexion.

Three important features of traumatic spondylolisthesis of the axis are the high incidence (79%) of associated injury of the head and of the cervical spine at other levels, the low incidence (6.5%) of neurologic damage, and the low incidence of nonunion (5.5%). The presence of head injury, and especially of facial injury, has proved to be a reliable indicator of a lesion of the upper cervical spine, with the predominance of wounds in the apical and frontal regions of the skull confirming hyperextension and axial loading as the mechanism of injury.

Fractures of other parts of the cervical spine occurred in more than a third of this series of patients. Most of these were upper cervical lesions such as arch fractures of C1 and C3 and avulsion fractures of C2 and C3, providing further evidence for hyperextension as the mechanism of injury. Multiple fractures of the cervical spine occurred in nine patients; most were of the compression type, but there were four fractures of the odontoid, an uncommon association. Six of nine fractures of the spine below the neck were of the compression type, again suggestive of injury from axial loading.

The low incidence of neurologic damage in this injury results from the lack of distraction force during hyperextension and the enlargement of the spinal canal and nerve root foramina. It is gratifying that of the eight patients with neurologic deficits, six recovered completely. A 9-year-old boy who was left with residual shoulder weakness had sustained a flexion injury and, in addition to fractures of the axis, had compression injuries of the third and fourth cervical vertebrae with rupture of the interspinous ligament. His neurologic deficit may well have been caused by this second injury. Another boy with a Brown-Séquard lesion had a residual spastic gait. Paralysis caused by traumatic spondylolisthesis of the axis has been reported, but tetraplegia or even tetraparesis is exceedingly uncommon.[40]

Spontaneous union of this fracture is usual, occurring in 94.5% of this series, and showing no correlation with the initial displacement or angulation. The majority of fractures healed with some displacement and it seemed that anatomic reduction was not necessary, or even advantageous, to achieve union of the fractures. Reduction was, however, attempted in most patients. Only a few anatomic reductions were achieved and in a large percentage there was no change in position between injury and union. Gross displacement responded to mild traction in extension, but this treatment should be used with great caution under close observation to avoid "iatrogenic hangings." The degree of ligamentous instability is difficult to determine, and excessive traction could reproduce the mechanism of judicial hanging. Conservative treatment yields a high incidence of union

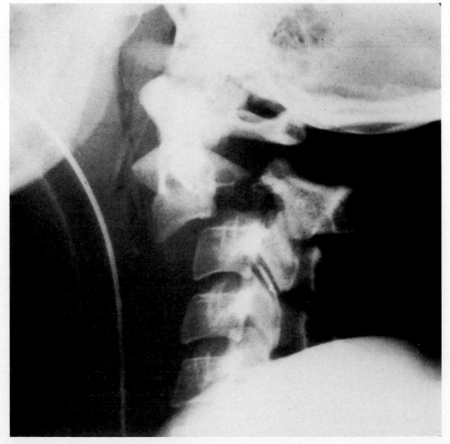

**Fig. 29–9** Traumatic spondylolisthesis of C2 with marked displacement.

with no difference between the results in patients walking early in a halo appliance and those treated in traction for six weeks. The duration of traction and bed rest did not influence fracture healing, and only one failure of union occurred in the 47% of patients who were allowed up in less than two weeks. With the use of a halo cast, or the newer halo vest, or halo-pelvic brace, even individuals with unstable fractures can be treated successfully as outpatients.

The fracture classification was based on angulation and displacement as features of instability likely to lead to nonunion, but the only correlation that could be obtained was that angulation of more than 11 degrees occurred in six of seven patients (85%) with nonunion. Angulation is not necessarily a determinant of nonunion, but is commonly present in fractures that fail to unite. Primary surgical treatment is not indicated. An anterior fusion of C2–3 is preferred for established nonunion or for segmental instability. This approach, unlike a posterior fusion, avoids incorporation of the atlas and thus preserves some rotational movement by sparing the atlantoaxial articulation.

## References

1. Cunningham DJ: The articulations or joints: The atlanto occipital and atlanto axial joints, in Robinson A (ed): *Textbook of Anatomy*, ed 6. London, Oxford University Press, 1931, pp 322–324.

2. Grogono BJS: Injuries of the atlas and axis. *J Bone Joint Surg* 1951;36B:397–410.

3. Jackson H: The diagnosis of minimal atlanto-axial subluxation. *Br J Radiol* 1950;23:672–674.

4. Martel W: The occipito-atlanto-axial joints in rheumatoid arthritis and ankylosing spondylitis. *Am J Roentgenol Radium Ther Nucl Med* 1961;86:223–240.

5. Steel HH: Anatomical and mechanical considerations of the atlanto–axial articulations. *J Bone Joint Surg* 1968;50A:1481–1482.

6. Spence KF Jr, Decker S, Sell KW: Bursting atlantal fracture associated with rupture of the transverse ligament. *J Bone Joint Surg* 1970;52A:543–549.

7. Dunbar HS, Ray BS: Chronic atlanto–axial dislocations with late neurologic manifestations. *Surg Gynecol Obstet* 1961;113:757–762.

8. Hamilton AR: Injuries of the atlanto–axial joint. *J Bone Joint Surg* 1951;33B:434–435.

9. Kahn EA, Yglesias L: Progressive atlanto–axial dislocation. *JAMA* 1935;105:348–352.

10. Mixter SJ, Osgood RB: Traumatic lesions of the atlas and axis. *Ann Surg* 1910;51:193–207.

11. Watson-Jones R: *Fractures and Joint Injuries*, ed 4. Baltimore, Williams and Wilkins, 1955, vol 2, p 190.

12. Wadia NH: Myelopathy complicating congenital atlanto-axial dislocation: A study of 28 cases. *Brain* 1967;90:449–472.

13. Wortzman G, Dewar FP: rotatory fixation of the atlantoaxial joint: Rotational atlantoaxial subluxation. *Radiology* 1968;90:479–487.

14. Coutts MB: Atlanto-epistropheal subluxations. *Arch Surg* 1934;29:297–311.

15. Fielding JW, Cochran GVB, Lawsing JF III, et al: Tears of the transverse ligament of the atlas: A clinical and biomechanical study. *J Bone Joint Surg* 1974;56A:1683–1691.

16. Roy-Camille R, De La Caffiniere J–Y, Saillant G: *Traumatismes du rochis cervical supérieur C1–C2*. Paris, Masson, 1973, pp 11–18.

17. Werne S: Studies on spontaneous atlas dislocation. *Acta Orthop Scand*, 1957, suppl 23, pp 32–43.

18. Fielding JW: Cineroentgenography of the normal cervical spine. *J Bone Joint Surg* 1957;39A:1280–1288.

19. Schneider RC, Schemm GW: Vertebral artery insufficiency in acute and chronic spinal trauma: With special reference to the syndrome of acute central cervical spinal cord injury. *J Neurosurg* 1961;18:348–360.

20. Wittek A: Ein Fall von Distensionsluxation im Atlanto-epistropheal-Gelenke. *Munch Med Wochenschr* 1908;55:1836–1837.

21. Fiorranni-Gallotta G, Luzzatti G: Sublussazione laterale e sublussazione rotatorie dell'atlante. *Arch Ortop* 1957;70:467–484.

22. Grisel P: Enucléation de l'atlas et torticollis naso-pharyngien. *Presse Med* 1930;38:50–53.

23. Hess JH, Bronstein IP, Abelson SM: Atlanto-axial dislocations: Unassociated with trauma and secondary to inflammatory foci in the neck. *Am J Dis Child* 1935;49:1137–1147.

24. Norton WL: Fractures and dislocations of the cervical spine. *J Bone Joint Surg* 1962;44A:115–139.

25. Garber JN: Abnormalities of the atlas and axis vertebra—congenital and traumatic. *J Bone Joint Surg* 1964;46A:1782–1791.

26. Termansen NB: Hangman's fracture. *Acta Orthop Scand* 1974;45:529–539.

27. Williams TG: Hangman's fracture. *J Bone Joint Surg* 1975;57B:82–88.

28. Rothman RH: Hangman's fracture. Presented at the AAOS Symposium on Cervical Injuries, Dallas, Feb 25, 1978.

29. Haughton S: On hanging, considered from a mechanical and physiological point of view. *London, Edinburgh and Dublin Philosophical Magazine and Journal of Science* (4th series) 1866;32:23–34.

30. Judicial hanging. *Lancet* 1913;1:629.

31. Marshall JJ de Z: Judicial hanging. *Lancet* 1913;1:639–640.

32. Schneider RC, Livingstone KE, Cave AJE, et al: "Hangman's fracture" of the cervical spine. *J Neurosurg* 1965;22:141–154.

33. Paterson AM: Fracture of cervical vertebrae. *J Anat Lond* 1890;24:ix.

34. Marshall JJ de Z: Judicial executions. *Br Med J* 1888;2:779–782.

35. Wood-Jones F: The examination of the bodies of 100 men executed in Nubia in Roman times. *Br J Med* 1908;1:1736–1737.

36. Wood-Jones F: The ideal lesion produced by judicial hanging. *Lancet* 1913;1:53.

37. Vermooten V: A study of the fracture of the epistropheus due to hanging with a note on the possible causes of death. *Anat Rec* 1921;20:305–311.

38. DeLorme TL: Axis-pedicle fractures. *J Bone Joint Surg* 1967;49A:1472.

39. Cornish BL: Traumatic spondylolisthesis of the axis. *J Bone Joint Surg* 1968;50B:31–43.

40. Edgar MA, Fisher TR, McSweeney T, et al: Tetraplegia from hangman's fracture: Report of a case with recovery. *Injury* 1972;3:199–202.

# The Halo Orthosis in the Treatment of Cervical Spine Injury

Donald S. Pierce, MD

## History

The halo orthosis was first used on a body jacket by Perry and Nickel in 1959[1] for immobilization of patients with severe poliomyelitis and paralysis of the cervical musculature. It can be used for stability in patients who undergo fusion of the entire cervical spine. The halo ring offers a four-point fixation on the skull that is superior to any type of tong fixation, particularly in producing traction with flexion or extension. Since the mid-1960s, the halo device, mounted either on a cast or on a plastic body jacket, has been used to stabilize the cervical spine in the treatment of fractures, dislocations, infectious disease, neoplasms, and rheumatoid arthritis. The halo orthosis has also provided stabilization following laminectomy and in rare conditions, such as disappearing bone disease.[2-4] The method of attaching the metallic device that supports the halo has evolved from the bulky cast of the mid-1950s. While the cast is more appropriate to the poliomyelitis patient than to the insensate patient with cervical spine injury, it tends to produce pressure sores. Also, the weight loss after spinal injury necessitates repeated cast changes to maintain good body contact. The halo has evolved from a pelvic orthosis with long rods and pads on the thoracic area that supported the halo from the pelvis upward, to the present versatile, plastic vest with multiple configurations of metal rods. This great versatility and ease of application have made the halo a popular and effective way of immobilizing the cervical spine.

## Application

The muscle splint is important in the treatment of cervical spine disease. Spasm of the cervical muscles often maintains a fractured or dislocated spine in such a way as to prevent further dislocation of the injured segments. If muscle tone is obliterated with general anesthesia, a shift in bony alignment can occur to cause further neurologic damage. For this reason, the halo orthosis is generally applied with local anesthesia. A number of devices are available to support the patient's neck during the application of the halo itself. A cervical collar already in place may be left on and supported by pads beneath the occiput.

The halo ring comes in six sizes that will fit virtually any person, including young children. The circumference of the skull is measured just above the ears and the proper halo ring size for this measurement is found on the manufacturer's chart. The halo and pins are sterilized prior to application and all sizes should be available at the site of fitting. While the pins themselves have a very sharp point that penetrates the skin without skin incision, a guard prevents the pins from penetrating too deeply into the skull, unless they are improperly tightened. The patient's head should be supported either with a collar padded beneath the occiput, or it should be placed in one of the application devices attached to the table that will hold the halo itself. The appropriate ring-sized halo is then placed approximately 1 cm above the eyebrows and 1 cm above the tip of the ears and is held in place with blunt pins and base plates, two posterior and one in the midline over the forehead between the eyes. The pin configuration centers the ring on the patient's skull. It is extremely important that the ring be positioned just below the greatest circumference of the patient's skull so that any pressure on the ring will not cause the halo to slip upward and out of position.

Several predrilled and threaded holes in the ring where pins can be applied allow the pins to be placed in the best possible position. Anteriorly, the supraorbital nerve should be avoided. It can be located by palpating its foramen.

As the pins are being tightened down on the skin, the patient's eyes should be closed and opened to be certain that the skin of the forehead is not pulling on the eyelid and preventing the eye from closing or opening.

The skin in the pin area is prepared by first washing the patient's hair with sterile water and then with a Betadine solution. Generally, two anterior pins should be placed in an area of bare skin. No attempt should be made to place them behind the hairline, as the bone is extremely thin anterior to the ears and does not allow good anterior anchoring. Also, pins placed behind the hairline would go through the muscles of mastication and cause the patient pain on chewing.

The small punctate scars over the patient's eyebrows caused by the halo pins have never, in the author's experience, required plastic surgery. It is conceivable that major infection in the area could lead to scarring that would require plastic surgery; however, proper pin tract care should avoid this complication.

With the halo held in position, a 1.5-inch, 25-gauge needle should be placed directly through the appropriate pin position hole in the halo ring and 1% lidocaine injected into the skin. Using a 22-gauge needle, the subcutaneous tissue and galea should be infiltrated with the same local anesthetic. Epinephrine is not used because, with pressure from the pin, it could cause skin sloughing. If the patient's hair is thick or dirty, a small area where the posterior pins are to be placed should be shaved prior to the application of Betadine solution and local anesthetic.

The person applying the ring should wear sterile gloves and insert the sterile pins into the four holes while an assistant uses the holding base plates, which have been screwed gently against the skull, to keep the halo in position. Care should be taken to tighten opposite pins, left anterior/right posterior and right anterior/left posterior, until they have begun to seat themselves on the bone of the skull.

Once the pins are hand-tightened on the skull, the base plate and positioning pins are removed. The position of the halo is checked again to be sure that it is low over the eyebrows and along the tips of the ears. Then, a torque screw driver is used to tighten the pins to 5 in-lb of torque. At this point, the halo ring is stable on the skull. During tightening, the patient should not feel severe pain or extreme pressure. Morphine and diazepam may be given intravenously or intramuscularly if necessary to calm the patient or alleviate any pain. However, the patient should not be heavily sedated.

Once the ring has been secured, the upright posts are attached to the vest. Then, the posterior half of the thoracic vest is applied. Care should be taken to move the vest gently under the patient. Placing the posterior half of the vest under the patient can also be done before applying the halo. Since the uprights can be arranged in a variety of ways to support the halo, it is important to decide ahead of time, if possible, what methods of evaluation or treatment may be used with the halo. Then, the upright posts can be placed to allow access to the patient posteriorly or anteriorly. In the author's experience, models of the halo which allow removal of the anterior and posterior halves of the jacket have been the most effective. These have four short upright bars, a crossbar at each side, and short uprights to support the halo, thus allowing for traction to be applied to it vertically. The short uprights allow forward and backward translation of the halo and removal of the posterior or anterior shell for surgery.

Once the halo orthosis has been applied with the vest or with a body jacket, even the patient with quadriplegia may be seated in an upright position.

An ambulatory patient may walk while wearing the halo. It is possible to send such a patient home in the halo device with proper instructions after treating the injury itself.

## Uses

The halo, without the jacket or cast, may be used on a Striker Frame or in a Roger's traction device. It may be used for fracture reduction, dislocation reduction, and immobilization. It may also be used during a surgical procedure to stabilize the spine before, during, and after surgery.

## Indications

The halo orthosis is used to produce complete stability of the cervical spine and to facilitate reduction of a malaligned cervical spine. Johnson and associates[5] have found in testing various devices that the halo vest stabilizes the cervical spine most effectively. The halo device can be used effectively on ambulatory patients for whom surgery is not indicated to hold a fracture or dislocation in place. It may also be used when long-term stability is needed during healing after vertebral body removal and anterior or posterior fusion and wiring.

## Complications and Cautions

Paralyzed patients should be turned every two hours. Extreme care should be taken to make certain that skin care is given to insensate patients in the halo vest. It is possible, in most cases, to loosen the lower portion of the halo vest enough to give skin care underneath the vest. With a cast, a large amount of padding is necessary to prevent pressure sores over the iliac crests, sacrum, and particularly over the prominence of the dorsal spine and the medial borders of the scapulae. Gel pads are recommended.

In elderly patients, some sensory deprivation may be felt; therefore, patients over the age of 65 frequently do not tolerate halo fixation well. If complete immobilization of the cervical spine must be maintained, then it may be necessary to seek the advice of a psychiatrist to maintain the patient in an emotionally stable condition during the time the patient is required to wear the halo. If other methods are available, they are probably preferable in this particular age group. However, the halo should be tried if at all appropriate.

Pin tract infection may occur if proper pin tract care is not given. It is mandatory that the areas around the pins be cleansed with hydrogen peroxide at least three times a day, and antibiotic ointment should be placed around the base of the pin.

Pins should be tightened to 5 in-lb of torque at the time of application. The guards, which keep the pins from backing out, should be tightened at the time of the initial application. The next day, the pins and pin guards may have loosened and need to be tightened again. The pins should remain tightened at 5 in-lb of torque. After the second day, the pins should be left alone unless there is discomfort around them. Discomfort around the pin usually indicates slight loosening. Under these circumstances, the physician should see the patient immediately and should loosen the pin guards and tighten the pins only by hand, not to 5 in-lb of torque with a torque screw driver. Continued tightening of the pins to 5 in-lb of torque during the weeks or months after application of the halo device will cause penetration of the skull. Brain abscess has been reported under such circumstances.[6] If a pin tract becomes infected, it is necessary to remove the pin and to replace it using an adjacent hole in the halo ring. After sterilizing this hole with antiseptic solution, a new pin is placed in the same manner as the original pin.

The halo vest is an extremely adaptable device. When it is applied, care should be taken not to place the metal upright rods and horizontal crossbars in the areas where radiographs will be taken of the cervical spine. Polytomography and also computed tomography of the cervical spine using third- and fourth-generation CT scanners can be performed on patients wearing the halo device. Magnetic resonance imaging (MRI) is possible with the latest halos made of aluminum or graphite.

The vest itself is cut out in the chest area so that there is no pressure over female breasts and also to allow for external cardiac massage, if necessary.

Before giving general anesthesia, nasotracheal intubation is usually done using topical anesthetic and mild sedation while the patient is in the halo vest; no adjustment of the halo vest is necessary. Occasionally, it is necessary to use a fiberoptic laryngoscope, particularly in patients with rheumatoid arthritis, ankylosing spondylitis, or severe dislocation or subluxation in the cervical spine.

Patient and family should be carefully instructed in pin tract care and possible complications that might arise with the halo itself, such as pin loosening or pressure areas developing under the halo vest or halo cast. They should be told that it is possible to shampoo the patient's hair carefully using bland soap without additives, if the pin areas are treated with antibiotic ointment after the shampoo.

In the author's experience, there have been only two instances in which the patient did not tolerate the halo device. Both were elderly patients and the intolerance was a result of sensory deprivation. There is one reported instance of meningitis in a child from penetration of both tables of the skull by pins that were tightened repeatedly to 5 in-lb of torque after halo application.

## References

1. Perry JP, Nickel VL: Total cervical spine fusion for neck paralysis. *J Bone Joint Surg* 1959;41A:37–60.
2. Freeman GE Jr: Correction of severe deformity of the cervical spine in ankylosing spondylitis with the halo device: A case report. *J Bone Joint Surg* 1961;43A:547–552.
3. Nickel VL, Perry J, Garrett A, et al: The halo: A spinal skeletal traction fixation device. *J Bone Joint Surg* 1968;50A:1400.
4. Thompson H: The "halo" traction apparatus: A method of external splinting of the cervical spine after injury. *J Bone Joint Surg* 1962;44B:655–661.
5. Johnson RM, Hart DL, Simmons EF, et al: Cervical orthoses: A study comparing their effectiveness in restricting cervical motion in normal subjects. *J Bone Joint Surg* 1977;59A:332.
6. Victor DI, Bresnan MJ, Keller RB: Brain abscess complicating the use of halo traction. *J Bone Joint Surg* 1973;55A:635.

# Soft-Tissue Injuries of the Lower Cervical Spine

Edward J. Dunn, MD

Steven Blazar, MD

## Introduction

Most orthopaedists are familiar with the diagnosis and treatment of fractures and dislocations of the cervical spine. The frequency and extent of soft-tissue injuries and their treatment and prognosis may not be fully appreciated, however. To simplify, we will discuss extension injuries, which include acceleration (often called whiplash) injuries; and flexion injuries, which include deceleration injuries. Frequently, however, rotational and other forces are involved, producing a more complex injury pattern.

## Extension Injuries

Extension injuries of the neck are caused directly by trauma or indirectly in rear-end collisions by acceleration of the person's neck. Extension injuries of the neck caused by acceleration were first recognized as a clinical entity with the introduction of catapult-assisted lift-offs from aircraft carriers.[1] However, the greatest numbers of injuries are caused by automobile accidents.[2] In the 1950s there was a 20% incidence of rear-end collisions in motor vehicle accidents in North America. Studies done in the early 1960s estimated that 85% of all neck injuries requiring medical evaluation resulted from motor vehicle accidents and that 85% of these accidents were rear-end collisions.[3] Since there are more than 4 million automobile collisions annually, the rear-end collision and resultant soft-tissue injury to the neck constitutes a major health problem.

Just as extending the seat back to support the pilot's head has reduced the number of catapult injuries, the federal government's mandate that head restraints be placed in all cars manufactured after 1968 brought about an 18% reduction in complaints of neck injury following auto accidents.[3]

### Anatomy of the Anterior Cervical Spine

The skin, subcutaneous fascia, and platysma of the anterior neck are mobile. Beneath the platysma and embedded within the deep cervical fascia are the four superficial branches of the cervical plexus including the great auricular nerve, which supplies the area of the parotid gland and skin about the ear; the anterior cervical cutaneous nerve, which supplies the region around the hyoid bone; the lesser occipital nerve, which supplies the lateral occipital region; and the supraclavicular nerve, which supplies the skin over the clavicle and anterior trapezius.

Below the hyoid bone are the strap muscles. The sternocleidomastoid is the most prominent muscle of the neck and divides it into anterior and posterior triangles. The carotid sheath lies immediately adjacent to the sternocleidomastoid surrounded by its alar fascia. The deepest muscles lie along the anterior surface of the vertebrae, covering the lateral aspect of the vertebral bodies and filling the space between them and their adjacent transverse processes. These include the longus colli (a neck flexor) located most central and the longus capitus (a head flexor) just lateral to the longus colli. The sympathetic trunk lies directly over these muscles in a loose fascia.

**Ligaments of the Anterior Cervical Spine** A number of ligaments firmly bond the odontoid to the anterior rim of the atlas and occiput providing primary stability to the C1 and C1-C2 articulations of the occiput. The lower five cervical articulations between the second and seventh cervical vertebrae are similar anatomically. The anterior longitudinal ligament adheres closely to the midportion of the vertebral bodies. Although thin and transparent, the anterior longitudinal ligament is effective in limiting spine extension. The ligament is thickest over the disk spaces and blends in with the underlying anulus fibrosus, which is a dense fibrous structure bonded to the cartilaginous end plates. It effectively limits shear movements between the vertebrae and can be considered the largest ligament of the cervical spine.

The vertebral artery is the first branch of the subclavian artery. It passes directly to the costotransverse foramen of C6 and ascends through successive foramina to C1. It leaves the foramen at C1 running posteromedially to extend through the foramen magnum.

### Mechanism of Injury

Direct trauma to the head that produces sudden extension of the neck can produce injuries ranging from mild muscular strain to decapitation, depending on the location and type and amount of force.

In 1955, Severy and associates[4] began to document the forces observed in "whiplash" injury. Prior to that time, hyperflexion was thought to be the mechanism primarily responsible for the injuries sustained by victims of rear-end collisions. Using both anthropomorphic dummies and human volunteers, Severy and associates performed a series of controlled rear-end collisions using accelerometers and motion picture technique. The subject was seated without restraints in a stationary car struck from the rear by a car that was moving between 7 and 20 miles per hour. Most rear-end collisions that produce whiplash occur at these low velocities, the approximate average being 15 miles per hour. When the car is struck from the rear, it moves forward. As it does, the trunk of the occupant is moved forward by the seat upright. Without a headrest, the head is unsupported, so that in the first few milliseconds following impact, the occupant's trunk is moving forward in relation to the head. At the limit of stretch of soft tissues of the neck, the head falls backward and an extension strain is applied to the neck. When the tone of the anterior cervical muscles is overcome, the extension movement of the neck is resisted only by the anterior longitudinal ligament and fibers of the anulus. When the car stops accelerating, the head rebounds forward; this forward movement may be accelerated by contraction of the neck flexor muscles caused by induction of the stretch reflex. Severy and associates recorded head accelerations as great as 11.4 g and with such magnitudes, forces in excess of 45 kg (100 lb) were applied to the head.

Some additional observations by MacNab,[5,6] Ewing and Thomas,[1] Wickstrom and associates,[7] and Unterharnscheidt[8] further elucidate injury mechanisms. Although headrests may provide protection in this type of accident, if the headrest is set too low, the head is able to roll over the top of the headrest, producing even more hyperextension.

The usual automobile accident rarely produces unidirectional extension only. Some component of rotation generally occurs. This rotation can cause the maxilla to rotate away from the mandible, causing the mouth to fling open and producing the potential for temporomandibular strain. If the initial position is not the usual one (the head may be dropped forward as the driver is changing a radio program), a concertina effect may be produced initially rather than the extension-hyperacceleration.

The surprising data of Severy and associates demonstrated conclusively that these seemingly harmless low-speed rear-end collisions were capable of producing damaging forces to the head and neck. Laboratory proof of pathology is contained in studies by MacNab,[6] Wickstrom and associates,[7] Ewing and Thomas,[1] and Unterharnscheidt.[8]

MacNab[6] described acceleration-extension injuries sustained by monkeys strapped to a steel platform attached to two vertical guide rails; the platform was dropped from distances of 2 to 40 feet. Altering the height of the drop produced varying lesions. Muscle injuries were produced varying from slight tears of the sternomastoid to ruptures of the longus colli with associated retropharyngeal hematoma. Esophageal hemorrhage was seen as were disruptions in the cervical sympathetic plexus. One of the most interesting lesions seen was tearing of the anterior longitudinal ligament and separation of the disk from the associated vertebra. In Wickstrom and associates'[7] studies on primates using a propelled cart, brain damage was seen in 32%, spinal cord damage in 57%, nerve root damage in 0.7%, ligamentous injury in 11%, and disk injuries in 2.3%. Unterharnscheidt[8] tested monkeys in acceleration sleds; their torsos were restrained and their head and neck were unrestrained, producing a hyperextension force. With sled accelerations of over 140 g, traumatic transection of the spinal cord with rupture of the vertebral arteries and massive atlanto-occipital separations occurred. Although vertebral fracture dislocation was rare in all of these experiments, studies by Davis and associates[9] on patients who die in auto accidents as the result of craniospinal injuries demonstrated similar soft-tissue injuries and associated fractures and dislocations. Of course, the mechanisms of injury were unlikely to be pure extension or pure flexion. MacNab[5] also noted frequent apophyseal joint damage in the presence of an unremarkable radiographic picture. He noted minor mismatching of surfaces and tears of capsular fibers at the zygapophyseal joints.

## Clinical Syndromes

Now that experimental and pathologic evidence and the mechanism and types of injuries have been delineated, we will discuss the correlation of symptoms with these data.[10]

Females experience "whiplash" injuries much more often than males, perhaps because their smaller muscle mass is less able to withstand acceleration forces. Patients usually complain of some pain immediately following injury, although a delay of 24 to 48 hours is not unusual. Radiation of the pain is variable, but usually occurs after several days. The pain is frequently felt in the neck, shoulders or arms, or suboccipital region. Absence of pain in the neck does not preclude cervical soft-tissue injury. Occipital headaches are common and may radiate over the vertex or bitemporally. Retro-ocular pain is a known associated symptom. To date, there is no accurate way to relate the symptom to a particular anatomic site. Especially important is the lack of correlation between the persistent suboccipital pain and atlantoaxial pathology. Pain radiating down the arm does not necessarily indicate nerve root compression. It may be merely another variant of referred pain. MacNab[5] believes that the relatively frequent complaint of numbness in the ulnar distribution is secondary to scalenus spasm. The superficial branches of the cervical plexus lay in close apposition to the sternomastoid and may be stretched or injured along with the sternomastoid muscle. Relevant nerve innervation to the side of the face, neck, upper chest, and shoulder may be compromised by this mechanism. A positive Tinel's sign may be present over these nerves for several years following injury.

Retropharyngeal hematoma and pharyngeal edema can cause dysphagia. The early onset of dysphagia associated with anterior soft-tissue swelling on radiograph is of prognostic significance. Dysphagia that is delayed (more than one week) is usually emotional in origin.

Otologic and ocular symptoms with associated vasomotor responses have been well-described. Barre[11] in 1926 described a symptom complex seen with neck pain. The symptoms included headache, tinnitus, deafness, recruitment of loudness, diplacusis (difference of perception of sound in both ears, either in time or in pitch, so that one sound is heard as two), and dizziness with and without vertigo. Pharyngeal symptoms encompass the feeling of a lump in the throat or tickling in the lower throat. Ocular symptoms are usually manifested in blurred vision and posterior ocular pain. Barre believed that continued stimulation of elements of the posterior cervical sympathetic nervous system either at the level of the cervical nerve root or of the plexus accompanying the vertebral artery was responsible. Other authors have postulated stimulation of the peripheral sensory elements of C1 and C2 and compression of the vertebral artery and venous system as possible etiologies of the components of this syndrome. Raney and associates[12] were able to reproduce frontal headache, dizziness, and nausea after the injection of saline subcutaneously into the upper cervical area. Tissington-Tatlow and Bammer[13] noted reversible headaches, dizziness, tinnitus, and partial loss of hearing and vision on one side by changing the position of the head and neck in cases of vertebral artery compression by spondylotic spurs. Chrisman and Gervais[14] found that more than 20% of patients with cervical syndrome had an accompanying Barre syndrome.

Muscle ruptures are well documented in the literature[5,15,16] The sternocleidomastoid muscle is frequently involved. The muscle may partially or wholly rupture with resultant hemorrhage and edema. Anterior strap muscles may also be injured; in this injury patients complain of difficulty when getting out of bed as they attempt to lift the head from the pillow and activate the neck flexors. In some patients, a large tender mass may be palpable; they can also experience increased pain when tested against resistance.

Frankel[17] reported that following hyperextension injury, 15 of 40 patients had signs and symptoms consistent with strain of the temporomandibular joint. These symptoms included pain in the temporomandibular joint on opening the mouth, limited mouth opening, snapping of the jaw, and pain on chewing. Dental treatment designed to restore the bite and place the mandibular condyle into a concentric relationship with the temporal fossa was found to be effective.[18]

Hilliwell[19] described a patient who developed bilateral vocal cord paralysis and bilateral lateral rectus palsies after an acceleration injury to her neck. The patient also exhibited temporary loss of consciousness. He believed that intracranial shearing forces were responsible for injury to the sixth and tenth nerves.

Amnesia and loss of consciousness caused by concussion or possibly vertebral artery injury have also been reported.[20-22]

Harris and associates[15] reported a patient who sustained traumatic disruption of a cervical disk as a result of hyperextension injury. The reported clinical syndromes associated with acceleration injuries are consistent with our anatomic knowledge and the pathologic findings in experimental animals. These patients' symptoms are probably legitimate.[23]

### Radiographic Findings

Radiographic findings must be carefully interpreted. Loss of cervical lordosis can be seen even in normal patients when they lower their chin. According to Hohl,[24] however, a sharp reversal of cervical lordosis is a pertinent finding. Penning[25] reported on the incidence and etiologic significance of prevertebral hematoma in cervical spine injury. He found a wide range of prevertebral soft-tissue width from patient to patient, level to level, and flexion to extension. He recommended taking the upper limits of the normal values as a reference for abnormal width and found them to be 11 mm at C1, 6 mm at C2, 7 mm at C3, and 8 mm at C4 when the film was placed with the shoulders against the cassette.

When present, widening was maximal on the early radiographs (zero to three days). It was very pronounced in avulsion fractures of the vertebral bodies and in hyperextension sprains (with disruption of the anterior longitudinal ligament and disk) even if the spine had returned to its normal position (Figs. 31–1 and 31–2).

Widening decreased to normal in 50% of the cases after two weeks and in 90% of cases after three weeks. Fractures of the pedicles and articular or spinous processes did not produce prevertebral hematoma unless associated with fracture or dislocation of the vertebral bodies. The odontoid is an obvious exception. Changes were seen consistently only in the upper cervical region (C1-C4). Hematoma caused by rupture of associated blood vessels rather than edema or bleeding caused by rupture of the relatively avascular ligaments is proposed as the explanation for this soft-tissue swelling. One case of rebleeding was seen and was attributed to re-opening of the vessel

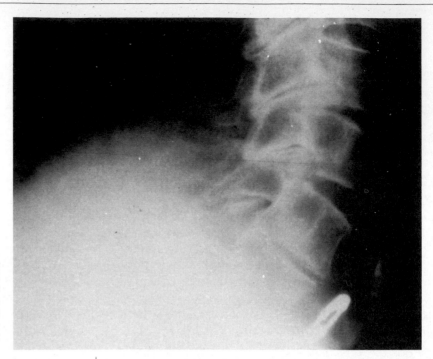

**Fig. 31–1** Disruptive hyperextension. Note opening of the disk space anteriorly and small avulsion fracture of the inferior aspect of the superior vertebral body, representing avulsion of the anterior longitudinal ligament. This injury may be an indication for anterior diskectomy and fusion and/or anterior plating for stabilization.

**Fig. 31–2** This patient sustained a disruptive hyperextension injury that left him quadriplegic. Radiographs at the time of admission show some anterior soft-tissue swelling at C6-C7. There is posterior subluxation of C6 on C7 and a small avulsion fracture of the anteroinferior portion of C6. It is likely that the patient sustained a hyperextension injury that resulted in tearing of the anterior and posterior longitudinal ligaments, disruption of the disk, at least partial tearing of the facet capsular ligaments, and a severe spinal cord injury.

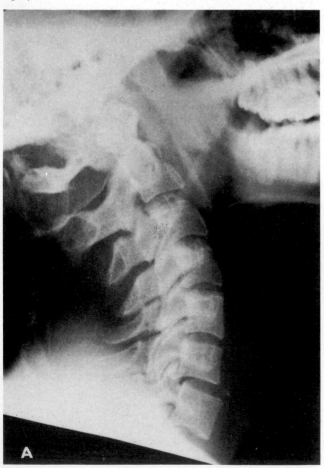

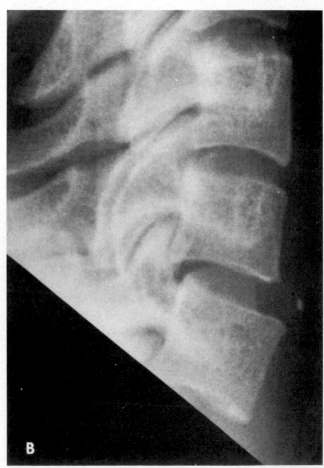

during extension radiographs. The reasssuring fact from Penning's work is that absence of prevertebral widening makes disruptive hyperextension injury very unlikely.

If present, degenerative changes should be duly noted as they may affect the prognosis. Hohl[24] has shown that restricted motion at one interspace, as documented by flexion and extension radiographic views, may also be prognostic, so these studies should be obtained.

## Treatment

The physician must realize that significant soft-tissue injury can occur in these acceleration injuries even in the absence of positive radiographic findings.

Obviously, clinical and radiographic assessment including flexion and extension views, myelography, and CT scanning when appropriate should be carried out. With the exception of the disruptive hyperextension injury, which may require halo immobilization or even surgical stabilization and fusion, the initial treatment will generally be nonsurgical. If muscle spasm is present, the milder cases may require rest and restriction of activity. The moderate cases may benefit from a well-fitting cervical collar, while the severe cases may require complete bedrest at home or in the hospital. Muscle relaxants may be helpful in breaking the cycle of spasm. Anti-inflammatory drugs will decrease the discomfort from muscle and joint injury. Severe pain may require analgesics and even narcotics. Traction may be used after a few days, but only if it relieves pain. It is contraindicated in those patients with accompanying temporomandibular joint symptoms. Chrisman and Gervais[14] showed that most patients with a Barre syndrome improved with these standard treatments at the same rate as was noticed in the treatment of their musculoskeletal complaint. In most cases, the patient should be able to return to work in one or two weeks. Instruction in neck-sparing routine, in which the patient avoids extension strains, is recommended.

MacNab[5] believes that if the patient's problems are severe enough to warrant a week of bedrest, then daily discomfort can be expected to last six weeks. If at the end of six weeks some discomfort persists all day long, intermittent discomfort may be expected for six months or a year. The patient must be told the expected duration of symptoms and the expected benefits of specific treatment. The patient must also be advised that the neck lesion and resultant discomfort are not sufficient to cause complete withdrawal from the activities of daily living. Most patients respond well to this program and improve to their own satisfaction. For patients with persistent referred pain, we have found transcutaneous nerve stimulation helpful occasionally. Patients with persistent radicular patterns may require surgical treatment if

myelography demonstrates nerve-root compression. A study by DePalma and Subin[26] supports this conclusion. Patients with spondylosis and discomfort persisting after prolonged conservative treatment may have an abnormality demonstrated on diskography and could benefit from diskectomy and fusion as shown by Roth and Whitecloud.[27]

Recent studies by Bogduk and Masland[28] and Dwyer and associates[29] have shown via facet injection techniques that the cervical zygapophyseal joint can be the site of local neck pain and nonradicular referred pain that is probably transmitted by the adjacent posterior primary rami. Some patients' pain has been relieved by anesthetic steroid injection into the offending facet joint. The duration of this relief has varied among patients. Whether or not a positive analgesic facet injection test is an indication for fusion to provide permanent pain relief has not been determined. When other treatments have failed to relieve pain, tricyclic antidepressants, such as amitriptyline, relieve some forms of chronic pain, possibly by blocking the reuptake of serotonin.[30]

Despite the passage of time and the available treatments, up to 12% of patients[5,31] may still have discomfort severe enough to prevent their return to work or enjoyment of leisure activity.

## Prognosis

Several long-term studies have pointed out that a significant number of patients have continuing symptoms following soft-tissue neck injuries. The incidence reported in these studies varies between 12% and 45% depending on the study and the length of follow-up. Persistent symptoms were most often intermittent neck ache, stiffness, and headache, but a few patients had radicular pain.

Greenfield and Ilfeld[32] studied short-term prognostic factors in 179 patients. They noted that shoulder pain and arm and hand pain indicated slower progress toward recovery and that when upper back pain and interscapular pain were present, a longer treatment program was needed. After seven weeks, only 37% of the patients were asymptomatic.

Several long-term studies have been reported that give us some guidelines for prognosis in this group of patients. Hohl[24] and Hohl and Hopp[33] found that complaints of interscapular pain, upper extremity pain, and numbness carried a poor prognosis, as did findings of a sharp cervical curve reversal, or restricted motion at one level on flexion/extension radiographs. They also noted that the incidence of recovery was better in men. Norris[34] found that the presence of objective neurologic signs, significant neck stiffness and muscle spasm, and/or preexisting degenerative changes[35] adversely affected the outcome. This latter finding is at variance with Hohl and Hopp's report.[33]

Hohl[36] also reported on radiographs taken an average of seven years after injury in one series of patients who had no prior etiologic evidence of disk disease; he found that 39% had developed disk disease at one or more levels. Available evidence indicated an expected incidence of 6% in this age group (mean age of 30 years), so it was postulated that the injury had started or accelerated the process of disc degeneration.

There was no statistical correlation between the development of degenerative changes and continued symptoms. In the studies of both Norris[34] and Hohl,[36] there was no indication that litigation, its absence, or its settlement influenced the long-term result.

### Medical, Legal, Psychoneurotic Considerations

Pain in the presence of initial negative radiograph and physical examination without objective stigmata of an identifiable organic lesion are associated with psychoneurosis, which has been repeatedly investigated and is often misunderstood. Gotten,[31] in 1956, studied 100 patients whose whiplash injuries prompted them to sue; their cases were settled by litigation. Overall, 88% were recovered and asymptomatic after settlement, while 12% needed further treatment (2% of whom eventually required surgery). The relation of symptoms to satisfaction with the settlement was investigated. About 80% (40 out of 49) of the patients who were satisfied with their settlement had no further symptoms or only minimal discomfort. Only 25% of those who were not satisfied with their claim experienced complete relief. Gotten observed a profound posttraumatic neurosis in his patients that included apprehension, nervous tension, and anxiety; he believed all of these reactions tended to worsen the neurosis and complicate the treatment. He believed that many of the patients were using the injury as an instrument of personal gain, for financial or psychosocial advantage. Gay and Abbott[37] believed that the significant soft-tissue injury somehow resulted in an insult to the patient's personality structure, causing protracted symptoms. Whether the resultant behavior was an emotional reaction to the accident or whether it revealed a predisposition to psychoneurotic behavior could not be definitely demonstrated. Leopold and Dillon[38] in 1960 argued that the emotional component of the symptom complex was integral to the whiplash patient, independent of litigation, concussion or physical injury, believing that injury to the head or neck had carried with it a strong, inherent, and subconscious meaning. MacNab[5] offered a different interpretation of possible litigation neurosis when he reported in his study of 266 patients that 45% continued to have complaints even after settlement. He pointed out that patients with associated injuries experienced normal healing times for these injuries. The symptomatic group in his study was comprised primarily of patients with hyperextension injuries, i.e., caused by motion that exceeds normal maximal extension of 60 to 75 degrees. Most asymptomatic patients had lateral or hyperflexion stress, i.e., had sustained an injury that allowed the normal range of neck motion. He hypothesized that hyperextension injuries produced some significant change causing a prolonged clinical course that was not seen with hyperflexion or lateral stress.

We should also recall that in both the long-term reports of Norris[34] and Hohl[24] there was no relationship seen between presence or settlement of litigation and ultimate relief of symptoms.

### Conclusion

The most injurious head deflection in an acceleration injury is hyperextension, which is motion that goes beyond the normal physiologic range. Even though sustained in low-velocity rear-end collisions, this acceleration injury can produce forces significant enough to produce musculoligamentous tears with resultant hemorrhage and even disk disruption and avulsion fractures of the vertebral bodies. In addition, the integrity of the apophyseal joints may be violated, leading to posttraumatic arthritis. Although most of these patients will improve in time with conservative treatment, some of them may require surgery for persistent radicular signs or demonstrable symptomatic disk degeneration. Up to 12% of the patients will continue to have symptoms despite conservative treatment and surgical therapy when indicated. There are data that suggest there is no preexisting psychological derangement in the majority of these patients and that there is no relation between the initiation or outcome of litigation and their ultimate health status. Development of an injury psychoneurosis and the role of postconcussion phenomena and sympathetic hyperactivity in producing a psychological reaction are not well understood at present.[39]

The use of a properly fitted headrest attached to the car seat to limit hyperextension will significantly decrease the development of symptomatic whiplash.

## Flexion Injuries

Because of the paucity of information in the literature on flexion and deceleration soft-tissue injuries, much of the material we will present is based on our own clinical experience.

Again, an anatomical review will help in better understanding these injuries and their treatment.

### Anatomy of the Posterior Cervical Spine

The occiput is joined to the atlas by a broad but thin posterior lateral occipital ligament. The ring of the atlas is joined to the lamina of the axis by the ligamentum flavum. The odontoid process has a pivotal position in the atlantoaxial joint. Most atlanto-axial ligaments are lax, permitting almost 90 degrees of rotation to both sides and 15 degrees of flexion and extension. The odontoid process and its integral ligaments, particularly the transverse ligament, are primarily responsible for stability at this joint. In flexion injuries, usually the odontoid process fractures before the ligaments give way. Pure shearing injuries, however, such as a violent blow to the back of the head, as described by Fielding and associates[40] can produce isolated transverse ligament ruptures.

Johnson and Southwick[41] published some exquisite anatomical drawings showing that the supraspinous and interspinous ligaments connect the spinous processes of the cervical vertebrae. Biomechanical trials indicated[41] that these ligaments consistently limited flexion and anterior horizontal displacement. The supraspinous ligaments are a continuation of the ligamentum nuchae, a fibrous midline intermuscular septum attached to the spinous processes and paracervical muscles. The ligamentum nuchae stretches from the external occipital protuberance to the spinous process of the seventh cervical vertebra. The paracervical muscles overlap and cross at the midline, are attached to the bifid spinous processes, and blend with the interspinous ligaments anteriorly. The fibers of the interspinous ligaments tend to run obliquely from the superior vertebra posteriorly to the next lower spinous process. At the facet joints is the capsular ligament, a short, thick fibrous structure the fibers of which are arranged perpendicularly to the plane of the facet joint. These fibers tighten when the facet glides forward or backward from mid position. The ligamentum flavum joins the lamina of one vertebra to the next. It is a thick, orange-yellow elastic ligament contained within the spinal canal. With age or degeneration, its elasticity may be lost, and with neck extension the ligament may protrude into the spinal canal and compress the spinal cord.

Lateral and deep to the superficial fascia is the trapezius muscle. The splenius capitis arises from the lower half of the ligamentum nuchae to attach deep to the sternomastoid on the occiput. The semispinalis capitis and cervicis is a long muscle group that originates from the articular processes of the fourth, fifth, and sixth cervical vertebrae and from the transverse processes of the upper five thoracic vertebrae. It has a thick insertion on the occipital bone and is pierced by the greater occipital nerve. There are also a group of small head extensors including the rectus capitis posterior (major and minor) and the superior and inferior capitis obliques, all attaching to the axis.

### Nature of Flexion Injury

Whereas the driver of a car struck from behind typically sustains an extension injury, the driver of a car that strikes a solid object head-on usually sustains a flexion-elongation injury, depending on the position of the head and neck at the time of impact.

Experimental and clinical evidence supports the fact that flexion forces on the cervical spine can produce a spectrum of injuries ranging from mild strain to spinal cord transection.[1,8,42,43] Of course, not all flexion injuries occur in motor vehicle accidents. Diving injuries, industrial accidents and other sports-induced trauma commonly produce flexion injuries. In low-velocity flexion accidents, because the chin strikes the chest when the full range of physiologic flexion has been reached, minimal soft-tissue damage occurs. Some of the most severe flexion injuries the authors see in patients surviving flexion injuries are teardrop injuries of the vertebral body, which result in spinal cord injury and quadriplegia. Alker and associates[42] evaluated cervical spine injuries in 312 victims of fatal traffic accidents and found a high proportion of flexion injuries involving the cranial cervical junction and upper two cervical segments.

A number of soft-tissue flexion injuries between these extremes may be encountered clinically. A flexion injury to the neck of a person already tensed in anticipation of an impending collision could produce stretching and partial tearing of muscle with resultant hemorrhage, inflammation, and muscle spasm. A traction injury to the greater occipital nerve could occur. Avulsion of the spinous process, also known as clay shoveler's fracture, can also result.

A more severe flexion injury could produce disruption of the interspinous ligaments, further separating the affected spinous processes (Fig. 31–3). If the capsular ligaments of the facet joints are injured, riding up of one facet on the other can occur. Further flexion can disrupt the capsular ligaments, stretch and rupture the posterior longitudinal ligament, and even disrupt the posterior aspect of the disk space itself. Using fresh unembalmed cadavers, Selecki and Williams[43] were able to demonstrate all of these lesions.

Information about some of the more severe flexion deceleration injuries also comes from studies of naval aviators.

Ewing and Unterharnscheidt[44] observed a high fatality rate in naval aviators who collided with water. Their analysis of the literature and the pilot's situation during a crash suggested that (1) the aviator's head and neck were unrestrained, permitting relative motion in a deceleration event between the restrained torso and the unrestrained head and neck; (2) the crash helmet shifted the center of gravity of the head-helmet mass superiorly and anteriorly, increasing the rotational moment of the head on the neck; (3) the crash helmet increased the normal weight of the head by 50% and therefore increased the force on the neck in a deceleration event; and (4) an analysis of

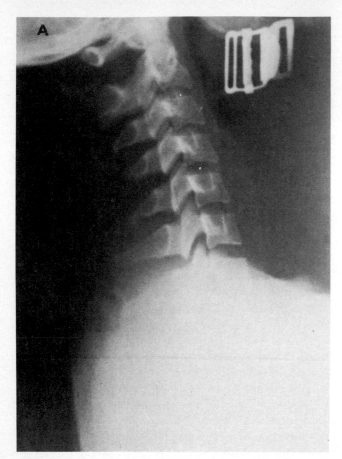
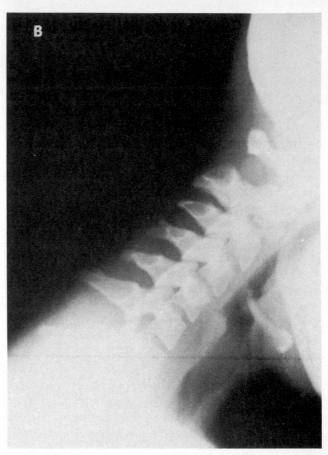

**Fig. 31–3** **A:** A 20-year-old female seen in the emergency room because of posterior neck pain, followng an auto accident in which she struck a car from behind. Initial radiographs in the emergency room were taken in traction and read as normal. No flexion/extension films were taken. **B:** Same patient seen two weeks later because of persistent discomfort. Flexion film shows localized kyphotic angulation at C6-C7, rotation of C6 on C7, anterior and superior displacement of inferior facet C6 (superior facets of C6-C7 joint), fanning of interspinous space C6-C7, anterior narrowing and posterior widening of the disk space, and an increase in the distance between the posterior cortex of the subluxated vertebral body and the anterior cortex of the articular masses of the subjacent vertebra. White's angle was greater than 11 degrees.

several factors involved revealed that stretch and flexion of the cranial cervical junction were important for mechanics of concussion. Jet aircraft thrown in the water from the deck of an aircraft carrier float for 60 seconds at most, and then sink at a minimum rate of 400 feet per minute. The pilot has two minutes at most to escape before being crushed by the water pressure. However, sudden deceleration from a head velocity of 25 miles per hour produces loss of consciousness often exceeding 60 seconds, obviously giving the pilot no practical time to escape. Several experiments were performed by Ewing and Thomas[1] and later by Unterharnscheidt[8] to determine the type of injuries sustained by human volunteers and rhesus monkeys in these deceleration situations. The torsos of both the human volunteers and the monkeys were completely restrained, but the head and neck were unrestrained. In the animal experiments, lesions ranged from subdural hemorrhage to hemorrhage and indentation of the spinal cord over the dens, to

complete cord transection. The injuries tended to occur at the cranial cervical junction. As described by Alker and associates,[42] this type of injury may be sustained in high-speed collisions. Shoulder restraint seat belts may be contributing factors.

Braakman and Penning[45] have classified flexion injuries as follows: distractive hyperflexion injuries (hyperflexion sprain, unilateral facet dislocation, and bilateral facet dislocation); and compressive hyperflexion injuries (anterior wedge compression, comminuted body fracture).

According to Babcock[46] and Braakman and Penning,[45] the distractive hyperflexion forces affect the soft tissues in the sequence we have previously described. While hyperflexion sprain results from pure distractive-flexion forces, unilateral facet dislocation is caused by these forces with rotation as an added vector (Fig. 31–4). A more forceful flexion can produce bilateral facet dislocation (Fig. 31–5). While distractive forces cause a predominance of soft-tissue injuries, the addition of axial loading changes the nature of the cervical spine injury. Axial compression frequently causes vertebral-body fracture, usually either a wedge or teardrop fracture. The presence of associated posterior soft-tissue injury depends on the extent to which flexion forces dominate compression forces. Bauze and Ardran[47] showed that the type of cervical spine injury suffered by a patient depends on the attitude of the head and neck at the time of impact, the point of impact, the direction and amount of force, and the continuing changing positions and force experienced before the patient comes to rest. We agree with Bauze and Ardran and remind the reader that our simple injury classification does not include all possible injury complexes.

### Radiographic Signs

Although many cervical spine injuries are easily detected by routine radiographs, there is often difficulty in radiographically detecting injuries limited to the soft tissues.[48] It is not uncommon for vertebrae to return to the normal position following these injuries. Subtle changes on standing radiographs must be appreciated, and in many instances dynamic flexion-extension films must be obtained with the physician's supervision to demonstrate pathology.[49] The study by Green and associates[50] of hyperflexion sprain identified six radiographic characteristics as follows: (1) a localized kyphotic angulation at the level of injury; (2) anterior rotation or displacement of the affected vertebra; (3) anterior and superior displacement of the superior facets of the involved interfacetal joints with respect to their contiguous inferior facets; (4) abnormal widening of the involved interspinous space (fanning); (5) anterior narrowing and posterior widening of the disk space; (6) increase in the distance between the posterior cortex of the subluxated vertebral body and the anterior cortex of the articular masses of the subjacent vertebra (Fig. 31–3). In most cases the first four characteristics are easily seen. In some patients with minimal injury, minor degrees of rotation as demonstrated on the lateral radiograph

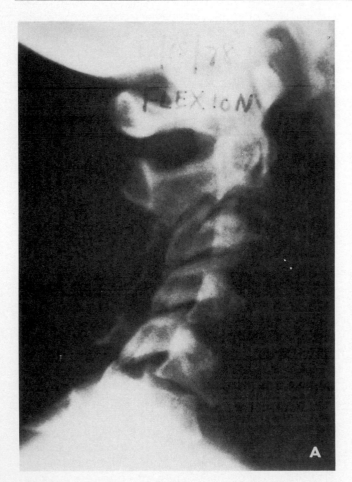
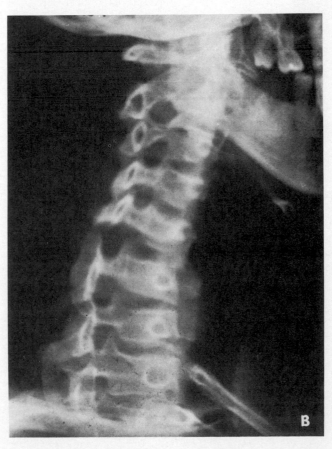

**Fig. 31–4** **A:** Lateral view. Unilateral facet subluxation; anterior portion of vertebral body displaced less than one-half the depth of the inferior vertebral body. Other characteristics are similar to those seen in hyperflexion sprain. **B:** Oblique view demonstrates foraminal widening and irregularity and reversal of shingling pattern of the articular masses.

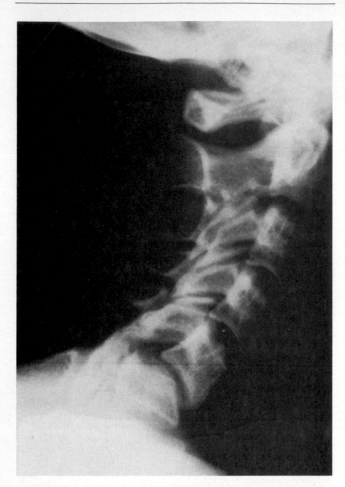

**Fig. 31–5** Lateral view demonstrates bilateral facet subluxation. All radiographic findings such as subluxation and fanning are accentuated.

may preclude an accurate measurement of the fifth and sixth characteristics. Localized kyphosis limited to the area of subluxation is characteristic of anterior subluxation and differentiates this entity from muscle spasm or the adoption of the military position that causes a diffuse reversal of the lordosis. Usually the affected vertebra is simply anteriorly rotated on the anterior inferior corner of the body. As the flexion force increases, more extensive soft-tissue damage occurs and anterior displacement may result. When the posterior section of the intervertebral disk tears and the vertebra subluxates, anterior narrowing and posterior widening of the intervertebral disk space may be seen. The localized widening of the space between the posterior cortical margin of the subluxated vertebral body and the anterior cortical margin of the subjacent articular masses is a more subtle and inconsistent radiographic sign. With the exception of the interspinous space at the C2-C3 level, the interspinous spaces are generally the same width when evaluated by a lateral radiograph. A severe flexion injury causes gross widening of the interspinous

space, producing a phenomenon called fanning. According to White and associates,[16] rotation measuring 11 degrees more than either adjacent vertebra or horizontal displacement of more than 3.5 mm are signs of instability (Fig. 31–6). Although the criteria for instability may not be met, any patient with signs of a flexion soft-tissue injury on radiograph should be closely evaluated at intervals for up to 12 weeks before being considered stable.

### Treatment

The patient who presents initially with what appears to be a strain of the posterior cervical spine should have a complete neurologic examination and radiographs including anteroposterior, lateral, oblique, and open-mouth odontoid views. If the radiologic examination is negative and the patient has intact neurologic function then supervised flexion/extension radiographs should be obtained (Fig. 31–7). If the patient presents initially with severe pain and spasm limiting flexion and extension, a short hospitalization with the administration of analgesics, anti-inflammatory agents, and muscle relaxants may be helpful. A soft collar or some other comfortable immobilizing device to provide pain relief while permitting soft-tissue healing should be used. As soon as is practicable, flexion/extension radiographs should be obtained. When appropriate, those patients with lesser injuries should have their collars removed, and they should begin gentle range of motion exercises and a neck muscle rehabilitation and strengthening program. It is not unusual for some patients to complain of persistent tension-like headaches when the collar is first removed. Some of these patients will respond to Fiorinal taken with the evening meal and at bedtime. A patient will occasionally develop persistent occipital pain. Occasionally these patients are helped by anesthetic blocks and even resection of the greater occipital nerve in those cases in which the anesthetic blocks were successful. Transcutaneous nerve stimulation may help those patients with well-localized persistent discomfort. New information on facet joint innervaton and diagnostic and therapeutic injection suggests that facet joint injury may be a source of chronic pain.[28,29] Amitriptyline, one of the tricyclic antidepressants, may also be helpful in producing some pain relief in chronic cases.[30]

Patients with radicular or long tract signs and symptoms could have disk protrusion secondary to a disk injury and should have a myelogram.

Some patients with symptoms and physical signs of recent injury have abnormalities on radiograph (Fig. 31–8) but do not meet White and associates' criteria of instability.[16] These patients should be treated in a brace that gives reasonable immobilization and prevents flexion, and they should be evaluated clinically

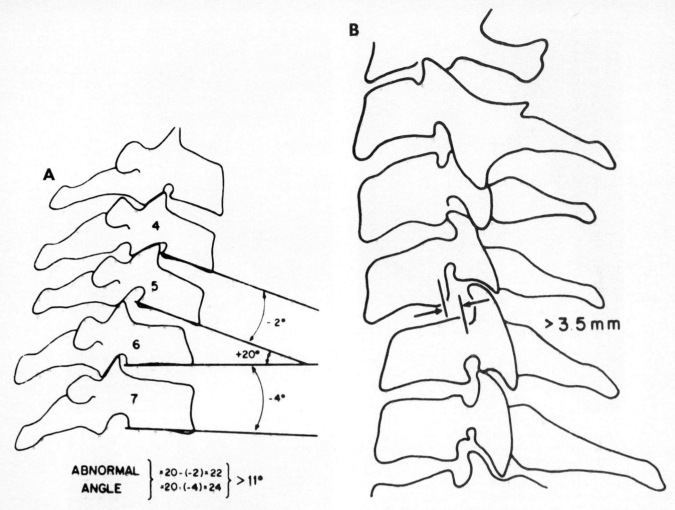

**Fig. 31–6** **A:** According to White and associates[16] and based on biomechanical testing of fresh cadaver specimens a rotational difference of more than 11 degrees in adjacent vertebra denotes instability. **B:** More than 3.5 mm of horizontal displacement of one vertebra in relation to an adjacent vertebra anteriorly or posteriorly denotes instability. (Reproduced with permission from White AA, Johnson RM, Panjabi MM, et al: Biomechanical analysis of clinical stability in the cervical spine. *Clin Orthop* 1975;109:85–95.

and radiographically at intervals over a 12-week period. Flexion/extension films to determine ultimate stability should be obtained at the end of the treatment period.

Surgical stabilization is generally reserved for those patients who demonstrate major instability based on White and associates' criteria. We have found as have others that the nonsurgical treatment of interspinous and capsular facet ligament injuries that surpass these criteria for instability on radiograph results in dangerous long-term disability in more than one third of the cases.[51]

For surgical stabilization we use a modified posterior wiring and fusion technique. Occasionally a patient will not meet White and associates' criteria for instability but nevertheless will have significant findings on flexion/extension films and persistent posterior pain. These patients may also be helped by a surgical stabilization.

Just as in the anterior extension acceleration injuries, as long as no bony or serious ligamentous injury is demonstrated, the great majority of these patients will improve with time. A small minority of patients will have no relief despite a careful consideration and application of the treatment measures described here. In patients with posterior ligamentous injury, anterior disk surgery can produce anterior and posterior instability. These cases, though rare, may require both an anterior and posterior cervical fusion to achieve stability (Fig. 31–7).

### Conclusion

There is good correlation among anatomic, biomechanical, radiographic, and clinical studies of flexion injuries. Flexion soft-tissue injuries do have specific radiographic characteristics that may be absent or subtle on plain radiographs that can be accentuated on flexion/extension radiographs. These flexion/

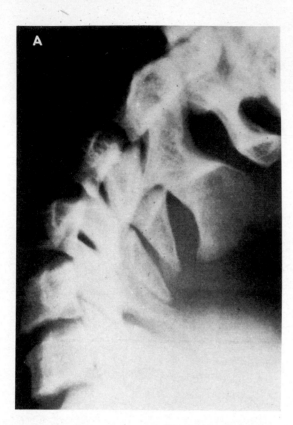

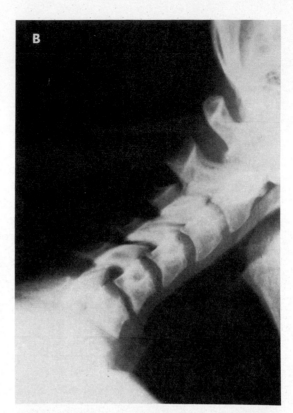

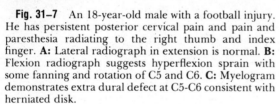

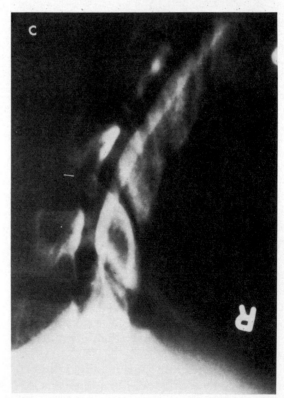

**Fig. 31–7**   An 18-year-old male with a football injury. He has persistent posterior cervical pain and pain and paresthesia radiating to the right thumb and index finger. **A:** Lateral radiograph in extension is normal. **B:** Flexion radiograph suggests hyperflexion sprain with some fanning and rotation of C5 and C6. **C:** Myelogram demonstrates extra dural defect at C5-C6 consistent with herniated disk.

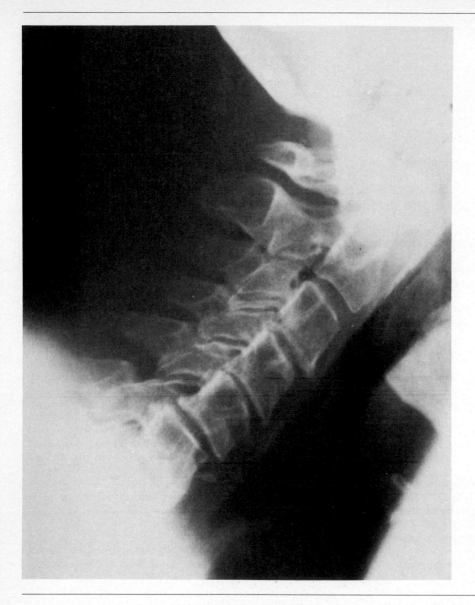

**Fig. 31–8** A 65-year-old male fell and struck the posterior aspect of his head in a shower producing a flexion injury. He has widening of interspinous space on this flexion view. Angulation of 8 degrees and horizontal displacement of 2 mm do not meet White and associates' criteria for instability.

extension radiographs should be obtained with the physician's supervision and should be repeated at a later date if initial pain and muscle spasm are prominent. Nonsurgical treatment modalities are similar to those used for extension injuries.

If angulation of greater than 11 degrees or horizontal displacement of greater than 3.5 mm is present, surgical stabilization is advised. The results of surgical stabilization have been good. Nevertheless, despite treatment a patient will occasionally be left with persistent discomfort.

### References

1. Ewing CL, Thomas DJ: Human head and neck response to impact acceleration. Naval Aerospace Medical Research Laboratory Monograph, No. 21, August 1971.
2. Kelsey JL, White AA, Pastides H, et al: The impact of musculoskeletal disorders on the population of the United States. *J Bone Joint Surg* 1979;61A:959–963.
3. O'Neill B, Haddon W, Jr, Kelley AB, et al: Automobile head restraints—frequency of neck injury claims in relation to the presence of head restraints. *Am J Public Health* 1972;62:399–406.
4. Severy DM, Mathewson JH, Bechtol CO: Controlled automobile rear end collisions, an investigation of related engineering and medical phenomena. *Can Serv Med J* 1955;11:727.
5. MacNab I: The "whiplash syndrome." *Orthop Clin North Am* 1971;2:389–403.
6. MacNab I: Acceleration injuries of the cervical spine. *J Bone Joint Surg* 1964;46A:1797–1799.
7. Wickstrom JK, Martinez JL, Rodriguez R, et al: Hyperextension and hyperflexion injuries to the head and neck of primates, in Gurdjian ES, Thomas LM (eds): *Neckache and Backache*. Springfield, Ill, Charles C Thomas, 1970, pp 108–119.
8. Unterharnscheidt F: Traumatic alterations in the Rhesus monkey undergoing -GX impact accelerations. *Neurotraumatology* 1983;6:151–167.
9. Davis DD, Bohlman HH, Walker AE, et al: The pathological findings in fatal craniospinal injuries. *J Neurosurg* 1971;34:603–613.

10. Braaf MM, Rosner S: Whiplash injury of the neck: Symptoms, diagnosis, treatment, and prognosis. *NY State J Med* 1958; 5:1501–1507.

11. Barre JA: Sur on syndrome sympathetique cervicale posterior, et sa cause frequent: L'arthrite cervicale. *Rev Neurol* 1926;45:1246.

12. Raney AA, Raney RB, Hunter CR: Chronic post traumatic headache and the syndrome of cervical disk lesion following head trauma. *J Neurosurg* 1949;6:458.

13. Tissington-Tatlow WF, Bammer HG: Syndrome of vertebral artery compression. *Neurology* 1957;F:331.

14. Chrisman OD, Gervais RF: Otologic manifestations of the cervical syndrome. *Clin Orthop* 1962;24:34–39.

15. Harris WH, Hamblen DL, Ojemann RG: Traumatic disruption of cervical inter-vertebral disc from hyperextension injury. *Clin Orthop* 1968;60:163-167.

16. White AA, Johnson RM, Panjabi MM, et al: Biomechanical analysis of clinical stability in the cervical spine. *Clin Orthop* 1975;109:85–95.

17. Frankel VH: Temporomandibular joint pain syndrome following deceleration injury to the cervical spine. *Bull Hosp Joint Dis* 1969;26:47.

18. Ernest EA III: The orthopedic influence of the TMJ apparatus in whiplash: Report of a case. *Gen Dentistry* 1979;27(2):62–64.

19. Helliwell M: Bilateral vocal cord paralysis due to whiplash injury. *Br Med J* 1984;288:1876–1877.

20. Carpenter S: Injury of neck as cause of vertebral artery thrombosis. *J Neurosurg* 1961;18:849.

21. Coburn DF: Cerebral artery involvement in cervical trauma. *Clin Orthop* 1962;24:61–63.

22. Schneider R, Schemm G: Vertebral artery insufficiency in acute and chronic spinal trauma. *J Neurosurg* 1961;18:348.

23. Braaf MM, Rosner S: Whiplash injury of neck, fact or fancy. *Int Surg* 1966;46:176–182.

24. Hohl M: Soft tissue injuries of the neck in automobile accidents. *J Bone Joint Surg* 1974;56A:1675–1682.

25. Penning L: Prevertebrae hematoma in cervical spine injury: Incidence and etiologic significance. *AJR* 1981;136:553–561.

26. DePalma AF, Subin DK: A study of the cervical syndrome. *Clin Orthop* 1965;38:135.

27. Roth D, Whitecloud T, personal communication, 1986.

28. Bogduk N, Masland A: Cervical zygo-apophyseal joints as a cause of neck pain. Presentation at the 14th Annual Meeting Cervical Spine Research Society, Palm Beach, Fla, Dec. 10-13, 1986.

29. Dwyer A, Aprill C, Thalcott J, et al: Referred pain patterns from stimulation of the cervical zygo-apophyseal joints. Read before the 14th Annual Meeting Cervical Spine Research Society, Palm Beach, Fla, Dec. 10-13, 1986.

30. Lance JW: Causes of headache, in *Mechanism and Management of Headache*, ed. 4. London, Boston, Butterworth Scientific, 1982, p 38.

31. Gotten N: Survey of one hundred cases of whiplash injury after settlement of litigation. *JAMA* 1956;162:865–867.

32. Greenfield J, Ilfeld FW: Acute cervical strain evaluation and short term prognostic factors. *Clin Orthop* 1977;122:196-200.

33. Hohl M, Hopp E: Soft tissue injuries of the neck: II. Factors influencing prognosis, abstracted. *Orthop Trans* 1978;2:29.

34. Norris SH: The prognosis of neck injuries resulting from rear end vehicle collisions. *J Bone Joint Surg* 1983;65:9.

35. Friedenberg ZB, Miller WT: Degenerative disc disease of the cervical spine: A comparative study of asymptomatic and symptomatic patients. *J Bone Joint Surg* 1963;45A:1171–1178.

36. Hohl M: Soft tissue neck injuries, in Cervical Spine Research Society (ed): *The Cervical Spine*. Philadelphia, JB Lippincott Co, 1983.

37. Gay JR, Abbott KH: Common whiplash injuries of the neck. *JAMA* 1953;152:1698–1704.

38. Leopold RL, Dillon H: Psychiatric considerations in whiplash injuries of the neck. *Pa Med J* 1960;63:385–389.

39. Farbmann AA: Neck sprain, associated factors. *JAMA* 1973;223:1010–1015.

40. Fielding JW, Cochran GVB, Lansing JF, et al: Tears of the transverse ligament of the atlas: A clinical and biomechanical study. *J Bone Joint Surg* 1974;56A:1683.

41. Johnson R, Southwick W: Surgical approaches to the spine, in Rothman RH, Simeone FA (eds): *The Spine*. Philadelphia, WB Saunders, 1982, pp. 67–93.

42. Alker GJ, Oh YS, Leslie EV, et al: Post mortem radiology of head/neck injuries in fatal traffic accidents. *Radiology* 1975;114:611-F.

43. Selecki BR, Williams HBL: Injuries to the cervical spine and cord in man. Australia Medical Association Medical Monograph, No. 7. South Wales, Australia Medical, 1970.

44. Ewing CL, Unterharnscheidt F: Neuropathology and cause of death in US naval aircraft accidents. Read before the Aerospace Medical Panel Specialists Meeting, Copenhagen, Denmark, April 1976.

45. Braakman R, Penning L: The hyperflexion sprain of the cervical spine. *Radiol Clin Biol* 1968;3:309–320.

46. Babcock JL: Cervical spine injuries. *Arch Surg* 1976;3:646–651.

47. Bauze RJ, Ardran GM: Experimental production of forward dislocation in the human cervical spine. *J Bone Joint Surg* 1978;60B:239–245.

48. Scher AT: Overdistraction of cervical spine injuries? *S Afr Med J* 1981;59(18)639–641.

49. Webb JK, Broughton RB, McSweeney T, et al: Hidden flexion injury of cervical spine. *J Bone Joint Surg* 1976;58B:332–337.

50. Green JD, Hartle TS, Harris JH: Anterior subluxation of the cervical spine: Hyperflexion sprain. *Am J Neuroradiol* 1981;2:243–250.

51. Waters RL, Adkins RH, Nelson R, et al: Cervical spinal cord trauma evaluation and nonoperative treatment with Halo-vest immobilization. *Contemp Orthop* 1987;14:35–45.

# Update on the Evaluation of Instability of the Lower Cervical Spine

Augustus A. White III, MD

Manohar M. Panjabi, PhD

## Introduction

A frequently recurring clinical challenge in the treatment of the lower cervical spine is to avoid both undertreatment and overtreatment of possible unstable conditions. As the medical profession develops and changes, quality of care, cost control, and malpractice issues are taking on increasing importance as factors to be considered in the treatment of patients. In this current context, the evaluation and management of certain conditions of the cervical spine have become critical clinical issues. The clinician is frequently required to evaluate the "whiplash patient," the football player with severe neck injuries, the gymnast, the wrestler, the diver, the auto accident victim with a fracture, the patient with a malignancy, and the patient with any variety of spontaneous or posttraumatic neurologic problems. This discussion presents a systematic checklist approach to the evaluation of clinical stability of the lower cervical spine; a review of cogent, recent developments in this area; a review of some of the interesting research; and clinical questions to be answered in the future.

Clinical instability is defined as the loss of the spine's ability under physiologic loads to maintain its patterns of displacement, so as to avoid initial or additional neurologic deficits, incapacitating deformity, and intractable pain. Physiologic loads are those incurred during activity considered normal or routine by the patient. Intractable pain is defined as pain that cannot be controlled by non-narcotic drugs. Clinical instability can occur as a result of trauma, disease, surgery, or some combination of the three. The patterns of displacement, or kinematics, have been evaluated physiologically and in the context of component ablation, excessive motion, and abnormal patterns of motion.

## A Checklist Approach to the Evaluation of Clinical Stability in the Lower Cervical Spine

The various departments of anesthesiology of the major teaching hospitals of Harvard Medical School recently proposed and agreed to use certain basic routine standards of care during the administration of general anesthesia.[1] The standards are found essentially in a checklist of certain monitoring procedures and other basic practices, such as the required presence of certain medical personnel in the room at all times. Although this "checklist" or "protocol" approach may run counter to tradition, it may well represent the next major era in clinical medicine. This topic should no doubt be discussed and debated at length. What follows is only a brief presentation of the background rationale, contents, and use of the checklist for the systematic evaluation of lower cervical spine stability.

### Radiographic Interpretations

A more detailed discussion of this topic has been presented elsewhere.[2-4] Several basic points will be reviewed here. All linear measures on regular clinical radiographs of the spine are magnified. By adopting standard distances, more meaningful measurements can be made. The relative positions of the roentgen source, the spine, and the film determine the magnification of the image. Increases in the distance between the spine and the film cause the greatest increase in magnification. The recommendation is to use a fixed distance of 1.83 m (72 in) from roentgen source to film and a spine-to-film distance of 0.36 m (14 in). This distance will accommodate most shoulders and give a 24% magnification. The checklist guidelines are based on these suggested distances. Some ratio/percentage guidelines will be offered as a control for variation resulting from changes in these distances.

### Muscle Forces

The role of the muscles in maintaining clinical stability remains obscure. Most likely at the time of injury, the muscles offer no protection through splinting because of the neurologic constraints on reaction time. In the less acute situation and against the normal range of physiologic loading, the muscles do not play a significant role. For example, in patients with polio who have total paralysis of cervical muscles, there is no loss of clinical stability as long as the bony and ligamentous structures remain intact.[5] It is thus possible to assess clinical instability without full knowledge of the exact role of the muscle forces exerted. It must be acknowledged, however, that our knowledge and evaluation can be refined through a better understanding of muscle activity in the injured spine.

### Anatomy

The anatomy of the lower cervical spine important to clinical stability is depicted in Figure 32–1. Going from front to back, we note that the most important anterior structure is the intact anulus fibrosus. Its strong attachment to the vertebral bodies by Sharpey's fibers embedded in the bone is a very important source of stability. The posterior longitudinal ligament is a well-developed structure that provides considerable stability. In the posterior segment, the joint capsules and articulations are the most important source of stability. The yellow ligament (ligamentum flavum) is a well-developed structure that is elastic in the physiologic range, but at the extremes of motion it provides some stability.

### Biomechanics

Experiments have been carried out on cervical spine segments in high-humidity chambers using physiologic loads to simulate flexion and extension.[2]

The experimental arrangement is shown in Figure 32–2. The ligaments were cut in sequence from posterior to anterior in some motion segments and from anterior to posterior in others. The failure point was defined as the point at which the upper vertebra suddenly rotated at least 90 degrees. The anterior elements were defined as the posterior longitudinal ligament and all structures anterior to it. The posterior elements were defined as all structures behind the posterior longitudinal ligament (Fig. 32–1). These experiments suggest that if a motion segment has all of its anterior elements and one additional structure, or all of its posterior elements and one additional structure, it will probably remain stable under physiologic loads. To provide some clinical margin of safety, it is suggested that any motion segment in which all the anterior elements or all the posterior elements are either destroyed or unable to function should be considered potentially unstable. Therefore, these experiments show that the

**Fig. 32–1** Diagrammatic view of anatomy designed to show separation of anterior and posterior elements, and the sequence in which the ligaments were transected. Going from the anterior to the posterior direction, they were sectioned in alphabetical order as labeled (A to I). Conversely, when going from posterior to anterior, they were sectioned in reverse order (I to A). (Reproduced with permission from White AA, Southwick WO, Panjabi MM: Clinical instability in the lower cervical spine: A review of past and current concepts. *Spine* 1976;1:15–27.)

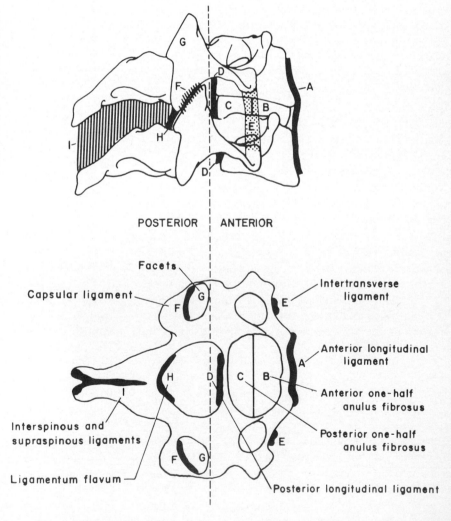

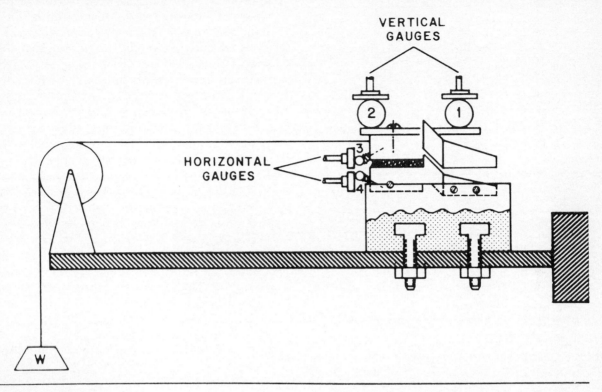

**Fig. 32–2**  The experimental arrangement: The vertical displacement balls (1 and 2) are fixed to a plate attached to the superior end plate of the upper vertebral body; the horizontal displacement balls (3 and 4) are fixed to orthopaedic screws and driven into the upper and lower vertebrae, respectively. The figure shows the motion segment arranged for the simulation of flexion. For a construction to be studied in extension, the segment would have to be turned 180 degrees. (Reproduced with permission from Panjabi MM, White AA, Johnson RM: Cervical spine mechanics as a function of transection of components. *J Biomechanics* 1975;8:327–336, Pergamon Press, Ltd.)

anatomic structures important in maintaining clinical stability are either all of the anterior elements and one posterior element, or all of the posterior elements and one anterior element.

### Clinical Considerations

A number of important clinical studies have considerable bearing on the analysis of clinical stability of the lower spine. These studies are reviewed in more detail elsewhere.[2] Briefly, the overall incidence of dislocations from nonsurgically treated, unstable cervical spine fractures is 10%. Although there are exceptions, a distinct correlation exists between neurologic deficit and the radiographic appearance of the traumatized spine.[6] If the trauma is severe enough to cause a neurologic deficit, the important components of the spine have generally been rendered unstable. Unilateral facet dislocations tend to be stable injuries, and bilateral facet dislocations are unstable injuries. Multiple-level laminectomy with or without facetectomy may lead to instability in the lower cervical spine. When facetectomy has been performed or when laminectomy has been combined

with diskectomy, the probability of instability is even greater.

### The Checklist

A standard checklist for the diagnosis of clinical instability in the lower cervical spine is presented in Table 32–1. The purposes of the checklist are to insure that all relevant clinical questions are asked and to provide standard objective criteria for prospective clinical studies. The items are weighted according to the investigator's judgment of their relative importance. The list, therefore, is designed to provide some checks and balances. The checklist also provides a mechanism for assigning a partial weight where a criterion is uncertain for a specific patient. Following is a review of cogent information about the use of the checklist.

The patient is evaluated according to each relevant item. All items will not be relevant for each patient. If the numbers assigned to the checked items total 5 or more, the spine should be considered clinically unstable. It is recommended that when the evaluation of a given item cannot be made with certainty, the value

**Table 32–1
Diagnostic checklist**

| Elements | Point Value | Individual Clinical Value* |
|---|---|---|
| Anterior elements destroyed or unable to function | 2 | _____ |
| Posterior elements destroyed or unable to function | 2 | _____ |
| Relative sagittal plane translation > 3.5 mm† | 2 | _____ |
| Relative sagittal plane rotation > 11 degrees | 2 | _____ |
| Positive stretch test | 2 | _____ |
| Cord damage | 2 | _____ |
| Root damage | 1 | _____ |
| Abnormal disk narrowing | 1 | _____ |
| Dangerous loading anticipated | 1 | _____ |

*A total of 5 points or more = unstable.
†Or a translation > 20% of the anteroposterior diameter of the involved vertebra.

for that criterion should be divided by two and added to the other points.

**Status of Anterior and Posterior Elements** The evaluation of the anterior and the posterior elements is based on clinical history, review of radiographs, interpretation of flexion-extension roentgen views, and the results of the stretch test, when available. A history of disk removal does not necessarily indicate that all of the anterior elements are destroyed, but this situation may be suspected, since there is a probability of disruption and weakening of the anulus when it is even partially removed by surgery, degenerative disease, or trauma. A separation of the vertebral end plate after an extension injury, as described by Taylor[7] or a transverse fracture of the vertebral body, as described by Marar,[8] may result in either the destruction or loss of functional ability of the anterior elements. Patients with bilateral facet dislocations are likely to be unstable. Beatson[9] showed that with bilateral facet dislocations, virtually all of the anterior elements and all of the posterior elements are destroyed. With regard to posterior elements, it is wise to assume that bilateral pedicle fractures or bilateral facet and lamina fractures have negated all support provided by the posterior elements.

**Radiographic Measurements** The measurement of translation is shown in Figure 32–3. This method takes into account variations in magnifications and is most accurate when there is a tube-to-film distance of 1.83 m (72 in). A sagittal plane translation of more than 3.5 mm under these conditions is considered abnormal and 2 points should be assigned in the checklist. To eliminate the possible error imposed by variation in technique (i.e., roentgen source-spine-film distance), one can use as an alternative to the 3.5-mm criterion, the percent of translation in relation to the anteroposterior diameter of the vertebral body (Fig. 32–3).[10] When the sagittal plane translation is more than 20% of the anteroposterior diameter of the vertebral body, it should be considered abnormal, and 2 points are assigned.

In children 7 years of age or younger the radiographic interpretation for sagittal-plane translation is decidedly different.[11] It is therefore unwise to interpret cervical spine radiographs of young children in this age group without a knowledge of some of the normal findings that may falsely appear to be pathologic.

There is no magnification problem when measuring rotation. Note that 11 degrees of rotation means 11 degrees greater than the amount of rotation at the motion segment above or below the segment in question. This standard of comparison takes into account the normal rotation between motion segments. The angles between these vertebral bodies are dictated largely by the existing lordosis and muscle spasm. Angular measurements are shown in Figure 32–4. They are significant when measured on either flexion-extension or resting lateral radiographs.

**The Stretch Test** The validity of the concept has been supported by laboratory studies and clinical observations.[12,13] The actual procedure is as follows:

(1) Perform the test under the supervision of an attending physician.

(2) Apply traction through secure skeletal fixation or a head halter. If the latter is used, a small portion of gauze sponge between the molars improves comfort.

(3) Place a roller under the patient's head to reduce frictional forces.

(4) Place the film a standard distance from the patient's neck. The tube film distance is 1.83 m (72 in).

(5) Take an initial lateral radiograph.

(6) Add weight up to 15 lb. If initial weight was 15 lb, omit this step.

(7) Increase traction by 10-lb increments. Take a lateral radiograph and measure it as shown.

(8) Continue by repeating Step 7 until either one third of body weight or 65 lb is reached.

(9) After each additional weight application, check the patient for any change in neurologic status. The test is stopped and considered positive should this occur. The radiographs are developed and read after each weight increment. Any abnormal separation of the anterior or posterior elements of the vertebrae is the indication of a positive test. There should be at least five minutes between incremental weight applications; this will allow for the developing of the film, necessary neurologic checks, and creep of the viscoelastic structures involved.

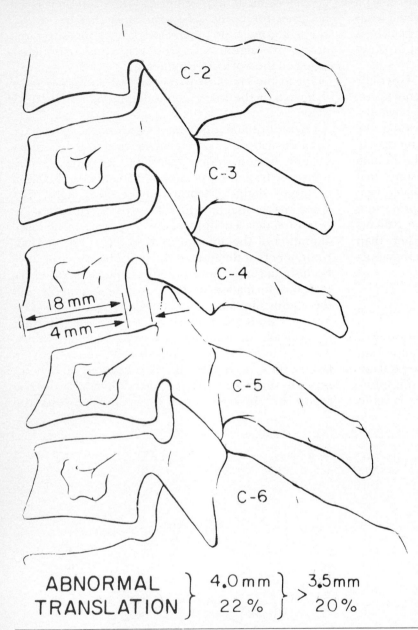

C-2

C-3

C-4

18 mm

4 mm

C-5

C-6

ABNORMAL TRANSLATION } 4.0 mm } > 3.5 mm
22 % } 20 %

**Fig. 32–3** The method of measuring translational displacement. A point at the posteroinferior angle of the lateral projection of the vertebral body above the interspace in question is marked. A point at the posterosuperior angle of the projection of the vertebral body is also marked. The distance between the two in the sagittal plane is measured (arrows). A distance of 3.5 mm or greater is suggestive of clinical instability.

Basically, the displacement patterns of the test spine are measured under carefully controlled conditions to identify any abnormalities in these patterns, which may be indicative of ruptured ligaments. Biomechanically, the spinal cord can tolerate considerable displacement in the axial direction. Thus, in the acute clinical situation, a test employing displacement in the axial direction is probably safer than the horizontal-plane displacement that occurs with flexion extension test movements.

**Cord or Nerve-Root Damage** As discussed previously, clinical evidence of spinal cord damage indicates probable spinal instability. Evidence of root involvement is, however, a less definitive indicator of clinical instability. For example, a unilateral facet dislocation

may cause enough foraminal encroachment to produce root symptoms, but not enough ligament damage to render the motion segment unstable.

**Disk Space Narrowing** Bailey[14] noted that in the traumatized spine there may be narrowing of the disk space at the level of the damaged functional spinal unit. Thus, it is believed that in a young person whose other disks are normal, this finding indicates disruption of the anulus fibrosus and a probable destabilizing influence on the involved motion segment.

**Dangerous Loading Anticipated** The final consideration involves the important individual variation in physiologic load limitations, especially with regard to differences in habitual activities. The clinician should attempt to estimate the magnitude of load that a particular patient's spine can be expected to sustain after injury. Examples of dangerous anticipated loads include those sustained by an interior lineman on a professional football team, a sumo wrestler, or a high-platform diver.

Anticipating dangerous loads can be especially helpful when other available criteria are inconclusive. In situations in which a particular life style obviously exposes the patient to large physiologic loading, the desirability of surgical fusion is greatly increased. The strength of ligamentous healing in the human spine is not known. It is reasonable to assume that arthrodesis provides better stability than healed ligaments do. The fusion may be thought of as protection against large anticipated loads. Some active patients would be better served by a fusion rather than depending on ligamentous healing to withstand anticipated loads.

### Discussion

There is statistically significant evidence to suggest that the size of the spinal canal is an important prognosticator of the likelihood of neurologic damage in cervical spine trauma.[15] Exactly how this information should be included in the evaluation is yet to be determined. It is suggested that another point be given for a cervical spinal canal that has a narrow anteroposterior diameter. Linear measurement errors are significant. However, it is reasonable, based on the work of Eismont and associates[15] to add 1 point to the checklist if the sagittal anteroposterior diameter in the lower cervical spine is less than 15 mm.

Occult unstable injuries of the cervical spine have been described.[16–18] The characteristics of this injury include flexion injury, transient neurologic symptoms, separation of posterior elements, subluxation of facets, slight vertebral compression, slight disk-space narrowing, and loss of lordosis. In order for extensive delayed dislocations to occur, mechanical alteration of the anterior and posterior ligamentous components at the time of the initial injury must have been significant. The alteration is failure or extensive plastic deformation of the posterior ligaments and the anulus fibrosus. This injury will usually be positive on a stretch test; however, a stretch test may not be available or it may fail to show the instability. Thus, it is necessary to look for the characteristics listed above, especially in the presence of a mild, cervical vertebral-body compression fracture. The report by Herkowitz and Rothman[18] suggests the

**Fig. 32–4**   The angulation between C5 and C6 is 20 degrees, which is more than 11 degrees greater than that at either adjacent interspace. The angle at C4 and C5 measures 2 degrees, and the one at C6 and C7 measures 4 degrees. The finding of abnormal angulation is based on a comparison of the interspace in question with either adjacent interspace. This comparison allows for the angulation present because of the normal lordosis of the cervical spine. We interpret a difference of 11 degrees or greater from that of either adjacent interspace as evidence of clinical instability.

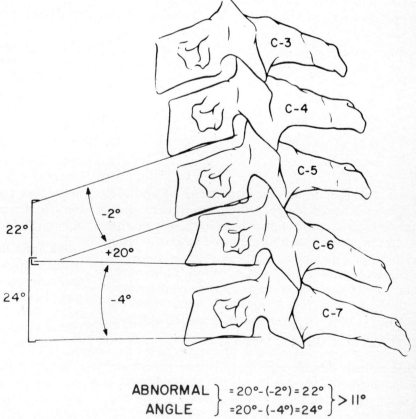

$$\begin{array}{l} \text{ABNORMAL} \\ \text{ANGLE} \end{array} \Big\} \begin{array}{l} = 20° - (-2°) = 22° \\ = 20° - (-4°) = 24° \end{array} \Big\} > 11°$$

existence of an even more challenging entity. The investigators present six patients in whom initial evaluation showed neither bony nor soft tissue involvement; after three weeks, however, all six had radiographic evidence of instability. The patients did not have stretch tests, which might have exposed the injury. These reports emphasize the care that must be taken in evaluating neck injuries and the absolute necessity of careful follow-up. The following suggested follow-up schedule should assure that the clinician will diagnose any delayed instability.

(1) The schedule begins after the termination of initial treatment, surgical or nonsurgical; that is, after removal of brace, cast, completion of bedrest, and initial physical therapy.

(2) After termination of initial treatment, the patient should be seen at three weeks, six weeks, three months, six months, and one year.

(3) If the appropriate clinical evaluation is carried out on this schedule, all early and late complications should be recognized in time for treatment. Whenever possible, radiographic techniques should be standardized for purposes of comparison.

The long-term effect of laminectomy is an important topic of discussion in regard to cervical spine instability. Surgeons are currently more aware of the importance of the lamina to the stability of the cervical spine. A ten-year follow-up of 40 children who had laminectomies showed that 40% of the patients required stabilization for unstable injuries and progressive deformity.[19] In this milestone study, a distinguished neurosurgeon emphasizes the liability of inauspicious laminectomy. Another recent study of cervical spine fractures documents the association between progressive deformity and increased incidence of second operations following laminectomy.[20]

A recent study of 52 patients with cervical spine injury states that only one case of instability was detected and that three other patients who fulfilled the criteria of clinical instability were symptom-free.[21] It is concluded that the criteria (>3.5 mm of sagittal plane translation, >11 degrees of rotational difference from either adjacent vertebra) alone cannot establish the indications for surgical intervention. The investigators state that the dislocations were reduced partially or completely in traction with Crutchfield tongs for an average of 7.9 weeks, and then a plastic collar was applied so as to continue immobilization for a total of 3.5 months. Therefore, all patients were treated adequately nonsurgically and then evaluated for instability. It appears from the information given that most of these patients were treated successfully with prolonged immobilization. The "criteria for instability" were then applied, and it was determined that four patients met them but that three were neurologically sound and pain-free. Apparently the investigators did not utilize the checklist

as recommended. As presented here, it is intended to be used to determine which patients need surgery or prolonged immobilization.

As previously delineated, in the checklist system clinical instability is defined as one of the following: intractable pain, major deformity, or neurologic deficit. Thus, by definition most of the patients in this study, having been treated with traction and immobilization, were not unstable, so the checklist need not be applied. One of the patients met two of the checklist criteria and had a complete neurologic recovery after a posterior cervical fusion. The assertion by the investigators that the "criteria" cannot establish the indications for surgical intervention is an example of the failure to use a common definition of instability and a failure to separate the treatment of instability from its diagnosis. An unstable or potentially unstable spine does not necessarily have to be treated surgically, but it must be adequately managed until it is no longer unstable.

Analysis of spinal instability is becoming more complex. Previous work has concentrated mainly on sagittal plane displacements and rotations. Future studies will study frontal and horizontal plane motions. In addition to abnormal ranges of motion, various types of abnormal quality of motion are being investigated in the lumbar spine.[22] Changes in the patterns and distribution of instantaneous axes of rotation may be an indication of instability. It may also be that changes in the normal coupling patterns are a manifestation of instability. Paradoxical motion may also be associated with instability. Paradoxical motion occurs when there are typical flexion patterns at a functional spinal unit when the overall motion is extension, or when the converse situation exists. Abnormal loading patterns may also be involved in spinal instability. The assumption that abnormal loads are associated with abnormal motion patterns is a reasonable hypothesis to explain some of the pain associated with instability.

There is a great need for additional knowledge; however, at present the checklist is useful because it includes several objective factors to help the clinician identify and appropriately manage instability in the lower cervical spine. Carefully designed clinical and experimental studies will greatly improve the clinician's ability to evaluate and manage this challenging problem. Such a project is being undertaken under the auspices of the Cervical Spine Research Society.

## Summary

Clinical instability of the cervical spine should be diagnosed accurately in order to avoid both unnecessary treatment and the serious consequences of inadequate treatment. A systematic method for evaluation utilizing a checklist is suggested.

The checklist is based on biomechanical analysis, anatomic analysis, experimental data and clinical studies. The elements of the checklist include (1) evaluation of anatomic components; (2) static radiographic measurements of sagittal plane displacements; (3) a dynamic (stretch test) evaluation of displacements; (4) evaluation of neurologic status; and (5) a consideration of future anticipated loads to the spine. Based on an analysis of these elements and an assignment of numerical values to each, the stability or instability of the spine can be determined. This systematic checklist approach is recommended as a useful method for evaluating clinical instability, given the currently available knowledge.

This methodology and current knowledge about the complex problem of spinal instability have certain limitations. Progress will come with more biomechanical experimental studies and controlled prospective clinical studies.

## References

1. Eichorn JH, Cooper JB, Cullen DJ, et al: Standards for patient monitoring during anesthesia at Harvard Medical School. *JAMA* 1986;256:1017–1020.
2. White AA, Southwick WO, Panjabi MM: Clinical instability in the lower cervical spine: A review of past and current concepts. *Spine* 1976;1:15–27.
3. White AA, Panjabi MM: *Clinical Biomechanics of the Spine.* Philadelphia, Toronto, JB Lippincott Co, 1978.
4. White AA, Panjabi MM, Posner I, et al: Spinal stability: Evaluation and treatment, in American Academy of Orthopaedic Surgeons *Instructional Course Lectures, XXX.* St Louis, CV Mosby, 1981, pp 457–482.
5. Perry J, Nickel VL: Total cervical spine fusion for neck paralysis. *J Bone Joint Surg* 1957;41A:37.
6. Riggins RS, Kraus JF: The risk of neurological damage with fractures of the vertebrae. *J Trauma* 1977;17:126.
7. Taylor AR: The mechanism of injury to the spinal cord in the neck without damage to the vertebral column. *J Bone Joint Surg* 1951;33B:543.
8. Marar BC: Hyperextension injuries of the cervical spine: The pathogenesis of damage to the spinal cord. *J Bone Joint Surg* 1951;42A:327.
9. Beatson TR: Fractures and dislocations of the cervical spine. *J Bone Joint Surg* 1963;45B:21.
10. Wilkins RH, Rengachary SS: *Neurosurgery.* New York, McGraw Hill Book Co, 1985, vol 3, chap 284.
11. Catell HS, Filtzer DL: Pseudo-subluxation and other normal variations of the cervical spine in children. *J Bone Joint Surg* 1963;47A:1295.
12. Panjabi MM, White AA, Keller D, et al: Stability of the cervical spine under tension. *J Biomech* 1978;11(4):189–197.
13. White AA, Johnson RM, Panjabi MM, et al: Biomechanics of the axially loaded cervical spine: Development of a safe clinical test for ruptured cervical ligaments. *J Bone Joint Surg* 1975;57A:582.
14. Bailey RW: Observations of cervical intervertebral disc lesions in fracture and dislocations. *J Bone Joint Surg* 1963;45A:461.
15. Eismont FJ, Clifford S, Goldberg M, et al: Cervical sagittal spinal canal size in spine injury. *Spine* 1984;9:663–666.
16. Webb JK, Broughton RBK, McSweeny T, et al: Hidden flexion injury of the cervical spine. *J Bone Joint Surg* 1976;58B:322.
17. Mazur JM, Stauffer ES: Unrecognized spinal instability associated with seemingly "simple" cervical compression fractures. *Spine* 1983;8:687–693.
18. Herkowitz HN, Rothman RH: Subacute instability of the cervical spine. *Spine* 1984;9:348–357.
19. Mayfield JK, Erkkila JC, Winter RB: Spine deformity subsequent to acquired childhood spinal cord injury. *J Bone Joint Surg* 1981;63A:1401–1411.
20. Dorr LD, Harvey JP Jr, Nickel VL: Clinical review of the early stability of spine injuries. *Spine* 1982;7:545–550.
21. Alpar EK, Karpinski M: Late stability of the cervical spine. *Acta Orthop Trauma Surg* 1985;104:224–226.
22. Gertzbein SD, Seligman J, Holtby R, et al: Centrode patterns and segmental instability in degenerative disc disease. *Spine* 1985;10:257–261.

## Acknowledgment

This work was supported by Grant AM-25601 from the National Institutes of Health, United States Public Health Service.

# Index